Microbial Toxins

VOLUME III

BACTERIAL PROTEIN TOXINS

Microbial Toxins

Editors: Samuel J. Ajl
Alex Ciegler
Solomon Kadis
Thomas C. Montie
G. Weinbaum

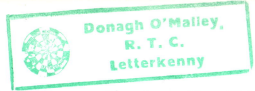
Microbial Toxins

VOLUME III

BACTERIAL PROTEIN TOXINS

Edited by

Thomas C. Montie   Solomon Kadis

Department of Microbiology   Research Laboratories
The University of Tennessee   Albert Einstein Medical Center
Knoxville, Tennessee   Philadelphia, Pennsylvania

Samuel J. Ajl

Research Laboratories
Albert Einstein Medical Center
Philadelphia, Pennsylvania

1970

ACADEMIC PRESS • NEW YORK AND LONDON

ACADEMIC PRESS, INC.
111 Fifth Avenue, New York, New York 10003

United Kingdom Edition published by
ACADEMIC PRESS, INC. (LONDON) LTD.
Berkeley Square House, London W1X 6BA

LIBRARY OF CONGRESS CATALOG CARD NUMBER: 78-84247

PRINTED IN THE UNITED STATES OF AMERICA

Contents

1A. Nature and Synthesis of Murine Toxins of *Pasteurella pestis*

THOMAS C. MONTIE AND SAMUEL J. AJL

1B. Site and Mode of Action of Murine Toxin of *Pasteurella pestis*

SOLOMON KADIS AND SAMUEL J. AJL

2. Streptolysin O

SEYMOUR P. HALBERT

3. Streptolysin S

Isaac Ginsburg

4. Erythrogenic Toxins

Dennis W. Watson and Yoon Berm Kim

5. Staphylococcal α-Toxin

John P. Arbuthnott

6. The Beta- and Delta-Toxins of Staphylococcus aureus

Gordon M. Wiseman

7. Enterotoxins

MERLIN S. BERGDOLL

8. Staphylococcal Leukocidin

A. M. WOODIN

Addendum — Production of Test Toxin of P-V Leukocidin

R. ELSWORTH AND K. SARGEANT

9. Anthrax Toxin

RALPH E. LINCOLN AND DONALD C. FISH

List of Contributors

Numbers in parentheses indicate the pages on which the authors' contributions begin.

SAMUEL J. AJL *(1, 39), Research Laboratories, Albert Einstein Medical Center, Philadelphia, Pennsylvania*

JOHN P. ARBUTHNOTT *(189), Department of Microbiology, The University of Glasgow, Glasgow, Scotland*

MERLIN S. BERGDOLL *(265), Food Research Institute and Department of Food Science and Industry, University of Wisconsin, Madison, Wisconsin*

PETER F. BONVENTRE *(415), Department of Microbiology, University of Cincinnati College of Medicine, Cincinnati, Ohio*

R. ELSWORTH *(357), Microbiological Research Establishment, Porton, Wiltshire, England*

DONALD C. FISH *(361), Process Development Division, U.S. Army Biological Laboratories, Fort Detrick, Frederick, Maryland*

ISAAC GINSBURG *(99), Laboratory for Microbiology, Faculty of Dental Medicine, Alpha Omega Research and Post Graduate Center, The Hebrew University, Jerusalem, Israel*

SEYMOUR P. HALBERT *(69), Department of Pediatrics, University of Miami School of Medicine, Miami, Florida*

ROBERT J. HECKLY *(473), School of Public Health, Naval Biological Laboratory, University of California, Berkeley, California*

CHARLES E. JOHNSON *(415), The Proctor and Gamble Company, Miami Valley Laboratories, Cincinnati, Ohio*

SOLOMON KADIS *(39), Research Laboratories, Albert Einstein Medical Center, Philadelphia, Pennsylvania*

EVANGELIA KAKLAMANIS *(493), Queen Alexandra Hospital, Athens, Greece*

YOON BERM KIM *(173)*, *Department of Microbiology, University of Minnesota Medical School, Minneapolis, Minnesota*

MARGUERITE M. LECADET *(437)*, *Institut de Biologie Moléculaire de la Faculté des Sciences de Paris, Service de Biochimie Cellulaire, Paris, France*

RALPH E. LINCOLN *(361)*, *Process Development Division, U.S. Army Biological Laboratories, Fort Detrick, Frederick, Maryland*

THOMAS C. MONTIE *(1)*, *Department of Microbiology, The University of Tennessee, Knoxville, Tennessee*

K. SARGEANT *(357)*, *Microbiological Research Establishment, Porton, Wiltshire, England*

LEWIS THOMAS *(493)*, *New York University School of Medicine, New York, New York*

DENNIS W. WATSON *(173)*, *Department of Microbiology, University of Minnesota Medical School, Minneapolis, Minnesota*

GORDON M. WISEMAN *(237)*, *Department of Medical Microbiology, University of Manitoba Medical School, Winnipeg, Canada*

A. M. WOODIN *(327)*, *Sir William Dunn School of Pathology, University of Oxford, Oxford, England*

Preface

The scope and objective of this treatise on microbial toxins have been presented in the Preface to Volume I. The second and third volumes are related to the first since they all deal with bacterial protein toxins. Whereas the emphasis of Volume I is on general problems and approaches, Volumes II and III are designed to give as complete a picture as possible of each specific toxin in question.

Since the number of bacterial protein toxins to be included is rather large, practical considerations dictated that they be distributed in two volumes. Many of these toxins have been studied intensively and much is known about them; research on others is of recent vintage and the researches are essentially in a developmental stage. Consequently, one consideration was to attain a comparatively even distribution within the two volumes of these two rough categories of toxins.

The second criterion for including these toxins in either Volume II or III was based on any general features that any of them may have in common. Thus, it will be noted that Volume II contains most of the bacterial protein toxins that are often referred to, on the basis of their physiological effects, as neurotoxins. Of course, a number of other toxins whose mode of action can by no stretch of the imagination be confined to the nervous system are also described in Volume II.

The classification of the bacterium producing the particular toxin was also taken into account. In instances in which protein toxins are produced by two or more species belonging to a particular bacterial genus, the toxins have been grouped together. Thus, the clostridial toxins will be found in Volume II and the staphylococcal and streptococcal toxins as well as those elaborated by the genus *Bacillus* have been assigned to and compose the bulk of Volume III since many of these proteins are considered to be cytolytic toxins as discussed by Dr. Bernheimer in Volume I.

The final chapter of this volume deals with the toxins of *Mycoplasma*. The mycoplasma do not possess rigid cell walls and are in many other ways quite different from bacteria. Nevertheless, these organisms have been examined in many textbooks of bacteriology and have been classified traditionally with the bacteria. Thus we chose to include the protein toxins produced by mycoplasma in this volume. Quite recently, long after the decision was made to have a chapter written on the toxins of *Mycoplasma*, the mycoplasma were given an official, separate classification in the order Mycoplasmatales under the class Mollicutes, and are now on a taxonomic basis distinct from bacteria, fungi, and viruses.

The cooperation and patience of the contributors to the present volume are greatly appreciated. We also extend our thanks and gratitude to the staff of Academic Press for their encouragement and expert assistance.

Contents of Other Volumes

    L. Joe Berry

Release of Vasoactive Agents and the Vascular Effects of Endotoxin
    Lerner B. Hinshaw

Addendum—The effects of Endotoxins in the Microcirculation
    B. Urbaschek

Endotoxin and the Pathogenesis of Fever
    E. S. Snell

The Mechanism of Action of Endotoxin in Shock
    Stanley M. Levenson and Arnold Nagler

Effects of Lipopolysaccharide (Endotoxins) on Susceptibility to Infections
    Leighton E. Cluff

Role of Hypersensitivity and Tolerance in Reactions to Endotoxin
    Louis Chedid and Monique Parant

AUTHOR INDEX-SUBJECT INDEX

Volume VI: Fungal Toxins Edited by
    S. Kadis, A. Ciegler, and S. J. Ajl

Section A *Aspergillus* Toxins

    Aflatoxins and Related Compounds
        E. B. Lillehoj, A. Ciegler, and R. W. Detroy
    Ochratoxin and Other Dihydroisocoumarins
        P. S. Steyn
    Miscellaneous *Aspergillus* Toxins
        Benjamin J. Wilson

Section B *Penicillium* Toxins

    Yellowed Rice Toxins
    a. Luteoskylin and related compounds (rugulosin, etc.)
        Penicillium islandicum; P. rugulosum, P. tardum, and
        P. brunneum, P. variabile, etc.
    b. Chlorine-containing peptide
        P. islandicum
    c. Citrinin
        P. citrinum, etc.
    Mamoru Saito, Makoto Enomoto, and Takashi Tatsuno
    d. Citreoviridin

Kenji Uraguchi
The Rubratoxins, Toxic Metabolites of *Penicillium rubrum* Stoll
    M. O. Moss
Patulins, Penicillic Acid, and Other Carcinogenic Lactones
    A. Ciegler, R. W. Detroy, and E. B. Lillehoj
Cyclopiazonic Acid and Related Toxins
    C. W. Holzapfel
Miscellaneous *Penicillium* Toxins
    a. Decumbin
    b. Puberulum
    c. β-Nitropropionic acid
    Benjamin J. Wilson

AUTHOR INDEX–SUBJECT INDEX

Volume VII: Algal and Fungal Toxins Edited by
    S. Kadis, A. Ciegler, and S. J. Ajl

Section A Algal Toxins

    The Dinoflagellate Poisons
        Edward J. Schantz
    Blue-Green and Green Algal Toxins
        John H. Gentile
    Toxins of Chrysophyceae
        Moshe Shilo

Section B Fungal Toxins, Toxins of *Fusarium*

    F-2 (Zearalenone) Estrogenic Mylotoxin from *Fusarium*
        C. J. Mirocha, C. M. Christensen, and G. H. Nelson
    Alimentary Toxic Aleukia
        A. Z. Joffe
    Toxin-Producing Fungi from Fescue Pasture
        Shelly G. Yates
    12,13-Epoxy Trichothecenes
        James R. Bamburg and Frank M. Strong
    Toxins of *Fusarium nivale*
        Mamoru Saito and Takashi Tatsuno

Section C

    Rhizoctonia Toxin (Slaframine)
        H. P. Broquist and J. J. Snyder

Microbial Toxins

VOLUME III
BACTERIAL PROTEIN TOXINS

Nature and Synthesis of Murine Toxins of *Pasteurella pestis*

THOMAS C. MONTIE AND SAMUEL J. AJL

I. Introduction

Implication of a toxin in the plague began to appear as early as 1928 when observations on the symptoms and pathology of the disease led Dieudonne and Otto (1928) to suggest that potent toxic substances were liberated by *Pasteurella pestis* during infection. McCrumb *et al.* (1953) found that antibiotics were unsuccessful in preventing death if administered 36–48 hours after infection. Autopsied patients whose organs and blood were sterile showed strong evidence of toxemia, further substantiating the idea that infection with *P. pestis* causes primarily a "toxic" death.

Studies have been conducted for a number of years to isolate, purify, and characterize the mouse-toxic components of *P. pestis*. The more recent isolation of two protein-toxic components has provided a *modus operandi* for investigations concerned with the nature of toxicity as related to similar active sites on these proteins and to the structural requirements of the molecules for toxicity. Knowledge of the nature of the toxic components also is needed to fully understand their relationship to the physiology and structure of the *P. pestis* cell, and to aid in elucidation of specific factors influencing toxin synthesis.

The need for obtaining purified toxin preparations is a prerequisite not only for experiments centered on determining any unique chemical properties responsible for toxicity, but also in studies concerned with determination of the mode or modes of action of the toxins in the mammalian cell. It is hoped that such studies taken together may shed light on the intriguing and basic question of why certain proteins which are produced and located inside a bacterial cell and which possibly serve some specific function, become extremely toxic to certain mammalian cells once they are released from their native environment.

II. Purification and Properties

A. Isolation and Purification

For over half a century it has been recognized that *P. pestis* contains "toxic" materials. For many years it has also been known that these materials along with other antigens are bound in some manner to the *P. pestis* cell. Early workers soon realized that the problem of obtaining these toxic materials centered on releasing them from the cells. A bibliography and discussion of much of the early plague toxin work can be found in Pollitzer's excellent monograph "Plague" (Pollitzer, 1954). Some of the important early findings are summarized below.

One of the earliest investigations was carried out by Lustig and Galeotti (1897, 1901). They extracted the plague bacillus with 1% potassium hydroxide and then neutralized with acetic acid, obtaining a flocculent white nucleoprotein. This material was both toxic and antigenic.

Rowland (1910, 1911) extracted agar-grown plague cultures with sodium sulfate following killing of the organisms with chloroform. These "nucleoprotein" extracts were fatal to rats within 18 hours at dosages from 0.05 to 0.1 mg. Such materials extracted with salt solutions also provided immunity to rats.

In later work two important points were noted by Girard and other French workers (Girard and Sandor 1947; Ramon *et al.*, 1947). First, although the toxin was found inside the cell (endotoxin in location), it resembled other exotoxins in not possessing the glucolipoid complex found in the endotoxins of numerous other gram-negative microorganisms. In addition, the toxin material was further characteristically similar to the classic exotoxin protein substances in being easily toxoided and showing thermolability. It is noteworthy in this early work that the substance responsible for killing was probably similar to the purified toxin obtained in more recent years, since the killing times reported of about 6–36 hours are in agreement with killing times of purified toxin protein.

Baker and co-workers (1947, 1952) took the first important steps in purifying the murine toxin. Plague bacilli that had been dried and lysed with acetone were extracted in excess 2.5% sodium chloride saturated with toluene at room temperature for 24 hours. After centrifugation the cell residue was again extracted with a smaller volume of sodium chloride. The combined supernatant material was dialyzed followed by concentration *in vacuo* to one-third the volume. Ammonium sulfate (pH 7.5) was added to give a final concentration of 0.3 saturation. This precipitate was designated fraction IA. The supernate was made to 0.4 saturation and the collected precipitate designated fraction IB. The supernate from this fraction contained the toxin (fraction II). It was found in additional experiments that the toxin could be precipitated at ammonium sulfate saturation between 0.55–0.67 providing the original extract was fractionated without concentration. The LD_{50} for fraction II, which contained almost all the mouse toxin material, was 0.6–0.8 μg. It had been obtained from extracts with LD_{50}'s of 8–10 μg. The toxin, however, was heavily contaminated with a nontoxic antigen. Fractions IA and IB were further purified. Both fractions contained various cell surface-located antigens. Fraction IB contained the so-called envelope antigen. Further attempts to purify the toxin resulted in 50–75% loss in toxicity.

Englesberg and Levy (1954) subsequently developed a casein hydrolyzate (Difco casamino acids)–glucose–mineral salts medium for production of large quantities of toxin from two avirulent strains of *P. pestis*. Strain EV 76 was a better toxin producer than strain A 1122 (an EV mutant), and these authors believed the amount of toxin produced correlated with the greater amount of splenic and hepatic damage induced by EV 76 *in vivo*. More luxuriant and rapid growth occurred with both strains at 30° than at 37°C. Less growth at 37°C probably reflected the need of most *P. pestis* cells for additional nutritional requirements at 37°C. Similarly, additional requirements at 37°C have been demonstrated for strain Tjiwidej at the Albert Einstein Laboratories. Of specific significance is that the Englesberg and Levy work showed that the proportion of toxin to soluble antigen was much greater at 30°C than at 37°C.

The growth curves showed that after 2 days, cell yield was at its maximum (5.6 × 10⁹ cells/ml). This was followed by gradual lysis and toxin release until the latter reached a maximum in the soluble medium by the seventh day (Englesberg and Levy, 1954). Attempts by these authors to apply the Baker *et al.* (1952) ammonium sulfate procedure proved unsuccessful; first, because of the resulting loss in toxicity, and second, loss of efficiency due to the dilution of the toxin in the medium resulted in very little precipitation at lower ammonium sulfate concentrations. These problems were overcome by saturating the supernatant medium with ammonium sulfate in the cold for 24 hours to precipitate total protein. Protein was collected, dialyzed, and concentrated by evaporation and ly-ophilization in the cold. This toxin preparation contained 10.8–11.6% nitrogen and gave an LD_{50} between 1 and 2 μg. It was quite stable in a lyophilized form. This material contained a number of proteins, but apparently it was relatively free of some soluble antigens as well as agar- and medium-contaminating protein encountered by Baker and co-workers.

Ajl *et al.* (1955) at Walter Reed Army Institute of Research began a series of extensive investigations to obtain the toxic component in a pure form from the avirulent strain Tjiwidej. This strain was first described in detail by Otten (1936) and was used extensively for human vaccination in Java and South America (Grasset, 1942). The initial steps of Baker and co-workers (1952) were utilized and toxin was extracted from acetone-dried cells with 2.5% sodium chloride. These steps were followed by ammonium sulfate precipitation between 0.2 and 0.6 saturation and isoelectric precipitation at pH 4.7 to separate toxin from the soluble envelope substance. The resulting preparation was further submitted to treatment with manganese chloride for removal of nucleic acids, methyl alcohol precipitation to concentrate protein and remove extraneous materials, and absorption of toxin to calcium phosphate gel with elution to separate further the toxin from the envelope substance. Lipid materials were removed by chloroform extraction. The final material had an LD_{50} of 2.6 μg for 16–18 gm Swiss albino mice exhibiting a 7-fold increase in toxicity from the starting material. Five of these purification steps, however, from the isoelectric precipitation step through the chloroform extraction procedure, yielded only a 2-fold increase in specific activity, and a decrease in total toxic units of 4 to 5 times. Apparently, some destruction or modification of the toxin molecule resulted from these purification procedures, since only a few contaminating antigens were detected in the analytical centrifuge and immunological assays.

Paper electrophoresis was employed as an adjunct to the chemical purification. Further purification was achieved with some preparations, although yields were low and toxicity loss was still a problem. Data for material obtained from these procedures showed that the toxin was protein in nature and exhibited the following characteristics: nitrogen content 14%; heat inactivated above 56°C; isoelectric point of 4.7; $s_{20,w}$ 2.73; molecular weight of 70,000–74,000; no detectable carbohydrate or capsular antigen. The molecular weight has since been revised in view of the value of 120,000 obtained by estimation with Sephadex and the $s_{20,w}$ values between 7 and 8 S obtained by a number of centrifugations of different preparations isolated by gel filtration (Montie *et al.*, 1966b, 1968b). From some recent studies carried out by us at the Albert Einstein Laboratories it appears that the Walter Reed material must have been partially depolymerized, possibly during the treatments with organic solvents (see later discussion on subunit composition). A molecular weight of 72,000 could be accounted for by loss of two 24,000 molecular weight subunits.

Some of the results obtained from paper electrophoresis experiments suggested that a number of purification steps might be omitted to avoid denaturation, and that material obtained by ammonium sulfate fractionation could be processed directly by paper electrophoresis (Ajl *et al.*, 1958). The crude toxin fraction, which was obtained between 35 and 70% saturated ammonium sulfate, was passed through a continuous flow, hanging curtain electrophoresis apparatus developed by Karler (1955). The first two passes were in a Veronal buffer, 0.01 ionic strength (pH 8.6), with subsequent passes in maleate buffer, 0.01 ionic strength (pH 6.0). After the final passage, a 17-fold purification of the toxin was achieved. This final material exhibited only one band against crude rabbit antisera in the Oudin reaction and had an intraperitoneal LD_{50} for 14-18 gm Swiss albino mice of 0.7 μg and an intravenous LD_{50} of less than 0.2 μg (Ajl *et al.*, 1958). Similar results were obtained with toxin from virulent strains of *P. pestis* by Spivack and Karler (1958). A reduction of from 8-10 antigens to 3 in the final product took place. The intravenous LD_{50} of 5-15 μg in the crude extract was reduced to 0.1-0.3 μg. Toxin from the attenuated strain EV76 behaved similarly in every way tested to the toxin isolated from the highly virulent strain 195/P.

Analysis of the Walter Reed toxin (Bent *et al.*, 1957) showed that it contained 18 amino acids but no peculiar or unusual component. A high percentage of glutamic and aspartic acids accounted for the isoelectric point reported of 4.7. Nineteen monovalent and divalent elements were detected. The significance of the presence of a large number of metals remains to be determined, but the occurrence of such a wide variety of metals suggests that most of them were coincidentally bound by the toxin. However, the metal binding capability of toxic protein may in itself be important (Montie *et al.*, 1968a).

Work at Albert Einstein in 1962-1963 (Kadis *et al.*, 1966) was directed toward modifying the continuous flow electrophoresis procedure to facilitate the production of purified plague toxin in milligram batch quantities. A fine glass bead bed was substituted for the paper medium. The beads were packed in a methylmethacrylate cell utilizing the apparatus and general methodology of Winsten *et al.* (1963). Protein precipitated between 35 and 70% saturation was used as starting material. The best toxin preparations obtained by this method had an LD_{50} of 2 μg but contained three to six additional impure proteins as assayed by acrylamide gel electrophoresis (Montie *et al.*, 1964).

During investigations examining the effects of temperature and trypto-

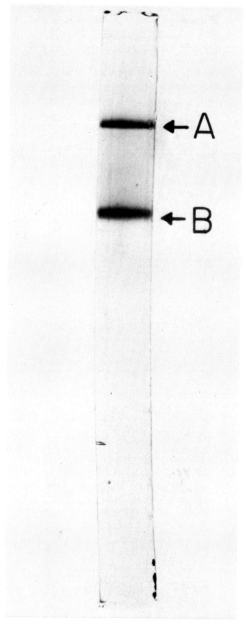

FIG. 1. Acrylamide gel electrophoresis of toxin A and toxin B. Upper band = toxin A; lower band = toxin B. Origin at the top of the gel; proteins migrate toward the positive pole (bottom of gel).

phan regulation on the level of toxin protein in the cell, it was found that the mouse toxin activity of *P. pestis* resided in two distinct protein antigenic components separable by acrylamide gel electrophoresis (Montie *et al.*, 1964). The intraperitoneal LD_{50} of protein eluted from the sliced gel sections were approximately 1 μg. The slower moving component of large molecular weight was designated toxin A and the faster moving component, toxin B (Fig. 1). Toxin B, as judged by mobility on acrylamide gels and amino acid analysis, is very similar or the same as toxic protein isolated at Walter Reed (Montie *et al.*, 1966b).

Studies involving purification of toxins A and B proteins showed that the two toxins are separable primarily on the basis of the difference in their molecular size and that size difference accounted for their separation by acrylamide gel electrophoresis (Montie *et al.*, 1966b). Previous techniques involving separation primarily by charge might account for failure to observe toxin A in earlier preparations (Ajl *et al.*, 1958). However, the presence of toxin A in these preparations should have been observed since this toxin gives a very distinctive Ouchterlony band against crude rabbit antisera (Fig. 2). Another explanation for failure to isolate two proteins previously could lie in the relative instability of toxin A compared to toxin B; in particular, instability to lyophilization has been suggested (Montie *et al.*, 1966b). A third possibility is that we are dealing with a mutation in a structural gene for toxin B polypeptide resulting in a new gene producing toxin A polypeptide. This latter possibility, however, seems unlikely. Other avirulent strains of *P. pestis* should be examined for their toxin A content in order to determine if toxin A resulted from an infrequent mutation, or whether it is an unresolved component of all *P. pestis* cells.

The two toxic proteins have been separated by gel filtration on acrylamide or Sephadex columns from crude 35-70% ammonium sulfate preparations or from preparations obtained by glass bead electrophoresis (Montie *et al.*, 1966b). Sephadex G-100 or G-200 equilibrated in 0.1 *M* potassium phosphate buffer (pH 7.0) have been used successfully to isolate milligram quantities of toxin A or B. The purity of each toxin estimated by densitometry ranges from 80 to 95% and consequently allows for isolation on a semipreparative basis using larger columns. It has been difficult to obtain protein preparations with an LD_{50} below 2 μg by this procedure, and evidence for some protein denaturation during the column run and during lyophilization of the purified product is indicated. Apparently the toxin proteins become much more susceptible to denaturation upon purification.

More recently, another purification procedure has been utilized based on the potential resolving power achieved by acrylamide gel electropho-

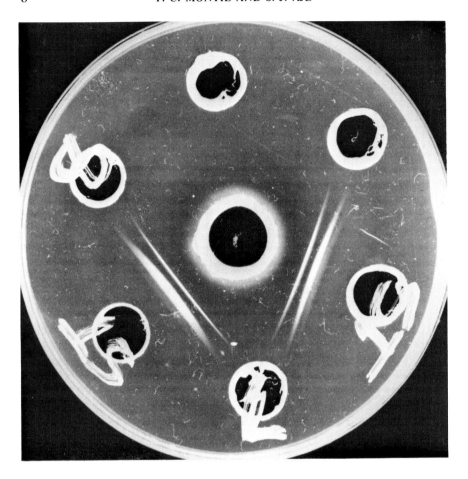

FIG. 2. Immunoprecipitin reactions of toxin A and toxin B. Inner band = toxin B; outer band = toxin A. Inner well = crude rabbit antiserum; outer wells (ST) = toxin samples.

resis. Employment of a large gel medium in a Büchler preparative gel electrophoresis apparatus has facilitated isolation of purified toxin A and B (Montie and Montie, 1969). Preparations of each toxin of approximately 100% purity as judged by acrylamide gel assay have been obtained. Toxins A and B have been isolated with an LD_{50} of 0.5 to 1.0 μg (I. P.).

B. CHEMISTRY AND STRUCTURE OF THE TWO TOXINS

1. AMINO ACID COMPOSITION

Amino acid analyses have been carried out on both toxins (Table I). These data indicated that toxins A and B are very similar in amino acid

TABLE I

AMINO ACID COMPOSITION OF TOXINS A AND B[a]

Amino acid	Moles of each amino acid per 100 moles amino acid residue[b]		Calculated number of amino acid residues per molecule	
	Toxin A	Toxin B	Toxin A (mol. wt. = 240,000)	Toxin B (mol. wt. = 120,000)
Arginine	4.27	3.99	58.7	26.8
Histidine	2.06	2.40	31.8	18.6
Lysine	5.52	5.14	91.1	42.1
Tyrosine	3.01	2.70	39.8	17.9
Phenylalanine	3.68	3.17	53.4	23.0
Cystine	0.90	0.95	9.0	4.7
Methionine	2.36	2.16	38.0	17.4
Serine	4.93	5.13	112.5	58.2
Threonine	5.32	5.82	107.0	58.6
Leucine	7.34	7.48	134.1	57.0
Isoleucine	5.00	4.63	91.4	42.4
Valine	6.11	5.94	85.6	34.8
Glutamic acid	8.93	8.99	145.5	73.3
Aspartic acid	9.61	9.66	175.6	87.8
Glycine	9.00	8.27	288.0	109.2
Alanine	8.47	9.59	228.5	129.5
Proline	4.99	4.68	104.1	48.9

[a]These data from Montie *et al.* (1966b).

[b]Values are the average of two determinations on each of three separate samples of each toxin.

composition (Montie *et al.*, 1966b). The protein samples analyzed contained up to 15% impurities. These impurities might account for any of the larger differences observed between toxins A and B such as alanine, glycine, or histidine content. Inaccuracy of analyses for amino acids present in small amounts such as histidine could further contribute to apparent discrepancies between the composition of the two toxins.

A comparison of amino acid molar ratios reported for the Walter Reed plague toxin (Bent *et al.*, 1957) with those for toxin B using lysine as the base 1.0 revealed a high degree of similarity between the two proteins. A comparison of samples from the two preparations also showed identical immunodiffusion and acrylamide gel bands, further confirming their identity (Montie *et al.*, 1966b).

Tryptophan determinations were performed on the toxin protein using the Spies and Chambers (1949) procedure (Montie *et al.*, 1966b). It was found that toxin B had approximately 33% less tryptophan than toxin A (approximately 7 residues/120,000 mol. wt. for toxin B and 10 residues/120,000 mol. wt. for toxin A). Samples containing approximately equal amounts of each toxin gave intermediate tryptophan values. Unpublished findings from our laboratories using the method of Fischl (1960) confirm a lower tryptophan content in toxin B than A or in an A plus B mixture. These data are in agreement with results from fluorescence assay at 350 mμ. Both the Spies and Chambers and Fischl methods were used following digestion of the toxins with minimal amounts of pronase. These results agreed with those obtained with nondigested protein.

Ultraviolet spectra of isolated toxin protein preparations have offered another means for comparison (Montie et al., 1966b). The patterns in the 250-330 mμ area were quite similar and gave typical protein spectra. From the 220-230 mμ wavelengths, toxin B repeatedly showed greater absorption per milligram protein when compared to toxin A. The authors tend to regard these latter results as a reflection of differences in the secondary and tertiary structure, interpeptide bonding, and degree of sulfhydryl group ionization. These interactions may be due in part to the size difference between the two toxic protein components, allowing for varied interactions between side chains. Peaks for tryptophan are evident at 293 mμ, but no differences between toxin A and B were observable at this wavelength, probably because the height of this shoulder is influenced to a large extent by absorption in the 280 mμ region, reflecting the larger number of tyrosine residues.

2. INTERACTION OF SULFHYDRYL GROUP REAGENTS WITH THE TOXINS

Our studies on the nature of the two protein toxins produced by *P. pestis* showed that both were denatured by relatively low concentrations of typical broad spectrum protein denaturants (Montie et al., 1966a). For example, urea at a concentration of 1-3 M inhibited toxicity approximately 75% (Montie et al., 1966a).

We then sought to employ more selective denaturants which are known to attack proteins at specific amino acid sites. In the course of studying the effects of a tryptophan binding agent, 2-hydroxy-5-nitrobenzyl bromide, it was found that it inhibited the expression of toxicity. It was further noted that the effects of this reagent were variable. The compound 2-hydroxy-5-nitrobenzyl bromide binds tryptophan primarily, but it has been reported to react with sulfhydryl groups (Horton and Koshland, 1965). To test this latter possibility, solutions containing both toxins were treated with various concentrations of sulfhydryl reagents known to react specifically with thiols. These included N-ethylmaleimide (NEM), *p*-chloromercuribenzoate (CMB), and iodoacetamide. All three reagents proved to be inhibitors of toxicity (Montie et al., 1966a). Toxicity was more sensitive, on a molar inhibitor basis, to CMB (2.5-10.0 μmoles) or iodoacetamide (15-25 μmoles) than to NEM (30-60 μmoles). However, toxicity was more consistently inhibited with NEM than with CMB or iodoacetamide. In this connection, Hardman and Yanofsky (1965) concluded that NEM forms a more stable linkage than CMB with tryptophan synthetase A because NEM binding was not reversed with reducing agents. The difference in relative inhibition of each compound probably relates to its charge and size which influenced the degree of penetration into the toxin proteins.

By separation of the toxins by gel filtration, enough of each protein was obtained to test the reaction of toxin A or B individually. NEM or CMB inhibited the toxicity of each toxin at concentration levels required to reduce the toxicity of both proteins when present together in solutions. Subinhibitory concentrations of CMB or NEM altered the structure of only toxin B as indicated by immunological assay. The precipitin band of toxin B completely disappeared, whereas toxin A band was unaffected except at much higher concentrations. Further confirmation of this effect on toxin B was demonstrated by disc electrophoresis assay showing a similar loss of the toxin B protein band. These results were obtained with CMB-treated toxin preparations, dialyzed to remove the CMB, or with nondialyzed solutions. A severe alteration of the native structure of toxin B was indicated by these and other experiments where unsuccessful attempts were made to isolate CMB-treated toxin B by gel filtration, or to isolate or identify a toxin B protein previously tagged with CMB-^{14}C by disc electrophoresis (Montie *et al.*, 1966a).

The method of Boyer (1954) was used to measure the reaction of CMB with toxin by measuring mercaptide formed as indicated by an increase in optical density at 255 mμ. Some reaction was immediate, but in some instances a rather sluggish reaction also occurred. Swenson and Boyer (1957) attributed this phenomenon to either the qualitative difference in reaction of various sulfhydryl groups or to the presence of certain masked sulfhydryl groups. The addition of 0.5% urea did not increase the reaction rate with toxin or the total number of sulfhydryl groups reacting over a period of time. However, preliminary experiments indicated an immediate reaction of toxin with CMB in 5 M urea (Montie *et al.*, unpublished data).

Zak *et al.* (1964) showed that 1-10% lithium bromide increased the rate and extent of the reaction of an azomercurial with either β-lactoglobulin, ovalbumin, or bovine plasma albumin. These results were attributed to a change in tertiary and possibly some secondary structures in these proteins, since Mandelkern and Roberts (1961) showed that lithium bromide changes the optical rotation of ribonuclease. Addition of as little as 0.5% lithium bromide initiated a rapid reaction of increased magnitude between a mixture of A plus B toxin and CMB. Approximately three times as many sulfhydryl groups reacted in the treated sample as in controls. When toxins A and B were titrated individually in lithium bromide, a 6- to 8-fold increase in available reactive sites was revealed with toxin A, and a 3-fold increase with toxin B (Montie *et al.*, 1966a).

As assayed by the titration technique, native toxin B was more susceptible to CMB than native toxin A protein, but with both toxins, results indicated that action of lithium bromide resulted in exposure of certain formerly unavailable sulfhydryl groups which became available to react with CMB. Both the exposed and also the more buried thiols probably play an important part in the native structure of plague toxin.

Hellerman *et al.* (1965) found silver ion to be a useful tool for elucidating the mechanism of sulfhydryl inhibition of amino acid oxidase. Although we were able to partially inactivate toxin using organic sulfhydryl reagents, the addition of 0.6–1.0 μmoles of silver nitrate partially precipitated the protein with a concomitant decrease in toxicity (Montie *et al.*, 1966a). It was observed by disc electrophoresis and immunoprecipitin techniques that again toxin B was altered structurally, since it no longer appeared as a discrete band. When both the supernatant fluid and the precipitate were tested for activity, it was found that the redissolved precipitate was completely inactivated, but toxin contained in the supernatant fluid retained partial activity.

Because a completely inactivated toxin preparation was obtained using Ag^+, attempts were made to reverse this inhibition with glutathione. The almost totally dissolved precipitate obtained after treatment with 6 μmoles of Ag^+ for 30 minutes and an identically treated suspension were reacted with 0.125 M glutathione, incubated for 1 hour, and injected into mice. The denatured soluble and the precipitate toxins were partially reactivated by the glutathione (Montie *et al.*, 1966a).

The striking inhibitory effect of Ag^+ at low concentrations on toxicity and the reversal by glutathione are particularly significant results. This is in contrast to the higher concentrations necessary for inhibition and less consistent effects of the other sulfhydryl reagents. From these data it is not immediately possible to relate the toxicity of these proteins to a special site needed for toxicity; it is possible to emphasize that certain sulfhydryl groups must be available to retain total toxicity in the toxin molecules. Whether toxicity is lost through a general rearrangement of the molecule or whether these sites are needed to combine with a physiological receptor in the mouse remains to be determined.

3. IMMUNOLOGICAL PROPERTIES

The two toxins A and B have been shown to initiate formation of distinctive immunoprecipitin bands in the Ouchterlony reaction when assayed against crude rabbit antisera (Montie *et al.*, 1964). Adjacent bands do not show any interaction, indicating a heterogeneity in the protein antigenic sites. Further work is required in this area to show whether the toxins contain different antigenic sites. Monospecific antisera to each toxin are required, and cross reactivity tests should be made.

In the Ouchterlony plate, toxin A migrates more slowly than toxin B, the former appearing as the outer band (Fig. 2). The concave shape of the precipitin band A suggested an antigen of greater molecular weight than the antibody (see Kabat and Mayer, 1961). The innermost band—representing toxin B—was observed as a straight or slightly convex precipitin band, suggesting a lower molecular weight than the corresponding antibody. This suggested difference in toxin molecular weights was later confirmed by Sephadex and ultracentrifuge studies.

4. PHYSICAL PROPERTIES

Molecular weights for the toxins have been estimated by filtration through Sephadex after the method of Andrews (1965). Using a series of standard proteins, elution volumes of each protein versus its molecular weights were plotted. Molecular weights of toxins A and B elution volumes were extrapolated from the standard plot made from data obtained on Sephadex G-200 (Montie *et al.*, 1966b). The latter data were in agreement with the Sephadex G-100 data. Toxin B was found to have an estimated molecular weight of 120,000 and toxin A 240,000. These results are in general agreement with $s_{20,w}$ values of 7.8 S for toxin B and 10.8 S for toxin A (Montie *et al.*, 1968b).

5. SUBUNIT COMPOSITION

The characteristics of mouse toxins A and B were found to be quite similar in their amino acid composition and their reaction with certain sulfhydryl reagents and other denaturants, as well as their specific toxicity to mice. Other evidence, such as the failure of adjacent Ouchterlony bands to intercept and the difference in tryptophan content, suggested that a few differences may never the less exist between these molecules. The overall picture, however, favored the suggestion that the two toxins contain similar or the same active sites required for toxicity. An approach to the problem of isolating a common toxic component was initiated by attempts to dissociate these proteins (Montie *et al.*, 1968a,b).

Extensive work reported in the literature suggested that proteins of over 100,000 molecular weight very likely consists of subunits. The presence in nature of a similar polymeric form (toxin A) of the B toxin suggested that both proteins are built from some of the same structural components. Attempts to convert toxin A to toxin B using mercaptoethanol, urea, and other dissociating agents resulted in denaturation of the toxin and complete disappearance of gel electrophoresis bands. No toxin B was detectable.

Dissociation of both toxins was achieved using both citric and acetic acids (pH 2.5).However, some denaturation and reaggregation occurred. These characteristics of acid subunits complicated detailed study of this system. Dissociation with acetic acid is enhanced by the presence of a chelating agent such as EDTA (Montie *et al.*, 1968a). A preliminary report of toxin dissociated by acid into subunits of 6000–10,000 molecular weight (Montie *et al.*, 1968a) as determined by Sephadex estimation has not been substantiated because of an unusual interaction of citric acid with toxin subunits. This interaction resulted in retarded subunit movement through molecular sieving columns.

Sodium dodecyl sulfate (SDS) was found to be a more successful dissociating agent for obtaining stable and biologically active subunits (Montie *et al.*, 1968b). Toxin was dissociated with SDS after the method of Shapiro *et al.* (1967). The latter method was employed originally to determine the molecular weight of virus subunits by acrylamide gel electrophoresis. SDS disrupts hydrogen and hydrophobic bonds at the same time saturating proteins with the SDS negative charge so that separation by gel electrophoresis is based on relative size rather than charge. Toxic protein was treated with a 1% SDS solution at 37°C for 3 hours followed by dialysis for 16 hours against 0.1% SDS in 0.01 M sodium phosphate buffer (pH 7.1). In initial electrophoretic studies we assayed toxin with the SDS-treated standards, serum albumin monomer and dimer and ribonuclease. Toxin A or B gave a single polypeptide band of the same electrophoretic mobility as ribonuclease, suggesting a molecular weight of 12,000. Ribonuclease, however, tends to travel somewhat more slowly than predicted from its molecular weight. More recently, ribonuclease was replaced by other standards such as cytochrome c and chymotrypsin or trypsin, which give more valid mobilities in the low molecular weight range. These results indicate a molecular weight for toxin subunits closer to 24,000. Since the accuracy of the method decreases for proteins with molecular weights below 24,000 (Shapiro *et al.*, 1967), an estimated size for the toxin subunits between 12,000 and 24,000 seems more justified. An estimate of 24,000 molecular weight would be in agreement with a minimum molecular weight unit of 12,000 based on one cysteine residue per polypeptide chain estimated from amino acid analyses (Montie *et al.*, 1966b).

In further confirmation that the toxins were composed of small subunits, toxin A or B was treated with 1% SDS and then 0.1% SDS under standard conditions as described for the electrophoresis experiments. This solution was subjected to ultracentrifugation. Toxin A or B in SDS showed single identical peaks with sedimentation coefficients of 1.4 S. Ribonuclease in SDS (0.1-1%) gave a peak sedimenting at 1.6 S. Toxin A was submitted to standard SDS conditions, and S values were calculated for three different concentrations of protein diluted in 0.1% SDS and extrapolated to zero concentration. An $s_{20,w}^0$ of 1.67 was obtained.

In other experiments, treatment of toxin B with 0.1% SDS for 30 minutes at 27°C followed by ultracentrifugation resulted in the appearance of two distinct peaks. Protein was distributed approximately equally between an intermediate size subunit (2.5 S) and a peak sedimenting at 7.6 S. This suggested that very brief treatment with low concentrations of SDS was sufficient to induce partial dissociation of toxin B to an intermediate form, probably representing a dimer (Montie *et al.*, 1968b).

The electrophoresis and ultracentrifugation data taken together with the amino acid composition and molecular weights of the toxin polymers indicate that toxin B contains 5 or 10 subunits (or 10 polypeptide chains). Toxin A contains twice the number as B. All of the subunits appear to be of equal size.

The observation that higher concentrations of SDS induced complete conversion to stable subunits suggested the validity of assaying these units for biological activity. Toxin A and toxin B were treated with 1.0% SDS as previously described. The 1% SDS-toxin solution was dialyzed for 16 hours against 0.1% SDS, and following dilution, 0.5 ml samples were injected intraperitoneally into 20-gm mice for toxicity assays. Toxin A or B control LD_{50}'s were 3 μg compared to the SDS subunit value of 5 μg. Therefore, approximately 60% of the initial mouse toxic activity was retained in SDS subunits. Samples which were diluted 5-20 times in 0.1% SDS or water gave the same result. A mixture of toxins A and B also retained 60% activity after SDS treatment. SDS alone began to exhibit toxicity when 0.5 ml of a 0.5-1% solution was injected intraperitoneally.

The data showing retention of biological activity in small subunits after SDS treatment of toxin A or B seem quite remarkable. The possibility exists that the subunits reassociate to a biologically active aggregate in the mouse upon dilution. However, reaggregation seems unlikely since dilution of SDS subunits with water, or with various concentrations of SDS in which subunits remain dissociated, did not cause any variation in specific toxic activity. Also the small amount of protein finally injected after dilution and further dilution in the mouse would tend to shift the equilibrium toward monomer formation. Since SDS binds tightly to proteins, removal of SDS may be required to initiate reassociation.

It is interesting to note first, from the literature, that the subunits from a number of enzymes retain their activity if detergent solutions used for dissociation are not too concentrated (Steiner and Edelhoch, 1961; Klee,

1962). Second, a large number of structural protein polymers from mito-chondrial membrane, viral coats, and bacterial membranes appear partic-ularly susceptible to SDS (Goldberger *et al.*, 1961; Criddle *et al.*, 1962; Hersh and Schachman, 1958; Rosenberg and Guidotti, 1968; Weinbaum and Markman, 1966). Susceptibility of the large toxin proteins to deter-gent may indicate the structural nature of toxin as part of the *P. pestis* membrane (Montie and Ajl, 1964a).

6. IMMUNOLOGY — HOST RESPONSE

Warren *et al.* (1955) used the purified Walter Reed toxin (from strain Tjiwidej) to study the possible role of this antigen in immunity. *P. pestis* toxin was shown to produce antitoxin in rabbits when injected as a toxin-adjuvant mixture. This observation was verified by neutralization, hemagglutination, and complement fixation reactions. Antisera obtained remained stable for over a year when stored at −20°C or lyophilized.

The antitoxin did not react with envelope antigen, although it neutral-ized and fixed complement with toxins prepared from *P. pestis* strains EV, TRU, and A 1122. Also, antisera from other strains of human and rodent origin reacted with purified toxin. These reactions indicated that toxins derived from different strains of *P. pestis* have common antigenic structures.

Heat- or formaldehyde-inactivated toxin remained active in comple-ment fixation reactions and this complement fixation method was sug-gested for assay of total antigen in bacterial extracts.

Warren *et al.* (1955) found that hemagglutination provided a very sensi-tive method for measuring serum antitoxin levels in blood from persons contracting plague. Using sera obtained from patients following pneu-monic plague infection, high antitoxin levels were detected during the first 2 weeks after onset of the disease followed by a rapid decrease in titer during the third and fourth week of convalescence. In vaccinated hosts or infected hosts treated with antibiotics, a high and persistent titer of anti-toxin was not demonstrated.

The relationship of toxin to induction of immunity and its relationship to virulence of the bacterial cell in the disease process still remains ob-scure. Englesberg and co-workers (1954) compared the relative amounts of toxin and envelope antigen (fraction IA + IB) in six virulent and eight avirulent strains. Generally it was noted that virulent strains produced higher levels of toxin than avirulent strains. However, the toxin content of few avirulent strains was the same or slightly higher compared to some of the virulent strains. In contrast, the envelope antigen was always present in all of the virulent strains at a higher concentration than in the avirulent strains. Chen (1965) concluded from these studies that although death in plague is due to processes initiated by the toxin, high toxicity alone is not enough to render an organism virulent.

None the less, death from *P. pestis* infection seems to be initiated by a toxic action. However, toxin per se is probably not essential for active immunization. The prevention of pathogenicity depends mainly on the control of bacterial growth in host tissues during the crucial first stage of infection. In this regard, the establishment of a bacterial population (i.e., virulence) seems to depend primarily on the presence of fraction I antigen associated with phagocytosis resistance and the VW complex associated with ability of *P. pestis* to multiply in the host. A number of other antigens including the L, PF, antigen 4, "pH 6," and the "specific polysaccharide" all may play a role in the antigenic structure of the disease. For a discussion of this subject, see reviews by Chen (1965), Surgalla (1960), and Burrows (1962).

It appears therefore, that the relationship of plague murine toxin to the disease parallels the situation of a number of other toxins in that the role of the toxin in the disease remains complex and undefined.

7. ADDITIONAL PROPERTIES AND PROBLEMS: ENDOTOXIC NATURE; DETECTION OF A GUINEA PIG TOXIN; SYNERGISTIC EFFECTS

For many years, investigators referred to the plague toxin as a classic endotoxic substance, primarily because of its location within the bacterial cell. This was a descriptive and thus useful term; but with the characterization of "true endotoxins" as substances containing large amounts of lipopolysaccharide, application of this term to plague murine toxin was not consistent. Purification and characterization of the mouse toxin has provided no evidence for the presence of lipopolysaccharide in highly purified material. However, analyses of any material so far purified have not ruled out the possibility, for example, of attachment of a single carbohydrate or fatty acid residue. Proof for this type of covalently bonded residue would be very difficult to obtain in view of the possibility of slight amounts of contamination contributing to the analyses.

Walker (1967), in a recent review, referred to plague murine toxin as a lipopolysaccharide—in other words, an endotoxic substance. In particular, a suggestion was made, in part prompted by an earlier suggestion of Montie *et al.* (1964), that toxin A might possibly contain a lipid component that could partly explain its decreased electrophoretic mobility relative to toxin B (Fig. 1). Since that time, it has been shown that the decreased mobility of toxin A in 7% acrylamide gels was primarily due to its large molecular weight (240,000), which in turn resulted in a molecular sieving effect (Montie *et al.*, 1966b). In this regard all the proteins obtained from the 35-70% crude toxin fraction are partially separable by molecular sieving procedures.

Walker (1967) also referred to the action of digitonin and deoxycholate on toxin A, previously reported by Montie and Ajl (1965), as evidence for its lipoprotein nature. Additional experiments showed that this reaction is apparently only a loose binding of these steroids to the toxin and that this binding does not reduce toxicity of toxin A; in fact, it may stimulate the toxicity. The steroid-binding effect which causes selective disappearance of toxin A stained band in acrylamide gels is completely reversible by dialysis (Montie *et al.*, 1966a). With respect to lipid content, Kadis, Trenchard, and Ajl (unpublished data) have found no evidence for the presence of lipopolysaccharide in more highly purified toxin using 2-keto-3-deoxy-octonate (KDO) as the marker for endotoxinlike material.

Further suggestions that death in mice may be due to contaminating endotoxin in the plague toxin seem highly unlikely since murine toxin preparations of close to 100% purity and protein content have been obtained with LD_{50}'s of approximately 1 μg. Accepting a value of 20% impurity would mean only 0.2 μg of endotoxin could be present. Endotoxins are not lethal for mice except at levels of over 100 μg. Therefore, the possibility that death in mice is caused partially or entirely by contaminating endotoxin is not a valid experimental hypothesis unless evidence for more highly lethal endotoxic substances is revealed.

The possibility of a separate guinea pig toxin or toxins has been reported by a number of investigators (see Walker, 1967). Walker believes that the true nature of toxin is probably an unstable complex of soluble protein toxin and lipopolysaccharide. The synergistic toxic effects which resulted from combining previously nontoxic or slightly toxic DEAE-cellulose fractions (Cocking *et al.*, 1960) are the basis for the theory that a complex of this nature is the true plague toxin. The results of these authors seem to indicate that death of guinea pigs is caused primarily by components other than or in addition to the plague murine toxin.

Recently Stanley and Smith (1967) have attempted to further isolate and examine the components of the guinea pig toxin. Fractions A, B, and C were obtained from strain EV 76 after extraction of the organisms with sodium dodecyl sulfate (SDS) to release guinea pig toxin from the cell. The SDS extract was further fractionated on DEAE-cellulose columns. Fraction A from the column was fractionated additionally on Sephadex G-25 columns and on another DEAE-cellulose column to separate fractions A_1, A_2, and A_3. Fraction B was further fractionated on Sephadex G

200 and hydroxyapatite, giving fractions D, F, and G. Fractions A_2 and G in mixtures were found to be most toxic for guinea pigs. Fraction A_2 was toxic at 400 μg and G at 3.1 mg after mixing each with a nontoxic dose (15 mg) of crude B and crude A (4.2 mg), respectively, before injection into guinea pigs. Fraction G was the most active fraction containing approximately 50% of the original activity in total fraction B. Cellulose acetate electrophoresis of fraction G showed two major and two minor protein bands and immunodiffusion gave two bands, one corresponding to murine toxin antigen. Fractions A_2 and G showed no bands specifically correlating with guinea pig toxicity, although one band (in gel diffusion) was common to both fractions. Both fractions were mainly protein in nature containing small amounts of lipid and carbohydrate. These latter results seem to rule out the possibility of a typical lipopolysaccharide toxicity for guinea pigs since the preparation contained only a small percentage of lipid and carbohydrate.

Research has continued at the Hooper Foundation (see Walker, 1967) investigating the effects of a phenol-extracted endotoxin on higher animals. The data reported using the phenol-extracted material show that the LD_{50} for a 300-gm guinea pig is at the level of 30–50 mg injected intraperitoneally. The soluble protein containing mouse toxin gave an LD_{50} for guinea pigs of 275 mg. The mouse lethality of the latter preparation, if calculated, was approximately 30 μg. The conclusion that mouse toxin is relatively nontoxic for other animals seems warranted and thus confirms previous reports (Rust *et al.*, 1963). To be valid, however, these comparisons should be made using more highly purified mouse toxin, since the soluble protein preparations, judging by the LD_{50}, contained very small amounts of active mouse toxin. Moreover, such large amounts of endotoxin are required to kill a mouse (3 mg) or a guinea pig (30–50 mg) that the question is raised of availability of this amount of toxin during *P. pestis* infection. This same question is raised concerning the Stanley and Smith (1967) synergistic toxin.

One of the major problems in both these studies is the lack of purity and delineation of the toxic components. With respect to endotoxin, much controversy exists with regard to the chemical nature of these substances and the components required for toxicity. The protein guinea pig toxin or toxins, although partially separated, require additional identification of the active components. Both of the above-mentioned studies consequently are difficult to evaluate. The very nature of the problem of examining and identifying naturally occurring, biologically active complexes is quite difficult. However, much research is required in this area, and various approaches are needed to be able to explain completely the very interesting problem of the cause of toxic death following *P. pestis* infection. It is possible that a number of toxic factors will prove important.

III. Assay Systems

A. BIOLOGICAL ASSAY SYSTEMS

The method of choice for detection of toxic protein per se has been the intraperitoneal injection of samples into 16- to 18-gm female Swiss albino mice. This method is fast, relatively inexpensive, reasonably sensitive, and quite accurate. Crude cell extracts or more highly purified material can be assayed for toxin in this manner. As far as we can observe, mouse assay is specific for mouse toxic protein showing no interference from any impurities present in a given preparation. Brief heating (e.g., 60°C for 30 minutes) will destroy mouse toxicity of crude or purified preparations underlining the specificity of the assay. Six mice are injected per dilution, and an effort is made to span the LD_{50} range by injecting a series of dilutions. The stability of the toxin in liquid enables storage in the refrigerator so that further injections of a given sample can be made following initial toxicity estimations. A more precise toxic level can then be pinpointed between the original concentration dilutions. The number of dead mice per dilution is recorded generally after 24 hours. Mice die as early as 7 and 9 hours and occasionally between 24 and 48 hours. The LD_{50}, expressed in micrograms Lowry protein required to kill 50% of the mice, is averaged from the dilutions. The method of Reed and Muench (1938) is used to calculate the LD_{50} more precisely.

Intravenous routes for injection also have been used on occasion. The sensitivity of assay is increased 8- to 10-fold and mice begin dying generally 4–7 hours after injection (Montie *et al.*, unpublished data). However, the increased labor involved in tail vein injection limits the usefulness of this technique for routine assay.

A modified method of Lowry (Oyama and Eagle, 1956) has been used to measure protein content of a given toxin preparation. The LD_{50} values generally are based on these determinations. Bovine serum albumin (Pentex, crystallized) serves as a standard, and consistent but relative protein values are obtained. The percentage Lowry protein (per milligram of dry weight) has been useful as a routine indicator of the quality of a given preparation with respect to the presence of nonproteinaceous materials. Since the Lowry method is based on the number of aromatic amino acids present in each protein, and because this number will vary to some extent among proteins, the method is not valid for absolute protein weight determinations. Absolute values are obtained by determination of total nitrogen on carefully dried samples.

B. IMMUNOLOGICAL ASSAY SYSTEMS

1. OUCHTERLONY DOUBLE DIFFUSION

The Ouchterlony technique (Ouchterlony, 1949, 1968) has been used with success as a routine assay employing a variety of toxin preparations. A qualitative estimate can be made of the presence and degree purity of toxins A and B in a given sample. The agar plates routinely used are 6 cm in diameter. The gel bed is composed of 1% Noble agar (Difco) in 0.05 M phosphate buffer (pH 7.3) and 0.85% physiological saline. Merthiolate (1 ml/100 ml agar solution of a 1:1000 dilution of concentrate) is added to prevent contamination. Crude rabbit antiserum (0.3 ml) is placed in the center well and 0.15 ml of toxin sample is placed in the outer wells. Plates are incubated at room temperature for 1–4 days. Plates a few weeks old that have hardened provide a more satisfactory agar bed because diffusion and penetration of the gel by antisera and toxin is faster, and therefore, precipitin bands are usually visible within 1–2 days. Separate bands are always discernible for toxins A and B, when present, providing the antisera are of good quality.

This gel diffusion technique has proved useful in providing a semiquantitative estimate of the degree of denaturation of toxin by chemical agents such as guanidine hydrochloride and urea (Montie *et al.*, 1966a). Loss of toxin biological activity correlated well with loss in the intensity of the toxin precipitin band.

There are some disadvantages to this technique, however. Toxin protein, as has been previously discussed does not serve as good antigenic material (Warren *et al.*, 1955), at least not under the conditions used routinely to prepare antisera in rabbits (Ajl *et al.*, 1955; Kadis *et al.*, 1963). Therefore, not only is the level of antitoxin very low, but its composition may vary considerably with each preparation. As a result relatively large amounts of concentrated antisera are needed for routine use.

Another problem inherent in the method itself remains in the difficulty in clearly distinguishing various antigens when, for example, more than seven to eight antigens are present. This is particularly the case when, in some instances, maximum band appearance requires a few days incubation. Some bands appearing earlier begin to break up after a few days, introducing an array of multiple bands which complicates interpretation. In such cases the identity of unknown toxin bands based on fusion with adjacent standards remains questionable.

A final disadvantage may lie in the lack of sensitivity of this technique. Fifty to 100 μg of crude protein are required per well in order to attain an adequate reaction. This disadvantage, however, may be minimized by reducing the size of the agar bed and the distance between antigen–antisera wells, providing that band detection remains definitive.

2. VERTICAL GEL DIFFUSION

This technique was used successfully with plague murine toxin. Ajl *et al.* (1958) employed the Oudin technique (Oudin, 1948) and the Ouchterlony method to assay for purity of toxin obtained from continuous flow paper electrophoresis. The Oudin technique involves diffusing toxin through a layer of agar gel containing rabbit antisera in vertical tubes. The antisera can be either dissolved in the agar or layered beneath the agar at the bottom of the tube for the double diffusion technique. An added advantage of the tube method over the plate method is that precipitin bands are better resolved and therefore readily distinguished.

This technique may be less desirable for routine work since it requires somewhat more skill and effort to properly set up the tube system. Also the advantage of identification of unknown antigens by lateral fusion is not possible, so that comparisons with standards must be made on the basis of relative band migration from the origin.

C. ACRYLAMIDE GEL ELECTROPHORESIS

Toxins A and B have been isolated and identified by a number of procedures. Of the various electrophoretic methods for separation and identification, cellulose acetate, starch electrophoresis, and acrylamide gel electrophoresis have been utilized. Disc electrophoresis as modified from Ornstein and Davis (1962) has proven most reliable and fast for routine assay of toxin preparations. Elimination of the sample and spacer gels improved the efficiency of the method with no appreciable loss in resolution. Electrophoresis run times of 20–30 minutes followed by staining with amido black and overnight destaining or electrophoretic destaining result in the appearance of amido black-stained toxin bands. The toxin bands are usually two of the major bands present and are readily distinguished by their electrophoretic mobilities. The percentage of each toxin present is relative to the amount of amido black-stained protein present. Band density is easily measured with a Photovolt densitometer equipped with recorder and integrator.

Accurate records of each preparation can be made for later reference. For the past 5 years, we used the acrylamide method in conjunction with mouse intraperitoneal assay to evaluate each toxin sample. From 1 to 5 μg of toxin can be detected in more purified samples. In our laboratory this has proven superior to the antigen–antibody diffusion methods which requires a constant supply of good quality antisera for a standardized reaction. Small amounts of impurities not detectable by immunoassay can be observed in acrylamide gel electrophoresis. In addition, as in the case of the Ouchterlony reaction, the extent of toxin denaturation can be semi-quantitatively correlated with loss of amido black-stained bands (Montie *et al.*, 1966a).

IV. Toxin Synthesis and Metabolism

A number of investigations have been devoted to defining cultural conditions for growth of *P. pestis* as related to general nutritional requirements and to synthesis of various antigens. In particular, studies of the synthesis of virulence antigens have indicated the complexity of the question concerned with why certain *P. pestis* cells are capable of initiating infection and disease (Burrows, 1962).

Studies of the synthesis of plague murine toxin have been sporadic, partly due to the rather difficult problem of defining precisely what was being synthesized, i.e., the chemical nature of plague murine toxin. This aspect has been discussed in the first part of this chapter. Another problem that arises in studies of toxin synthesis concerns application of an appropriate assay system for detection of toxin in cell extracts. This is particularly true in the case of plague murine toxin, since it is tightly bound in the cell until released by autolysis or some other physicochemical procedure. Consequently, changes in toxin levels may not be only directly dependent on cultural conditions and genetic considerations, but also on the relationship of these factors in determining the overall anatomical structure of *P. pestis*. As a result, the method chosen for measuring toxin levels will depend on the interrelationship of toxin to cellular structure.

Misconceptions concerning total toxin cellular levels can and do arise by relying too heavily on results obtained by extracting toxin using a single physical or chemical method. To illustrate the profundity of such problems, one need only turn to the literature on penicillinase synthesis (see papers by Lampen, 1967a,b). Here, a very thorough study of what initially appeared to be examination of synthesis of a single simple exoprotein evolved into quite complex studies concerning the role of membrane-bound intermediate penicillinase serving as precursor pencillinase. The interrelationship of penicillinase release to the structure of the cell surface remains to be clarified.

A. Requirements for Growth, Nutritional Effects, and Antigen Synthesis

In our laboratories we have made a beginning in understanding the relationship of toxin to the *P. pestis* cell by demonstrating how extreme shifts in toxin levels can be initiated. The patterns that emerge following these metabolic shifts should help us to identify and understand those factors responsible for changes in the relative toxin content of a cell as well as understanding regulation of *P. pestis* protein synthesis in general. Many studies concerned with antigen levels in virulent and avirulent cells have shown that cultural-environmental conditions markedly influence the antigenic pattern in *P. pestis*. Although correlative explanations and cause and effect relationships with respect to the influence of cultural conditions have been slow in forthcoming, some of these investigations will be briefly reported in view of their possible significance with regard to toxin synthesis in strain Tjiwidej.

Many studies have been reported concerning the nutrition and requirements for growth of various strains (virulent and avirulent) of *P. pestis*. Much of the early nutritional work is reviewed by Pollitzer (1954). It became apparent that *P. pestis* could not sustain rapid growth on a mineral salts-glucose medium. Furthermore, such factors as the size of inoculum and growth temperature were variable factors that could not be ignored in establishing nutritional requirements. It was soon evident in many of the strains studied that the amino acid phenylalanine was an absolute requirement. Also, some source of organic sulfur such as (a) cysteine; (b) cystine and methionine; or (c) methionine and thiosulfate was found to be a minimal requirement (Rao, 1939; Douderoff, 1943; Englesberg, 1952). The addition of other amino acids to the minimal media increased the growth rate and total cell yields. Synthetic and semisynthetic media were employed containing the full complement of amino acids found in casein (Berkman, 1942; Rockenmacher *et al.*, 1952; Hills and Spurr, 1952). Hills and Spurr (1952) reported the additional requirement for vitamins in a minimal medium as the growth temperature was raised. A mixture of 22 amino acids were required if biotin and pantothenate were omitted at 36°C. A number of chemically defined media have since been suggested and employed (Higuchi and Carlin, 1958; Brownlow and Wessman, 1960).

Surgalla (1960) compared some of the growth properties of virulent and avirulent strains. A lethal effect of glucose or mannitol on *P. pestis* cells under certain conditions was observed with virulent, but not avirulent strains (Wessman *et al.*, 1958). Brownlow and Wessman (1960) substituted xylose for glucose to avoid the glucose effect. Pirt *et al.* (1961)

showed that substituting galactose for glucose prevented acid formation and accounted for larger cell yields.

The interrelationship between Ca^{2+} and Mg^{2+}, virulence, temperature, and growth rate has been studied by a number of investigators. Virulent *P. pestis* strains require Ca^{2+} for growth at 37°C, but cultures soon became dominated with avirulent cells since Ca^{2+} repressed virulence antigen (VW) production. Lack of Ca^{2+} (with added Mg^{2+}) resulted in stasis of virulent cells which possessed the genetic potential of producing virulence antigens (Brubaker and Surgalla, 1964). Magnesium ion potentiated a Ca^{2+} deficiency in the medium and promoted growth of avirulent cells (Higuchi and Smith, 1961). Brubaker and Surgalla (1964) observed that Ca^{2+} deficiency at 37°C affected the process of normal cross wall formation and induced enlarged cells of virulent (but no avirulent) *P. pestis*. These morphological changes were later confirmed by the experiments of Gadgil *et al.* (1966). Brubaker and Surgalla (1964) also showed that regardless of the Ca^{2+} concentration, massive lysis of cells occurred at 1.2×10^{-3} M Mg^{2+}. If the Mg^{2+} concentration was raised 2- to 4-fold, no lysis occurred provided 2.5×10^{-3} M Ca^{2+} was present. At low concentrations of Ca^{2+} (3×10^{-4} M to 1.2×10^{-3} M) and with 0.01 M Mg^{2+}, neither significant growth nor lysis occurred. Magnesium ion addition prevented lysis, induced VW production, but did not permit growth of virulent cells. This work indicates that the level of virulence protein antigens is very rapidly changed under varying cultural conditions. It is of further interest that these changes are in some way related to significant morphological changes.

B. TEMPERATURE EFFECTS AND TOXIN CELLULAR LEVELS

All of these ion interactions are related to culture temperature since they are only demonstrable at 37°C. Other, more specific, effects of temperature on toxin cellular levels have been reported. It was noted in the Brubaker and Surgalla studies (1964) that a VW^+ avirulent mutant (relatively rare) exhibited apparent deficiences in antigens F, Q, and T (toxin) synthesis at 37°C, although in this particular mutant there was no effect of varying Ca^{2+} to magnesium oxalate. These antigens were detected by gel diffusion. Englesberg and Levy (1954) also showed decreased toxin levels at 37°C in an avirulent strain A 1122 but not in avirulent EV 76 as assayed by decreased total LD_{50}'s. Fukui *et al.* (1960), experimenting with the virulent Alexander strain showed that toxin was always present in cells grown at 5°, 26°, or 37°C, whereas antigens F, V, and W were absent at the two lower temperatures. Again, assay was by the immunodiffusion technique. Goodner (1955) found that EV 76 organisms grown at 37°C were 62 times as lethal per cell (assayed by injection) as those grown at 26°C, the optimum for vegetative multiplication. It can be concluded from such temperature studies that growth temperature is intimately related to regulation of protein levels in *P. pestis* cells.

In our laboratories it was observed that toxin levels in strain Tjiwidej were lower at 37°C compared to 25° or 27°C as assayed by mouse injection. This decreased level of toxin at 37°C was noted in spheroplasts as well as whole cells (Montie and Ajl, 1964a). In line with earlier observations, there appeared to be an increased nutritional requirement at 37°C. Enzymic casein hydrolyzate is preferred over synthetic medium containing five amino acids or casamino acids. Also, much higher concentrations of casein hydrolyzate are required at 37°C relative to 27°C to sustain rapid growth. Higher inocula concentrations are also needed to initiate growth at 37°C (Leon *et al.*, unpublished data).

Temperature shift experiments have indicated that toxin levels can increase or decrease over short time periods relative to 27° or 37°C temperatures, respectively. These observations suggest that control is allocated to a precise point where a turn on–turn off mechanism can function. It is very likely that at the same time toxin synthesis is being reduced that other antigens are being synthesized. Pirt *et al.* (1961) showed that V (virulence) antigen was not detected in organisms grown at 28°C. At 37°C maximum V antigen content was attained.

Decrease in relative toxin content has been observed by assay on acrylamide gels after short-term and long-term experiments. The loss of toxin A protein band always coincided with an increased LD_{50} of the sonicated or alumina-ground extracts. Also, crude 37°C ribosome preparations containing adsorbed toxin showed large decreases in toxin content relative to 27°C ribosomes (Montie and Ajl, 1964a, Leon *et al.*, unpublished data). Experiments with cell-free, amino acid incorporating systems have shown that the 37°C system is less active in incorporating phenylalanine-^{14}C into proteins precipitable by hot TCA.

These results taken together suggest the possibility that a specific inhibition of toxin protein synthesis in strain Tjiwidej occurs at 37°C. Another factor affecting the toxin level may be increased turnover at the higher temperature. Lability of cell envelope containing toxin has been observed under a number of conditions at 37°C. Increased metabolism observed at 37°C may be reflecting a greater requirement for amino acids and consequently this need may induce toxin–membrane turnover. It is interesting to speculate that loss of the ability of Tjiwidej to synthesize toxin at high temperatures (animal body temperature) relates in some manner to its lack of virulence.

C. SPECIFICITY OF TRYPTOPHAN ANALOGS ON TOXIN CELLULAR LEVELS

Before evidence was found indicating a difference in tryptophan content between toxin A and B, some earlier studies (Montie and Ajl, 1964b) showed that toxin synthesis could be separated from total protein synthesis not only by growth at high temperatures, but also by the addition of tryptophan analogs to culture media. A number of inhibitors were tested, but only the tryptophan analogs showed this selectivity as a specific inhibitor of toxin synthesis (Fig. 3). A number of investigators have previously reported the selective action of tryptophan analogs on protein synthesis (Mach *et al.*, 1963; Pardee and Prestidge, 1958; Thang *et al.*, 1963). With these findings it has become increasingly clear that tryptophan analogs and the tryptophan level itself can regulate protein synthesis in a number of defined ways, in addition to their roles in end product inhibition as elucidated by Moyed (1960).

In *P. pestis*, 4-methyltryptophan (4-MT) showed the most inhibition of growth and toxin synthesis of the five tryptophan analogs tested (Fig. 3). The results with 5-fluorotryptophan (5-FT) were quite interesting, since 5-FT gave little growth inhibition during short-term experiments (4–6 hours) but showed very significant decreased toxin levels. After longer-term experiments in which very dilute suspensions of cells were exposed to 5-FT for 8–11 hour periods, it was found that extracts of analog-treated cells showed a 3- to 4-fold increase in LD_{50} compared to controls (Montie *et al.*, 1964). The decrease in toxin activity in extracts from sonic-treated

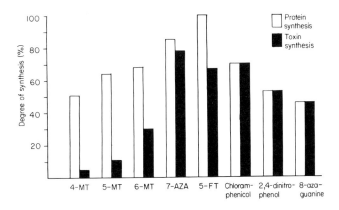

FIG. 3. The selective action of tryptophan analogs on toxin formation. Analogs were added to a final concentration of 20μg/ml. Chloramphenicol, 2,4-dinitrophenol, and 8-azaguanine concentrations were 1, 10, and 40 μg/ml, respectively. Degree of synthesis in treated cells is relative to the control cells taken as 100% (Montie and Ajl, 1964b).

cells following short-term or longer-term experiments correlated with a decrease in amount of toxin A band in the acrylamide gel assay. A band coinciding with electrophoretic mobility of toxin B remained present even during long-term experiments.

The addition of small amounts of L-tryptophan prevented inhibition by a 20-fold excess of analogs such as 4-MT. Since Moyed and Friedman (1959) with *Escherichia coli* and Ames (1964) using *Salmonella typhimurium* reported permease competition between tryptophan and its analogs, indole was employed in our studies as an antagonist in an attempt to avoid possible permease competition (Montie and Ajl, 1964b). Data in Table II show that indole partially reversed the effects of three tryptophan analogs. Both protein and toxin inhibition were prevented by concentrations of indole lower than the analog level. Indole by itself became inhibitory at levels required to obtain complete reversal. Shikimic acid completely prevented the selective effect of 4-MT but only partially prevented growth inhibition. In contrast, anthranilic acid plus 4-MT produced a synergistic inhibitory effect (Table II). The different effects of shikimic and anthranilic acids remain to be explained. In view of the action of 4-MT on the synthesis of anthranilate in mutants of *E. coli* (Trudinger and Cohen, 1956), one would expect anthranilate to be a better antagonist than shikimate. However, it is interesting that these authors also reported an anthranilate–4-MT inhibitory synergisim using various *E. coli* strains.

Recently, Jensen (1969) has reported a somewhat parallel situation between anthranilate and 5-methyltryptophan in *Bacillus subtilis*. These experiments may shed light on the anthranilate effects in *P. pestis*. In *B. subtilis*, although L-tryptophan or indole overcame 5-MT inhibition, anthranilate was a very poor antagonist. Anthranilate was found less effective at higher concentrations, suggesting that in *B. subtilis* as in *E. coli* (Gibson and Yanofsky, 1960), anthranilate may inhibit indole glycerol-3-phosphate synthetase at higher concentrations. This inhibition may relate to the susceptibility of macromolecular aggregates of the tryptophan enzymes (Whitt and Carleton, 1968).

Jensen also found that with the addition of histidine and anthranilate, complete antagonism of 5-MT occurred. He suggested that the combined effect may reflect the ability of histidine to spare 5-phosphoribosyl 1-pyrophosphate (PRPP) (a multifunctional metabolite marking a metabolic branch point leading to both histidine and tryptophan), consequently increasing the level of PRPP as substrate available to phosphoribosyl transfer.

As another indicator of tryptophan analog effect, the total tryptophan content of *P. pestis* cellular protein, was measured by the method of Spies and Chambers (1949). An inverse correlation was found between the de-

TABLE II

INDOLE, ANTHRANILIC ACID, AND SHIKIMIC ACID AS ANTAGONISTS OF
THE ACTION OF TRYPTOPHAN ANALOGS ON TOTAL PROTEIN AND TOXIN SYNTHESIS[a]

Sample	Protein formed (mg)	LD_{50} (μg protein)
Control	11.5	40
4-Methyltryptophan	5.3	60–80
4-Methyltryptophan + indole	8.9	40
Control	5.9	30
5-Methyltryptophan	4.3	60
5-Methyltryptophan + indole	5.7	40
Control	17.1	50
5-Fluorotryptophan	15.1	70
5-Fluorotryptophan + indole	15.9	60
Control	11.3	<40
4-Methyltryptophan	6.7	50
Anthranilic acid	12.1	<40
4-Methyltryptophan + anthranilic acid	4.1	>60
Control	9.9	<40
4-Methyltryptophan	4.7	60
Shikimic acid	8.3	40
4-Methyltryptophan + shikimic acid	4.9	40

[a] This table was compiled from results given in Montie and Ajl (1964b).

gree of analog inhibition and the tryptophan content of cell protein. Decreases of tryptophan content of 20–30% were observed in analog-treated cell protein compared to controls. Tryptophan levels increased in cell protein in cells treated with indole and 4-MT together compared to protein from 4-MT cells.

In some preliminary experiments evidence was found that membrane toxin of spheroplast envelopes showed more sensitivity to inhibition by analogs (Montie *et al.*, 1964). These results suggested initially that the membrane toxin was inhibited to a greater degree than cytoplasmic toxin, and that this correlated with the absence in analog-treated extracts of toxin A, a possible membrane toxin. Data obtained following examination of alkaline extracts of spheroplast envelopes showed the presence of a slow-moving electrophoretic band corresponding to toxin A (Montie *et al.*, 1964). The location of toxin A exclusively in the cell envelope must be further confirmed using other separation techniques. In recent years results from experiments with various kinds of cell envelopes and their protein components as well as viral coat proteins have emphasized the likelihood of obtaining artificial protein polymeric aggregates after extraction followed by acrylamide electrophoresis in weak alkaline systems. Therefore, earlier conclusions showing toxin A primarily in the membrane fraction and toxin B primarily of cytoplasmic origin must be considered tentative until not only is membrane protein examined by a variety of methods, but also it is conclusively shown that toxin B is not readily removed from membrane during cell breakage.

It was concluded from the tryptophan experiments that the formation of tryptophanless protein accounted for continued protein synthesis in tryptophan-depleted cells. In addition, the cellular tryptophan level may determine the quantity and quality of protein made in *P. pestis*. Although the Tjiwidej strain synthesizes at least a minimal required amount of tryptophan (added tryptophan does not seem to stimulate synthesis of toxin or protein), a shift in this apparently delicate tryptophan balance influences protein metabolism and toxin synthesis.

D. Location and Bound Nature of *P. pestis* Toxin

It has been observed by a number of workers that the murine toxin is intracellular and that it can be released following lysis or autolysis of the organisms (Englesberg and Levy, 1954; Goodner *et al.*, 1955; Warren *et al.*, 1955). Cocking *et al.* (1960) submitted *P. pestis* grown *in vivo* to sonic oscillation. They found that toxicity for mice resided primarily in the extract with a minority of the activity remaining in the cell residue. The possibility that certain breaking procedures might lead to erroneous conclusions about toxin distribution in growing organisms prompted the use of spheroplasts instead of whole organisms to demonstrate location of active toxin in the cell (Montie and Ajl, 1964a).

Actively growing cells were converted to spheroplasts with either penicillin or glycine. At least 10% of total activity was found to be associated with the envelope fractions, whereas the remainder resided in the cytoplasmic fraction. Ribosomal fractions contained an insignificant amount of toxin. This is at variance with some of our more recent findings which showed that large amounts of toxin are adsorbed to once-washed ribosomes obtained from soluble extracts of alumina-ground whole cells. The latter toxin is readily removed by high speed centrifugation through a sucrose cushion.

When washing the envelope fraction, it was found that significant amounts of protein, toxin, and RNA were removed during these procedures. It was attempted to maintain envelope integrity by modifying the fractionation procedure (Montie and Ajl, 1965). A final step involving homogenization with a Teflon pestle to induce weakening of the spheroplast structure was eliminated and a lyophilization procedure was substituted. Also, the total number of washings was reduced. These changes in procedure resulted in a shift of the percentage distribution of total cell toxin so that toxin in the envelope fraction increased to 20-30%. There were concomitant decreases in the protein weight and total toxic activity of the cytoplasmic fraction.

Along with observations of the fragility of spheroplast envelopes to washing, the former data suggested that in addition to possible adsorbed cytoplasmic protein, some envelope protein and bound toxin was being released from disrupted spheroplast envelopes. Further evidence supporting this suggestion was found. It was demonstrated that certain enzymes of the citric acid cycle and of the electron transfer system including NADH oxidase were associated with the membrane fraction. Using NADH oxidase activity as a membrane marker, a comparison was made of toxin distribution in spheroplast fractions prepared by homogenization and by lyophilization. The cytoplasmic fraction of the homogenized extracts contained considerable enzymatic activity, whereas the lyophilized extracts exhibited almost no activity in the cytoplasmic fraction. Some enzymatic activity began to appear in the wash fractions of the lyophilized envelopes. The ready release of membrane marker enzyme added support to the concept of a very fragile *P. pestis* envelope. Also, part of the protein and toxin that appeared in the cytoplasmic and membrane wash fractions was actually derived from the membranes. The membrane system of *P. pestis* may be comparable to that of *Azotobacter agilis* (Pangborn *et al.,* 1962). Release of NADH oxidase from isolated *Azotobacter* membranes has been correlated with selective disintegration of the more labile intracytoplasmic membranes but not the peripheral membrane.

Salton (1967a) has reported findings with *Micrococcus lysodeikticus* membranes, showing that very carefully controlled washing is required to keep membranes intact. Release of a specific ATPase, a membrane component, can be achieved by selective washing of *M. lysodeikticus* membranes (Whitside and Salton, 1969).

Envelopes of gram-negative bacteria have been reported to be much more susceptible than gram-positives to washing with low salt concentrations, especially in the absence of an adequate concentration of divalent cations (Salton, 1967b). This sensitivity is reflected in the fragility of *P. pestis* envelopes. Isolated *P. pestis* envelopes were disrupted by various means to examine the relationship of the toxin to the envelope of the *P. pestis* cell (Montie and Ajl, 1964a). An envelope suspension subjected to sonic vibration increased significantly in specific toxic activity compared to the original suspension. Addition of Mg^{2+} to such suspensions protected the isolated membranes against disruption by sonic treatment. The

LD_{50} of released protein decreased approximately threefold below the initial envelope bound protein. These data suggested that the potential toxic activity of bound toxin cannot be adequately expressed until the toxin is solubilized.

When isolated envelopes were incubated with trypsin, most of the protein released by trypsin was nontoxic. Since trypsin will not hydrolyze native toxin, these findings suggested that the toxin may be bound in some manner which makes it inaccessible to trypsin action.

Isolated membranes were also susceptible to partial dissolution by sodium deoxycholate or alkaline aqueous solvents (pH 8-10). As in the case of short sonic treatments, soluble proteins that had been removed from the envelopes showed a higher specific toxic activity than the original envelope material. These data argue against the importance of a complex as the ultimate mouse toxin in *P. pestis*. On the contrary, these results suggest that mouse-toxic protein must be released from a complex before it assumes full toxicity.

Results from such *in vitro* experiments may help to more fully understand the sequence of events during autolysis and possible enzymatic release of toxin at the end of the growth cycle in liquid culture. In addition, such parallels could be further extended to the mammalian system where autolysis occurs and toxic death ensues toward the termination of bacterial population growth. With respect to the autolytic process, Goodner (1955) studied the lysis of *P. pestis* with deoxycholate and concluded that very active mouse toxin was released by deoxycholate and other bile salts from whole cells or autolysates. These authors suggested the possibility that deoxycholate brings about the conversion of a poorly toxic substance or a precursor into an active toxic substance. This finding and hypothesis are in agreement with our results and interpretations of the effects of deoxycholate on release and activation of envelope toxin (Montie and Ajl, 1964a).

A number of Russian workers have investigated the possible relationship between the toxin and certain enzymatic activity and enzyme location. Kanchukh *et al.* (1963) found that catalase appeared in the 0.4–0.7 ammonium sulfate fraction which contained the toxin. In repeated fractionation, the maximum quantity of catalase was precipitated at 0.5 saturation. The electrophoretic mobilities of catalase and toxin were similar, although the catalase was less acidic than the toxin and precipitated at a higher pH. Yaromyuk and Domaradskii (1962) reported the presence of an F antigen responsible for fibrinolytic activity in *P. pestis*. This antigen is apparently bound to the cell envelope and was extracted with a 15% urea solution or with 0.5 M potassium thiocyanate (pH 7.7). The F factor and toxicity were not bound to the same substance.

E. *P. pestis* AND LYSOGENY

Related to the problem of autolysis of *P. pestis* and toxin release is the possible role of phage-induced lysogeny. Smith (1961) made a survey of 54 strains of *P. pestis* (virulent and avirulent) and reported failure to detect lysogeny among these strains. This would suggest that autolysis of *P. pestis* in liquid culture at any temperature is not phage induced.

V. Summary Remarks

The bacterium *Pasteurella pestis* produces protein extremely toxic to mice and rats and was designated the murine toxin. Initially, at the Walter Reed Laboratories, a single toxic protein (toxin B) was isolated and characterized (Ajl *et al.*, 1958). During the past 8 years, at the Albert Einstein Laboratories, a second toxic protein (toxin A) has been isolated and the properties and molecular weights of both toxins have been examined in some detail (Montie *et al.*, 1964; Montie *et al.*, 1966b). Toxin A (240,000 mol. wt.) is approximately twice the molecular weight of toxin B (120,000 mol. wt.). The molecular weights and similar amino acid content suggested that toxin A is merely a dimer of toxin B. This relationship is further emphasized by their similar specific toxic activities for 16–18 gm mice, the presence of sensitive sulfhydryl groups, denaturation of both toxins by urea and guanidine hydrochloride, and similar ultraviolet spectra in the 250 to 300 mμ range. Arguing against the simple dimer hypothesis is the following evidence: a significant difference in tryptophan content between toxin A and B; toxin A and B Ouchterlony bands do not intercept; toxin B shows greater specific absorption in the far ultraviolet; only toxin A forms an unstable complex with digitonin or deoxycholate. Both proteins when examined for subunit components were found to be dissociated with sodium dodecyl sulfate into small subunits of the same molecular weight (12,000–24,000). These subunit preparations retained 50–60% of the toxicity of the original preparation. This would suggest that only a small portion of the parent macromolecule may be required to react with a receptor site in the mouse or rat. The possibility remains that the toxins reaggregate after dilution and reinjection into mice. This possibility is very difficult to disprove, but it seems unlikely since dilution with aqueous solvents with or without SDS did not affect the comparative LD$_{50}$'s of these solutions. Also, dilution would tend to shift the equilibrium toward dissociation.

All of the evidence taken together indicates that the toxins are composed of the same size subunits, 5 or 10 in number, depending upon the number of polypeptide chains per subunit. The different properties exhibited by both toxins may reflect a difference in a particular subunit or particular subunits in terms of their amino acid content. These differences in properties may further indicate conformational variation between the polypeptide chains of each toxin complex.

The difference in tryptophan content relates to experiments showing selective inhibition of toxin synthesis by the addition of certain tryptophan analogs. Since the average polypeptide chain in *P. pestis* contains only a few tryptophan residues at most, those proteins containing the highest number of tryptophan residues may have the least number of molecules formed under tryptophan-limiting conditions induced by accumulated analogs. The observation that toxin A is primarily absent in analog extracts as noted by assay in acrylamide gels agrees with the latter hypothesis, since this protein appears to contain a relatively higher amount of tryptophan compared to toxin B. The question remains whether or not toxin B formed under these conditions is functional.

The most likely alternative explanation would provide that the tryptophan analogs are incorporated into polypeptide chains preventing synthesis of viable toxin. Evidence favoring this explanation has increased in recent years. The incorporation of tryptophan analogs into protein has been reported by a number of laboratories (Barbour and Pardee, 1966; Ezekiel and Carlson, 1967; Lark, 1969).

Incorporation of amino acid into toxins A and B in a cell-free system has been demonstrated. It is hoped that this approach may be used to elucidate specific factors involved in regulation of toxin synthesis. In the case of the high temperature effect on toxin synthesis, some indications of alterations in the pH 5 fraction have been detected.

Induction of toxin deficiency may be a product of a more general metabolic imbalance. Metabolic rates, growth, and growth requirements are increased at 37°C. Under these conditions, cells may express an immediate need for free amino acids, and donations from pool amino acids may be insufficient. A high turnover rate of certain proteins including toxin may take place, and further, may result in the observed condition of a weakened cell envelope in 37°C whole cells or in spheroplasts. Thus autolysis in old cells at 27°C may relate to protein turnover, although toxin is not reduced to amino acids at 27°C as may be the case with 37°C cells.

REFERENCES

Ajl, S. J., Reedal, J. S., Durrum, E. L., and Warren, J. (1955). *J. Bacteriol.* 70, 158.
Ajl, S. J., Rust, J. H., Jr., Hunter, D., Woebke, J., and Bent, D. F. (1958). *J. Immunol.* 80, 435.
Ames, G. F. (1964). *Arch. Biochem. Biophys.* 104, 1.

Andrews, P. (1965). *Biochem. J.* 96, 595.

Baker, E. E., Sommer, H., Foster, L. E., Meyer, E., and Meyer, K. F. (1947). *Proc. Soc. Exptl. Biol. Med.* 64, 139.

Baker, E. E., Sommer, H., Foster, L. E., Meyer, E., and Meyer, K. F. (1952). *J. Immunol.* 68, 131.

Barbour, S. D., and Pardee, A. B. (1966). *J. Mol. Biol.* 20, 505.

Bent, D. F., Rosen, H., Levenson, S. M., Lindberg, R. B., and Ajl, S. J. (1957). *Proc. Soc. Exptl. Biol. Med.* 95, 178.

Berkman, S. (1942). *J. Infect. Diseases* 71, 201.

Boyer, P. D. (1954). *J. Am. Chem. Soc.* 76, 4331.

Brownlow, W. J., and Wessman, G. E. (1960). *J. Bacteriol.* 79, 299.

Brubaker, R. R., and Surgalla, M. J. (1964). *J. Infect. Diseases* 114, 13.

Burrows, T. W. (1962). *Brit. Med. Bull.* 18, 69.

Chen, T. H. (1965). *Acta Trop.* 22 (2), 97.

Cocking, E. C., Keppie, J., Witt, K., and Smith, H. (1960). *Brit. J. Exptl. Pathol.* 41, 460.

Criddle, R. S., Bock, R. M., Green, D. E., and Tisdale, H. (1962). *Biochemistry* 1, 827.

Dieudonne, A., and Otto, R. (1928). *In* "Handbuch der Pathogenen Mikroorganismen" (W. Kolle, R. Kraus, and P. Uhlenhuth, eds.), p. 179. Fischer, Jena.

Douderoff, M. (1943). *Proc. Soc. Exptl. Biol. Med.* 53, 73.

Englesberg, E. (1952). *J. Bacteriol.* 63, 675.

Englesberg, E., and Levy, J. B. (1954), *J. Bacteriol.* 68, 57.

Englesberg, E., Chen, T. H., Levy, J. B., Foster, L. E., and Meyer, K. F. (1954). *Science* 119, 413.

Ezekiel, D. H., and Carlson, N. (1967), *Bacteriol. Proc.* p. 116.

Fischl, J. (1960). *J. Biol. Chem.* 225, 999.

Fukui, G. M., Lawton, W. D., Ham, D. A., Janssen, W. A., and Surgalla, W. A. (1960). *Ann. N.Y. Acad. Sci.* 88, 1146.

Gadgil, M. D., Ninbkar, Y. S., and Jhala, H. E. (1966). *Indian J. Pathol. Bacteriol.* 9, 323.

Gibson, F., and Yanofsky, C. (1960). *Biochim. Biophys. Acta* 43, 489.

Girard, G., and Sandor, G. (1947). *Compt. Rend.* 224, 1078.

Goldberger, R., Smith, A. L., Tisdale, H., and Bomstein, R. (1961). *J. Biol. Chem.* 236, 2788.

Goodner, K. (1955). *J. Infect. Diseases* 97, 246.

Goodner, K., Pannell, L., Bartell, P., and Rothstein, E. L. (1955). *J. Infect. Diseases* 96, 82.

Grasset, E. (1942). *Trans. Roy. Soc. Trop. Med. Hyg.* 34, 203.

Hardman, J. K., and Yanofsky, C. (1965). *J. Biol. Chem.* 240, 725.

Hellerman, L., Coffey, D. S., and Neims, A. H. (1965). *J. Biol. Chem.* 240, 290.

Hersh, R. T., and Schachman, H. K. (1958). *Virology* 6, 234.

Higuchi, K., and Carlin, C. E. (1958). *J. Bacteriol.* 75, 409.

Higuchi, K., and Smith, S. L. (1961). *J. Bacteriol.* 81, 605.

Hills, G. M., and Spurr, E. D. (1952). *J. Gen. Microbiol.* 6, 64.

Horton, R. E., and Koshland, D. E. (1965). *J. Am. Chem. Soc.* 87, 1126.

Jensen, R. A. (1969). *J. Bacteriol.* 97, 1500.

Kabat, E. A., and Mayer, M. M. (1961). "Experimental Immunochemistry," 2nd ed., p. 86. Thomas, Springfield, Illinois.

Kadis, S., Ajl, S. J., and Rust, J. H., Jr. (1963). *J. Bacteriol.* 86, 757.

Kadis, S., Montie, T. C., and Ajl, S. J. (1966). *Bacteriol. Rev.* 30, 177.

Kadis, S., Trenchard, A., and Ajl, S. J. Unpublished data.

Kanchukh, A. A., Losera, N. L., Norosed'tev, N. N., Kolesnikova, L. I., and Gubarev, E. M. (1963). *Ukr. Biokhim. Zh.* 35, 700.

Karler, A. (1955). *Federation Proc.* 14, 233.

Klee, W. A. (1962). *Biochim. Biophys. Acta* 159, 562.

Lampen, J. O. (1967a). *J. Gen. Microbiol.* 48, 249.

Lampen, J. O. (1967b). *J. Gen. Microbiol.* 48, 261.

Lark, K. G. (1969). *J. Bacteriol.* 97, 980.

Leon, S. A., Montie, T. C., and Ajl, S. J. Unpublished data.

Lustig, A., and Galeotti, G. (1897). *Deut. Med. Wochschr.* 23, 227 and 289.

Lustig, A., and Galeotti, G. (1901). *Brit. Med. J.* I, 206.

McCrumb, F. R., Jr., Mercier, S., Robic, J., Bouillat, M., Smadel, J. E., Woodward, T. E., and Goodner, K. (1953). *Am. J. Med.* 14, 284.

Mach, B., Reich, E., and Tatum, E. L. (1963). *Proc. Natl. Acad. Sci. U.S.* 50, 175.

Mandelkern, L., and Roberts, D. E. (1961). *J. Am. Chem. Soc.* 83, 4292.

Montie, T. C., and Ajl, S. J. (1964a). *J. Gen. Microbiol.* 34, 249.

Montie, T. C., and Ajl, S. J. (1964b). *J. Bacteriol.* 88, 1467.

Montie, T. C., and Ajl, S. J. (1965). *J. Albert Einstein Med. Center* 13, 141.

Montie, T. C., and Montie, D. B. (1969). *J. Bacteriol.* 100, 535.

Montie, T. C., Montie, D. B., and Ajl, S. J. (1964). *J. Exptl. Med.* 120, 1201.

Montie, T. C., Montie, D. B., and Ajl, S. J. (1966a). *Arch. Biochem. Biophys.* 114, 123.

Montie, T. C., Montie, D. B., and Ajl, S. J. (1966b). *Biochim. Biophys. Acta* 130, 406.

Montie, T. C., Heffler, S., and Ajl, S. J. Unpublished observations.

Montie, T. C., Montie, D. B., and Ajl, S. J. (1968a). *Bacteriol. Proc.* 68, 96.

Montie, T. C., Montie, D. B., Leon, S. A., Kennedy, C. A., and Ajl, S. J. (1968b). *Biochem. Biophys. Res. Commun.* 33, 423.

Montie, T. C., Montie, D. B., and Ajl, S. J. Unpublished data.

Moyed, H. S. (1960). *J. Biol. Chem.* 235, 1098.

Moyed, H. S., and Friedman, M. (1959). *Bacteriol. Proc.* p. 107.

Ornstein, L., and Davis, B. J. (1962). "Disc-electrophoresis," preprint. Distillation Prod. Ind., Rochester, New York.

Otten, L. (1936). *Indian J. Med. Res.* 24, 73.

Ouchterlony, O. (1949). *Acta Pathol. Microbiol. Scand.* 26, 516.

Ouchterlony, O. (1968). "Handbook of Immunodiffusion and Immunoelectrophoresis." Ann Arbor Sci. Publ., Ann Arbor, Michigan.

Oudin, J. (1948). *Ann. Inst. Pasteur* 75, 30.

Oyama, V. F., and Eagle, H. (1956). *Proc. Soc. Exptl. Biol. Med.* 91, 305.

Pangborn, J., Marr, A. G., and Robrish, S. A. (1962). *J. Bacteriol.* 84, 669.

Pardee, A. B., and Prestidge, L. S. (1958). *Biochim. Biophys. Acta* 27, 330.

Pirt, S. J., Thackeray, E. J., and Harris-Smith, R. (1961). *J. Gen. Microbiol.* 25, 119.

Pollitzer, R. (1954). "Plague," World Health Organ. Monograph Ser. No. 22. World Health Organ., Switzerland.

Ramon, G., Girard, G., and Richou, R. (1947). *Compt. Rend.* 224, 1259.

Rao, M. S. (1939). *Indian J. Med. Res.* 27, 75.

Reed, L. J., and Muench, H. (1938). *Am. J. Hyg.* 27, 493.

Rockenmacher, M., Howard, A. J., and Elberg, S. S. (1952). *J. Bacteriol.* 63, 785.

Rosenberg, S. A., and Guidotti, G. (1968). *J. Biol. Chem.* 243, 1985.

Rowland, S. (1910). *J. Hyg.* 10, 536.

Rowland, S. (1911). *J. Hyg.* 11, Suppl. I, 11, 20.

Rust, J. H., Jr., Cavanaugh, D. C., Kadis, S., and Ajl, S. J. (1963). *Science* 142, 408.

Salton, M. R. J. (1967a). *Trans. N.Y. Acad. Sci.* [2] 29, 764.

Salton, M. R. J. (1967b). *Ann. Rev. Microbiol.* 21, 417.

Shapiro, A. L., Vinuela, E., and Maizel, J. V., Jr. (1967). *Biochem. Biophys. Res. Commun.* 28, 815.

Smith, D. A. (1961). *Nature* **191**, 522.

Spies, J. R., and Chambers, D. C. (1949). *Anal. Chem.* **22**, 1229.

Spivack, M. L., and Karler, A. (1958). *J. Immunol.* **80**, 441.

Stanley, J. L., and Smith, H. (1967). *Brit. J. Exptl. Pathol.* **48**, 124.

Steiner, R. F., and Edelhoch, H. (1961). *J. Biol. Chem.* **83**, 1435.

Surgalla, M. J. (1960). *Ann. N.Y. Acad. Sci.* **88**, 1136.

Swenson, A. D., and Boyer, P. D. (1957). *J. Am. Chem. Soc.* **79**, 2174.

Thang, M. N., Williams, F. R., and Grunberg-Manago, M. (1963). *Biochim. Biophys. Acta* **76**, 572.

Trudinger, P. A., and Cohen, G. N. (1956). *Biochem. J.* **62**, 488.

Walker, R. V. (1967). *Current Topics Microbiol. Immunol.* **41**, 23.

Warren, J., Walz, U., Reedal, J. S., and Ajl, S. J. (1955). *J. Bacteriol.* **70**, 170.

Weinbaum, G., and Markman, R. (1966). *Biochim. Biophys. Acta* **124**, 207.

Wessman, G. E., Miller, D. J., and Surgalla, M. J. (1958). *J. Bacteriol.* **76**, 368.

Whitside, T. L., and Salton, M. R. J. (1969). *Bacteriol. Proc.* p. 43.

Whitt, D. D., and Carlton, B. C. (1968). *J. Bacteriol.* **96**, 1273.

Winsten, S., Friedman, H., and Schwartz, E. E. (1963). *Anal. Biochem.* **6**, 404.

Yaromyuk, G. A., and Domaradskii, I. V. (1962). *Dokl. — Biochem. Sect.* (*English Transl.*); *Chem. Abst.* **57**, 6405.

Zak, R., Curry, W. M., and Dowben, R. M. (1964). *Anal. Biochem.* **10**, 135.

Site and Mode of Action of Murine Toxin of
Pasteurella pestis

SOLOMON KADIS AND SAMUEL J. AJL

I. Introduction

Plague has been known for over 2000 years as a most deadly and devastating infectious disease. The first satisfactory evidence relating to the prevalence and destructive capacity of this disease concerns a pandemic that occurred during the reign of Emperor Justinian in the 6th century A.D. It was reported to have spread "to the ends of the habitable world," lasted for 50 to 60 years and killed a total of approximately 100 million people (Pollitzer, 1954). In the 14th century, plague—then referred to as the "black death" because of its tendency to produce cyanosis in its terminal stages—was responsible for the death of a quarter of the population of Europe and spread not only through Europe but also into the Middle East, China, and India. Since that time, no major outbreaks of comparable catastrophic magnitude have arisen until relatively modern times. In the epidemic that started in Hong Kong in 1894, it has been estimated that approximately 95% of those who became infected succumbed. During the past five or six decades, there has been a remarkable decline in the incidence of human plague. Although there have been reports of occasional epidemics and sporadic cases in various parts of the world, plague is now considered a rare disease. However, the possibility still exists that social and ecological conditions could be right for another major outbreak.

The causative agent of plague, the bacterium *Pasteurella pestis*, was discovered independently by Yersin (1894) and Kitasato (1894) at Hong Kong in 1894. Shortly thereafter, Ogata (1897), Simond (1898), and Gauthier and Raybaud (1902, 1903) were mainly responsible for formulating the concept that plague is primarily a disease of certain species of rodents and that the bacilli are transmitted from one rodent to another and from rodents to man by the bites of infected fleas. This was definitely proved to be correct by the British Plague Research Commission (1906).

Despite the long history of plague as a major epidemic disease, very little is known about how *P. pestis* causes injury and death. However, many investigators have suggested that the release of toxin from the bacillus is the primary factor involved. This was based on clinical observations. The formation of lesions in the lymph glands and lungs in bubonic and pneumonic plague, respectively, is accompanied by central nervous system symptoms, such as prostration, restlessness, and sometimes incoordinate movements and delirium, as well as by high fever, high pulse rate, and weakness of the heart. Many clinicians considered these symptoms to be indicative of toxemia. Muller (1898) believed that plague toxins act directly on the myocardium or on the vasomotor center in the medulla oblongata. Rowland (1910) suggested that plague victims could die from cardiac failure while the bacilli were still confined to the lymph glands. Observations by Dieudonne and Otto (1928) were likewise indicative of toxemia and a remote action of plague toxin. These investigators found that fetuses carried by mothers infected with plague exhibited hemorrhages and degenerative changes in their internal organs, but no plague bacilli could be detected. This toxin concept was given additional credence by the findings of McCrumb *et al.* (1953) that antibiotics administered 36–48 hours after the onset of the disease failed to save patients despite the fact that, on autopsy, their blood and organs were sterile. Overall postmortem examinations revealed that these plague victims exhibited typical symptoms of so-called "toxic deaths."

Clinical substantiation of toxemia, however, does little more than to perhaps limit the scope of involvement of the ten or more antigens known to be present in fully virulent *P. pestis* organisms (Crumpton and Davies, 1956; Lawton *et al.*, 1960). Even if it were vigorously demonstrated that toxin liberated by *P. pestis* following infection was primarily or solely responsible for the multitude of biochemical and pathophysiological changes that take place in the host's cells and tissues, questions concerning which of the toxins known to be produced by *P. pestis* are associated with plague pathogenesis and whether the combined action of two or more of these toxins culminates in death must be answered.

The bacterium *P. pestis* produces several distinct toxins. The most extensively studied of these is the soluble protein toxin that is lethal for mice and rats and not for a number of other animals tested and is consequently referred to as the murine toxin. Plague murine toxin has been found to consist of two toxic proteins (see Chapter 1A of this volume by Montie and Ajl). The protein toxin or toxins lethal for guinea pigs (Keppie *et al.*, 1957; Cocking and Smith 1958; Smith *et al.*, 1960) has been fractionated by Cocking *et al.* (1960) and by Stanley and Smith (1967). None of the fractions was by itself toxic for guinea pigs in large amounts, but mixtures of the various fractions were toxic in much smaller concentrations indicating synergistic actions. Investigations on the properties of the guinea pig toxin or toxins have already been described by Montie and Ajl (see Chapter 1A of this volume). Since very little has been done on the mechanism of action of these toxic products, they will not be discussed in this chapter.

A lipopolysaccharide endotoxin first isolated from *P. pestis* cells by Davies (1956) was found to be similar in chemical composition to the endotoxins produced by most gram-negative bacteria (Ellwood, 1968). Since partially purified plague murine toxin that has been shown to be contaminated with lipopolysaccharide endotoxin has been used for many of the studies conducted with the protein toxin, it has been often difficult to ascertain whether the results obtained were due primarily to the action of the lipopolysaccharide or the protein. This has been especially perplexing insofar as the effects exerted by the heterogeneous preparations are amazingly similar to those routinely observed with bacterial lipopolysaccharide material. A comprehensive review of *P. pestis* lipopolysaccharide endotoxin is not within the province of this chapter; reference will be made to studies on the endotoxin when they relate to investigations involving plague murine toxin.

The first two sections of this chapter will deal primarily with the *in vitro* effects of the murine toxin of *P. pestis* on an enzymatic level. Special emphasis has been placed on the effect of the toxin on the function of mitochondria. Some of this work has been reviewed previously (Kadis *et al.*, 1966a). The following two sections will be concerned with the pathological and physiological changes resulting from toxin administration to toxin-susceptible animals. It is hoped that any correlations existing between the *in vitro* and *in vivo* studies will become apparent as well as any discrepancies which warrant future experimental scrutiny.

II. Cell and Tissue Oxidative Metabolism

A. INHIBITION OF KETO ACID OXIDATION

The first extensive studies on the mode of action of the murine toxin of *P. pestis* at an enzymatic level were initiated by Ajl *et al.* (1958a). Investigations were conducted on the effect of toxin purified by chemical and electrophoretic procedures (Ajl *et al.*, 1955) on the oxidation of a number of substrates by cell-free bacterial extracts, as well as by crude mouse liver homogenates. It was shown that whereas the oxidation of α-ketoglu-tarate and pyruvate, the two α-keto acids tested, was inhibited by 75% -95%, the toxin exerted little, if any, effect on the oxidative metabolism involving succinate and citrate. Similar results were obtained when toxin inactivated by heating or treatment with formalin was added to actively respiring cell-free extracts of bacteria. This finding indicates, at least on a cursory examination, that the inhibition of α-keto acid oxidation has little relevance to the *in vivo* action of the toxin. However, a subsequent section of this chapter (III,A) will include a discussion of experiments in-volving inhibition of mitochondrial respiration only by plague murine toxin that is active *in vivo* and an explanation for the apparently paradox-ical effects of inactivated toxin on crude cell-free extracts, on one hand, and mitochondrial preparations, on the other.

The inhibition of α-keto acid oxidation by crude cell-free bacterial ex-tracts and mouse liver homogenates can be reversed by the addition of excess nicotinamide adenine dinucleotide (NAD). Since it was known that the oxidation of pyruvate to acetylcoenzyme A (CoA) and carbon dioxide and the oxidation of α-ketoglutarate to succinyl-CoA and carbon dioxide required the participation of NAD-dependent dehydrogenases, the possibility existed that the toxin by acting as an NAD cleaving en-zyme could interfere with these reactions by depriving them of the neces-sary intact NAD molecules. In an earlier study, Ajl *et al.* (1956) found that NAD, when incubated with purified toxin, was split by a phosphate-dependent reaction into at least two components, one of which was nico-tinamide monoucleotide. This enzymatic cleavage of NAD did not take place in the presence of nicotinamide—a well-known inhibitor of NAD-ase (Zatman *et al.*, 1953)—or partially purified antitoxin γ-globulin. It was also shown that the NAD levels of erythrocytes of intoxicated mice were considerably reduced when compared with control animals.

The toxin used for studying the enzymatic degradation of NAD as well as the inhibition of α-keto acid oxidation behaved as a homogeneous pro-tein in ultracentrifugal and electrophoretic analyses (Ajl *et al.*, 1955) but exhibited at least two and often three or more individual zones of precipi-tation by the Oudin and Ouchterlony gel diffusion precipitation reactions. When serologically homogeneous toxin was obtained (Ajl. *et al.*, 1958b), it was found that whereas the characteristic of inhibition of α-keto acid oxidation remained, the activity of NAD disappeared and was recovered in a different protein fraction with electrophoretic mobility similar to that of the toxin.

Other studies on the ability of plague murine toxin to inhibit α-keto acid oxidation (Vasil'eva and Domaradskii, 1963; Vasil'eva, 1967) revealed a suppression of pyruvate oxidation by liver homogenates prepared from mice injected subcutaneously with toxin. However, following the daily administration of thiamine for 15–20 days at a dose of 4 μg, the pyruvate oxidation of liver homogenates increased above the control level, and the inhibitory effect of the toxin was eliminated. It has been established that thiamine pyrophosphate, α-lipoic acid, CoA, and NAD are among the major components involved in the reactions responsible for the oxidative decarboxylation of pyruvate as well as α-ketoglutarate. There is therefore some rationale for assuming that thiamine may play a role in the inhibition by the toxin of pyruvate oxidation. However, the finding (Vasil'eva, 1967) that pantothenate, a constituent of the CoA molecule, when injected subcutaneously into mice stimulates the oxidation of pyruvate in liver homogenates of control mice but inhibits its oxidation in homogenates of intoxicated animals is not readily explainable. Additional studies of a more definitive nature are needed to elucidate the significance of these observed effects of thiamine and pantothenate.

III. Action of Toxin on Mammalian Mitochondria

A. Effect on Respiration and Oxidative Phosphorylation

In order to determine the action of the murine toxin of *P. pestis* at a higher level of organization from the standpoint of enzymatic structure and closer to what might be expected to occur in an animal while still maintaining an *in vitro* system, investigations were undertaken to study the effect of the toxin on mitochondria, the active sites of energy production and transduction. This toxin is known to be lethal for the mouse and the rat, but not for the rabbit, chimpanzee, dog, and monkey. Initial studies on mitochondrial respiration by Packer *et al.* (1959) suggested that a close correlation existed between the ability of the toxin to inhibit the mitochondrial respiration of certain animal species and their susceptibility to the *in vivo* action of the toxin (see Table I). Although the toxin inhibited the oxidation of α-ketoglutarate, β-hydroxybutyrate, glutamate, and malate by heart mitochondria isolated from the rat and the mouse, it had little or no effect on these respiratory activities of similar preparations obtained from the rabbit. Subsequent experiments by Rust *et al.* (1963) also demonstrated that the toxin exerted no inhibitory effect on the respiration of heart mitochondria from the toxin-resistant chimpanzee, dog, and monkey. The endogenous respiration by rat and mouse heart mitochondria, unlike that occurring in the presence of specific substrates, was not diminished by the addition of toxin. Other purified biological agents such as bovine serum albumin, representing another protein, and the Vi and O lipopolysaccharide antigens of *Escherichia coli* and *Salmonella typhosa*, respectively, had no effect on the exogenous respiration of heart mitochondria from toxin-susceptible animals.

The action of the toxin on mitochondrial respiration was found to vary not only with regard to the species of animals from which the mitochondria were prepared but also the organ from which they were derived. Rat brain mitochondrial respiration was not altered by the toxin, but the respiration of rat and rabbit liver mitochondria was inhibited to the same extent as that of rat heart mitochondria (Kadis *et al.*, 1963).

The ability of the toxin to inhibit mitochondrial respiration was shown by Packer *et al.* (1959) to be specifically associated with its toxicity *in vivo* (Table I). When the toxin was heated to 100°C for 45 minutes or toxoided with formalin, it no longer retained its capacity to inhibit rat heart mitochondrial respiration. This finding contrasts sharply with the observed effect of inactivated toxin on crude cell-free bacterial extracts and liver homogenates (see Section II,A). The apparent discrepancy is explained by Ajl *et al.* (1958a) in the following manner. In the case of the crude extracts or homogenates, the inhibition of α-keto acid oxidation is a reflection of the chance interaction of the toxin or the toxoid with randomly dispersed enzyme molecules. The active portion of the molecule is not destroyed by heating or treatment with formalin. However, when the mitochondrion with its relatively complex structure is involved, the toxin must have not only that part of the molecule that interacts with the enzyme but also that portion that enables it to be effectively oriented within the structure of the mitochondrion before the toxin can exert its inhibitory effect.

The question as to why the toxin is unable to inhibit the respiration of intact mitochondria isolated from the heart of the rabbit and the other toxin resistant animals tested is a most intriguing one. Perhaps the most obvious reason is that the membranes of these mitochondria can in some way exclude the toxin. If this were the case, then the addition of toxin to disrupted rabbit heart mitochondria should result in an inhibition of respiration comparable to that observed with intact rat or mouse heart mitochondria. Kadis *et al.* (1963) found that this is what occurred when toxin was added to rabbit heart mitochondria that had been incubated with deoxycholate or subjected to sonic oscillation.

Studies have also been conducted on the effect of the toxin on oxidative phosphorylation. Packer *et al.* (1959) found that the respiration by rat heart mitochondria with α-ketoglutarate as substrate was stimulated 12-

and 7-fold in the absence and presence of toxin, respectively, upon the addition of the phosphate acceptor adenosine diphosphate (ADP). This indicated the initiation of oxidative phosphorylation. The rate of respiration during phosphorylation was the same in both experiments as was the phosphorus to oxygen ratio calculated from the amounts of ADP added and oxygen consumed.

TABLE I

EFFECT OF PLAGUE TOXIN, VI AND O ANTIGENS, AND
BOVINE SERUM ALBUMIN ON THE RESPIRATION OF HEART MITOCHONDRIA[a]

Source of mitochondria	Additions	Oxygen consumed (μmoles/liter/second)	Inhibition (%)
Rat heart	None	0.72	—
	Boiled plague toxin (2.5 mg)	0.66	8.3
	Bovine serum albumin (2.5 mg)	0.72	0.0
	O antigen (2.5 mg)	0.65	9.7
	Plague toxin (1.0 mg)	0.24	66.7
Rabbit heart	None	0.41	—
	Vi antigen (2.5 mg)	0.41	0.0
	O antigen (2.5 mg)	0.50	0.0
	Plague toxin (2.5 mg)	0.44	0.0

[a]This table was compiled from results reported by Packer *et al.* (1959).

Neubert and Merker (1965), however, observed that the toxin not only inhibited the oxidation of α-ketoglutarate by rat heart mitochondria *in vitro* but also exerted an uncoupling effect on oxidative phosphorylation as indicated by reduced phosphorus/oxygen ratios. It should be noted that these investigators admittedly used toxin preparations that were by no means the purest available and the experimental conditions were rather extreme. Similar effects could be observed on mitochondria isolated from hearts of rats injected with high doses of toxin. There was evidence for a pronounced inhibition of α-ketoglutarate oxidation and to a smaller degree, an uncoupling effect could be demonstrated. Liver mitochondria obtained from toxin-treated rats did not exhibit an uncoupling of oxidation from the phosphorylating reactions.

B. ABILITY OF TOXIN TO INDUCE MITOCHONDRIAL SWELLING

The most conspicious function of the respiratory chain of mitochondria is the aerobic regeneration of adenosine triphosphate (ATP) from ADP and inorganic phosphate; that is, the conversion of the oxidation-reduction energy of electron transport into the chemical energy of

ATP. Energy is, however, also provided for two primary transport processes in which mitochondria are involved; namely, the translocation of
ions and the uptake and extrusion of water, referred to as swelling and
contraction, respectively. Raaflaub (1953a,b) was the first to suggest that
mitochondria can undergo a passive volume change that is dependent
upon the osmotic pressure of the suspending medium as well as an active
change that requires respiration or high energy compounds. The studies
on swelling to be described subsequently will refer to the active process.

As already indicated, Kadis *et al.* (1963) suggested that the toxin does
not inhibit the respiration of intact heart mitochondria from toxin-resistant animals because these mitochondria are capable of excluding the
toxin. Since it has been proposed (Hunter *et al.*, 1959) that at least one
type of mitochondrial swelling, known as electron transport-dependent
swelling, depends upon increased membrane permeability that ceases
short of osmotic rupture of the mitochondrion, an attempt was made to
determine whether the toxin exerts any effect on mitochondrial swelling
and its relationship to the effect on mitochondrial respiration. Kadis and
Ajl (1963), using a method involving measurement of changes in the absorption of light in the visible region (520 mμ) by suspensions of mitochondria as a measure of changes in mitochondrial volume, reported that
the murine toxin of *P. pestis* was capable of inducing swelling in isolated
rat heart mitochondria (Table II). Rat brain mitochondria exhibited only
slight spontaneous swelling, and this was not affected by the addition of
toxin (Kadis *et al.*, 1963). Thus, the toxin was found to induce swelling
only in those mitochondria where the toxin had previously been found to
inhibit exogenous respiration. Since inhibition of mitochondrial respiration was not tested under the same conditions as swelling, it is not at all
certain whether inhibition of respiration occurs under the conditions that
are optimal for swelling. Evidence was also obtained to indicate that only
toxin that is toxic *in vivo* can exert the *in vitro* swelling effect (Kadis and
Ajl, 1963). Neither heat-denatured toxin nor mixtures of toxin and antitoxin induced swelling, whereas normal rabbit serum plus toxin promoted
swelling to the same extent as toxin alone.

The mechanism of toxin-induced swelling was investigated by determining the effect of the addition of certain inhibitors of electron transport
or high energy intermediate-supported swelling, such as cyanide (Lehninger and Ray, 1957), azide (Hunter *et al.*, 1959), and 2,4-dinitrophenol
(Tapley, 1956). Each of these agents prevented completely the swelling
caused by relatively low concentrations of toxin. Figure 1 represents typical results obtained with 2,4-dinitrophenol. Swelling promoted in the
presence of large concentrations of toxin was only partially prevented by
each of the inhibitors tested. It is conceivable that high concentrations of

TABLE II
EFFECT OF TOXIN ON SWELLING OF HEART,
LIVER, AND BRAIN MITOCHONDRIA[a]

Source of mitochondria	Condition of mitochondria	Net change in optical density at 520mμ of experimental minus control[b]
Rat heart	Incubated with 2.0 mg toxin	0.325
	Incubated with 0.5 mg toxin	0.210
Rabbit heart	Incubated with 2.0 mg toxin	0.025
	Incubated with 0.5 mg toxin	0.020
Rat liver	Incubated with 2.0 mg toxin	0.243
	Incubated with 0.5 mg toxin	0.120
Rabbit liver	Incubated with 2.0 mg toxin	0.235
	Incubated with 0.5 mg toxin	0.170
Rat brain	Incubated with 2.0 mg toxin	0.020

[a]This table was compiled from results reported by Kadis and Ajl (1963) and by Kadis *et al.* (1963).

[b]Change in optical density at 520 mμ recorded at end of 30-minute incubation period.

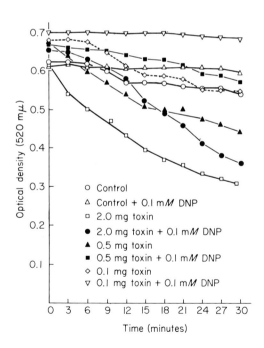

FIG. 1. Effect of 2,4-dinitrophenol on toxin-induced swelling of rat heart mitochondria. From Kadis and Ajl (1963).

toxin exerted a damaging effect on the mitochondrial membranes, thereby resulting in elimination of electron transport. As can be noted from Fig. 1, a small but consistent degree of spontaneous swelling characterized by an initial short lag period occurs when rat heart mitochondria, for example, are incubated in an appropriate medium. The swelling curves show that the lag period is eliminated in the presence of toxin alone and restored by the addition of cyanide, azide, or 2,4-dinitrophenol. This elimination of the lag period by a swelling agent and its restoration by the inhibitors is characteristic of electron transport-dependent swelling.

Although mitochondrial swelling can be induced by a wide variety of chemical and biological agents, Lehninger (1959) showed that only ATP together with Mg^{2+} is necessary for the reversal of swelling. Kadis and Ajl (1963) found that swelling of rat heart mitochondria induced by plague murine toxin could likewise be reversed by ATP plus Mg^{2+}.

C. Effect on Mitochondrial Ion Accumulation

Isolated mitochondria can actively accumulate a number of ions (including K^+, Ca^{2+}, Sr^{2+}, Mn^{2+}, and Mg^{2+}) by a respiration-dependent process (Lehninger et al., 1967). It has been suggested (Brierly et al., 1963; Chappell and Greville, 1963; Gamble, 1957; Vasington, 1963) that alterations in the integrity of mitochondria may influence their ability to retain ions that have been accumulated. Some of the observed volume changes of mitochondria appear to be related to reversible changes in the semipermeability of the inner membrane and some biological agents are able to render the semipermeable membrane "leaky" (Parsons, 1965). Since the murine toxin of P. pestis has been shown to induce mitochondrial swelling, studies were initiated to determine the effect of the toxin on the accumulation of ions by mitochondria and its relationship to the swelling effect (Kadis et al., 1965a). It was shown that the accumulation of Ca^{2+} and inorganic phosphate (P_i) by rat heart mitochondria in the presence of succinate (Table III), as well as α-ketoglutarate, β-hydroxybutyrate or malate as respiratory substrate was inhibited by the toxin to a significant extent. When the toxin was inactivated by treatment with formalin, the inhibitory effect was no longer evident. Evidence was presented to show that the ability of the toxin to inhibit the oxidation of the substrates employed was not responsible for the results obtained from the ion accumulation experiments. Mitochondria can transport ions by an ATP-supported pathway in the absence of respiration as well as by a respiration-dependent process. The toxin inhibited the former as readily as the latter. Additional experiments also revealed that the toxin had no ef-

TABLE III

INHIBITION BY TOXIN OF Ca^{2+} AND P_i UPTAKE
BY RAT HEART MITOCHONDRIA AND REVERSAL BY EDTA[a]

Components present in addition to complete system	Ca^{2+} taken up ($m\mu moles/$ mg protein)	P_i taken up ($m\mu moles/$ mg protein)	Inhibition	
			Ca^{2+} taken up (%)	P_i taken up (%)
Succinate	896	562	—	—
Succinate + 2.0 mg toxin	473	292	47.2	48.0
15 m*M* ATP	578	338	—	—
15 m*M* ATP + 2.0 mg toxin	261	172	54.8	49.1
Ascorbate + TMPD	1028	602	—	—
Ascorbate + TMPD + 2.0 mg toxin	410	265	61.5	55.9
Succinate + EDTA				
Succinate + EDTA + 2.0 mg toxin	1065	668	—	—
	879	550	17.5	17.6
Ascorbate + TMPD + EDTA	1365	803	—	—
Ascorbate + TMPD + EDTA + 2.0 mg toxin	1130	697	17.2	13.2

[a]This table was compiled from results reported by Kadis *et al.* (1965a).

fect on the respiration of rat heart mitochondria in the presence of tetra-methylphenylenediamine (TMPD), which involves the part of the electron transport system between cytochrome c and oxygen; but, nevertheless, it inhibited the uptake of Ca^{2+} and P_i supported by this segment of the electron transfer chain.

The relationship between the ability of the toxin to induce swelling and its effect on ion accumulation was studied by incubating untreated and toxin-treated rat heart mitochondria with ethylenediaminetetraacetic acid (EDTA) at a concentration (10^{-4} *M*) which has been found to prevent swelling (Tapley, 1956) without inhibiting Ca^{2+} uptake (Vasington and Murphy, 1962). Kadis *et al.* (1965a) found that this concentration of EDTA reduced to a considerable extent the inhibitory effect of the toxin on the uptake of Ca^{2+} and P_i in the presence of succinate as respiratory substrate (Table III) as well as in the presence of ascorbate and TMPD. These observations suggested that the EDTA, by preventing the swelling induced by the toxin, enables the mitochondria to retain the ions that have been accumulated in the mitochondrial lumen. However, the amounts of Ca^{2+} and P_i accumulated per milligram of protein by the controls were somewhat greater in the presence of EDTA than in its absence, indicating that EDTA may exert an overall stabilizing effect on the mitochondrial membrane.

D. Effect on Electron Transport System

The studies by Packer *et al.* (1959) on plague murine toxin involving the inhibition of respiration of isolated heart mitochondria from toxin-susceptible animals have been extended in an effort to locate the inhibitory site. Initial findings by Kadis *et al.* (1965b) suggested that the effect of the toxin on mitochondrial respiration was exerted somewhere in the electron transfer chain. The inhibition by the toxin of rat liver as well as rat heart mitochondrial respiration in the presence of four different substrates (α-ketoglutarate, β-hydroxybutyrate, glutamate, and succinate) and with ADP as phosphate acceptor was not relieved by the addition of 2,4-dinitrophenol. In this respect, the murine toxin of *P. pestis* does not act like the antibiotic oligomycin, a classic inhibitor of phosphorylating oxidation. Lardy *et al.* (1958) showed that when phosphorylating electron transport is blocked by oligomycin, the inhibition of respiration can be alleviated by 2,4-dinitrophenol.

From the schematic diagram of the respiratory chain in Fig. 2, it can be noted that the cytochromes are among the major components of the electron transport system. In order for electrons to be transferred from reduced nicotinamide adenine dinucleotide (NADH) or succinate to oxygen, the terminal electron acceptor, each of the cytochromes must remain in a reduced state. Kadis *et al.* (1965b) attempted to obtain a general indication of the site of action of plague murine toxin in the electron transport system by examining the absorption spectra of toxin-treated mitochondrial suspensions and determining whether any alteration could be observed in one or more of the absorption peaks corresponding to specific cytochrome components.

Both absolute and difference spectra were obtained with rat heart and liver mitochondria. From Fig. 3, which illustrates the difference spectrum of a toxin-treated rat heart mitochondrial preparation incubated in the presence of α-ketoglutarate, it is apparent that at the wavelengths in the visible region, corresponding to cytochromes a (604 mμ), b (shoulder at 564 mμ), and c (550 mμ), characteristic decreases in absorbancy occur. This indicates that the cytochromes of the mitochondria in the experi-

$$NADH \longrightarrow FP_1 \longrightarrow CoQ \longrightarrow cyt\ b \longrightarrow cyt\ c_1 \longrightarrow cyt\ c \longrightarrow cyt\ a \longrightarrow cyt\ a_3 \longrightarrow O_2$$
$$Succinate \longrightarrow FP_2$$

Fig. 2. Schematic diagram of the electron transport system. Abbreviations: cyt = cytochrome, FP = flavoprotein, NADH = reduced nicotinamide adenine dinucleotide, CoQ = coenzyme Q.

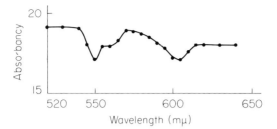

FIG. 3. Difference spectrum of the cytochrome components of rat heart mitochondria incubated with plague murine toxin in the presence of α-ketoglutarate as substrate. From Kadis *et al.* (1965b).

mental cuvette which have been incubated with toxin are oxidized compared to the mitochondria in the reference cuvette which have not been exposed to the action of the toxin. When rat liver mitochondria were employed, similar decreases in absorbancy with either β-hydroxybutyrate or succinate as substrate were noted. These results suggest that the toxin exerts its effect on the electron transport system in the region between NADH or succinate and cytochrome b.

This has been further substantiated by experiments involving the use of TMPD, which can serve as a mobile electron carrier between ascorbate and members of the respiratory chain and has been found to act between cytochrome c and oxygen (Howland, 1963). It was found that the oxidation of ascorbate by rat heart and liver mitochondria in the presence of TMPD or cytochrome c as carriers was not affected by the addition of toxin, indicating that the toxin does not act on the area of the electron transfer chain between cytochrome c and oxygen.

In an initial attempt to determine whether the murine toxin of *P. pestis* exerts its inhibitory effect by inactivating enzymes in the region between NADH or succinate and cytochrome b, the effect of the toxin on NADH dehydrogenase was studied (Kadis *et al.*, 1965b). The activity of this enzyme — assayed by the reduction of ferricyanide according to the method of Minakami *et al.* (1962) in rat liver and heart mitochondria as well as in electron transport particles from rat heart — is not affected by the toxin. This finding suggested that the toxin might not act on individual enzymes but on complexes of two or more respiratory carriers representing limited segments of the electron transfer chain.

Four such complexes have been isolated from beef heart mitochondria and obtained in highly purified form. Complex I corresponds to the NADH-CoQ reductase of Hatefi *et al.* (1962a), which catalyzes the oxidation of NADH by CoQ_1. Complex II refers to the succinic CoQ reductase of Ziegler and Doeg (1962), which catalyzes the reduction of CoQ_2, and, to a considerably lesser extent, CoQ_{10} by succinate. Complex III is the reduced CoQ-cytochrome c reductase of Hatefi *et al.* (1962b) that catalyzes the reduction of cytochrome c by reduced CoQ. Complex IV is the cytochrome oxidase system (Griffiths and Wharton, 1961; Fowler *et al.*, 1962) that catalyzes the oxidation of reduced cytochrome c by molecular oxygen.

Studies by Kadis and Ajl (1966) on the effect of the toxin on the enzymatic activity of these complexes have shown that incubating toxin with purified NADH-cytochrome c reductase, from which NADH-CoQ reductase and CoQ-cytochrome c reductase are derived (Hatefi *et al.*, 1961), results in the inhibition of the enzymatic activity of this complex. Likewise, the NADH-cytochrome c reductase of electron transport particles prepared from heavy beef heart mitochondria (ETP_{II}) is inhibited to the same degree by the toxin. Similar results have been obtained when the effect of the toxin on the NADH-CoQ reductase activity of purified Complex I and ETP_{II} particles was investigated.

Attempts were made to determine whether the inhibition by the toxin of the enzymatic activity of Complex I results from the alteration of the function of one or more of the individual components of this complex, namely, NADH dehydrogenase flavoprotein, nonheme iron, and CoQ_{10}. A characteristic property of NADH dehydrogenase isolated by various means is its ability to catalyze the rapid reduction of ferricyanide by an amytal-insensitive reaction (Hatefi *et al.*, 1962b). It was found by Kadis and Ajl (1966) that the murine toxin of *P. pestis* had no effect on the NADH-ferricyanide reductase activity exhibited by purified complex I or by ETP_{II} particles. This suggests that the toxin has no effect on the NADH dehydrogenase activity of complex I and confirms the results of previous investigations with mitochondrial suspensions (Kadis *et al.*, 1965b). Additional evidence indicating that the toxin has no effect on the flavoprotein moiety of the NADH-CoQ reductase enzyme complex stems from the observations of the difference spectra of toxin-treated Complex I. These experiments revealed that flavoprotein is as readily reduced in the presence of toxin as in its absence. Electron paramagnetic resonance spectroscopy of Complex I showed that the $g = 1.94$ signal exhibited by the nonheme iron component is not modified by the addition of toxin. Likewise, the toxin does not have any effect on the CoQ_{10} of Complex I.

E. Interaction of Toxin with Mitochondrial Structural Protein

As already noted, although the murine toxin of *P. pestis* exerts its inhibitory effect on the electron transport system by inhibiting the

NADH-CoQ reductase activity of Complex I, it had no discernible effect on any of the major components of this complex. Consequently, it was suggested by Kadis *et al.* (1966b) that the inhibition of the enzymatic activity exhibited by Complex I manifests itself as a result of the alteration by the toxin of the structural configuration of the multienzymatic unit of a mitochondrion.

When this concept was formulated, there were reports (Green *et al.*, 1961; Criddle *et al.*, 1962) of the isolation and purification from beef heart mitochondria of a nonenzymatic protein that was claimed to be homogeneous and to satisfy various criteria for a structural protein. These preparations, as well as those obtained by the modified Richardson *et al.* (1964) procedure, were found to exist as water-insoluble polymers at neutral pH and could be resolved into their monomeric units under conditions of high pH or in the presence of anionic detergents. The monomers were found to form one-to-one water-soluble complexes with cytochromes a, b, and c_1 (Criddle *et al.*, 1962), as well as with cytochrome c (Edwards and Criddle, 1966a) and with myoglobin (Edwards and Criddle, 1966b). The polymers, however, could bind with micellar phospholipids (Richardson *et al.*, 1964), orthophosphate, and nucleotides (Hultin and Richardson, 1964).

In a preliminary report, Montanaro and Sperti (1965) showed that the monomeric units of this structural protein could interact with crystalline diphtheria toxin. Studies were initiated to determine whether the murine toxin of *P. pestis* could interact with beef heart mitochondrial structural protein by measuring the solubility of the structural protein following incubation of both proteins at pH 11.0 and gradual adjustment of the pH to 8.0. It was found (Kadis *et al.*, 1966b) that the protein content of the water-washed precipitates forming at pH 8.0, because of the insolubility of the structural protein at this pH, decreased as the concentration of the toxin in the incubation mixture was increased. This was not observed with heat-inactivated toxin or with various concentrations of bovine serum albumin or when the toxin was incubated with structural protein at pH 8.0; that is, under conditions where the structural protein exists as a polymer.

These data suggest that the toxin can interact with the structural protein monomers and thus prevent them from forming polymers at neutral pH. This could occur if the toxin, by exerting proteolytic activity, were capable of splitting the monomers into their constituent peptides or if the toxin could act as an exopeptidase. However, no evidence has as yet been obtained to indicate that the toxin can behave in this manner. An alternative explanation is that the toxin is able to bind with the structural protein to form complexes.

If binding of the two proteins did occur, it would be reasonable to expect that the bound portion of the toxin might not be able to exert its toxic activity *in vivo*. Thus, the toxin that has interacted with structural protein should exhibit a higher LD_{50} for toxin-susceptible mice than the noninteracted toxin control. Kadis *et al.* (1966b) showed that although the toxin maintained at pH 11.0 had a slightly higher LD_{50} than that at pH 8.0, the LD_{50} of the toxin incubated with structural protein increased above the pH 11.0 control as the dry weight ratio of the structural protein to toxin in the incubation mixture was increased. When the ratio of structural protein to toxin was 10:1, a 10–15-fold increase in the LD_{50} of the toxin was observed. At a 20:1 ratio of structural protein to toxin, the LD_{50} of the toxin was so high that it was considered for all practical purposes to be nonlethal for mice. Experiments with purified toxin B, one of the two protein components of the murine toxin of *P. pestis* (see Montie *et al.*, 1964), gave essentially the same results as those with toxin preparations containing mixtures of toxin A and toxin B. No such elevation in the LD_{50} of the toxin was observed when it was incubated with polymeric structural protein or with bovine serum albumin.

Investigations involving the effect of interacting structural protein with toxin at pH 11.0 on the antigenic components of the toxin, as ascertained by the double diffusion precipitation reaction in agar, revealed that at exactly that ratio of structural protein to toxin at which the toxin had lost its toxicity *in vivo*, the band for toxin B could not be observed. When the toxin was incubated with polymeric structural protein or with bovine serum albumin, the toxin B band remained intact. The band for toxin A, however, could not be detected even when the ratio of structural protein to toxin was very low or when the toxin was incubated with bovine serum albumin. These results suggest that the specificity of the interaction of toxin with structural protein somehow resides with toxin B.

Since many of the studies concerning the effect of the murine toxin of *P. pestis* on various mitochondrial energized processes (see Sections IIIA,B,C,D) were conducted with rat heart mitochondrial preparations, it was deemed necessary to determine whether the toxin can interact with structural protein isolated and purified from this source. Experiments carried out in the same manner as those with beef heart mitochondrial structural protein indicated that this toxin is indeed capable of interacting with rat heart mitochondrial structural protein. This interaction, however, is not as effective as that between the toxin and the beef heart mitochondrial structural protein. For example, samples containing beef heart mitochondrial structural protein and toxin in a ratio of 20:1 give an LD_{50} of greater than 200, whereas with rat heart mitochondrial structural protein, this same ratio gives an LD_{50} of 30. However, the general pattern of events is essentially the same with the structural protein obtained from both of these sources.

The obvious question that arose concerned the nature of the interaction that had occurred between the toxin and the structural protein. As already indicated, it had been reported that monomeric beef heart mitochondrial structural protein forms water-soluble complexes with cytochromes a, b, and c_1 (Criddle *et al.*, 1962), as well as with cytochrome c (Edwards and Criddle, 1966a). In order to determine whether a complex can be formed between the murine toxin of *P. pestis* and beef heart mitochondrial structural protein, Kadis *et al.* (1967) employed procedures involved in the "reconstitution" experiments of Criddle *et al.* (1962). Ultracentrifugal analyses of solutions of toxin B alone, structural protein alone, and equimolar ratios of both proteins showed that a single sedimentation peak was exhibited in each case. The sedimentation coefficient of the solution containing both the toxin and the structural protein was intermediate in value between that of the toxin B alone and that of the structural protein alone. The studies by Criddle *et al.* (1962) involving complex formation between structural protein and cytochromes a, b, and c_1 yielded similar results. The same findings were obtained when the molar ratio of structural protein to toxin was 2:1. This indicates either that one molecule of toxin can bind more than one molecule of structural protein or that structural protein, when complexed with toxin B, can bind a second molecule of structural protein.

IV. Pathology

The first extensive observations of the pathological changes occurring in toxin-susceptible mice and rats that had succumbed to the administration of the murine toxin of *P. pestis* were made by Schar and Meyer (1956), who amplified the preliminary findings of Schar and Thal (1955). Mice injected intravenously with more than 2 LD_{50} of a toxic fraction precipitating between 35 and 70% saturation with ammonium sulfate (fraction II of Baker *et al.*, 1952) died within 2-4 hours, whereas death ensued 10-30 hours after the injection of 1 LD_{50}. No striking macroscopic or microscopic effects were noted postmortem in animals that had succumbed to the toxin within the first 10 hours. Some of the most evident gross changes included distention of the blood vessels, especially the veins of the subcutis and the vessels of the peritoneum and mesenterium, and the presence of exudates in the peritoneal and pleural cavities. The pathological changes revealed upon microscopic examination were restricted almost exclusively to the vascular system. Passive hyperemia of the internal organs was most prominent. The endothelial cells of the blood vessels in the lungs were swollen and protruded into the lumen.

In animals that died or were sacrificed 16-24 hours after injection of toxin, the subcutaneous and abdominal vessels were distended and a peritoneal exudate was present, but not to the same extent as in the animals that had died or were sacrificed earlier. The most pronounced macroscopic change concerned the appearance of the liver. In over 50% of the animals that survived 1 LD_{50} of the toxin, many yellow spots were observed either only near the margin of the liver or covering the whole surface of the organ. Evidence of petechial bleeding was found in the intestine and in the mesenterium. The intestinal contents of more than 50% of the rats examined were blood stained, but in mice this was a rare occurrence.

The organs of these animals exhibited more pathological changes upon microscopic examination than did those of animals that had died within the first 10 hours after toxin administration. Liver cell death characterized by karyorrhexis was noted as early as 10 hours after the injection of toxin, but by 16–24 hours the liver was studded with many necrotic foci. The spleen exhibited hyperemia and hyperplasia of the pulp, but occasionally the reticular elements were necrotic. Evidence for epithelial degeneration in the tubuli of the kidneys consisting either of cloudy swelling or fatty degeneration in varying degrees of severity was always obtained. However, in the heart and brain only insignificant alterations were observed. Likewise, the adrenal glands did not show any histological changes except passive hyperemia.

Neubert and Merker (1965) made electron microscopic observations of the livers and hearts of rats sacrificed 18 hours after the injection of a non-lethal dose ($\frac{1}{2}$ LD_{50}) of a partially purified plague murine toxin preparation. In the liver, fatty infiltration as well as a fragmentation of the endoplasmic sacs and an early stage of mitochondrial swelling were evident. Structural changes in the heart were virtually negligible.

The most characteristic local reaction was edema formation (Schar and Meyer, 1956). Edema appeared in the subcutis as early as 1–2 hours and within 24 hours, depending on the concentration of the toxin solution, local skin necrosis developed. Increased permeability of the capillaries of the subcutis at the site of toxin injection was demonstrated. If Evans blue dye was injected intravenously 2–3 hours after the subcutaneous administration of the toxin, a distinct blueish hue appeared in the skin where the toxin was injected.

The subcutaneous tissue when examined histologically exhibited signs of edema a few hours after toxin injection but contained only a few leukocytes. However, within 16 hours the edematous area was surrounded and penetrated mostly by polymorphonuclear leukocytes but also by a few lymphocytes. Decay of cell nuclei of the subcutaneous tissue and degeneration of the adjacent muscle fibers could also be observed. When skin necrosis occurred, hemorrhages were always present in and around the dead tissue.

Tissue reaction in the lungs following intranasal instillation of the toxin was manifested initially by the appearance of edema in the interstitium around the smaller bronchi and in the adventitiae of smaller arteries and arterioles and later on was accompanied by leukocytic infiltration. The endothelial cells, especially of the small arteries, were found to be swollen and protruded into the lumen of the blood vessels. When high concentrations of toxin were used, tissue necrosis and hemorrhages were observed.

Schar and Meyer (1956) noted that the pathological findings in mice and rats after injection of toxin resemble closely those following infection with virulent plague bacilli. Cocking *et al.* (1960) reported that the lesions resulting from injection of mice and rats with toxic products obtained by subjecting *P. pestis* cells to sonic oscillation followed by low speed centrifugation to remove predominately cell wall material according to the procedure of Smith *et al.* (1960) were similar to those caused by infection and also to the findings of Schar and Meyer (1956). These investigators also showed that in guinea pigs the changes produced by injection of their toxic material were similar to those resulting from plague infection.

The toxin used by Schar and Meyer (1956) in all of the studies was obviously not homogeneous. These preparations were found previously by Baker *et al.* (1952) to be contaminated heavily with atoxic soluble antigens. In addition, Larrabee *et al.* (1965) isolated a lipopolysaccharide-protein complex from fraction II of Baker *et al.* (1952) which was shown to be similar to the phenol-extracted lipopolysaccharide obtained from *P. pestis* cells by Davies (1956). Kadis *et al.* (1968) carried out heptose and 2-keto-3-deoxyoctolonate (KDO) determinations on phenol-extracted toxic fractions precipitating between 35 and 70% saturated ammonium sulfate and found that this material contained 20% or more lipopolysaccharide. Studies have also been carried out on the pathological changes produced by purified *P. pestis* lipopolysaccharide endotoxin in mice and guinea pigs (Walker *et al.*, 1966) as well as in monkeys (Walker, 1968). The changes observed, which were indicative of failure of regulation of the peripheral blood circulation, were similar to those observed by Schar and Meyer (1956). In the subsequent section of this chapter (Section V) it will be shown that Schar and Meyer (1956) concluded from their physiological observations that the murine toxin of *P. pestis* acted mainly on the peripheral vascular system and the liver to produce hemoconcentration and shock. It thus seems conceivable that the findings of Schar and Meyer (1956) could be due, at least partially, to the lipopolysaccharide contained in their preparations.

Burrows (1963) casts doubt on the overall significance of the pathological changes following toxin injection. He emphasizes that the negligible visible pathological changes occurring in animals dying rapidly from administration of comparatively large doses of the toxin show that death can result without the development of pathological changes that have been described in animals dying at longer time intervals after the injection of smaller amounts of the toxin or from plague infection. This led him to suggest that "these changes may in fact not themselves be responsible for death but consequences of the earlier occurrence of a more fundamental lesion in a vital system." A similar concept has been formulated by Neubert and Merker (1965). These investigators point out that their finding that the inhibition by the toxin of mitochondrial function was found only with heart mitochondria, whereas only minor changes occurred with liver mitochondria is surprising since electron microscopic observations revealed pronounced structural changes in the liver but not in the heart. They believe that these results may indicate a more specific action of the toxin on the heart.

V. Physiological Studies

A. Electrocardiographic Changes

The investigations of Packer *et al.* (1959), described previously (Section III,A) involving the inhibition by highly purified preparations of the murine toxin of *P. pestis* of exogenous mitochondrial respiration, showed that a correlation existed between the toxicity of the toxin *in vivo* and its *in vitro* effect on mitochondria and led to the hypothesis that the inhibition of mitochondrial respiration may be an explanation for its action *in vivo*. Since rat and mouse heart mitochondria were affected by the toxin, it was assumed that alterations in the myocardial physiology of these intoxicated animals might be expected which could possibly be detected by electrocardiographic measurements. Rust *et al.* (1959), Ajl and Rust (1960), and Rust *et al.* (1963) reported that elevations occurred in the S–T segment of the electrocardiogram of a rat within 60 minutes after the injection of $0.25-10$ LD_{50} of toxin and prior to changes in hemotocrit or blood pressure (see Fig. 4). In animals surviving sublethal doses of the toxin, the initial electrocardiographic alterations were no longer evident after 24–48 hours or after the animals had recovered completely. Similar changes did not occur in the electrocardiograms of rats dying from hemorrhagic shock, hypoxia, or intoxication with glucose or *E. coli* endotoxin. Electrocardiograms from the toxin-resistant rabbit did not show any abnormality, even when the toxin was administered in amounts up to 50 mg per kilogram of body weight.

Rats infected with plague bacilli were also examined for the development of aberrant electrocardiograms (Rust *et al.*, 1960). Electrocard-

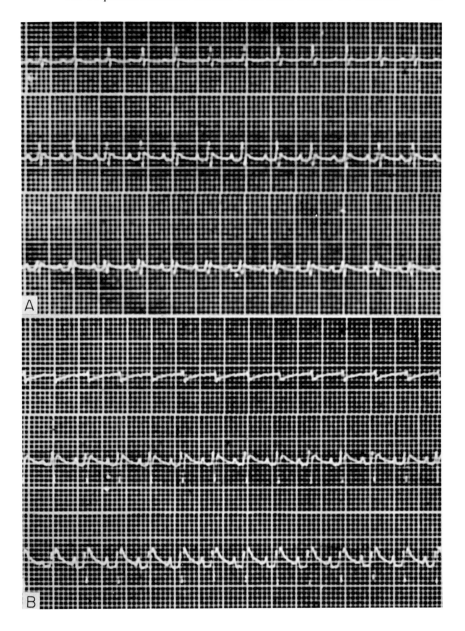

FIG. 4. Three-lead electrocardiograms recorded from a normal rat (A) and from a rat injected with plague murine toxin (B). From Rust *et al.* (1963).

iographic alterations similar to those obtained after injection of plague murine toxin were noted following infection with 10^6 bacterial cells, a toxic dose which killed the animals within 24 hours. However, rats infected with 10^3 bacilli, a nontoxic dose, failed to show cardiac changes at any stage of the disease from infection to death.

Additional examinations of the electrocardiographic patterns of rats after injection of the murine toxin of *P. pestis* were made by Hildebrand *et al.* (1966) who used toxin preparations that were purified by chromatography on DEAE-cellulose columns following treatment with ammonium sulfate between 0.35 and 0.70 saturation. Abnormalities in the electrocardiograms that preceded or accompanied the persistently noted drop in systemic arterial pressure to shock level were observed in only 50% of the animals receiving toxin. These alterations consisted of an elevation of the S-T segment and transient inversion of the P wave. An elevation of the S-T segment was also noted in 30% of the animals during the control period before the injection of the toxin. It was surmised that this electrocardiographic change was induced by a slight degree of asphyxia due to secretion of viscous mucus in the upper respiratory tract. Consequently, the conclusion was reached that elevation of the S-T segment was not indicative of a specific toxic effect on the heart muscle. Persistent pathological changes in the electrocardiogram such as lowering of the S-T segment, inversion of the T wave, and ectopic beats were always observed after the systemic arterial pressure had reached shock level and were never found in the control electrocardiogram.

B. BLOOD AND CIRCULATORY SYSTEM

1. HEMOCONCENTRATION

Schar and Thal (1955) and Schar and Meyer (1956) reported that when rats and mice were injected intravenously with large doses (5 or more LD_{50}) of plague murine toxin (fraction II of Baker *et al.*, 1952) the blood pressure dropped to shock levels within 2-4 hours (see Section V,B,2 for further details) and this was accompanied by an increase of 25-35% in the number of erythrocytes per cubic millimeter. Measurements of plasma volume revealed that the increase in the concentration of erythrocytes was caused by a loss of plasma. However, if shock did not develop within a few hours, hemoconcentration was not significant even though the animals were moribund. Similar findings were obtained by Krupenina (1964) who showed that intraperitoneal injection of crude toxin preparations to rats provoked hemoconcentration and reduction of the circulating blood volume chiefly at the expense of plasma discharge into the interstitial spaces.

2. BLOOD PRESSURE

A number of investigators have noted that the behavior of the arterial and venous blood pressure in animals injected with a lethal dose of plague murine toxin is very characteristic. Schar and Meyer (1956) observed that after a short initial increase, the arterial pressure remained at a constant level for 1–2 hours and then dropped within 30 minutes to shock level. The intoxicated rats died following this precipitous decline in arterial blood pressure. The central venous pressure remained very low until just before death, when a moderate increase was observed.

Essentially the same results were obtained by Hildebrand *et al.* (1966). The toxin preparations employed by Schar and Meyer (1956) were, as pointed out on several previous occasions, undoubtedly contaminated with lipopolysaccharide endotoxin. Since a drop in blood pressure is one of the characteristic physiological manifestations of the action of endotoxin, it might be suspected that the findings of Schar and Meyer (1956) could be due, at least partially, to endotoxin present in their toxin samples. However, the purified toxin of Hildebrand *et al.* (1966) was shown to contain only trace amounts of carbohydrates measured by the anthrone test, and this may rule out the participation of endotoxin in their experiments. These investigators also showed that the effects of injection of crude toxin were similar to those of purified toxin and developed after a significantly shorter time than after injection of comparable lethal doses of purified toxin.

In this connection it is pertinent to note that experiments on dogs, animals that have been found to be resistant to the action of plague murine toxin (Rust *et al.*, 1963) and only rarely exhibit symptoms associated with plague infection (Pollitzer, 1954), showed that intravenous injection of large amounts of fraction II of Baker *et al.* (1952) (approximately 40 mg per kilogram of body weight) produced a prolonged sustained drop in arterial blood pressure (Walker, 1967). This pronounced decrease in blood pressure could be blocked by the administration of small increments of crude plague murine toxin or by an atoxic protein extracted from the nontoxigenic TRU strain of *P. pestis* by the same method employed to obtain toxin. Neither the TRU protein nor bovine serum albumin injected by themselves lowered blood pressure. These results are certainly indicative of the involvement of the *P. pestis* lipopolysaccharide endotoxin. The reversal of the observed effects by nontoxic protein could be due to the binding of the lipopolysaccharide to the protein, thus diminishing the effective concentration of the lipopolysaccharide.

If future experiments should indeed reveal that highly purified preparations of plague murine toxin that have definitely been demonstrated to be free of lipopolysaccharide give the same results as those obtained with the crude preparations, then we will be faced with the fact that plague murine toxin is a most unusual toxic protein. In other words, it will behoove us to explain why a protein exerts practically the same physiological, pathological, and biochemical effects heretofore associated with lipopolysaccharide endotoxins and why the protein produces these alterations in animals that are resistant to its action as well as those that are susceptible.

Hildebrand *et al.* (1966) attempted to uncover the mechanism responsible for circulatory failure caused by plague murine toxin. The fall in systemic arterial pressure to shock level following injection of the toxin was neither preceded nor accompanied by a substantial rise in the systemic right ventricular pressure as is the case in anaphylactic shock or anaphylactoid reactions, indicating that the toxin-induced drop in systemic arterial pressure is not due to pulmonary vasospasm resulting in decreased filling of the left ventricle and reduced ventricular output.

Hildebrand *et al.* (1966) also observed that a brief initial rise in left atrial pressure, systolic right ventricular pressure, and central venous pressure after injection of toxin was followed by a steady and gradual fall below control level. In conjunction with this, it was found that there was a gradual decrease in stroke volume of the heart that was reflected in a decrease in arterial and right ventricular pressure after the initial increase. After a short initial increase, venous blood return from the inferior vena cava decreased steadily while the volume of extremities increased. It was concluded from the results of these experiments that the major factor in the pathogenic mechanism responsible for circulatory failure induced by plague murine toxin is decrease in venous return resulting in reduced cardiac output. Since circulatory failure was also observed when toxin was injected into decapitated rats, it was suggested that the action of the toxin was not mediated through the central nervous system. It was concluded that the decrease in venous return was caused by a direct action of the toxin on peripheral vascular elements.

It has also been reported that there was no indication that the toxin induced circulatory collapse by interfering with adequate ventilation of the lungs, adequate oxygenation of the blood, delivery of oxygen to the tissues, or its use in the tissues. Krupenina (1964), however, reported that rats injected with crude preparations of plague murine toxin develop severe circulatory hypoxia reminiscent of the impaired hemodynamics characteristic of shock. The decrease in oxygen consumption by the tissues and the presence of nongaseous acidosis indicated that tissue hypoxia was concomitant with plague intoxication. It was suggested, however, that the leading role was played by the circulatory type of hypoxia.

Krupenina (1963) studied the activity of several enzymes that were believed to participate simultaneously in the oxidation–reduction processes of tissues during plague intoxication. Mitochondria were isolated from the heart, liver, and kidney of rats 4 hours after the intraperitoneal injection of 3 LD_{50} of crude plague murine toxin as well as from control animals. The administration of toxin resulted in a slight suppression of the activity of succinic dehydrogenase and that of cytochrome oxidase in all of the tissues investigated. The activity of catalase, however, was somewhat increased. No change in the activity of these three enzymes was noted in *in vitro* experiments involving the addition of the toxin to heart, liver, and kidney mitochondria isolated from normal animals.

C. Liver Function

Schar and Meyer (1956) observed that mice and rats that did not succumb within the first 10-16 hours after intravenous injection of 1 LD_{50} of plague murine toxin developed severe jaundice within 48 hours. The blood of some animals without apparent icterus contained abnormal amounts of bilirubin. Liver function tests performed on animals that survived 1 LD_{50} of the toxin for more than 10 hours showed retention of bromsulfalein, whereas during the first few hours after administration of the toxin, bromsulfalein retention was not significant.

Another interesting finding that pointed to an early deterioration of liver function was that when livers of mice injected intravenously with 10 LD_{50} of toxin were removed from the animals 2 hours after toxin administration, homogenized, extracted, and analyzed for glucose content, only minute quantities of glucose were obtained from these livers as compared with those from control animals. Actually, the amount of glucose extractable from livers of intoxicated mice was significantly smaller than the amount of glucose obtained from normal mouse livers inactivated by heat immediately after removal. Since no glycogen is transformed into glucose and since it was also shown that blood sugar concentration falls to shock levels within 2-3 hours after intravenous administration of several LD_{50} of toxin, it was concluded that the inhibition of enzymatic processes was the underlying principle of the action of plague murine toxin. However, no indication was given as to which enzymes or coenzymes might be affected by the toxin.

Kratinov and Kharkova (1960, 1961a) reported that during plague intoxication experimentally produced by the injection of an autolyzate of the avirulent EV strain of *P. pestis* or fraction II obtained from virulent strain No. 65 into mice, rats, or guinea pigs induced glycogenolysis in the liver accompanied by hyperglycemia and lacticemia. During fatal intoxication, hyperglycemia changes into hypoglycemia. The extent of these disturbances of carbohydrate metabolism is dependent upon the severity of the toxicosis and the particular susceptibility to the toxin of the species of rodent studied. In highly sensitive mice and rats, the derangements in carbohydrate metabolism are considerably more pronounced than they are in the highly resistant guinea pigs.

In addition, it was shown (Kratinov and Kharkova, 1960) that under the effects of the toxin there is a decrease in the absorption of glucose by the rabbit small intestine. Because of this, the alimentary glycemic response is depressed during the intoxication. Experiments with the intravenous injection of glucose showed that during toxicosis the glucose tolerance of the organism is reduced.

Comparative studies on the effects of crude *P. pestis* toxin preparations on hepatic metabolism of phosphate were conducted on animals sensitive and resistant to the toxin (Domaradskii *et al.*, 1960). Intraperitoneal injection of the toxin into mice induced a reduction of the activities of acid and alkaline phosphatase and of ATPase and an accumulation of ATP in the liver. The rates of incorporation of phosphorus-32 into ATP in the livers of toxin-treated mice and guinea pigs do not differ from those observed in the livers of healthy animals. In both animal species, the toxin does not affect the capacity of liver homogenates to bind inorganic phosphate. No attempt was made to elucidate the significance of these findings.

D. Increased Sensitivity to Histamine During Plague Intoxication

A number of Russian investigators have observed that following injection with crude preparations of plague murine toxin, animals exhibit increased sensitivity to histamine. Kratinov and Kharkova (1961b) reported that as early as 1 hour after intraperitoneal administration of 16–25 LD_{50} of fraction II to mice, the injection of histamine induced pronounced glycogenolysis in the liver and hyperglycemia resulted instead of hypoglycemia, which was found to be characteristic of the terminal stage of plague toxemia.

Domaradskii and Klimova (1962) found that in *in vitro* experiments the addition of large amounts of fraction II to histaminase preparations obtained from lungs of rats by dialysis depressed significantly the histaminase activity. These investigators thus suggested that the increased sensitivity to histamine following toxin administration was caused by the increase in histamine levels resulting from the inactivation of the regulatory enzyme histaminase by the toxin. Subsequent studies (Domaradskii and Krupenina, 1963) revealed that this hypothesis was untenable and investigations were initiated to determine the effect of plague murine toxin administration on the histaminopexic (histamine binding) effect exhibited by whole citrated blood obtained from rats and guinea pigs. There was no difference between the capacity of the blood of either species to bind histamine. A marked reduction in the histaminopexic effect of the blood was observed 4 hours and even 18 hours following the injection of fraction II to these animals. In experiments *in vitro*, no depression of the histaminopexic effect of the blood by the toxin was noted. Since it was also observed that the blood of adrenalectomized rats that were not injected with toxin exhibited no histaminopexic effect, it was concluded that during plague infections, the murine toxin released caused a depressed formation by the adrenal glands of histamine-binding substances present in normal blood.

The physiological changes described above are similar to those produced by lipopolysaccharide endotoxin. The toxin preparations employed were undoubtedly contaminated with endotoxin, and the amounts of toxin injected were surprisingly large. Moreover, these changes were observed in both toxin resistant and susceptible animals. Consequently, it seems apparent that the increased sensitivity to histamine noted during intoxication with plague murine toxin was due primarily, if not exclusively, to the lipopolysaccharide endotoxin present in the plague murine toxin preparations.

ACKNOWLEDGMENTS

The research conducted by the authors of this chapter was supported by grants from the National Science Foundation (GB-7873) and the National Institute of Allergy and Infectious Diseases, United States Public Health Service (AI-03866), and a contract (NR136-754) from the Office of Naval Research.

REFERENCES

Ajl, S. J., and Rust, J. (1960). *Ann. N.Y. Acad. Sci.* **88**, 1152.
Ajl, S. J., Reedal, J. S., Durrum, E. L., and Warren, J. (1955). *J. Bacteriol.* **70**, 158.
Ajl, S. J., Rust, J., Jr., Woebke, J., and Hunter, D. H. (1956). *Federation Proc.* **15**, 581.
Ajl, S. J., Woebke, J., and Rust, J., Jr. (1958a). *J. Bacteriol.* **75**, 449.
Ajl, S. J., Rust, J., Jr., Hunter, D., Woebke, J., and Bent, D. F. (1958b). *J. Immunol.* **80**, 435.
Baker, E. E., Sommer, H., Foster, L. E., Meyer, E., and Meyer, K. F. (1952). *J. Immunol.* **68**, 131.
Brierly, G. P., Murer, E., and Green, D. E. (1963). *Science* **140**, 60.
British Plague Research Commission. (1906). *J. Hyg.* **6**, 421.
Burrows, T. W. (1963). *Current Topics Microbiol. Immunol.* **37**, 59.
Chappell, J. B., and Greville, G. D. (1963). In "Methods of Separation of Subcellular Structural Components" (J. K. Grant, ed.), pp. 39–65. Cambridge Univ. Press, London and New York.

Cocking, E. C., and Smith, H. (1958). *Abstr. 7th Intern. Congr. Microbiol., Stockholm, 1958*, p. 86. Almgvist and Wiksell, Uppsala.

Cocking, E. C., Keppie, J., Witt, K., and Smith, H. (1960). *Brit. J. Exptl. Pathol.* **41**, 460.

Criddle, R. S., Bock, R. M., Green, D. E., and Tisdale, H. (1962). *Biochemistry* **1**, 827.

Crumpton, M. J., and Davies, D. A. L. (1956). *Proc. Roy. Soc.* **B145**, 109.

Davies, D. A. L. (1956). *Biochem. J.* **63**, 105.

Dieudonne, A., and Otto, R. (1928). *In* "Handbuch der pathogenen Mikroorganismen" (W. Kolle, R. Kraus, and P. Uhlenhuth, eds.), pp. 179-412. Fischer, Jena.

Domaradskii, I. V., and Klimova, I. M. (1962). *Byul. Eksperim. Biol. i Med.* **53**, 69.

Domaradskii, I. V., and Krupenina, V. I. (1963). *Byul. Eksperim. Biol. i Med.* **55**, 48.

Domaradskii, I. V., Klimova, I. M., and Perevalova, L. G. (1960). *Vopr. Med. Khim.* **6**, 288.

Edwards, D. L., and Criddle, R. S. (1966a). *Biochemistry* **5**, 583.

Edwards, D. L., and Criddle, R. S. (1966b). *Biochemistry* **5**, 588.

Ellwood, D. C. (1968). *Biochem. J.* **106**, 47P.

Fowler, L. R., Richardson, S. H., and Hatefi, Y. (1962). *Biochim. Biophys. Acta* **64**, 170.

Gamble, J. L., Jr. (1957). *J. Biol. Chem.* **228**, 955.

Gauthier, J. C., and Raybaud, A. (1902). *Compt. Rend.* **54**, 1497.

Gauthier, J. C., and Raybaud, A. (1903). *Rev. Hyg.* **25**, 426.

Green, D. E., Tisdale, H. D., Criddle, R. S., Chen, P. Y., and Bock, R. M. (1961). *Biochem. Biophys. Res. Commun.* **5**, 109.

Griffiths, D. E., and Wharton, D. C. (1961). *J. Biol. Chem.* **236**, 1850.

Hatefi, Y., Haavik, A. G., and Jurtshuk, P. (1961). *Biochim. Biophys. Acta* **52**, 106.

Hatefi, Y., Haavik, A. G., and Griffiths, D. E. (1962a). *J. Biol. Chem.* **237**, 1676.

Hatefi, Y., Haavik, A. G., and Griffiths, D. E. (1962b). *J. Biol. Chem.* **237**, 1681.

Hildebrand, G. J., Ng, J., von Metz, E. K., and Eisler, D. M. (1966). *J. Infect. Diseases* **116**, 615.

Howland, J. L. (1963). *Biochim. Biophys. Acta* **77**, 419.

Hultin, H. O., and Richardson, S. H. (1964). *Arch. Biochem. Biophys.* **105**, 288.

Hunter, F. E., Jr., Levy, J. F., Fink, J., Schutz, B., Guerra, F., and Hurwitz, A. (1959). *J. Biol. Chem.* **234**, 2176.

Kadis, S., and Ajl, S. J. (1963). *J. Biol. Chem.* **238**, 3472.

Kadis, S., and Ajl, S. J. (1966). *J. Biol. Chem.* **241**, 1556.

Kadis, S., Ajl, S. J., and Rust, J. H., Jr. (1963). *J. Bacteriol.* **86**, 757.

Kadis, S. Trenchard, A., and Ajl, S. J. (1965a). *Arch. Biochem. Biophys.* **109**, 272.

Kadis, S., Cohen, M., and Ajl, S. J. (1965b). *Biochim. Biophys. Acta* **96**, 179.

Kadis, S., Montie, T. C., and Ajl, S. J. (1966a). *Bacteriol. Rev.* **30**, 177.

Kadis, S., Trenchard, A. V., and Ajl, S. J. (1966b). *J. Biol. Chem.* **241**, 5605.

Kadis, S., Urbano, C., and Ajl, S. J. (1967). *Bacteriol. Proc.* p. 88.

Kadis, S., Trenchard, A. V., and Ajl, S. J. (1968). Unpublished data.

Keppie, J., Smith, H., and Cocking, E. C. (1957). *Nature* **180**, 1136.

Kitasato, S. (1894). *Lancet* **II**, 428.

Kratinov, A. G., and Kharkova, N. M. (1960). *Vopr. Med. Khim.* **6**, 603.

Kratinov, A. G., and Kharkova, N. M. (1961a). *Byul. Eksperim. Biol. i Med.* **51**, 63.

Kratinov, A. G., and Kharkova, N. M. (1961b). *Zh. Mikrobiol., Epidemiol. i Immunobiol.* **32**, 135.

Krupenina, V. I. (1963). *Izv. Irkutsk. Nauchn. Issled. Protivochumn. Inst. Sibri i Dal'n. Vost.* **25**, 109.

Krupenina, V. I. (1964). *Byul. Eksperim. Biol. i Med.* **7**, 33.

Lardy, H. A., Johnson, D., and McMurray, W. C. (1958). *Arch Biochem. Biophys.* **78**, 587.

Larrabee, A. R., Marshall, J. D., and Crozier, D. (1965). *J. Bacteriol.* **90**, 116.

Lawton, W. D., Fukui, G. M., and Surgalla, M. J. (1960). *J. Immunol.* **84**, 475.

Lehninger, A. L. (1959). *J. Biol. Chem.* **234**, 2465.

Lehninger, A. L., and Ray, B. L. (1957). *Biochim. Biophys. Acta* **26**, 643.

Lehninger, A. L., Carafoli, E., and Rossi, C. S. (1967). *Advan. Enzymol.* **29**, 259.

McCrumb, F. R., Jr., Mercier, S., Robic, J., Bouillat, M., Smadel, J. E., Woodward, T. E., and Goodner, K. (1953). *Am. J. Med.* **14**, 284.

Minakami, S., Ringler, R. L., and Singer, T. P. (1962). *J. Biol. Chem.* **237**, 569.

Montanaro, L., and Sperti, S. (1965). *Biochim. Biophys. Acta* **100**, 621.

Montie, T. C., Montie, D. B., and Ajl, S. J. (1964). *J. Exptl. Med.* **120**, 1201.

Muller, H. E. (1898). *Denkschr. Akad. Wiss. Wien Mat. Kl.* **66**, 174.

Neubert, D., and Merker, H. J. (1965). *In* "Recent Advances in the Pharmacology of Toxins" (H. W. Raudonat, ed.), pp. 9-26. Proc. 2nd Int. Pharmocol. Meeting, Vol. 9. Pergamon Press, Oxford.

Ogata, M. (1897). *Zentr. Bakteriol.* **21**, 769.

Packer, L., Rust, J. H., Jr., and Ajl, S. J. (1959). *J. Bacteriol.* **78**, 658.

Parsons, D. F. (1965). *Intern. Rev. Exptl. Pathol.* **4**, 1.

Pollitzer, R. (1954). "Plague," World Health Organ. Monograph Ser. No. 22. World Health Organ., Geneva, Switzerland.

Raaflaub, J. (1953a). *Helv. Physiol. Pharmacol. Acta* **11**, 142.

Raaflaub, J. (1953b). *Helv. Physiol. Pharmacol. Acta* **11**, 157.

Richardson, S. H., Hultin, H. O., and Fleischer, S. (1964). *Arch. Biochem. Biophys.* **105**, 254.

Rowland, S. (1910). *J. Hyg.* **10**, 536.

Rust, J. H., Jr., Goley, A., F., Baker, H. J., and Ajl, S. J. (1959). *Bacteriol. Proc.* p. 95.

Rust, J. H., Jr., Goley, A. F., Randall, R., Ajl, S. J., and Cavanaugh, D. C. (1960). *Bacteriol. Proc.* p. 108.

Rust, J. H., Jr., Cavanaugh, D. C., Kadis, S., and Ajl, S. J. (1963). *Science* **142**, 408.

Schar, M., and Meyer, K. F. (1956). *Schweiz. Z. Allgem. Pathol. Bakteriol.* **19**, 51.

Schar, M., and Thal, E. (1955). *Proc. Soc. Exptl. Biol. Med.* **88**, 39.

Simond, P. L. (1898). *Ann. Inst. Pasteur* **12**, 625.

Smith, H., Keppie, J., Cocking, E. C., and Witt, K. (1960). *Brit. J. Exptl. Pathol.* **41**, 452.

Stanley, J. L., and Smith, H. (1967). *Brit. J. Exptl. Pathol.* **48**, 124.

Tapley, D. F. (1956). *J. Biol. Chem.* **222**, 325.

Vasil'eva, Z. I. (1967). *Vopr. Med. Khim.* **13**, 124.

Vasil'eva, Z. I., and Domaradskii, I. V. (1963). *Izv. Irkutsk. Nauchn. Issled. Protivochumn. Inst. Sibri i Daln. Vost.* **25**, 106.

Vasington, F. D. (1963). *J. Biol. Chem.* **238**, 1841.

Vasington, F. D., and Murphy, J. V. (1962). *J. Biol. Chem.* **237**, 2670.

Walker, R. V. (1967). *Current Topics Microbiol. Immunol.* **41**, 23.

Walker, R. V. (1968). *J. Infect. Diseases* **118**, 188.

Walker, R. V., Barnes, M. G., and Higgins, E. D. (1966). *Nature* **209**, 1246.

Yersin, A. (1894). *Ann. Inst. Pasteur* **8**, 662.

Zatman, L. J., Kaplan, N. O., and Colowick, S. P. (1953). *J. Biol. Chem.* **200**, 197.

Ziegler, D. M., and Doeg, K. A. (1962). *J. Biol. Chem.* **97**, 41.

CHAPTER 2

Streptolysin O*

SEYMOUR P. HALBERT

I. Introduction

That streptococci can cause several types of hemolysis on blood agar plates has been known since the early part of the century, and this fact served as the basis for early classification of these microorganisms. Most human infections were shown to be due to strains capable of producing completely clear lytic zones, i.e. β hemolysis. Todd (1932, 1938) and Weld (1935) demonstrated that two distinct hemolytic toxins were synthesized by most strains; one became inactive on exposure to oxygen (streptolysin O); the other was soluble or extractable from microorganisms grown in serum (streptolysin S). Todd (1932) demonstrated that streptolysin O was clearly antigenic and that inhibition of hemolysis furnished a clinically useful tool for studying the immune responses of patients with streptococcal disease. The recognition of two distinct streptococcal hemolytic agents helped to clarify the mechanisms of lysis in blood agar plates. Although most β-hemolytic streptococcal strains synthesize both lysins, surface colonies bring about hemolysis primarily through the mediation of streptolysin S, since the streptolysin O becomes oxidized, while deep colonies are hemolytically active through both. Some naturally

*The author's research was supported in part by research grants from the National Institutes of Health, The American Heart Association, and the Office of Naval Research.

occurring and some mutant strains have been described which are capable of producing only one of these hemolytic toxins (Bernheimer, 1948; Li, 1955).

Since these early observations, a large literature has accumulated concerning the oxygen-labile streptolysin O. Measurement of the antibody response to this streptococcal product has indeed proven invaluable in the diagnosis and analysis of streptococcal disease and some of its various complications. However, in spite of the very wide clinical use of this diagnostic procedure, progress in understanding the chemistry and pathogenic significance of streptolysin O has been relatively slow and difficult, to a large extent since it appears to be secreted in rather low concentrations into culture media. Substantial information has accumulated nonetheless, and this review will summarize the present state of our knowledge about this toxin, with emphasis being placed on the experimental, rather than clinical aspects.

II. Synthesis of Streptolysin O

Early work on streptolysin O was often carried out with culture filtrates prepared from organisms grown in very complex media, such as Todd-Hewitt broth (Hewitt and Todd, 1939). The presence of large molecular weight peptides derived from the medium made purification very difficult, but Bernheimer *et al.* (1942) showed that streptolysin O can be synthesized in a chemically defined medium. Excellent yields have also been obtained in small molecular weight media prepared by dialysis (Halbert *et al.*, 1955a,b), by Sephadex filtration (Holm, 1967), or by ultrafiltration through Ioplex (Amicon) membrane units (Halbert *et al.*, 1968). Other media containing minimum concentrations of large molecular weight substances have been used with satisfactory streptolysin yields (Alouf and Raynaud, 1965; Boszormenyi *et al.*, 1967). In general, it appears that increased growth of the microorganisms is accompanied *pari passu* by increased streptolysin yields (Halbert *et al.*, 1955a; Bernheimer, 1948). However, Slade and Knox (1950), as well as Fuvessy *et al.* (1967) obtained evidence that in certain media, addition of cysteine and ascorbic acid results in enhanced streptolysin O production without a concomitant growth increase. This was not the experience of the present author with the C203S strain of streptococcus using cysteine as an additive (Halbert *et al.*, 1955a). There is general agreement that optimum concentrations of glucose are essential for the satisfactory synthesis of streptolysin O, and that the resulting acids, particularly lactic, must be neutralized if decreased yields or destruction are to be avoided (e.g., Boszormenyi *et al.*,

1967). The peak of streptolysin O synthesis usually occurs between 6 and 12 hours after inoculation, and in many studies, the titers dropped rapidly following this time (e.g., Fuvessy *et al.*, 1967).

Although streptolysin O is usually produced by batchwise cultures in liquid medium (e.g., Gualandi *et al.*, 1965), continuous cultivation of the microorganisms may result in good yields (Ogburn *et al.*, 1958). Veress *et al.* (1964) applied this latter method for streptolysin O production on a relatively large scale. Using a 3-liter effective growth volume, they obtained an hourly yield of 5 liters of culture containing between 900 and 1000 hemolytic units, and 10^{12} organisms/ml. It may be pointed out that the very large scale fermentations employed by several pharmaceutical companies for the production of streptokinase are often associated with the synthesis of substantial quantities of streptolysin O, which must be eliminated from the final product.

Streptolysin O is synthesized by most strains of group A, by many strains of group C and G streptococci, particularly those causing human infections, but not by organisms of other groups. All strains appear to produce a streptolysin O which is identical immunochemically and functionally. Although individual strains vary considerably in their quantitative ability to synthesize streptolysin O *in vitro*, no relationship between this property and serological type in the group A organisms has been found (Rantz *et al.*, 1948b; Todd, 1939; Inoué, 1959a).

In a few human infections, demonstrably caused by the group A streptococcus, the antistreptolysin O response has been absent or minimal during convalescence (Coburn and Pauli, 1935; Taranta, 1967). Some correlation has been observed in experimentally infected animals between the *in vitro* capabilities of the infecting strain and the antistreptolysin response which occurred *in vivo* (Inoué, 1959b). Interestingly, 18 of 20 strains of group A streptococcus from apparently normal healthy individuals, failed to produce streptolysin O in detectable quantities *in vitro*, while the majority of strains isolated from patients with active infection were readily capable of synthesizing this toxin (Inoué, 1959a). It is thus possible that the variation of streptolysin formation found among strains *in vitro*, also characterizes their behavior *in vivo*.

A number of other bacterial species are capable of synthesizing oxygen-labile hemolytic toxins with characteristics resembling streptolysin O. Todd (1934, 1941) demonstrated that streptolysin O, pneumococcal hemolysin, and tetanolysin, as well as *Clostridium welchii* θ-toxin were neutralized by a hyperimmune horse serum from an animal which had been immunized with a group A streptococcal streptolysin concentrate. More recently, Bernheimer and Grushoff (1967) demonstrated that *Bacillus cereus* and other members of this group synthesized a hemolysin closely resembling streptolysin O. The latter were also neutralized by hyperimmune horse antistreptolysin, but it was of interest that antistreptolysin O from human sera failed to show this immunochemical relationship. Relevant to this, Sugihara and Squier (1951) studied 30 patients with pneumococcal pneumonia, and failed to find a significant rise in antistreptolysin O titer during convalescence, although an antipneumolysin response is known to occur. The lack of immunochemical relation of staphylococcal α-toxin and streptolysin O was shown both experimentally (Todd, 1934), and in human patients (Robinson and Crawford, 1952; Westergren, 1948).

III. Purification and Chemistry

Streptolysin O is a heat-labile protein which can be reversibly oxidized and reduced (Neill and Mallory, 1926). Its biological activities, such as hemolysis and lethal toxicity, are apparent only in the reduced state. Reversible oxidation to inactivity can be accomplished by exposure to air or by treatment with a variety of mild oxidizing agents such as iodine, hydrogen peroxide, and potassium ferricyanide. While a number of organic and inorganic reducing agents have been found quite effective in reducing streptolysin O, the amino acid cysteine is most commonly used. Some evidence suggests that the oxidation–reduction system of the streptolysin molecule involves shifts between disulfide and sulfhydryl bonds (Smythe and Harris, 1940; Herbert and Todd, 1941). Streptolysin O has been reported to be rather unstable, but it is conceivable that some of this apparent instability may be due to the parallel synthesis of streptococcal proteinase in the culture medium (Elliott and Dole, 1947; Halbert et al., 1955a). This enzyme is active only in the reduced state, as is streptolysin O, and is known to rapidly destroy this toxin.

Although amino acid analyses of streptolysin O concentrates have been reported (Mesrobeanu et al., 1958; Pentz et al., 1964; Pentz and Shigemura, 1955), low activity of the preparations analyzed make it unlikely that the observed values relate to the streptolysin O molecule itself.

Appreciable progress has been made in the purification of this toxin by two groups (Halbert, 1958; Halbert and Auerbach, 1961; Alouf and Raynaud, 1962, 1967). In the author's laboratory, supernatant harvests from streptococcal growth in dialyzate medium were used. A sequence of purification steps involving precipitation with ammonium sulfate at 85% saturation, continuous flow electrophoresis, hydroxylapatite, and other chromatography, resulted in streptolysin preparations with hemolytic activities up to 225,000 hemolytic units per milligram of protein (Halbert and Auerbach, 1961). Immunochemical analysis of these fractions indicated that they were contaminated with trace quantities of at least one or two additional streptococcal antigens, one of the latter being identified as nicotinamide adenine dinucleotidase. Alouf and Raynaud (1967) have purified streptolysin O by freeze-thaw concentration of culture super-nates, precipitation with 70% saturated ammonium sulfate, batchwise adsorption of contaminants from DEAE-cellulose and column chroma-tography on Sephadex G-100. The most active preparations obtained by these investigators revealed a hemolytic potency approximately twice as great as above (Alouf and Raynaud, 1967). In attempting to estimate the molecular weight of the purified streptolysin O, the latter workers first re-ported a molecular size of less than 10,000 (Alouf and Raynaud, 1962), but subsequently, this figure was revised upward by data which suggested a value of approximately 80,000 (Alouf and Raynaud, 1967). It is con-ceivable that polymerization might have been involved in these discrep-ancies. The helpfulness of Sephadex G-100 as a purification step for the preparation of streptolysin O has been confirmed by the author (Halbert and Kiefer, 1968). During purification, streptolysin O usually converts al-most completely to the reversibly oxidized state unless special precau-tions are taken. Over 95-98% of the molecule may become oxidized. It has proven difficult to bring the oxidation process to completion, although Alouf (1966) has reported success.

Earlier attempts to determine the isoelectric point of streptolysin O with relatively impure preparations, had suggested a value between pH 4.0 and 4.5 (Smythe and Harris, 1940). Preliminary results with rather highly purified streptolysin fractions and isoelectric focusing procedures, have indicated some heterogeneity, with the isoelectric point of the major constituent being approximately pH 7.5. This value agrees fairly well with that found by Alouf (1969) (pH 7.1-7.3). However, when the samples were first dissolved in 1 M glycine, as recommended, the streptolysin O repeatedly revealed an isoelectric point of 5.8. The purified preparations are heat labile, being destroyed completely by exposure to 56° C for a period of 30 minutes. Concentrated solutions of such purified preparations are water-clear and nonviscous.

Purification of group C streptococcal streptolysin O indicates that it behaves identically to the group A toxin with regard to its elution and salt-ing out characteristics, electrophoretic properties, and hemolytic potency (Halbert, 1958; Halbert and Kiefer, 1968). The toxicity of each ap-pears completely equivalent in many systems (Halbert et al., 1961b, 1963a; Reitz et al., 1968a,b). Immunochemically, the two appear to be in-distinguishable, as judged by immunodiffusion techniques (Halbert, 1958; Halbert and Auerbach, 1961; Halbert and Keatinge, 1962).

Antisera raised to the reversibly oxidized or to the reduced form of streptolysin behaved similarly with regard to streptolysin O inhibiting and precipitating activities. It is conceivable that the reducing conditions in the tissues bring about an activation of the oxidized streptolysin prior to its functioning as an antigen. Only fragmentary attempts have been made to determine whether the reversibly oxidized molecule possesses immunological determinant groups distinct from those of the reduced molecule. The results were inconclusive because of the presence of small quantities of proteinase in the streptolysin concentrates employed which caused dissolution of the immune precipitates within the framework of the agar gel (Halbert *et al.*, 1955a).

IV. Lethal Toxicity

Intravenous injection of activated streptolysin is very rapidly lethal in the animals tested—mice, rabbits, and guinea pigs (Bernheimer, 1948, 1954; Herbert and Todd, 1941; Howard and Wallace, 1953a; Halbert *et al.*, 1961a,b). Death usually occurs within seconds or minutes, and is preceded by convulsions and nasal frothing. With several multiples of a lethal dose, death has been observed in mice almost instantaneously. The 50% lethal dose (LD_{50}) for this species is approximately 1–2 μg per 20-gm animal (100 μg/kg) with the most active preparations available (Halbert, 1963; Alouf, 1966). This represents approximately 150–400 hemolytic units per mouse, according to the unit employed. It is of interest that titrations of the lethal activity of streptolysin fractions tend to show sharp end points. In most instances, at dose levels which kill only a portion of the animals, death will occur very rapidly from the injection or survival will be indefinite. This "all or none" lethal property appears to be shared with some other rapidly acting bacterial toxins (Bernheimer, 1948). Intravenous injection of reversibly oxidized streptolysin is much less toxic than the reduced activated form, seven to eight times the amount of the latter being required for similar responses (Halbert *et al.*, 1961b). Since the reversibly oxidized group A and group C preparations tested were about 95% in that state, it is thus possible that some further reduction of the molecule occurred *in vivo*. Although careful studies have not been carried out, routes of administration other than intravenous are not nearly as lethal.

It has been reported that the mouse on a weight basis is about 30 times more resistant to the lethal effects of streptolysin O than the guinea pig or rabbit. (Howard and Wallace, 1953a). However, crude culture supernatant concentrates were used for these tests, and when rather highly purified preparations were employed, mice proved to be only about twice as resistant as rabbits (Halbert *et al.*, 1963a). The rabbit and mouse LD_{50} of a group A preparation were 50 and 100 µg/kg, respectively; or 8,000 and 16,000 hemolytic units/kg. The pattern of death was quite the same in both species, and similar ratios were seen with group C streptolysin in these two species. The naturally occurring anti-streptolysin O antibody from human sources neutralized the acute lethal effects of both streptolysins (Halbert et al., 1961b).

V. Pathology

Detailed investigations of the histopathologic changes induced by streptolysin O have been hampered by the tendency to an "all or none" response, i.e., the very short survival of animals given a small lethal dose, or the apparent lack of any appreciable effects (Barnard and Todd, 1940). However, several reports have indicated that this toxin produces cardiac lesions in instances where a relatively prolonged intoxication occurred. Partially purified streptolysin O in rabbits caused focal heart lesions of myocardial cell destruction within 24 and 40 hours, and scar tissue by 5 days (Halbert et al., 1961b). In an electron microscopic study by Waldman (1965) it was found that streptolysin O intoxication caused ultrastructural changes in myocardial cells in vivo. Pretreatment with a streptococcal preparation predisposed rabbits to the development of focal cardiac lesions when subsequently challenged with streptolysin O containing culture filtrates (Schwab et al., 1955). A good correlation was found between the factor producing the heart lesions and streptolysin O. Injection of a fraction of a group A streptococcal extracellular concentrate containing streptolysin O caused focal cardiac and liver lesions in rabbits, while other fractions devoid of this toxin failed to do so (Spira et al., 1968). A small dose of a streptolysin O containing concentrate greatly enhanced the severity of certain viral myocardial lesions when the two were administered simultaneously (Pearce, 1953, 1960).

VI. Cardiotoxicity

Electrocardiographic tracings in rabbits and mice given lethal intravenous doses of streptolysin O clearly revealed that the abrupt death of these animals was mediated by disruption of the heart function (Halbert et al., 1961b, 1963a,b; Halpern and Rahman, 1968). Several multiples of the LD_{50} produced complete disorganization of the cardiac cycle within as short a time as 2–4 seconds following the injection. This was roughly equivalent to the time required for the dose to reach the heart from the peripheral vein. Typical examples of these extremely rapid changes are shown in Fig. 1, while the bizarre and variable sequence of electrocar-

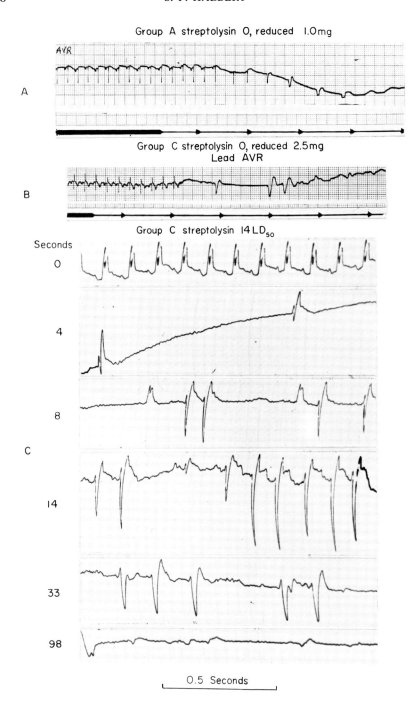

Group A streptolysin O, reduced 1.0 mg

Group C streptolysin O, reduced 2.5 mg
Lead AVR

Group C streptolysin 14 LD$_{50}$

0.5 Seconds

diographic events following smaller lethal doses are illustrated in Fig. 2. Nonlethal doses of streptolysin O produced temporary electrocardio-graphic changes in 9 of 13 rabbits studied, while controls receiving the reducing agent alone (cysteine) and several other purified streptococcal extracellular products never showed such effects. Electroencephalo-graphic tracings taken in parallel with the electrocardiograms revealed that alterations of the central nervous system patterns only occurred long after the heart had stopped functioning adequately and well after the blood pressure had fallen to almost zero (Halbert *et al.*, 1961b).

The extraordinarily rapid cardiac alterations in these lethally treated animals suggested that streptolysin O might liberate small molecular weight, physiologically active mediators. To explore this possibility *in vivo*, a study was carried out using drugs of known pharmacological activ-ity (Halbert *et al.*, 1963a). It was found that certain substances with anti-serotonin activity could protect animals against the acute lethal effects of this toxin (see Fig. 3). However, other antiserotonin drugs were without any effect, and no correlation was seen between this property and the streptolysin protective activity.

The possible role of intravascular hemolysis and plasma potassium in these cardiotoxic manifestations *in vivo* has also been investigated (Hal-bert *et al.*, 1963b). In those animals which died very acutely within 2.5 minutes, a significant elevation of potassium was found which was asso-ciated with very rapid hemolysis. For example, injection of approximately 3 LD_{50} of group A streptolysin into a rabbit, produced intravascular he-molysis of 38% of the erythrocytes within 1 minute, and an elevation of plasma potassium from 4.9 to 21.9 mEq/liter. The potential simple expla-nation that the acute lethal toxicity of streptolysin O is based on intravas-cular hemolysis, and potassium release from the latter affecting the heart, could not account for the *in vitro* findings described below, nor for the protective effects of various drugs *in vivo*. Furthermore, a number of dis-crepancies were found between the plasma potassium levels and the elec-trocardiographic findings during the *in vivo* studies. For example, in one instance (Fig. 4A), the intravascular hemolysis was virtually complete within 18 minutes without significant electrocardiographic changes, and only modest elevation of plasma potassium was observed at that time. However, 51 minutes after the injection, just prior to death and concomi-tantly with profound electrocardiographic changes, a striking elevation of

FIG. 1. Electrocardiogram changes in rabbits and mice receiving large lethal doses of acti-vated streptolysin O from group A and group C streptococci. The injection period is noted below each tracing on the left of A and B, which also indicates second intervals. A, B = rab-bits; C = mouse (time in seconds). (From Halbert *et al.*, 1961b, 1963a.)

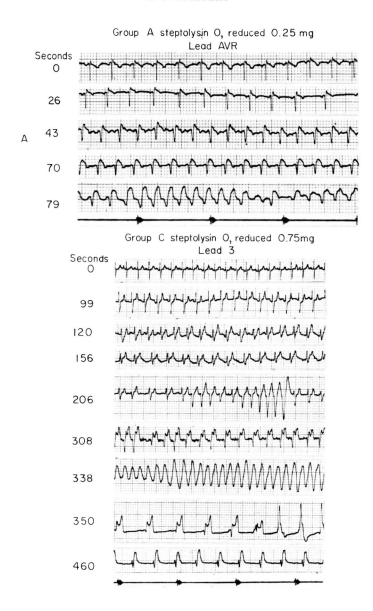

FIG. 2. Electrocardiogram changes seen in rabbits given small lethal doses of activated streptolysin O from (A) group A and (B) group C streptococci (time in seconds). (From Halbert *et al.*, 1961b.)

plasma potassium occurred without significant further hemolysis. The latter potassium must have been derived from some source other than erythrocytes. In Fig. 4B, a small amount of intravascular hemolysis was associated with only a relatively modest increase in plasma potassium (4.4–12.8 mEq/liter). In spite of these rather minor changes, the electrocardiogram was profoundly altered, and the animal succumbed within several minutes. In Fig. 4 C, an appreciable amount of hemolysis occurred (31%) with a concomitant increase in the plasma potassium level to 12 mEq/liter, the same level as in Fig. 4B. However, in this case no significant electrocardiographic changes were ever seen, and the animal survived.

The extreme susceptibility of the heart to the toxic effects of streptolysin O have been intensively studied *in vitro*, primarily in the isolated perfused beating heart in the absence of erythrocytes. The early studies by Bernheimer and Cantoni (1945, 1947); Cantoni and Bernheimer, (1945, 1947) demonstrated that the isolated amphibian (frog) heart was susceptible to this toxin in an unusual way. Perfusion of the first dose of activated toxin through the heart had no demonstrable effect, but after a brief washing, a second small dose produced rapid systolic contracture. The latter was reversible if the second dose were low, but irreversible if it were high.

Isolated perfused mammalian hearts proved extremely susceptible to the *direct* toxic action of streptolysin O, as demonstrated by Kellner *et al.* (1956), as well as by Vanecek (1955) and Coraboeuf and Goullet (1963). Guinea pig, rat, and rabbit hearts were shown to be equivalently affected. Unlike the amphibian heart, the first exposure of these beating hearts to streptolysin O produced cardiac standstill, usually within 2–3 minutes. As little as 5, 15, and 50 hemolytic units were able to cause cessation of rat, guinea pig, and rabbit hearts, respectively. Since the time required for passage of the streptolysin through the vascular system of the perfused heart was brief, 0.5–2 minutes, and since the most highly purified streptolysin presently available contains more than 250,000 hemolytic units/mg, it is clear that this substance is an extremely potent cardiotoxic agent.

The site of streptolysin O toxicity for the perfused guinea pig, rat, and rabbit heart has been considerably clarified by the elegant recent observations of Reitz, Prager, and Feigen (1968a,b). They convincingly showed that the toxic response consisted of two distinct mechanisms. One was atrial in origin, occurred earlier than the other, required larger amounts of streptolysin, manifested tachyphylaxis, and was due to the release of acetylcholine. The second phase was irreversible, was ventricular in origin, appeared to be due to disturbance of the conduction system, and probably

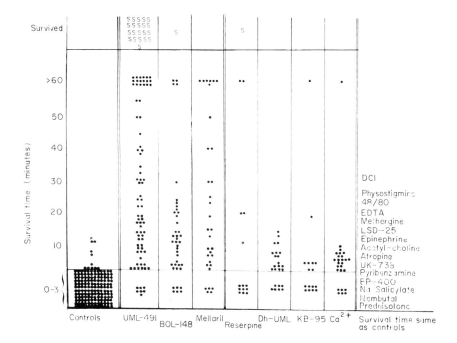

FIG. 3. Effects of various drugs on the acute lethal toxicity of streptolysin O. In all instances, the streptolysin challenge ($2 \times LD_{50}$) was administered intravenously at an appropriate interval following the intraperitoneal injection of the drug. Each point represents one mouse. s = survival time for at least 3 days. (From Halbert *et al.*, 1963a.)

Parasympathomimetics
    Physostigmine salicylate
    Acetylcholine chloride
Parasympathetic inhibitors
    Atropine sulfate
    n-Ethylnortropine benzhydryl ether HBr (UK-738)
Sympathomimetic
    Epinephrine
Sympathetic inhibitor (β receptors)
    Dichloroisoproterenol (DCI)
Antiserotonin agents
    d-Lysergic acid diethylamide tartrate (LSD-25)
    1-Methyl-*d*-lysergic acid butanolamide bimaleate (UML-491)
    Methylergonovine maleate
    d-Lysergic acid butanolamide bimaleate (Methergine)
    1-Methyldihydro-*d*-lysergic acid butanolamide tartrate (DH-UML)
    d-Bromolysergic acid diethylamide (BOL-148)
    The pyrazole derivative, 1-(*N*-methylpiperidyl-4')-3-phenylbenzylpyrazolone 5(KB-95)
Antihistamines
    Tripelennamine HCl (Pyribenzamine)
    9-(*N*-Methylpiperidyliden-4')thioxanthene maleate (BP-400)

accounted for the lethal effects *in vivo*. The early reversible and late irreversible effects are clearly evident in Fig. 5. It is of significance that normal ventricular strips exposed to high concentrations of streptolysin O contracted normally when driven electrically. Furthermore, ventricular strips obtained from hearts poisoned *in vitro* by streptolysin O, also contracted normally on electrical stimulation. Results indicating damage to the conduction system by streptolysin O were also obtained independently by Halpern and Rahman (1968) with the perfused rat heart. Goullet *et al.* (1963) have shown that contractions of electrically stimulated isolated ventricle strips were not inhibited by streptolysin O.

An antiserotonin drug shown to protect animals against the lethal toxicity of streptolysin O failed to afford protection against the toxic effects seen in the isolated perfused heart system (Reitz *et al.*, 1968a). Although considerable release of serotonin, as well as of some noradrenalin, rapidly occurred from perfused hearts intoxicated by streptolysin O *in vitro*, little or no histamine release was found (G. Feigen, 1968). A rapid leakage of potassium ions from the myocardial cells was also demonstrated in streptolysin O poisoned perfused hearts (G. Feigen and Neustaedter, 1967).

Very recent observations in the author's laboratory have shown that streptolysin O is highly toxic to isolated beating rat heart cells in tissue culture. Cessation of beating was virtually instantaneous, and cell membrane blebs were formed shortly thereafter. The toxicity was not prevented by an antiserotonin drug known to be protective against streptolysin O *in vivo* (Thompson and Halbert, 1969).

Tranquilizers
    Reserpine phosphate — a serotonin and catechol amine liberator
    Thioridazine HCl
    Mellaril [a phenothiazine derivative; 2 methylmercapto-10-(2(*n*-methyl-2-piperidyl)
    ethyl)phenothiazine HCl — This agent also possesses moderate antiserotonin activity.]
Histamine liberator
    48/80
Calcium ions
    Calcium gluconogalactogluconate
Calcium chelating agent
    Ethylenediaminetetraacetate (EDTA)
Corticosteroid
    Prednisolone phosphate
Analgesic, antipyretic
    Sodium salicylate
Anesthetic
    Sodium pentobarbital (Nembutal)

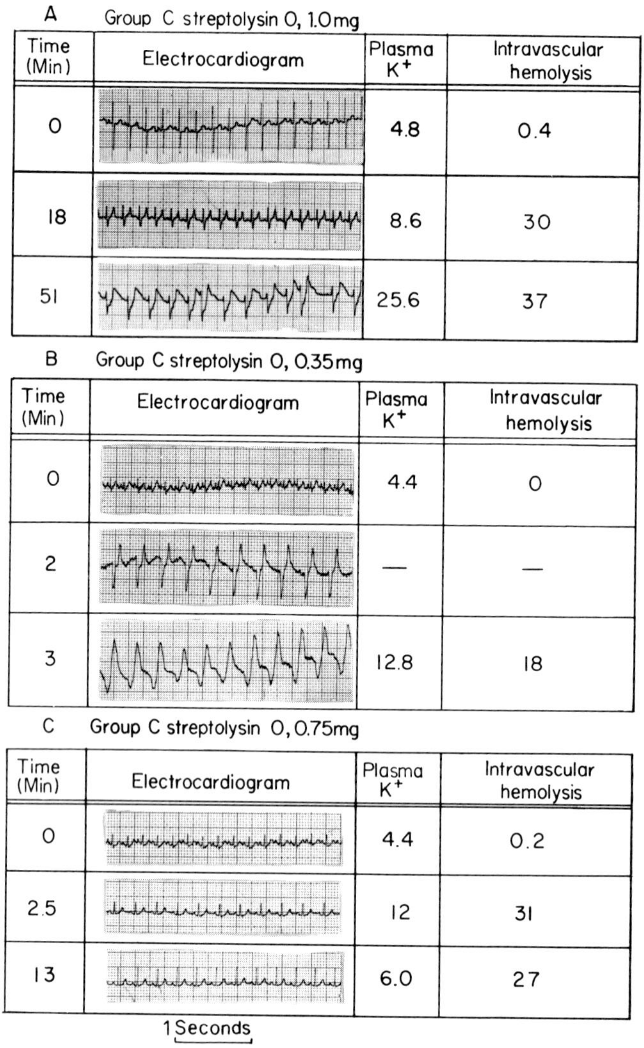

FIG. 4. Some discrepancies observed among the relationships of the plasma potassium elevation, percent intravascular hemolysis, and electrocardiographic changes in rabbit following a challenge dose of intravenous streptolysin O, time in minutes. (From Halbert *et al.*, 1963b.)

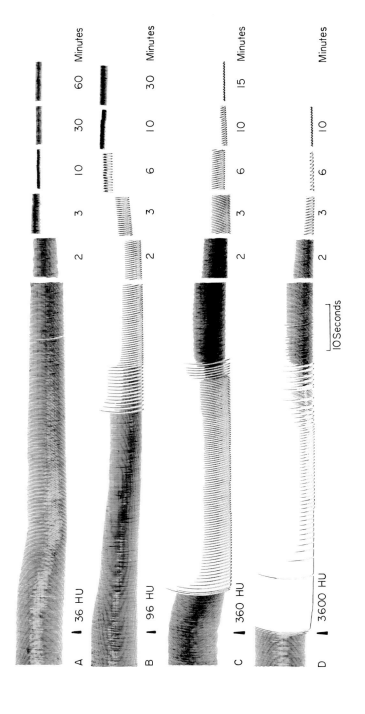

FIG. 5. The responses of 4 isolated perfused guinea pig hearts following challenge with different doses of group A streptolysin O. (From Reitz et al., 1968a.)

VII. Toxicity to Other Tissues

Intradermal injection of as little as 10–20 hemolytic units produced skin necrosis in guinea pigs and mice in a limited study carried out in the author's laboratory with partially purified streptolysin O (Halbert, 1968). Yellow areas of dermis death occurred in about 6 hours in these species, with relatively little edema and mild local erythema. Controls given the same amount of streptolysin O inactivated by cholesterol or by mild heat (56° C for 30 minutes) did not reveal significant lesions at the injection sites. Microscopically, the death of dermis cells was associated with an acute inflammatory reaction without any apparent damage to the elastic fibers. Of some interest was the "all or none" type of myofiber skeletal muscle destruction in adjacent areas, where smaller quantities of streptolysin O had presumably diffused. The completely healthy appearance of the unaffected skeletal muscle fibers, and the immediate neighboring dead fibers interspersed between them were clearly demonstrated by the Masson trichrome technique (Halbert, 1968). It was noted that many of the destroyed skeletal muscle fibers were in the process of being phagocytosed.

Investigations from G. Feigen's laboratory (1968) are possibly related to this finding. Using microelectrode recordings of mouse intercostal muscle preparations, it was shown that the random discharges of individual skeletal muscle fibers (miniature end plate potentials) were explosively increased in the presence of small quantities of streptolysin O. Normally, about 5–10 of these random discharges occur per second, but exposure of the skeletal muscle to streptolysin O caused a striking increase in the frequency of potential spikes, to as much as 500 per second. This may be compared to a factor in tetanus toxin described by G. Feigen and Peterson (1963) which increased the rate of such discharges approximately twofold.

The central nervous system was found to be highly susceptible to streptococcal culture supernates containing streptolysin O by intraventricular injection (Raskova and Vanecek, 1957). Similarly, such concentrates were shown to affect chemoreceptors (Vanecek and Raskova, 1956), uterine contractions, blood vessel constriction, and nerve conduction (Raskova, 1958). However, the undoubted complexity of the concentrates that were used (see Halbert and Keatinge, 1961; Halbert, 1963, 1964) makes it difficult to assign responsibility for these disturbances to streptolysin itself. Akatani (1961a,b) demonstrated that streptolysin O increased capillary permeability in rabbits and this effect was prevented by cholesterol and ACTH, but not by cortisone or antihistamines.

Curiously, streptolysin O concentrates have been reported to cause little effect on the synovial tissue of rabbits following intraarticular injection, although streptolysin S produced severe chronic arthritis (Weissmann *et al.*, 1963, 1965). These results were not confirmed by Ginsburg *et al.* (1968), who found severe arthritic lesions in rabbits given streptococcal extracellular concentrates devoid of streptolysin S but containing appreciable quantities of streptolysin O.

VIII. Cytotoxicity

Numerous studies have demonstrated the toxicity of streptolysin O for a wide variety of nucleated cells *in vitro*. Rapid changes were noted in mouse and rabbit polymorphonuclear leukocytes, extensive degranulation being seen in a matter of minutes (Bernheimer and Schwartz, 1960; Hirsch *et al.*, 1963; Zucker-Franklin, 1965). Macrophages also were highly susceptible (Fauve *et al.*, 1966) and it was noted here, too, that cell death tended to be "all or none." Even at high streptolysin O concentrations, a few cells appeared unaffected in the presence of the vast majority which were clearly killed. Leukocytes were about 100 times more resistant than erythrocytes to the destructive effects of streptolysin O. Ehrlich ascites tumor cells were destroyed by crude streptolysin O (Ginsburg and Grossowicz, 1960) and this effect was thought to be enhanced by proteinases (Ginsburg, 1959).

Platelets also are lysed by streptolysin O (Bernheimer and Schwartz, 1965a), as are lysosomes from a variety of mammalian cells (Weissmann *et al.*, 1963; Bernheimer and Schwartz, 1964). Bernheimer *et al.*, (Bernheimer and Schwartz, 1965b; Bernheimer and Davidson, 1965; Bernheimer, 1966) showed that certain pleuropneumonia-like organisms (mycoplasma) were susceptible to lysis by streptolysin O, but bacterial protoplasts of several species were not. A correlation was found between such sensitivity, and the presence of cholesterol in the cell membrane (Bernheimer, 1968) in agreement with other data suggesting this lipid molecule as a possible receptor site for streptolysin O. More primitive cells, such as free-living protozoa, and *Arbacia* eggs were unaffected by this toxin (Bernheimer, 1954).

IX. Hemolysis

Inasmuch as streptolysin O was first discovered as a result of its hemolytic activity, it is not surprising that this aspect of its toxicity has received some attention. Erythrocytes of many vertebrate species were found to be roughly equivalent in their susceptibility to destruction by streptolysin, with one exception, those of the mouse (Howard and Wallace, 1953b). The red cells of this species were roughly 30 times more resistant than the others tested, which included cells derived from the rabbit, man, guinea pig, dog, rat, hamster, ox, pig, cat, horse, sheep, goat, duck, pigeon, chicken, and frog. The last four were nucleated, but this did not significantly affect their susceptibility. The relative resistance of mouse erythrocytes to streptolysin O has been confirmed, together with the fact that the hemolysis titration curve was much flatter than that with rabbit erythrocytes (Halbert et al., 1963b; Petersen et al., 1966).

The kinetics of hemolysis have been investigated in detail. Certain quantitative aspects of streptolysin O hemolysis proved to be different from a number of other lytic agents, including the closely related pneumococcal hemolysin (Bernheimer, 1947). The latent period was relatively short at minimal hemolytic levels, but this decreased to very short intervals of less than 1 minute with increasing concentrations. Similarly, the rate of lysis increased very rapidly at high concentrations, so that lysis was almost instantaneously complete, once it started (Vargues, 1965; Alouf and Raynaud, 1968b).

The rate of hemolysis decreased with dropping temperature, and Bernheimer showed that the critical thermal increment (μ) of streptolysin showed two values; 43,000 between $0°$ and $15°C$, and 21,400 between $20°$ and $30°C$. In this respect, it resembled tetanolysin but none of the other hemolytic agents studied (Bernheimer, 1947). The hemolysis rate appeared to increase and then decrease, while the latent period increased, with increasing erythrocyte concentrations (Vargues, 1965; Alouf and Raynaud, 1968b). The latter authors analyzed such data mathematically and concluded that streptolysin O is fixed by the cells and is then "lost for further attack" on other erythrocytes. They also showed that lysis was inhibited in an isosmotic solution of sucrose when salts were absent.

In studying mechanisms of lysis, Alouf and Raynaud (1968b) demonstrated that reduced streptolysin was firmly bound by red blood cells at $0°C$, but that the reversibly oxidized form was not. The attachment of the reduced molecule was quite rapid and was practically independent of temperature. When such red cells containing fixed streptolysin O were brought from $0°$ to $37°C$, lysis was rapid and complete. Thus bound to the erythrocyte, streptolysin O proved to be unaffected by exposure to a sulfhydryl "poisoning" compound such as p-chloromercuribenzoate or to cholesterol. These data, similar to those obtained with pneumolysin (Cohen et al., 1942), suggest that streptolysin O fixes to the cholesterol molecules in the erythrocyte membrane by means of the sulfhydryl-dependent segment of the molecule. Alouf and Raynaud (1968b) also made the important observation that addition of antistreptolysin antibody can completely prevent subsequent lysis of red cells after reduced streptolysin O had become fixed to them at 0°C. Of interest was their observation that different antibodies varied considerably in their potency for neutralizing such erythrocyte-fixed streptolysin O. They suggested that these antibodies could be directed either against the fixation (f) or the toxic (t) sites of the streptolysin molecule, acting as distinct and unrelated determinants. Should this prove to be the case by means of absorption experiments, such information about the characteristics of antistreptolysin antibody formed in rheumatic fever might be of importance.

Alouf and Raynaud (1968a,b) estimated that about 1500 streptolysin O molecules sufficed to saturate the fixation site on the erythrocyte surface, and that about 360 molecules could cause irreversible lesions in a red cell. These figures indicated that streptolysin O was considerably more potent than several other bacterial or organic hemolytic agents which have been studied. As examples, staphylococcal α-toxin required about 13,000 molecules, while saponin glycosides (digitonin), fatty acids, polyenes, or detergents required from 2 million to several billion molecules for lysis of a single erythrocyte. At the electron-microscope level, streptolysin O was found to produce holes 500 Å in diameter in rabbit red cell membranes, while streptolysin S did not (Dourmashkin and Rosse, 1966).

It is common experience that red cell suspensions in buffered saline become somewhat resistant to streptolysin O on standing. Merucci et al. (1959) showed that this increased resistance also occurred in rabbit erythrocytes held at 4°C in their own serum.

X. Nonspecific Inhibitors

A. STEROIDS

It has long been known that cholesterol can inhibit streptolysin O hemolysis, as well as its lethal activities (Hewitt and Todd, 1939), and the reaction with cholesterol appears to be irreversible. Erythrocyte stroma is also known to be highly inhibitory to streptolysin O, as are lipid extracts from red cells (Alouf and Raynaud, 1968a; Petersen et al., 1966; Thiele et al., 1965). Delipidated stroma is not inhibitory, however, and only the cholesterol-containing fractions of the extracted stromal lipids are active in this regard. Similar findings were obtained with pneumolysin, a closely related hemolytic toxin (Cohen et al., 1942). These data further support the suggestion that streptolysin O attaches to the erythrocyte membrane via the cholesterol molecule. Badin and Barillec (1968) have speculated that the relatively small number of streptolysin molecules found to saturate the erythrocyte membrane may be caused by steric factors at the surface of the red cell, since the total amount of cholesterol there — and available to a small molecule such as digitonin — is known to be relatively quite large.

Some reports have suggested that phosphatides are also inhibitory to streptolysin O (Vella *et al.*, 1960; Hewitt and Todd, 1939), but more careful analysis has indicated this is not the case. Certain phosphatides have, however, been shown to potentiate the inhibitory action of cholesterol. This enhancing effect is thought to be mediated by the improved dispersion of cholesterol in aqueous menstruum (Petersen *et al.*, 1966; Thiele *et al.*, 1965). The earlier suspected inhibition of streptolysin O by phosphatides might be accounted for by this effect, as well as inhibition by trace contaminations with cholesterol.

Petersen *et al.* (1966) investigated the lipid content of human and mouse erythrocytes in an attempt to understand the relative resistance of the latter red cells to lysis. Streptolysin O fixation occurred equivalently at $0°$ C onto the cells of both species, and their cholesterol contents proved similar. The second phase of streptolysin hemolysis was thus involved in the resistance of mouse erythrocytes, and an unidentified lipid found in extracts of mouse, but not human red cells, was considered to be potentially responsible.

A careful comparison of the streptolysin O inhibitory activity of a number of steroids was carried out by Howard *et al.* (1953) and more recently by Badin and Barillec (1968). Of the large number of compounds tested, cholesterol and cholestanol were the most effective inhibitors. Correlation with molecular structure showed that inhibitory activity appeared to require a free β-hydroxyl group, no other polar group in the molecule, and an intact side chain of the sterol.

Despite the firm bond between cholesterol and streptolysin O, a brief report by Turner and Pentz (1950) indicated that the cholesterol-neutralized toxin is as antigenic as free streptolysin. On the other hand, antibody-neutralized streptolysin prevented an immune response in the doses used.

B. Nonspecific Inhibitors in Plasma

Although serum or plasma of man or other mammals contains considerable quantities of cholesterol, most of it is not usually available for inhibiting streptolysin O (Badin, 1968). When serum is contaminated with certain bacteria or is treated with acid or alkali, however, it becomes highly inhibitory. This appears to be due to the release of cholesterol from the lipoprotein complexes in some unknown manner so that its combining sites then become available to streptolysin (Packalen, 1948; Rozansky and Strauss, 1961; Inoué, 1960; Rudolph, 1962).

More detailed investigations of the antistreptolysin activity of "normal" human or animal sera has been carried out by several groups. In addition to antistreptolysin antibody (Halbert *et al.*, 1955a,b; Halbert and Keatinge, 1961), the normal lipoproteins of human serum have been shown to possess some inhibitory activity. β-Lipoprotein has been particularly implicated, and methods have been devised for the independent assay of the nonspecific β-lipoprotein inhibition, and the antistreptolysin activity in a given specimen. The lipoprotein inhibitors may be removed by treatment with heparin and calcium ions (Cabau and Badin, 1965a); by gel filtration, or by dextran sulfate precipitation (Killander *et al.*, 1965), and by isoamyl alcohol treatment of the serum (Badin and Barillec, 1969). In addition, inclusion of bovine serum albumin (fraction V) in the assay mixture, interfered with the nonspecific inhibitor, but not with antibody. In the latter technique, it was found that the effect was not due to albumin itself, but to a mucoprotein contaminant in commercial preparations of fraction V (Cabau, 1961; Cabau and Badin, 1959, 1961). Using these techniques in studies on the antistreptolysin activity of "normal" human sera, it was estimated that, on the average, about 40% of the total antistreptolysin titer may often be due to nonspecific lipoprotein inhibition (Badin, 1966; Winblad, 1966). As in the case of erythrocyte stroma, extraction of the lipids from human β-lipoprotein has revealed that only the cholesterol-containing fractions possessed streptolysin inhibitory properties (Badin and Barillec, 1968). Perez *et al.* (1964) studied the nonspecific inhibitor levels of rabbit and horse sera. In agreement with the authors experience, the former generally did not possess antistreptolysin activity, but 1 out of 8 specimens revealed a low titer which resided in the α- and β_1-globulin fraction. However, normal horses revealed a distribution of nonspecific and antibody antistreptolysin similar to that seen in man. Horses are often known to be spontaneously infected with group C streptococci.

Stollerman (1953) studied the nonspecific inhibition of experimentally induced hyperlipemic sera. Hypercholesterolemia evoked in rabbits by cholesterol feeding, resulted in sera which were intensely inhibitory to streptolysin O when the cholesterol levels reached 200–300 mg%. However, sera from alloxan diabetic rabbits or from those treated with a nonionic detergent were not inhibitory, despite a comparable elevation of serum cholesterol. It was suggested that the ratio of phospholipids to cholesterol was a critical factor in determining the availability of serum cholesterol to the combining site of streptolysin O.

C. Nonspecific Inhibitors in Disease States

It has been found that the nonspecific lipoprotein inhibitor of streptolysin O is strikingly increased in certain disease states, a fact which has been helpful diagnostically. Liver disturbances associated with jaundice often revealed very high nonspecific antistreptolysin O titer (Oker-Blom *et al.*, 1950; Badin *et al.*, 1962, 1966; Winblad, 1966; Hallen, 1963). Wahl *et al.* (1964) have shown that the serum of rabbits made cirrhotic by ligature of the bile duct also possessed high nonspecific antistreptolysin O titers.

Patients with active tuberculosis frequently revealed elevated levels of nonspecific inhibitors in their sera (Wahl and Cabau, 1958; Cabau *et al.*, 1962; Cabau, 1961; Cabau and Badin, 1965a). Badin *et al.* (1964) have found a striking elevation of the nonspecific titer in a patient with a simultaneous episode of rheumatic carditis and nephrosis. Most patients with rheumatic fever revealed antistreptolysin activity principally in their immunoglobulin fractions (Cabau and Badin, 1965a). Curiously, sera from patients with the nephrotic syndrome only rarely showed increased elevation of the nonspecific antistreptolysin titer, despite extreme degrees of cholesterolemia (Stollerman, 1953; Azzena *et al.*, 1959).

D. Paraprotein "Nonspecific" Antistreptolysin O

In several instances, extraordinarily high titers of antistreptolysin O activity have been recently detected in sera containing abnormal immunoglobulins. Badin and Cabau (1964) investigated the serum from a patient with an antistreptolysin O titer of 1,000,000. This may be compared with titers of 1000–2000, which represent the usual upper limits of intense post streptococcal infection responses. The inhibitory activity was solely associated with a rather homogeneous immunoglobulin G, not with lipoproteins; and the paraprotein did not inhibit staphylococcal α-toxin. The patient, suffering from a "collagen" type illness, had no evidence of preceding streptococcal infection and did not reveal elevated titers to several other streptococcal enzymes.

Similar results have been reported by other groups, sometimes in association with immunoglobulin diseases such as myeloma, but also in patients without obvious illness (Waldenstrom *et al.*, 1964; Mansa and Kjems, 1968; Zettervall *et al.*, 1966; Hallen, 1963). Mansa and Kjems (1965, 1968) have devised a special technique for identifying the streptolysin-inhibiting proteins by immunoelectrophoresis. None of the patients reported with these unique immunoglobulins have had obvious preceding streptococcal disease, but several of the investigators have speculated about the possibility that they may represent "monoclonal" antibodies. Seligmann *et al.* (1969) have shown that the antistreptolysin O activity of such a myeloma protein resided in the Fab fragments, and not the Fc fragment, of the molecule.

E. Other Nonspecific Inhibitors

Bernheimer (1947) demonstrated that a small nontoxic dose of strepto-lysin O given intravenously to mice makes them resistant to a sub-sequent lethal dose. This refractoriness lasted for about 2 days, and it was shown by Rowen and Bernheimer (1956) that this protection was due to the presence of a new or altered lipoprotein in the serum. This substance could be purified over 300-fold by flotation in a high speed centrifugal field. The resultant very low density lipoprotein differed quantitatively in its lipid composition from the counterpart obtained from normal serum (Rowen, 1963). Rowen and Wiest (1965) have also detected a new acute phase protein in the sera of mice given sublethal doses of streptolysin O. This protein, a slow α_2-globulin is distinct from the above inhibitory lipo-protein, as well as from C-reactive protein.

XI. Antistreptolysin Antibody

It is clear that the principal streptolysin inhibitor in the sera of patients convalescent from streptococcal disease is usually specific antibody. As pointed out above, its measurement for diagnostic purposes has proven of considerable value over several decades, both for the detection of clinical and subclinical streptococcal infections, as well as their nonsuppurative complications such as rheumatic fever and glomerulonephritis (e.g., Rantz et al., 1948a; Kwapinski and Snyder, 1962; Feinstein et al., 1964; Dunbar and Erwa, 1967; Ingestad and Winblad, 1963). It seems probable that subclinical exposure to streptococcal infection is extremely frequent, since antistreptolysin O antibody activity is almost universally present in normal human sera in many different populations. This specific activity increases in incidence and titer with age (Bonilla-Soto and Pomales-Le-bron, 1959; Hanson and Holm, 1961), and is transferred from mother to child (Hanson and Holm, 1961; Murray and Calman, 1953; Rozansky et al., 1960). Human antistreptolysin antibody has been found to be of the precipitating type by immunodiffusion methods (Halbert et al., 1955a,b; Halbert, 1964; Halbert and Auerbach, 1961), and it is found almost ex-clusively in fraction II γ-globulin, obtained by the Cohn procedures. Solu-tions of this γ-globulin in concentrations 10-12-fold greater than that found in normal human serum, have shown antistreptolysin O titers of 1500-3500 Todd units/ml (Halbert et al., 1955a; Streitfeld, 1960; G. Feigen, 1968). The antistreptolysin antibody from human sera has been more precisely localized primarily in the 7 S IgG immunoglobulins; no activity was found in the IgM fractions from these same specimens (Killander and Philipson, 1964; Breton *et al.*, 1961; Cabau and Badin, 1965b). Low levels of antistreptolysin O activity are found in human milk, especially during the early period of lactation (Kohler, 1968).

Although the diagnostic assay of antistreptolysin activity of human sera has been routine for several decades, adaptation of the microtiter plate procedure for this determination has been proposed (Edwards, 1964; Precechtel, 1966; Klein *et al.*, 1968), as well as such refinements as the use of precise 50% lysis end points (e.g., Kusama *et al.*, 1958). In addition, Vargues (1965) has developed an automated procedure for this purpose, and has used it to analyze the kinetics of neutralization of streptolysin O by antistreptolysin. This was shown to be a monomolecular reaction of the first order (Vargues, 1966; Trinquier and Morel, 1966).

XII. Clinical Significance of Streptolysin O

In spite of the considerable amount of information available about this toxin, as seen above, it is fair to state that the precise role of streptolysin O in the development of local suppurative lesions or in the evolution of streptococcal nonsuppurative sequelae is not clear. Its numerous toxic effects in experimental animals must be related to the infectious process in man if the observations are to be relevant. Only a few reports are available which are concerned with the transition from test animals to humans. Hamburger and Lemon (1953) showed that some patients with elevated antistreptolysin titer could develop severe enough acute streptococcal infections to be hospitalized. Quinn (1957) investigated this question directly in human patients by injecting streptolysin O concentrates into rheumatic and nonrheumatic subjects. Single intradermal doses of 8, 16, and 80 Todd combining units of reduced streptolysin O into adult normal volunteers resulted in severe local erythema and induration, with lymphangiitis, lymphadenitis, malaise, and fever, reaching a maximum by 2 days and gradually waning thereafter. The local lesions desquamated after 2 weeks, leaving permanent scars at the injection sites. Twenty children with active or inactive rheumatic fever were given intramuscular doses of 40–60 combining units of streptolysin O; 6 of the 20 developed severe systemic reactions, with febrile responses lasting up to 4–5 days. In one patient, an episode of arthritis ensued. Seventeen of the 20 developed local tenderness at the injection site as well. However, only one of the 55 nonrheumatic children developed similar systemic reactions. Analyses of the antistreptolysin responses to these injections failed to reveal any striking differences between the titers in the rheumatic and control groups. Since one streptolysin combining unit is equivalent to roughly 45 hemolytic units (Alouf, 1966), the doses used in this human study indicate that as little as 360 hemolytic units intradermally may cause severe local and systemic reactions.

In addition to these observations, there is certain circumstantial evidence which is compatible with the possible role of streptolysin O in the pathogenesis of rheumatic fever. Coburn and Pauli (1935) isolated 40 strains of group A streptococci from 38 patients with rheumatic fever. Twenty of these infections had been followed by a rheumatic fever recurrence, while the others had not. Comparison of the strains *in vitro* revealed that those which were "effective" in initiating such a recurrence, were also capable of synthesizing considerable quantities of streptolysin O, while most of the "noneffective" strains were not. These data have been indirectly supported by the observations of Taranta (1967) who analyzed the recurrence rate in rheumatic patients after proven streptococcal infections in relation to the antistreptolysin O response. In one group of 79 patients who failed to develop antistreptolysin O responses following infection, only one (1%) developed a rheumatic recurrence. However, of 26 patients with striking increases in antistreptolysin titer following the streptococcal infections, 9 (35%) had recurrences of rheumatic fever. Patients with intermediate rises in titer showed intermediate recurrence rates. Similar trends were seen in a smaller group of patients with previous rheumatic heart disease. It is of interest that those patients who failed to show elevations of antistreptolysin titer following proven streptococcal infection sometimes revealed rises in the titers of other streptococcal antibodies. This is reminiscent of the experimental data by Kirschner and Howie (1952) who produced cardiac lesions in rabbits by repeated streptococcal infections and found a correlation between such lesions and the rise in antistreptolysin O titer, but not the antihyaluronidase responses.

In a large study of patients without previous rheumatic fever (Stetson, 1954), a similar relationship was found between the intensity of the antistreptolysin O responses following streptococcal infection and the initiation of the first rheumatic attacks. Thus, of 856 patients with the smallest rise in titer following infection (0–120 units), only 0.8% developed rheumatic fever; while of the 545 with the highest rises (over 250 units), 5.5% showed this complication. Of the 553 patients with an intermediate antistreptolysin O increase (120–250 units) the incidence of rheumatic fever was also intermediate (3.6%). It is perhaps of some significance that rheumatic fever recurrences can be prevented by curing streptococcal infections in the early stages with sufficient penicillin. Enough penicillin must be given so that the antibody responses (including antistreptolysin O) will be stifled (Wannamaker *et al.*, 1951; Houser *et al.*, 1953; Massell *et al.*, 1951).

Coburn (1945) has reported that patients with several diseases associated with hypercholesterolemia (myxedema, diabetes, and nephrosis) are refractory to rheumatic recurrences, while those with hypocholesterolemia (hyperthyroidism) are prone to these attacks. He has also reported that diets inducing hypercholesterolemia have protected rheumatic patients against recurrences (Coburn and Moore, 1943). Although these studies have not yet been confirmed, it is intriguing to speculate about their possible relationship to the known inhibition of streptolysin O by plasma cholesterol under the circumstances described above.

A working hypothesis has been proposed which incriminates streptolysin O as the streptococcal factor responsible for the pathogenesis of rheumatic fever, which accounts for certain key characteristics of the illness (e.g., its latent period, its prolonged course after elimination of the streptococcal infection, and the presence of circulating antistreptolysin O) (Halbert et al., 1961a, 1961b). It has been postulated that during the streptococcal infection an abundance of streptolysin O (and other extracellular products) are released into the tissues and the circulation. The secreted streptolysin combines with antibody immediately and circulates as an antigen–antibody complex. An equilibrium becomes established between continued secretion of streptolysin and further development of antistreptolysin during the period of invasion by streptococci. Because of the well established, small, but definite *in vivo* dissociation of antigen–antibody complexes (e.g., Walter and Zipper, 1960), the streptolysin–antistreptolysin O complex could act as the source for the slow release of active streptolysin O. This latter, having a higher degree of predilection for certain tissues (e.g., heart, etc.) accumulates on or in the susceptible tissue cells until a toxic level is reached. At this point in time, the overt symptoms of rheumatic fever would begin. Symptoms and damage would continue as long as significant amounts of streptolysin-antistreptolysin complexes were present to supply a source of streptolysin. Several tests of this hypothesis are feasible but have not yet been performed.

REFERENCES

Akatani, I. (1961a). *Japan. J. Bacteriol.* **16**, 199.
Akatani, I. (1961b). *Japan. J. Bacteriol.* **16**, 281.
Alouf, J. E. (1966). Personal communication.
Alouf, J. E. (1969). Personal communication.
Alouf, J. E., and Raynaud, M. (1962). *Nature* **196**, 374.
Alouf, J. E., and Raynaud, M. (1965). *Ann. Inst. Pasteur* **108**, 759.
Alouf, J. E., and Raynaud, M. (1968a). *In* "Current Research on Group A Streptococcus" (R. Caravano, ed.), pp. 192–206. Excerpta Med. Found., Amsterdam.
Alouf, J. E., and Raynaud, M. (1967). *Compt. Rend.* **264**, 2524.
Alouf, J. E., and Raynaud, M. (1968b). *Ann. Inst. Pasteur* **115**, 97.

Azzena, D., Astengo, F., and Ghigliotti, G. (1959). *Ann. Sclavo* 1, 299.

Badin, J. (1966). *Pathol. Biol. Semaine Hop.* [N.S.] 14, 21.

Badin, J. (1968). *Compt. Rend.* 266, 2007.

Badin, J., and Barillec, A. (1968). *Ann. Biol. Clin.* (*Paris*) 26, 213.

Badin, J., and Barillec, A. (1969). *Ann. Biol. Clin.* (*Paris*) 27, 395.

Badin, J., and Cabau, N. (1964). *Rev. Rhumat.* 31, 17.

Badin, J., Cabau, N., Levy, C., and Cachin, M. (1962). *Ann. Biol. Clin.* (*Paris*) 10, 525.

Badin, J., Cabau, B., Herve, B., Guedon, J., and Slama, R. (1964). *Pathol. Biol. Semaine Hop.* [N.S.] 12, 995.

Badin, J., Saladin, F., and Barbier, S. (1966). *Transfusion* 9, 203.

Barnard, W. G., and Todd, E. W. (1940). *J. Pathol. Bacteriol.* 51, 43.

Bernheimer, A. W. (1947). *J. Gen. Physiol.* 30, 337.

Bernheimer, A. W. (1948). *Bacteriol Rev.* 12, 195.

Bernheimer, A. W. (1954). *In* "Streptococcal Infections" (M. McCarty, ed.), pp. 19–38. Columbia Univ. Press, New York.

Bernheimer, A. W. (1966). *J. Bacteriol.* 91, 1677.

Bernheimer, A. W. (1968). *Science* 159, 847.

Bernheimer, A. W., and Cantoni, G. L. (1945). *J. Exptl. Med.* 81, 295.

Bernheimer, A. W., and Cantoni, G. L. (1947). *J. Exptl. Med.* 86, 193.

Bernheimer, A. W., and Davidson, M. (1965). *Science* 148, 1229.

Bernheimer, A. W., and Grushoff, P. (1967). *J. Bacteriol.* 93, 1541.

Bernheimer, A. W., and Schwartz, L. L. (1960). *J. Pathol. Bacteriol.* 79, 37.

Bernheimer, A. W., and Schwartz, L. L. (1964). *J. Bacteriol.* 87, 1100.

Bernheimer, A. W., and Schwartz, L. L. (1965a). *J. Pathol. Bacteriol.* 89, 209.

Bernheimer, A. W., and Schwartz, L. L. (1965b). *J. Bacteriol.* 89, 1387.

Bernheimer, A. W., Fillman, W., Hottle, G. A., and Pappenheimer, A. W. (1942). *J. Bacteriol.* 43, 495.

Bonilla-Soto, O., and Pomales-Lebron, A. (1959). *Proc. Soc. Exptl. Biol. Med.* 102, 337.

Boszormenyi, J., Veress, A., and Fuvessy, I. (1967). *Acta Microbiol. Acad. Sci. Hung.* 14, 323.

Breton, A., Biserte, G., Beerens, H., Havez, R., and Boniface, L. (1961). *Arch. Franc. Pediat.* 18, 310.

Cabau, N. (1961). *Rev. Tuber. Pneum.* 25, 1469.

Cabau, N., and Badin, J. (1959). *Compt. Rend. Soc. Biol.* 43, 390.

Cabau, N., and Badin, J. (1961). *Ann. Inst. Pasteur* 100, 765.

Cabau, N., and Badin, J. (1965a). *Clin. Chim. Acta* 12, 508.

Cabau, N., and Badin, J. (1965b). *Pathol. Biol., Semaine Hop.* [N.S.] 13, 767.

Cabau, N., Badin, J., and Meyer, A. (1962). *Ann. Biol. Clin.* (*Paris*) 10, 543.

Cantoni, G. L., and Bernheimer, A. W. (1945). *J. Exptl. Med.* 81, 307.

Cantoni, G. L., and Bernheimer, A. W. (1947). *J. Pharmacol. Exptl. Therap.* 91, 31.

Coburn, A. F. (1945). *Am. J. Diseases Children* 20, 348.

Coburn, A. F., and Moore, L. V. (1943). *Am. J. Diseases Children* 65, 744.

Coburn, A. F., and Pauli, R. H. (1935). *J. Clin. Invest.* 14, 755.

Cohen, B., Halbert, S. P., and Perkins, M. E. (1942). *J. Bacteriol.* 43, 607.

Coraboeuf, E., and Goullet, P. (1963). *J. Physiol.* (*London*) 55, 232.

Dourmashkin, R. R., and Rosse, W. F. (1966). *Am. J. Med.* 41, 699.

Dunbar, J. M., and Erwa, H. H. (1967). *Bull. World Health Organ.* 37, 492.

Edwards, E. A. (1964). *J. Bacteriol.* 87, 1254.

Elliott, S. P., and Dole, V. P. (1947). *J. Exptl. Med.* 85, 305.

Fauve, R. M., Alouf, J. E., Delauney, A., and Raynaud, M. (1966). *J. Bacteriol.* 92, 1150.

Feigen, G. (1968). Personal communication.

Feigen, G., and Neustaedter, J. (1967). Personal communication.

Feigen, G. A., and Peterson, N. S. (1963). *J. Gen. Microbiol.* **33**, 489.

Feinstein, A. R., Stern, E. K., and Spagnoulo, M. (1964). *Am. Heart J.* **68**, 817.

Fuvessy, I., Boszormenyi, J., and Veress, A. (1967). *Acta Microbiol. Acad. Sci. Hung.* **14**, 335.

Ginsburg, I. (1959). *Brit. J. Exptl. Pathol.* **40**, 417.

Ginsburg, I., and Grossowicz, N. (1960). *J. Pathol. Bacteriol.* **80**, 111.

Ginsburg, I., Silberstein, Z., Spira, G., Bentwich, Z., and Boss, J. H. (1968). *Experientia* **24**, 256.

Goullet, P., Coraboeuf, E., and Breton, D. (1963). *Compt. Rend.* **257**, 1735.

Gualandi, G., Bizzini, B., Guyot-Jeannin, N., Alouf, J. E., and Raynaud, M. (1965). *Ann. Inst. Pasteur* **109**, 312.

Halbert, S. P. (1958). *J. Exptl. Med.* **108**, 385.

Halbert, S. P. (1963). *Ann. N.Y. Acad. Sci.* **103**, 1027.

Halbert, S. P. (1964). *In* "The Streptococcus, Rheumatic Fever and Glomerulonephritis" (J.W. Uhr, ed.), pp. 83–139. Williams & Wilkins, Baltimore, Maryland.

Halbert, S. P. (1968). *In* "Current Research on Group A Streptococcus" (R. Caravano, ed.). pp. 173–187. Excerpta Med. Found., Amsterdam.

Halbert, S. P., and Auerbach, T. (1961). *J. Exptl. Med.* **113**, 131.

Halbert, S. P., and Keatinge, S. (1961). *J. Exptl. Med.* **113**, 1013.

Halbert, S. P., and Keatinge, S. (1962). *Federation Proc.* **21**, 24.

Halbert, S. P., and Kiefer, D. (1968). Unpublished observations.

Halbert, S. P., Swick, L., and Sonn, C. (1955a). *J. Exptl. Med.* **101**, 539.

Halbert, S. P., Swick, L., and Sonn, C. (1955b). *J. Exptl. Med.* **101**, 557.

Halbert, S. P., Bircher, R., and Dahle, E. (1961a). *Biochem. Pharmacol.* **8**, 242.

Halbert, S. P., Bircher, R., and Dahle, E. (1961b). *J. Exptl. Med.* **113**, 759.

Halbert, S. P., Bircher, R., and Dahle, E. (1963a). *J. Lab. Clin. Med.* **61**, 437.

Halbert, S. P., Dahle, E., Keatinge, S., and Bircher, R. (1963b). *In* "Recent Advances in the Pharmacology of Toxins" (H. Rašková, ed.), pp. 437–452. Pergamon Press, Oxford.

Halbert, S. P., Holm, S. E., and Tompson, A. (1968). *J. Exptl. Med.* **127**, 613.

Hallen, J. (1963). *Acta Pathol. Microbiol. Scand.* **57**, 301.

Halpern, B. N., and Rahman, S. (1968). *Brit. J. Pharmacol.* **32**, 441.

Hamburger, M., and Lemon, H. M. (1953). *J. Lab. Clin. Med.* **42**, 140.

Hanson, L. A., and Holm, S. E. (1961). *Acta Paediat.* **50**, 7.

Herbert, D., and Todd, E. W. (1941). *Biochem. J.* **35**, 1124.

Hewitt, L. F., and Todd, E. W. (1939). *J. Pathol. Bacteriol* **49**, 45.

Hirsch, J. G., Bernheimer, A. W., and Weissmann, G. (1963). *J. Exptl. Med.* **118**, 223.

Holm, S. E. (1967). *Acta Pathol. Microbiol. Scand.* **69**, 264.

Houser, H. B., Eckhardt, G. C., Hahn, E. O., Denny, F. W., Wannamaker, L. W., and Rammelkamp, C. H. (1953). *Pediatrics* **12**, 593.

Howard, J. G., and Wallace, K. R. (1953a). *Brit. J. Exptl. Pathol.* **34**, 185.

Howard, J. G., and Wallace, K. R. (1953b). *Brit. J. Exptl. Pathol.* **34**, 181.

Howard, J. G., Wallace, K. R., and Wright, P. (1953). *Brit. J. Exptl. Pathol.* **34**, 174.

Ingestad, R., and Winblad, S. (1963). *Acta Pathol. Microbiol. Scand.* **57**, 455.

Inoué, A. (1959a). *Japan. J. Bacteriol.* **14**, 878.

Inoué, A. (1959b). *Japan. J. Bacteriol.* **14**, 936.

Inoué, A. (1960). *Japan. J. Bacteriol.* **15**, 285.

Kellner, A., Bernheimer, A. W., Carlson, A. S., and Freeman, E. B. (1956). *J. Exptl. Med.* **104**, 361.

Killander, J., and Philipson, L. (1964). *Acta Pathol. Microbiol. Scand.* **61**, 1.

Killander, J., Philipson, L., and Winblad, S. (1965). *Acta Pathol. Microbiol. Scand.* **65**, 587.

Kirschner, L., and Howie, J. B. (1952). *J. Pathol. Bacteriol.* **64**, 367.

Klein, G. C., Moody, M. D., Baker, C. N., and Addison, B. V. (1968). *Appl. Microbiol.* **16**, 184.

Köhler, W., and Dietel, K. (1968). *Z. Immunität. Allerg. Klin. Immunol.* **136**, 347.

Kusama, H., Ohashi, M., Shimazaki, H., and Fukumi, H. (1958). *Japan. J. Med. Sci & Biol.* **11**, 347.

Kwapinski, J. B., and Snyder, M. L. (1962). "The Immunology of Rheumatism," Appleton, New York.

Li, K. (1955). *J. Bacteriol.* **69**, 326.

Mansa, B., and Kjems, E. (1965). *Acta Pathol. Microbiol. Scand.* **65**, 303.

Mansa, B., and Kjems, E. (1968). *In* "Current Research on Group A Streptococcus" (R. Caravano, ed.), pp. 218–224. Excerpta Med. Found., Amsterdam.

Massell, B. F., Sturgis, G. P., Knobloch, J. D., Streeper, R. B., Hall, T. N., and Norcross, P. (1951). *J. Am. Med. Assoc.* **146**, 1469.

Merucci, P., Vella, L., and Zampiere, A. (1959). *Rend. Ist. Super. Sanita* **22**, 1085.

Mesrobeanu, L., Baldovin, C., Mihalco, F., and Mitrica, N. (1958). *Arch. Roumaines Pathol. Exptl. Microbiol.* **17**, 251.

Murray, J., and Calman, R. M. (Jan. 3, 1953). *Brit. Med. J.* pp. 13.

Neill, J. M., and Mallory, T. C. (1926). *J. Exptl. Med.* **44**, 241.

Ogburn, C. A., Harris, T. N., and Harris, S. (1958). *J. Bacteriol.* **76**, 142.

Oker-Blom, N., Nikkila, E., and Kalaja, T. (1950). *Ann. Med. Exptl. Biol. Fenniae (Helsinki)* **28**, 125.

Packalen, T. (1948). *J. Bacteriol.* **56**, 143.

Pearce, J. M. (1953). *Acta Pathol.* **56**, 13.

Pearce, J. M. (1960). *Circulation* **21**, 448.

Pentz, E. I., and Shigemura, Y. (1955). *J. Bacteriol.* **69**, 210.

Pentz, E. I., Kot, E., and Ferretti, J. J. (1964). *J. Bacteriol.* **88**, 497.

Perez, J. J., Wahl, R., and Boissol, C. (1964). *Ann. Inst. Pasteur* **106**, 380.

Petersen, K. F., Nowak, P., Thiele, O. W., and Urbashek, B. (1966). *Intern. Arch. Allergy Appl. Immunol.* **29**, 69.

Precechtel, F. (1966). *Z. Immunitaetsforsch., Allergie Klin. Immunol.* **30**, 391.

Quinn, R. W. (1957). *J. Clin. Invest.* **36**, 793.

Rantz, L. A., Randall, E., and Rantz, H. H. (1948a). *Am. J. Med.* **5**, 3.

Rantz, L. A., Boisvert, P. J., and Clark, W. H. (1948b). *Stanford Med. Bull.* **6**, 55.

Rašková, H. (1958). *In* "Pharmacology of Some Toxins," pp. 60–90. Publ. House Czech. Acad. Sci., Prague.

Rašková, H., and Vanecek, J. (1957). *Science* **126**, 700.

Reitz, B. A., Prager, D. J., and Feigen, G. A. (1968a). *J. Exptl. Med.* **128**, 1401.

Reitz, B. A., Prager, D. J., and Feigen, G. A. (1968b). *Federation Proc.* **27**, 226.

Robinson, J. J., and Crawford, Y. E. (1952). *Am. J. Clin. Pathol.* **22**, 247.

Rowen, R. (1963). *Proc. Soc. Exptl. Biol. Med.* **114**, 183.

Rowen, R., and Bernheimer, A. W. (1956). *J. Immunol.* **77**, 72.

Rowen R., and Wiest, M. A. (1965). *J. Exptl. Med.* **122**, 547.

Rozansky, R., and Strauss, M. (1961). *Bull. Res. Council Israel* **9**, 81.

Rozansky, R., Batat, A., and Bercovivi, B. (1960). *J. Immunol.* **84**, 54.

Rudolph, F. (1962). *Z. Immunitatsforsch.* **124**, 249.

Schwab, J. H., Watson, D. W., and Cromartie, W. J. (1955). *J. Infect. Diseases* **96**, 14.

Seligmann, M., Danon, F., Basch, A., and Barnard, J. (1968). *Nature* **220**, 711.

Slade, H. D., and Knox, G. A. (1950). *J. Bacteriol.* **60**, 301.

Smythe, C. V., and Harris, T. N. (1940). *J. Immunol.* **38**, 283.

Spira, G., Silberstein, Z., Harris, T. N., and Ginsburg, I. (1968). *Proc. Soc. Exptl. Biol. Med.* **127**, 1196.

Stetson, C. A. (1954). *In* "Streptococcal Infections" (M. McCarty, ed.), pp. 208–218. Columbia Univ. Press, New York.

Stollerman, G. H. (1953). *J. Clin. Invest.* **32**, 607.

Streitfeld, M. M. (1960). *Antimicrobial Agents Ann.* pp. 160–166.

Sugihara, C. Y., and Squier, T. L. (1951). *J. Allergy* **22**, 264.

Taranta, A. (1967). *Ann. Rev. Med.* **18**, 159.

Thiele, O. W., Petersen, K. F., and Nowak, P. (1965). *Biochim, Biophys. Acta* **106**, 427.

Thompson, A., Halbert, S. P., and Smith, U. (1970). *J. Exp. Med.* **131**, 745.

Todd, E. W. (1932). *J. Exptl. Med.* **55**, 267.

Todd, E. W. (1934). *J. Pathol. Bacteriol.* **39**, 299.

Todd, E. W. (1938). *J. Pathol. Bacteriol.* **47**, 423.

Todd, E. W. (1939). *J. Hyg.* **1**, 39.

Todd, E. W. (1941). *Brit. J. Exptl. Pathol.* **22**, 172.

Trinquier, E., and Morel, C. (1966). *Ann. Biol. Clin. (Paris)* **24**, 1155.

Turner, G. S., and Pentz, E. I. (1950). *Proc. Soc. Exptl. Biol. Med.* **73**, 169.

Vanecek, J. (1955). *Proc. 1st Conf. Fac. Pediat., Charles Univ., Prague*, p. 23.

Vanecek, J., and Raskova, H. (1956). *Arch. Exptl. Pathol. Pharmakol.* **229**, 1.

Vargues, R. (1965). *Ann. Biol. Clin. (Paris)* **23**, 10.

Vargues, R. (1966). *Ann. Inst. Pasteur* **110**, 373.

Vella, L., Sampieri, A., and Merucci, P. (1960). *Rend. Ist. Super. Sanita* **13**, 978.

Veress, A., Fuvessy, I., and Boszormenyi, J. (1964). *Ann. Immunol. Hung.* **7**, 63.

Wahl, R., and Cabau, N. (1958). *Rev. Rheum. et Maladies Osteoartic.* **25**, 433.

Wahl, R., Perez, J. J., Cayeux, P., and Derlot, E. (1964). *Ann. Inst. Pasteur* **106**, 388.

Waldenstrom, J., Winblad, S., Hallen, J., and Liungman, S. (1964). *Acta Med. Scand.* **176**, 619.

Waldman, G. (1965). *Acta Biol. Med. Ger.* **15**, 788.

Walter, H., and Zipper, H. (1960). *Proc. Soc. Exptl. Biol. Med.* **103**, 221.

Wannamaker, L. W., Rammelkamp, C. H., Denny, F. W., Brink, W. R., Houser, H. B., and Hahn, E. O. (1951). *Am. J. Med.* **10**, 673.

Weissmann, G., Keiser, H., and Bernheimer, A. W. (1963). *J. Exptl. Med.* **118**, 205.

Weissmann, G., Becher, B., Widermann, G., and Bernheimer, A. W. (1965). *Am. J. Pathol.* **46**, 129.

Weld, J. T. (1935). *J. Exptl. Med.* **61**, 473.

Westergren, A. (1948). *Acta Med.* **213**, 21.

Winblad, S. (1966). *Acta Pathol. Microbiol. Scand.* **66**, 93.

Zettervall, O., Sjoquist, J., Waldenstrom, J., and Winblad, S. (1966). *Clin. Exptl. Immunol.* **1**, 213.

Zucker-Franklin, D. (1965). *Am. J. Pathol.* **47**, 419.

CHAPTER 3

Streptolysin S*

ISAAC GINSBURG

*Supported in part by research grant BSS-CD-IS-2 EXT-1 from the U.S. Public Health Service.

99

I. Introduction

Since the discovery by Marmorek (1895) that filtrates of certain streptococcal cultures possess hemolytic activity toward red blood cells of various animal species, much work has been done on the hemolysins produced by streptococci. Todd (1938) was the first to demonstrate that
streptococci isolated from human sources produce two distinct hemolysins which he named oxygen-labile streptolysin O (SLO) to indicate its
sensitivity to oxygen, and oxygen-stable streptolysin S (SLS) to indicate
its stability to oxygen and its high solubility in serum. While SLO could be
found in supernates of streptococcal cultures grown in ordinary or defined
media (Todd, 1938; Bernheimer, 1949; Slade and Knox, 1950; Ginsburg
and Grossowicz, 1958) and was found to be immunogenic (Todd, 1938),
SLS was found only in cultures grown in the presence of serum and was
apparently nonimmunogenic. The zones of hemolysis found around streptococcal colonies grown on blood agar are produced by streptolysin S and
not by SLO, and the latter is readily oxidized by contact with air. It was
also found that oxygen-stable hemolysin could be "extracted" from
washed streptococci by serum protein fractions (Herbert and Todd, 1944;
Klinge, 1962a; Ginsburg *et al.*, 1963), by lecithovitelline from egg yolk as
well as by egg white, or by heated milk (Herbert and Todd, 1944).
Okamoto (1939) showed that yeast nucleic acid induced the formation of
potent hemolysin in growing streptococcal cultures as well as by washed
resting streptococci (Bernheimer and Rodbart, 1948; Egami *et al.*, 1950;
R. Ito *et al.*, 1948a,b). This hemolysin was found by R. Ito (1940a,b,c),
R. Ito *et al.* (1948a,b), Humphrey (1949a), and Bernheimer (1954) to
show a number of similarities to the serum hemolysin. None of these hemolysins were immunogenic. Schwab (1956a,b) showed that hemolytic
material can be obtained from washed group A streptococci subjected to
sonic vibrations for long periods of time. The hemolytic material was
named intracellular hemolysin (IH). It was found to be similar in certain
respects to the hemolysin produced in the presence of yeast RNA
(Schwab, 1956b). However, it was later reported (Schwab, 1960) that
IH is immunogenic in rabbits and thus may be different from SLS. The
picture became even more complicated when Weld (1934), Smith (1937),
Ginsburg and Grossowicz (1958), and Y. Taketo and Taketo (1967)
showed that washed streptococci hemolyzed red blood cells, but that no
extracellular hemolysin could be demonstrated. This hemolytic factor
was named cell-bound hemolysin (CBH) (Ginsburg and Grossowicz,
1958). The cell-bound factor which could be released from the streptococcal cells by certain detergents and serum albumin (Ginsburg and
Grossowicz, 1958) and by α-lipoproteins (Ginsburg *et al.*, 1963) was
named streptolysin D (D stands for detergents). It showed many similar

properties to the hemolysins produced by streptococci in the presence of serum or yeast RNA. A tabular comparison of some of the similarities and differences as reported for these hemolytic materials is given in Table I. A major problem to be solved is that quite unrelated materials appear to induce the formation by streptococci of a very similar if not identical hemolysin.

In view of the nonimmunogenicity of any of the different forms of the oxygen-stable hemolysin (Bernheimer, 1954; Ginsburg and Harris, 1964), the problem of whether streptococci are capable of producing a single oxygen-stable hemolytic factor with similar physical and biological properties remains to be solved. Also, the problem of whether "induction" of hemolytic activity in growing or resting streptococci by the different agents involves synthesis *de novo* or is due to the "extraction" of preformed hemolysin is still not fully clear. Some aspects concerning the nature, synthesis, and mode of action of the oxygen-stable hemolysis have been comprehensively reviewed by Bernheimer (1954), Okamoto (1962), Koyama *et al.* (1963), Klinge (1963), and by Ginsburg and Harris (1964). Because streptolysin S may exist in various forms (e.g., associated with different inducers or carriers) the description of the various forms of SLS will be given separately.

II. Definition of SLS Activity

The only known way to detect SLS activity is by determining its hemolytic action on red blood cells or through its cytotoxic effects on other mammalian cells (Ginsburg and Harris, 1964). One hemolytic unit (HU) of SLS is arbitrarily defined as the amount in 1 ml of sample that will hemolyze rabbit or human red blood cell suspensions [final concentration 0.7%, Bernheimer (1949), 2%, Ginsburg and Grossowicz (1958), or 3%, Koyama *et al.* (1963)] after 30 minutes of incubation at 37°C. The degree of hemolysis is determined by reading the optical density (OD) of hemoglobin at 540 mμ. The SLS potency is also expressed as hemolytic units per milligram dry weight (Bernheimer, 1949) or hemolytic units per OD unit at 260 mμ (Koyama and Egami, 1963). The dilutions of the hemolysin are usually made in saline buffered with phosphate ($\mu = 0.15$) (PBS), pH 7.4 (Bernheimer, 1949; Ginsburg and Grossowicz, 1958) or in a solution containing 0.078 M sodium chloride and 0.033 M sodium phosphate, pH 7.0 (Ishikura, 1962; Koyama and Egami, 1963). It was shown, however, (Ginsburg and Bentwich, 1964) that 1 HU titrated by the method described by Ginsburg and Grossowicz (1958) is roughly equivalent to 5 HU when titrated with the slightly hypotonic buffers described by Ishikura (1962) or Koyama and Egami (1963). Also, SLS activity (RNA hemolysin) was found to be influenced by the buffers employed. Thus 1 HU

TABLE I

AGENTS USED TO OBTAIN OXYGEN-STABLE HEMOLYSINS FROM GROUP A STREPTOCOCCI[a]

Hemolysin	Agents involved in formation	Chemical nature reported	Inhibition by	Selected references
Streptolysin S (SLS)	Whole serum, albumin, β-lipoprotein, lecithovitelline	Lipoprotein	Lecithin, β-lipoproteins	Weld (1934), Todd (1938), (Humphrey 1949a), Klinge (1962a), Ginsburg and Harris (1963, 1964)
Streptolysin S′ (SLS′)	RNA, RNA core, oligonucleotides, biosynthetic polynucleotides	Polynucleotide-polysaccharide-protein complex, oligonucleotide-polypeptide complex	Lecithin, trypan blue, Congo red, α-β-lipoproteins, papain, ficin	Okamoto (1939), Bernheimer (1949, 1954), Okamoto (1962), Koyama and Egami (1963), Ginsburg and Harris (1964), Koyama (1964)
Intracellular hemolysin (IH), ICH(S)	—	—	K⁺, lecithin antiserum	Schwab (1956a), A. Taketo and Taketo (1965)
Cell-bound hemolysin (CBH)	Sugars, Mg²⁺, sulfhydryl compounds	—	Trypan blue, tetracyclines, chloramphenicol, iodoacetic acid, sodium fluoride	Weld (1934), Smith (1937), Ginsburg and Grossowicz (1958), Ginsburg and Harris (1965)
Streptolysin D (SLD)	Sugars or amino acids, Mg²⁺, sulfhydryl compounds, serums, albumin, detergents (Tween, Triton)	Complex between albumin or detergents with protein	Lecithin, trypan blue, Congo red, whole serum, β-lipoproteins, papain, ficin	Ginsburg and Grossowicz (1958), Ginsburg and Harris (1964), A. Taketo and Taketo (1964b)

[a]Modified from Ginsburg and Harris (1964).

of RNA hemolysin determined in PBS was roughly equivalent to 3 HU when assayed in barbital–sodium chloride buffer (complement buffer, Kabat and Meyer, 1961). Assay of SLS in Tris HCl buffer usually yielded 2 HU (Ginsburg, unpublished data).

III. Streptococcal Strains Producing SLS

Most of the data on SLS have been derived from studies on streptococci belonging to group A according to Lancefield. Ginsburg and Grossowicz (1958) and Snyder (1960) have shown that over 95% of group A, C, and G strains tested (total of 200 strains) produced serum or RNA hemolysin. However, no SLS was produced by streptococcal strains of group B and D. Okamoto (1962) has shown that certain streptococcal strains belonging to groups E, H, and L also produced SLS in the presence of RNA. More data are needed, however, to determine whether the response of the streptococci to the RNA varies with the streptococcal groups other than group A.

The isolation of group A streptococcal strains capable of producing only SLO or SLS shed light on the phenomenon of hemolysis produced by hemolytic streptococci on blood agar. Herbert and Todd (1944) showed that strain Blackmore (type 11) produced only SLS. However, strain C203U (type 3), which is a mutant of strain C203S (Type 3), produced only SLO. When streaked on blood agar plates, colonies of strain Blackmore produced large hemolytic zones, while those of strain C203U produced very faint zones of slight hemolysis, it was concluded that SLS was responsible for hemolysis on blood agar.

IV. Multiple Forms of SLS

Since SLS can be formed by streptococci in the presence of different inducers, the properties of the different forms of oxygen-stable hemolysins will be described separately.

A. SERUM HEMOLYSIN

Weld (1934) showed that a potent hemolysin indistinguishable from the serum hemolysin described by Todd (1938) in growing cultures could be obtained by shaking washed streptococci with horse or human serum. A single batch of streptococci could be extracted at least 5 times, each time yielding approximately the same amount of hemolysin. The hemolysin, which according to Weld was found "upon" the streptococcal cells, was considered to be solubilized by the serum. Snyder (1960) studied the effect of sera from various species on the production of SLS by strain C203S. While sera of horses and dogs induced the formation of 300 HU/ml of SLS, sera of humans and monkeys formed 74 and 68 HU/ml, respectively. Sera of rabbit and guinea pigs under similar condition each formed only 15 HU/ml of SLS.

1. ROLE OF PROTEIN FRACTIONS

Herbert and Todd (1944) studied the nature of the serum hemolysin. Whole serum was found to be essential for the extraction of the hemolysin, while serum ultrafiltrates, purified pseudoglobulins, euglobulin, and albumin were inactive. SLS was not inactivated by dialysis, and dialyzed serum extracts could be dried *in vacuo* or lyophilized to form a light brown powder which is readily soluble in water. Under such conditions, SLS retained its full hemolytic activity over long periods of time. Ginsburg and Grossowicz (1958) and Ginsburg *et al.* (1963) showed that the low ionic strength supernatant fluid derived from human serum following dialysis against acetate buffer (pH 5.2; $\mu = 0.01$) yielded very high hemolytic activity from washed streptococci, indicating that the albumin fraction of the serum participated in the formation of the hemolysin. Ginsburg *et al.* (1963) further showed that both dialyzable and nondialyzable fractions participated in this reaction. The dialyzable fraction could be replaced by Mg^{2+}, glucose, and cysteine (see Section VII). Of the nondialyzable fractions, both albumin (Cohn fraction V) and α-lipoprotein (Cohn fraction IV-I) induced the formation of hemolysin from streptococci incubated with glucose Mg^{2+}, and sulfhydryl compounds. Albumin at 38 mg/ml induced approximately 80% of the hemolysin, and fraction IV-I at 4.2 mg/ml 20% of the hemolysin induced by whole serum (Table II). Thus, the serum hemolysin of the literature probably is largely the hemolysin induced by serum albumin. Further confirmation of the association of albumin and α-lipoprotein with the serum hemolysin was obtained by studies on the chromatography of human serum hemolysin on DEAE-cellulose. Linear gradient elution with potassium chloride was employed. Two peaks of hemolytic activity emerged from the column, with the maximum corresponding to 0.22 and 0.27 M potassium chloride (Fig. 1C). The first peak appeared just before the bulk of the albumin was eluted from the column. This appeared in the position at which lipid-rich fraction of serum proteins was found by Peterson and Sober (1960). This relationship seems reasonable, since α-lipoproteins have been found to induce hemolytic activity from streptococci (Ginsburg *et al.*, 1963). The second peak of hemolytic activity was associated with the descending limb of the albumin peak. Rechromatography of the first peak was not

TABLE II
ROLE OF PLASMA PROTEIN FRACTIONS IN HEMOLYSIN PRODUCTION[a]

Inducing agent[b]	Concentration of inducing agent	Hemolytic activity (HU/ml)
Human serum	50%	2700
Low ionic strength precipitate[c]	50% (of serum)	450
Low ionic strength supernatant fluid	50% (of serum)	2300
Fraction I	3.5 mg/ml	13
Fraction II	7.7 mg/ml	66
Fraction III	10.0 mg/ml	136
Fraction III-0	4.2 mg/ml	15
Fraction IV	11.0 mg/ml	84
Fraction IV-1	4.2 mg/ml	320
Fraction IV-5,6	1.7 mg/ml	90
Fraction V	38.0 mg/ml	1750

[a] From Ginsberg *et al.* (1963).

[b] Glucose, $MgSO_4 \cdot 7H_2O$, and cysteine HCl added to each agent at 1 mg/ml, except in the case of whole serum where only cysteine was added.

[c] Fraction obtained by dialyzing serum against acetate buffer (pH 5.2, $\mu = 0.01$).

successful because the hemolysin associated with this fraction could not be eluted from DEAE-cellulose column in active form. Rechromatography of the second hemolytic portion again showed that the fraction obtained with increasing molarity of the eluant showed progressive decreases in the amount of protein eluted, but progressive increases in hemolytic activity. The lowest amount of protein and the highest yield of hemolysin were obtained on eluting with 0.25 M potassium chloride (Fig. 1A). Treatment of this fraction with alcohol–ether yielded material giving considerable opalescence in aqueous suspension. In a different approach to the same question, fractions of fresh serum albumin were compared in their effectiveness in the induction of hemolysin by resting streptococci. The fraction of albumin eluted at 0.25 to 0.3 M potassium chloride under the same conditions induced the formation of larger amounts of hemolysin than did the fraction eluted at 0.175 M, although the OD ($280m\mu$) was substantially less (Fig. 2). It appears, therefore, that the fraction of albumin responsible for hemolysin induction is probably not associated with protein, but with other materials contaminating the albumin.

2. ROLE OF LIPIDS

Further studies on the role of fractions IV-I and V in this reaction revealed that treatment with ethanol–ether (3:1) or chloroform–methanol

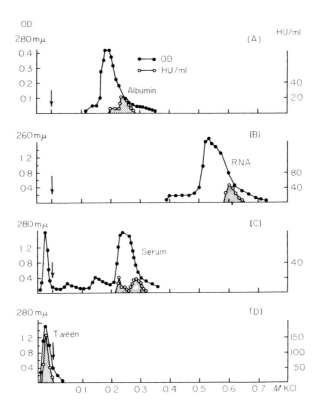

FIG. 1. Chromatography of several of the oxygen-stable streptococcal hemolysins on DEAE-cellulose in 0.01 M phosphate, pH 7.2. The vertical arrow indicates the beginning of elution with potassium chloride in linear gradient increase of concentration. The molarity of the potassium chloride is shown on the abscissa. A = albumin hemolysin, B = RNA hemolysin, C = "serum hemolysin," D = Tween 40 hemolysin. From Ginsburg and Harris (1963).

(2:1) completely destroyed the capacity of these fractions to produce hemolysin. However, the digestion of either albumin or α-lipoprotein with crystalline trypsin did not affect their hemolysin-producing capacity (Ginsburg and Harris, 1963).

Klinge (1962b) concluded that neither bound lipids nor lipoprotein participated in hemolysin formation. He based his conclusions on the findings that serum extracted with ether to which lecithovitelline was added failed to induce hemolysin from resting streptococci. These experiments, however, are open to question since Klinge did not employ serum lipoprotein but rather chose lecithovitelline from egg yolk as the attempted replacement for the lipoprotein fraction.

In another study (Ginsburg and Harris, 1963) on the relationship of the material in the first hemolytic peak eluted from DEAE-cellulose to lipoproteins, the serum hemolysin was chromatographed on glass powder columns according to the method of Carlson (1960). In this method, the α- and the β-lipoproteins are bound to the glass powder at pH 8.8, and the rest of the serum components are not adsorbed. The α- and β-lipoproteins can then be eluted at pH 9.6 and 9.8, respectively. Upon chromatography of serum hemolysin by this method, one part of the hemolytic material was not adsorbed to the column (probably the albumin hemolysin), while the other fraction was adsorbed and eluted at pH 9.6 (corresponding to the position of α-lipoproteins). The latter fraction con-- tained relatively little 280 mμ adsorbing material and a relatively large concentration of lipid (see Foster, 1960).

Hemolytic activity was not seen with lipid-free albumin or with the lipid fraction extracted from the albumin. In fact, the lipid extracted from albumin was found to inhibit the activity of the hemolysin induced by intact albumin, which agrees with the findings of Humphrey (1949a,b) on the presence of an SLS inhibitor in albumin (see Section VIII).

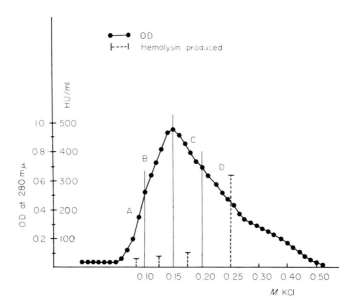

Fig. 2. The formation of hemolysin by fractions of human serum albumin obtained by elution from DEAE-cellulose. From Ginsburg and Harris (1964).

B. RNA Hemolysin

Okamoto (1939), Okamoto *et al.* (1941a), and Bernheimer and Rodbart (1948) demonstrated that formation of a hemolytic toxin by hemolytic streptococci was greatly enhanced by addition of yeast ribonucleic acid to the culture medium. The amount of hemolysin was found to be a function of the concentration of RNA, the optimal amount of RNA being approximately 1%. It was also found that the very small SLS content from the supernatant fluid of cultures grown in meat infusion broth was due to trace amounts of RNA extracted from the muscle.

Hosoya *et al.* (1949a,b), Bernheimer (1949), and Egami *et al.* (1950) have further demonstrated that the enhancement of hemolysin formation by yeast RNA could also be obtained by shaking resting streptococci with solutions containing a mixture of nucleic acids. This hemolysin was found by R. Ito (1940a,b,c), Bernheimer (1954), and Humphrey (1949b) to show a number of similarities to the serum hemolysin in that it was inhibited by lecithin, trypan blue, Congo red, papain, and chymotrypsin, but was uneffected by trypsin, pepsin, cholesterol, or by sera of animals injected with preparations of SLS.

Properties of RNA as Inducer of SLS

In detailed studies on the nature of the RNA hemolysin, it was shown that RNA preparations obtained from different sources — yeast, streptococci, liver (Bernheimer and Rodbart, 1948; Shoin *et al.*, 1955; Okamoto, 1962), wheat germ (Bernheimer and Rodbart, 1948), spleen (Egami *et al.*, 1950), muscle and Ehrlich ascites tumor cells (Okamoto, 1962), *Azotobacter vinelandii* (Tanaka *et al.*, 1958b), tobacco leaves (Bernheimer, 1954), and kidney (Bernheimer and Rodbart, 1948; Shoin *et al.*, 1955) — were all effective in the induction of hemolysin formation by streptococci. However, RNA derived from tobacco mosaic virus (TMV RNA) was only slightly active (Tanaka *et al.*, 1958; Bernheimer and Rodbart, 1948), while RNA derived from *Escherichia coli* and *Clostridium welchii* was inactive (Bernheimer, 1952). In contrast to ribonucleic acid, deoxyribonucleic acid (DNA) preparations had been shown to be entirely without effect (Bernheimer, 1952, 1954; Okamoto, 1962). More recently, Egami *et al.* (1950) have reported that both highly polymerized and depolymerized DNA preparations induced hemolytic activity in resting streptococci. Further studies by Bernheimer and Rodbart, 1948) and by Bernheimer (1949), Hosoya *et al.* (1949a,b), and Tanaka *et al.* (1958) have shown that following digestion of yeast RNA with pancreatic ribonuclease and precipitation with ethanol, the precipitate markedly increased hemolysin formation by streptococci. Bernheimer and Rodbart (1948) have further shown that the active fraction (AF) thus obtained was associated with the ribonuclease-resistant core and had approximately 100 times the activity of the starting material. The AF appeared to be a polynucleotide. Similar treatment of TMV–RNA made it totally inactive, while DNA treated with ribonuclease or by deoxyribuonuclease remained inactive.

The ultraviolet absorption spectrum of the RNA and AF showed a maximum absorption at 250 and 255 mμ, respectively. Egami *et al.* (1950) found that when a dialyzable fraction of yeast RNA digested with ribonuclease was incubated with washed streptococci, one portion of this material produced hemolysin which was nondialyzable, suggesting that the formation of hemolysin from this fraction involved polymerization of the fraction involved. The best preparation of the hemolysin produced with the AF by Bernheimer (1949) contained 60% polynucleotide; and of the remaining 40% a substantial portion was carbohydrate. There was no direct evidence that either the polynucleotide or the carbohydrate was essential for the toxic activity of the hemolysin since both these fractions were also isolated from supernatant fluids of a group A streptococcal mutant (strain C203U type 3) which did not produce SLS. Since papain and chymotrypsin destroyed the hemolysin, it seemed likely that protein or peptide was involved. This work has been reviewed in greater detail by Bernheimer (1949, 1954).

Very extensive studies on the chemical nature of the active fraction of RNA responsible for the induction of SLS have been carried out by several investigators in Japan. Tanaka *et al.* (1956a,b) hydrolyzed yeast RNA with weak alkali at 0°C and separated from the resulting mixture a fraction which precipitated at 25% acetone. This fraction, a polynucleatide, was several-fold more active than RNA in SLS induction. Further treatment with RNAse increased its potency. Alkaline hydrolysis resulted in cleavage of all internucleotide linkages of RNA with the formation of 2' and 3' mononucleotides. Also, some of the degradation products were probably oligonucleotides rich in adenine and guanine.

The effect of phosphatases on the SLS-inducing activity of the RNAase-resistant core and yeast RNA has been studied by Bernheimer and Rodbart (1948), Hosoya *et al.* (1949a,b), Heppel and Hilmoe (1952), Okamoto (1962), and Tanaka *et al.* (1958b). They showed that the RNA moiety involved in the SLS induction is relatively resistant to phosphodiesterase obtained from prostate, spleen, potatoes, and snake venom. Since prostatic phosphomonoesterase was not active, it was assumed that the terminal phosphomonoester linkage did not play a role in SLS formation.

The snake venom phosphodiesterase which hydrolyzed RNA into 5' mononucleotides did not lower the SLS-inducing capacity of RNA. However, a marked decrease in SLS-forming capacity occurred after treatment of RNA by RNAase T from Taka Diastase. This enzyme has been shown by Sato and Egami (1957) to release 3'-guanylic acid from RNA core.

Tanaka *et al.* (1957, 1958b) showed that polynucleotides synthesized from nucleoside diphosphate by a polynucleotide phosphorylase of *Azotobacter vinelandii* were highly effective in promoting SLS formation. PolyAGUC (1:1:1:1) was more active than yeast RNA, while poly-AGUC (1:0.5:1:1) had but negligible activity, and polyAU and polyAC were inactive. PolyGUC had good SLS-inducing capacity.

Sato-Asano *et al.* (1960) demonstrated that oligoguanylic acid from guanosine-2'3' cyclic phosphate showed SLS-inducing activity.

Ishikura (1961) showed that RNAase core I prepared from yeast RNA according to Tanaka (1958) was separated into two fractions by gel filtration through Sephadex and that SLS-forming activity was present only in the higher molecular weight fraction which was found to be rich in guanylic acid. More recently, Shugar and Tomersko (see Okamoto, 1962) found that synthetic poly guanylic acid had excellent SLS-inducing activity. It may be concluded that guanylic acid moiety of natural RNA plays an important role in the phenomenon of SLS induction. The reason for this effect, however, is still obscure.

C. DETERGENT HEMOLYSIN

Ginsburg (1958), Ginsburg and Grossowicz (1958), Ginsburg *et al.* (1963), and Ginsburg and Harris (1963) showed that a potent hemolytic factor was obtained by incubating washed group A streptococci with Tween 40, 60, or 80 (polyoxyethylene sorbitan mono palmitate, stearate, or oleate, respectively), Triton X-205 (octylphenol polyethylene oxide), or with trypan blue (Ginsburg and Harris, 1965) (see Section X). The hemolysin which was named streptolysin D (D stands for detergent) (Ginsburg and Grossowicz, 1958) showed many properties similar to those of the serum and RNA hemolysins (Table I). Streptococcal strains (e.g., C-203U) incapable of producing RNA or serum hemolysin also failed to produce detergent hemolysin. Chromatography of the Tween and Triton hemolysins on DEAE-cellulose and carboxymethylcellulose revealed that neither of these hemolysins were absorbed to the columns, nor were Tween or Triton alone (Fig. 1D) (Ginsburg and Harris, 1963).

D. CELL-BOUND HEMOLYSIN

Various strains of group A streptococci possess a cell-bound hemolysin (CBH) (Weld, 1934; Smith, 1937) which can be demonstrated by the incubation of red blood cells of various animal species with washed streptococci in the presence of glucose, Mg^{2+}, and sulfhydryl compounds (Ginsburg and Grossowicz, (1958); Ginsburg and Harris, 1965). Under such conditions, hemolysis occurs within a short time although no extracellular hemolysin can be demonstrated in supernatant fluids of the incubation mixture or in extracts of streptococci disrupted by sonic oscillation. Streptococci possessing CBH activity have been found to cause distinct cytopathogenic changes in a variety of mammalian cells *in vitro* (Ginsburg, 1959); Ginsburg and Grossowicz, 1960). The hemolytic as well as the cytopathogenic effect caused by the washed streptococci can be abolished by a variety of metabolic inhibitors and by factors known to inhibit RNA, serum, and detergent hemolysins (See Section VII). Streptococcal strains producing RNA and serum hemolysin possess CBH activity and the inhibition of CBH activity always results in the inhibition of the formation of the other forms of the oxygen-stable hemolysin. Strain C 203U, which does not produce RNA or serum hemolysins, also does not show any CBH activity. A source of difficulty in the comparison of the two forms of the hemolysin stems from the fact that while RNA, serum, or the detergent hemolysins are estimated in solution, CBH must be determined in the presence of streptococci, under conditions in which it is not possible at present to eliminate entirely the effect of continued synthesis of the CBH (see Section VII).

E. INTRACELLULAR HEMOLYSIN

Schwab (1956a,b) has demonstrated that group A streptococci subjected to sonic oscillation released an hemolytic factor which was designated intracellular hemolysin (IH). The hemolytic activity of IH increased rapidly during sonification and after 60 minutes not more than 1% of the cells remained intact. The amount of IH released steadily increased with the time of sonic treatment. Very little hemolytic activity remained in the cell debris following sonification. It was also found that treatment of IH with acid activated the hemolysin. The author suggested that IH is probably part of the cell structure and that the increase of hemolytic activity following treatment at low pH may be due to dissociation of hemolysin-inhibitor complex. This hemolysin can be readily distinguished from SLO by virtue of the failure of various reagents which are known inhibitors of SLO to influence its activity. Establishing the distinction or identity of the IH and the RNA hemolysin was more difficult. Both hemolysins were similarly inhibited by lecithin, Ca^{2+}, and rabbit serum. Also, both hemolysins demonstrated similar stability and kinetic properties. However, it was possible to distinguish between the two hemolysins by the different susceptibilities of sheep and rabbit red cells. Also, the production of significant amount of IH in strains which produced very little SLS further supports their distinct nature. More recently, Schwab (1960) has shown that serum from rabbits immunized with an extract of sonically disrupted group A streptococci contained an antibody specific for IH, suggesting in fact that IH is distinct from SLS.

Further insight into the problem of the intracellular hemolysin was recently given by A. Taketo and Taketo (1964a, 1965). Cell-free extracts prepared from hemolytic streptococci contained two distinct intracellular hemolysins, the one termed intracellular streptolysin O (ICH-O) and the other intracellular streptolysin S (ICH-S). The incubation of cell-free extracts with an oligonucleotide fraction resulted in the formation of an oligonucleotide–streptolysin S complex. It was concluded that the *in vitro* formation of the RNA hemolysin was due to a transfer of a hemolytic group to the oligonucleotide (see Section VI). The relationship between the ICH-S described by A. Taketo and Taketo (1964a, 1965) to the intracellular hemolysin IH described by Schwab (1956a) is not yet clear. Although Schwab's hemolysin was differentiated from RNA hemolysin on the basis of the effect of Na^+ and K^+ and their relative activity on sheep and rabbit erythrocytes, close resemblance was noted between the two hemolysins in many other properties. Since Schwab's hemolysin has not yet been purified, and since the possibility of transfer of the hemolysin to oligonucleotide has not yet been examined, it is not possible to compare the hemolysin directly with ICH-S. However, it seems not unlikely that Schwab's hemolysin is in fact an intracellular form of SLS.

The relationship of CBH to IH and ICH-S is not clear, although CBH resembles IH and ICH-S in some respects. Extensive sonification of streptococci failed to release CBH activity. (Ginsburg and Grossowicz, 1958). Further work on this problem will shed more light on the interrelationships among the intracellular hemolysins.

V. Chemical Nature of the Hemolytic Moiety of SLS

In considering the possible relationships among the hemolysins produced by serum, albumin, detergents, or RNA, the problem is narrowed by the indications that albumin hemolysin constitutes the greater part of serum hemolysin (Ginsburg *et al.*, 1963); Ginsburg and Harris, 1963). Thus, the question of whether the streptococcus produced one or more oxygen-stable hemolysins is largely that of whether the hemolysin produced by RNA and by albumin (or detergents) are the same or different. Among the properties which are similar in the case of RNA hemolysin, albumin hemolysin, and CBH are the destruction of hemolytic activity by papain, chymotrypsin, but not by trypsin or pepsin (Bernheimer, 1949; Okamoto, 1962; Ginsburg *et al.*, 1963), suggesting that the hemolytic group is a peptide or protein.

Koyama and Egami (1963, 1964) and Koyama (1963, 1964), have employed DEAE-cellulose to isolate RNA-core hemolysin. SLS preparation eluted from the column at salt concentration above 0.6 M had a specific activity of 100,000 hemolytic units per optical density unit at 260 mμ. Analysis for base composition by paper chromatography after acid hydrolysis showed a base ratio similar to that of the oligonucleotide effective in hemolysin formation, i.e., rich in guanine and poor in pyrimidine content. Also, such a SLS preparation was found to contain 2 moles of amino acid (leucine equivalent) per mole of nucleotide (guanylic acid equivalent). The oligonucleotide fraction used to induce SLS formation contained only 0.8 mole of amino acids. These results indicated a definite increase of amino acids in the hemolysin preparation. In further studies incorporation of ^{14}C amino acids was carried out using a hydrolyzate of ^{14}C Chlorella protein. Zone electrophoresis of the labeled hemolysin indicated the presence of radioactivity in the fraction with high hemolytic activity. The labeled hemolysin was further purified by chromatography on DEAE-cellulose (Fig. 3). The ^{14}C-labeled SLS was hydrolyzed in acid,

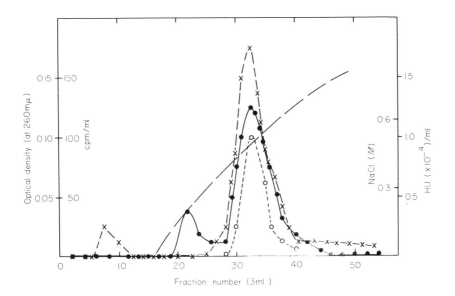

FIG. 3. DEAE-cellulose column chromatography of purified ^{14}C-labeled streptolysin S'. Solid circles = optical density at 260 mμ; open circles = hemolytic activity; crosses = radioactivity; broken line = concentration of sodium chloride. DEAE-cellulose column: 1 × 15 cm; 0.01 M phosphate buffer at pH 7.0; temperature: 4°C. From Koyama and Egami (1964).

and an amino acid analysis performed with an automatic amino acid analyzer reveal the presence of 12 amino acids (Table III). It is of interest that SLS had a high content of glutamic acid and serine but lacked cystine, methionine, and aromatic amino acids. Similar amino acid analysis of the oligonucleotide used to induce the SLS revealed only trace amounts of glycine and ammonia. Like the unlabeled RNA hemolysin, the ^{14}C-labeled SLS was inactivated by Nagarse and 8 M urea, but not by trypsin or by 6 M guanidine (see Section Xc).

More recently, Bernheimer (1967) studied the molecular weight of the RNA hemolysin by the method and principles of gel filtration described by Andrews (1964) using Sephadex G-75 columns. He found that the SLS had an effluent volume which corresponded on an Andrews plot to a molecular weight of 12,000. The sedimentation coefficient of the SLS on sucrose gradient determined with an ultracentrifuge had an $s_{20,w}$ of 2.4

TABLE III

AMINO ACID COMPOSITION OF HYDROLYZATES OF STREPTOLYSIN S[a]

	Amino acid residues per 30 O.D. 260 mμ (μmoles)		
	Streptolysin S		Oligoribo-nucleotide[b]
Amino acid	Prep. 1[b]	Prep. 2[c]	
Aspartic acid	0.088	0.080	0
Threonine	0.047	0.037	0
Serine	0.170	0.157	0.011
Glutamic acid	0.322	0.275	0
Proline	0.025	0.022	0
Glycine	0.439	0.275	0.341
Alanine	0.062	0.055	0
½ Cystine	—	—	—
Valine	0.044	0.050	0
Methionine	0	0	0
Isoleucine	0.059	0.050	0
Leucine	0.029	0.027	0
Tyrosine	0	0	0
Phenylalanine	0	0	0
Lysine	0.043	0.027	0
Histidine	0.023	0.014	0
Arginine	0	0	0
Tryptophan	—	—	—
Ammonia	3.16	2.38	2.55

[a]From Koyama (1963).
[b]36-hour hydrolyzate at 110°C.
[c]24-hour hydrolyzate at 105°C.

suggesting a molecular weight of the order of 20,000. Since, according to Koyama (1963), the molar ratio of polypeptide to oligonucleotide of highly purified SLS was 0.3 the molecular weight of the polypeptide moiety was calculated to be of the order of 2800. It should, therefore, consist of about 28 amino acids residues. The small size of the active moiety may therefore account for its inability to induce the formation of neutralizing antibodies (see Section XVII). These results clearly demonstrated that the RNA hemolysin is composed of a polynucleotide moiety and a polypeptide which is probably responsible for the hemolytic activity (see Section VI).

VI. SLS — a Carrier–Hemolysin Complex

From the foregoing considerations, it appears that quite unrelated substances — serum albumin, α-lipoprotein, RNA, detergents, and trypan blue — can induce the formation of hemolysin from streptococci and that the chromatographic patterns of the various forms of the hemolysins on DEAE-cellulose actually reflect the behavior of the inducing agents rather than the hemolysins induced by them (Fig. 1). This hypothesis was further strengthened by the findings of Ginsburg and Harris (1963), Koyama and Egami (1964), and of A. Taketo and Taketo (1964b). Ginsburg and Harris (1963) showed that when both RNA and albumin hemolysin were mixed with either Tween or Triton and the mixture chromatographed on DEAE-cellulose, hemolytic activity was eluted from the column in two peaks. One peak was associated with the Tween or Triton (Fig. 1), while the other was associated with the albumin or RNA at their expected position of elution from DEAE-cellulose (at 0.25 M and 0.6 M potassium chloride, respectively). Since no trace of either albumin or RNA could be found associated with the Tween or Triton passing through the column, it was concluded that Tween or Triton had bound part of the hemolytic activity previously associated with the albumin or RNA. It was further shown (Ginsburg and Harris, 1963) that RNA could bind hemolytic activity originally associated with albumin and vice versa. The amount of hemolysin transferred depended on the relative concentration of the RNA and albumin in the reaction mixture. These results were confirmed recently by A. Taketo and Taketo (1964b) using a transfer system between ^{14}C-labeled RNA hemolysin and Tween. Further experiments showed that electrophoresis of RNA, albumin, and Tween hemolysins on agar had migration rates typical of the carrier molecules, and that when either albumin or RNA hemolysin were mixed with Tween or Triton and subjected to electrophoresis, hemolytic activity was found only at the position of Tween or Triton (Figs. 4 and 5).

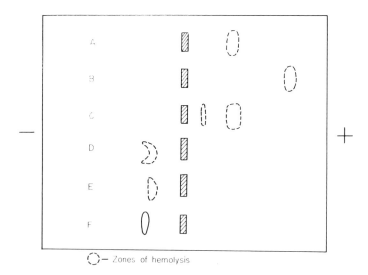

○— Zones of hemolysis

FIG. 4. Zone electrophoresis of hemolysins on agar block at 40 V/cm for 6 hours in 0.01 *M* barbital acetate buffer, pH 8.6. Following electrophoresis, a layer of agar containing sheep red blood cells was poured on the agar block and allowed to harden. Hemolytic zones appeared after incubation at 37°C for 2 hours. A = albumin hemolysin, B = RNA core hemolysin, C = horse serum hemolysin, D = Tween hemolysin, E = Triton hemolysin, F = Dextran. From Ginsburg and Harris (1964).

These experiments suggested that streptolysin S probably existed as a carrier–hemolysin complex and that the distribution of the hemolytic group (peptide) among available carriers depended on the concentration of the different carriers and on their affinities for the hemolytic moiety (Ginsburg and Harris, 1963). To further substantiate the concept of the carrier–hemolysin complex structure of SLS, these authors showed that the hemolytic activity of any complex could be destroyed by either inactivating the hemolytic moiety (see Section X) or by destroying the carrier molecule — at low pH in the case of the albumin hemolysin and at high pH in the case of the RNA hemolysin (Ginsburg and Harris, 1964). Other experiments have shown that RNA hemolysin could be destroyed by a ribonuclease of *Aspergillus*. The hemolytic moiety became resistant to the ribonuclease when the former was transferred to albumin or Tween, indicating that the integrity of the carrier molecule is essential for hemolytic activity. These experiments also indicated that the hemolytic moiety decays very rapidly when the carrier molecules are destroyed or altered and that free hemolysin probably does not exist as such. The experiment involving the transfer of the hemolysin from one carrier to another and the similar degree of inhibition of all the hemolysins by the same inhibitors all lead to the conclusion that a single hemolytic group (a peptide) synthesized by streptococci can be bound to a variety of carriers which have affinity for the active group.

In the transfer of the hemolytic group from one carrier molecule to another, the distribution of this moiety between the carriers involved would depend on the relative affinities of the carriers for the hemolytic group and the relative concentrations of the carriers. It is not possible at present to assign relative values of average affinity of binding sites of the respective carriers for the hemolytic moiety. However, certain relative differences among the carriers have been suggested by chromatographic and electrophoretic data (Ginsburg and Harris, 1963). These data suggest that Tween and Triton have greater affinity for the hemolytic moiety than do RNA and albumin, and that with respect to the last two, RNA has a greater affinity than albumin. However, it may be presumed that both have a greater affinity for the hemolytic moiety than has the streptococcal component in its original cell-bound form (Ginsburg and Grossowicz,

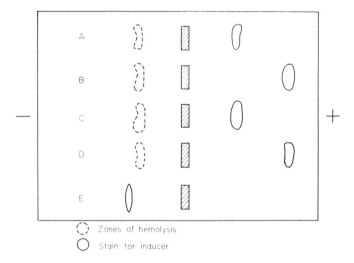

Fig. 5. Effect of detergents on the electrophoresis of hemolysins on agar. Albumin and RNA hemolysin were mixed with Tween 40 (2 mg/ml) or Triton X-205 (2 mg/ml) and subjected to electrophoresis at 40 V/cm for 6 hours. Following the appearance of hemolytic zones, the agar-red blood cell layer was removed and the agar block was stained with amido black (for albumin hemolysin), pyronin (for RNA hemolysin), sudan black (for Tween hemolysin) or bismuth nitrate and potassium iodide (for Triton hemolysin). A = albumin hemolysin + Tween 40, B = RNA hemolysin + Tween 40, C = albumin hemolysin + Triton X-205, D = RNA hemolysin + Triton X-205, E = dextran. From Ginsburg and Harris (1964).

1958; Ginsburg *et al.*, 1965; A. Taketo and Taketo, 1964b). Thus, these molecular species, if present in suspensions of streptococcal cells, become recognized as carriers.

A new light is also shed on the cell-bound hemolysin and its relation to the various forms of hemolysin described. It may be assumed that during the growth of streptococci in media devoid of any of the carriers mentioned above, the hemolysin is synthesized and is found closely associated with the bacterial cell (probably bound to some constituent of its surface in an as yet unknown manner). Upon the addition of red blood cells there is a transfer of hemolytic material from the bacterial cell to the red blood cell (Ginsburg and Harris, 1965). The transfer of significant amounts of this material is inhibited by the same metabolic poisons and antimetabolites that inhibit the induction of hemolysin by the various carriers. Also the interaction between the hemolysin and red blood cell involved an analog carrier which is present in the cell membrane of the red blood cell.

Upon the addition of a substance, which has greater affinity for this hemolysin than that of the streptococcal cell component involved, the hemolysin is released from the cells to form a complex with this substance. The transfer and the continued production of the material to be transferred is energy dependent (see Section VII). As to the chemical nature of the carrier essential for this process, at least four families of compounds may be involved in the induction or binding of hemolysin — (1) lipids, phospholipids, or fatty acids, (2), the polynucleotides of RNA, (3) substituted oxyethylene polymers such as Triton and Tween, and (4) trypan blue. The only common basis for binding of a peptide by the substances of these four classes, which can be suggested at present, is hydrogen binding. Further work should, however, be performed to establish the nature of the carrier hemolysin complexes.

VII. Synthesis of SLS by Streptococci

In the early phase of the research on SLS, it had already become apparent that formation of the hemolysin by streptococci is not dependent on autolysis and that in the absence of an adequate carrier only traces of hemolysin were released following disruption of streptococci by sonic oscillation or by other devices (Bernheimer, 1949; Okamoto, 1962). When it became recognized that quite unrelated materials (carriers) could induce the formation from streptococci of a very similar hemolysin, the question arose whether the carriers and other co-factors participated in the synthesis *de novo* of the hemolysins or only served to extract preformed hemolysin from the cells. Despite the striking similarity in the hemolytic moiety of SLS obtained by the various inducers, the optimal conditions for formation of the different forms of SLS by resting and by growing streptococci vary to some extent. Therefore, the consideration of this problem will be dealt with separately.

A. FORMATION *in Vitro*

1. FORMATION BY GROWING CELLS

Role of Fermentable Sugars. Bernheimer (1949) showed that streptococci grown in semidefined medium yielded only small amounts of RNA hemolysin over most of the logarithmic part of the growth curve as compared with the stationary growth phase. However, Weld (1934) emphasized the importance of employing young cultures for maximal production of serum hemolysin. Ginsburg *et al.* (1963) showed that production of albumin and Tween hemolysin took place during the logarithmic phase of growth with maximal concentration of the hemolysin being attained at the end of this phase. This apparent discrepancy concerning the optimal time of production was later resolved (see below). Bernheimer and Rodbart (1948) also showed that of the numerous mono-, di-, and trisaccharides, hexahydric alcohols, and miscellaneous hexose derivatives tested, only maltose, and to a lesser extent glucosamine, proved effective as energy sources in SLS formation by growing streptococci, provided the medium also contained glucose. As little as $1/64,000 M$ of maltose was effective in SLS production, provided the initial concentration of glucose was $1/360$ M and an excess of RNA core fraction was present. Maximum yield of streptolysin (1500 to 3000 units per milliliter of culture) was obtained when the initial maltose concentration was approximately $1/20,000 M$. Higher concentrations sometimes depressed the hemolysin yield. Maltose was not effective when the medium was deficient in RNA and destruction of maltose by α-glucosidase markedly depressed hemolysin formation (Bernheimer and Rodbart, 1948).

The inability of growing streptococci to utilize glucose for SLS synthesis is puzzling. Since maltose has also been shown to be superior to glucose as the chief energy source in the production of diphtheria toxin (Strom, 1935), the role of maltose in the formation of SLS seems to be specific. Although the streptococci utilized either maltose or glucosamine as a source of energy, Bernheimer and Rodbart (1948) questioned whether they do so in the presence of relatively high concentrations of glucose. The authors raised the possibility that maltose and glucosamine were not oxidized but were used instead as units from which larger molecules were synthesized.

Okamoto (1964) studied the formation of SLS by growing streptococci in broth containing 0.8% RNA core to which 0.01–0.8% glucose were added. He found that maximal SLS titers were obtained in the presence of 0.005% glucose. Higher concentration of glucose markedly depressed hemolysin formation and caused the pH of the cultures to drop below 5.0. Resting streptococci obtained from cultures grown in the presence of 0.8% glucose have almost lost their ability to produce SLS. Such cocci regained their SLS-producing capacity when transferred to plain broth. Since the final pH of cultures grown in the presence of maltose also dropped below 5.0, but the capacity of the cocci to produce high amounts of SLS was not lost, the authors postulated that the inhibitory effect of glucose on SLS formation by growing streptococci might be due to glucose effect in enzyme synthesis, and not to the killing effect of low pH.

2. Formation by Resting Cells

The fact that large amounts of hemolysin could be obtained by resting streptococci simplified the conditions of studies and allowed a better insight into the mechanism of formation of the various forms of hemolysins.

a. Role of Energy Sources and Mg^{2+}. Bernheimer (1949) and Okamoto (1962) showed that in addition to RNA core (AF) or oligonucleotides, an energy source (maltose, glucosamine), K^+, and PO_4^{3-} were essential for maximal hemolysin formation by resting streptococci. Also, glucose, when used in sufficiently large concentrations, served as an energy source for the formation of high yields of SLS.

Weld (1934), Bernheimer (1949), and Ginsburg *et al.* (1963, 1965) have shown that a single batch of streptococci can be used many times for the production of high amounts of SLS provided optimal amounts of RNA core (albumin or Tween), an energy source, Mg^{2+}, and sulfhydryl compounds were present (Ginsburg *et al.*, 1965) (Table IV).

Bernheimer (1949) showed that during the formation of SLS by resting streptococci, 70% of the glucosamine disappeared in 90 minutes and 65% of the amino sugar was converted to lactic acid. There was a direct relationship between hemolysin yield and the quantity of glucosamine fermented. His findings indicate that the cocci were actively metabolizing when SLS appeared in the medium and that this process is energy dependent.

Ginsburg *et al.* (1963) showed that washed streptococci incubated with either glucose, glucosamine, or glucosaminic acid and Mg^{2+} yielded relatively high amounts of RNA hemolysin. However, glucosamine and glucosaminic acid were ineffective in promoting the formation of Tween or albumin hemolysin. No explanation for this phenomenon was given.

Ginsburg and Grossowicz (1958) and Ginsburg *et al.* (1965) studied

TABLE IV

ROLE OF MALTOSE, Mg^{2+}, AND CYSTEINE IN THE PRODUCTION OF
CELL-BOUND HEMOLYSIN AND RNA-INDUCED HEMOLYSIN[a]

Included in incubation mixture			Hemolytic activity	
Maltose	Mg^{2+}	Cysteine	Cell-bound hemolysin (units/ml)	RNA hemolysin[b] (units/ml)
−	−	−	30	0
+	−	−	35	5
−	+	−	40	0
−	−	+	150	150
+	+	−	650	500
+	−	+	1250	2250
−	+	+	2560	650
+	+	+	3000	2500

[a]From Ginsburg et al. (1965).
[b]100 μg/ml of RNA-resistant core added to all tubes. Maltose, cysteine, Mg^{2+} at final concentration as indicated in Table II.

the formation of the cell-bound hemolysin by resting group A streptococci. They found that the demonstration of hemolytic activity by washed streptococci was dependent on the same co-factors which participated in the formation of RNA, albumin, and detergent hemolysin. Very little CBH was obtained in the absence of maltose, Mg^{2+}, or cysteine (see below) or a combination of maltose and Mg^{2+}. Maximal hemolytic activity of CBH was obtained when all three co-factors were present (Table IV). Some differences between CBH and RNA hemolysin formation was, however, found. When streptococci were incubated with Mg^{2+} and cysteine in the absence of maltose, the streptococci yielded 80% of the hemolytic titer obtained by a mixture of maltose, Mg^{2+}, and cysteine, but only 25% RNA hemolysin was obtained compared with the control (Table IV).

It was also shown that glucose could be effectively replaced by other sugars fermented by the strain used or by a mixture of 22 amino acids. However, adenosine triphosphate (ATP) or intermediates of the glycolytic and tricarboxylic acid cycles (glyceraldehyde, phosphoglyceric acid, pyruvate, lactate, acetate, citrate, ketoglutarate, malate, and succinate) were all ineffective (Ginsburg and Grossowicz, 1958).

b. *Role of Sulfhydryl Compounds.* Ginsburg and Grossowicz (1958), Ginsburg and Bentwich (1964), and Ginsburg et al. (1965) studied the kinetics of the formation of the albumin, serum, and RNA hemolysins by resting streptococci. They showed that cysteine, thioglycolic acid, glutathione, and thiomalic acid markedly increased up to fivefold the yield of all hemolysins in the presence of optimal concentrations of glucose and Mg^{2+}. Maximal hemolytic activity in the presence of cysteine was attained after 20 minutes at 37°C. In the absence of sulfhydryl compounds, 50–60 minutes were needed to reach maximal value which were much lower than those attained in the presence of sulfhydryl compounds. The total yield of hemolysin was dependent on the absolute concentration of cysteine in the system, the optimal concentration of cysteine being 0.001 M in the case of albumin, RNA, or CBH. Similar results were obtained with glutathione but not with ascorbic acid. The role of cysteine in the formation of the hemolysin is not clear, but it probably acts as a donor of sulfhydryl groups essential for still unknown processes rather than as a reducing agent.

c. *Effect of Temperature on Formation.* Bernheimer (1949) studied the effect of temperature on the formation of RNA hemolysin by resting streptococci (strain C203S type 3). He showed that no hemolysin was produced below 15° or above 40°C. Between 20° and 37°C, SLS formation proceeded without lag and was linear for the first 30–50 minutes. Calculation of the Arrhenius constant using the linear rate of formation of SLS at 21.8 and 29.9°C yielded in two successive experiments, values of 37,000 and 34,500 calories per mole, respectively. Further studies (Ginsburg *et al.*, 1963) have shown that when RNA, albumin, or Tween were added to resting streptococci preincubated at 37°C for 10 minutes and then chilled to 10°C, no trace of hemolysin was produced. However, continued incubation at 37°C with the carrier molecules and other diffusible components caused the production of large amounts of hemolysin. From these experiments it is apparent that the hemolysin which appears in incubation of streptococci with Tween, albumin, or RNA is not simply extracted from the organisms but is probably synthesized by the streptococci under the conditions of such incubation.

d. *Effect of Metabolic Poisons on Formation.* Further evidence of the dependence of SLS production on cellular metabolism was shown in experiments with enzyme poisons (Bernheimer, 1949; Hayano, 1952; Ginsburg and Grossowicz, 1958). Table V shows that all ten substances employed inhibited RNA hemolysin formation by resting streptococci. The most potent inhibitors were mecuric chloride (3×10^{-6} M), arsenite (3×10^{-5} M), iodoacetic acid (4×10^{-5} M), and dinitrophenol (5×10^{-5} M). It is notable that the first three are sulfhydryl poisons. The inhibition by iodoacetate (10^{-3} M) could not be reversed by 5×10^{-2} M cysteine (Ginsburg and Grossowicz, 1958). Since SLS formation occurs anaerobically (Bernheimer, 1949), and since SLS formation was also found to be prevented by inhibitors of the aerobic metabolism — namely, malonate, cyanide, and azide — it appears that these substances affect metabolic processes in addition to those involved in respiration. None of the enzyme poisons studied (Table V), at the concentrations indicated, were found to inhibit hemolysis of red blood cells by SLS.

e. Effect of Antibiotics. The formation of RNA, albumin, Tween, and the cell-bound hemolysins have been shown to be strongly inhibited by chlormaphenicol (10^{-5} M), tetracyclines (10^{-6}-10^{-8} M), streptomycin (10^{-3} M), and sulfathiazol (10^{-3} M) (Hayano, 1952; Younathan and Barkulis, 1957; Ginsburg and Grossowicz, 1958; Ginsburg *et al.*, 1965). However, penicillin G, although a potent bacteriostatic agent for growing streptococci, was completely inert up to a concentration of 10^{-3} M (Younathan and Barkulis, 1957; Ginsburg and Grossowicz, 1958). The ratio of the concentration of antibiotics required for growth inhibition to the concentration required for 50% inhibition of SLS formation was less than 4×10^{-6} in the case of penicillin, 1.6×10^{-2} in the case of streptomycin, 1.25 in the case of chloramphenicol, and 500 in the case of the tetracyclines (Hayano, 1952).

Tetracylines have great avidity for several cations (Albert, 1953). It was shown, however, that preincubation of aureomycin ($1 \times 10^{-6} M$) with Mg^{2+}, Fe^{2+}, Mn^{3+}, or sodium molybdate ($5 \times 10^{-5} M$) did not reverse its inhibitory effect; Cu^{2+} at $5 \times 10^{-5} M$ was found to cause almost complete inhibition of the production of SLS (Younathan and Barkulis, 1957).

The inhibitory activity of aureomycin was reversed by cysteine. No such effect of cysteine was obtained with terramycin (Hayano, 1952). However, Ginsburg and Bentwich (1964) could not reverse the inhibitory effect of aureomycin on SLS formation by cysteine.

TABLE V

EFFECT OF ENZYME POISONS ON FORMATION OF
STREPTOLYSIN S[a]

Enzyme poison	Molar concentration producing approximately 50% inhibition of streptolysin S formation
Sodium malonate	3×10^{-2}
Potassium cyanide	2×10^{-2}
Sodium fluoride	1.5×10^{-2}
Sodium azide	5×10^{-3}
Sodium arsenate	2×10^{-3}
Sodium selenite	5×10^{-4}
Dinitrophenol	5×10^{-5}
Sodium iodoacetate	4×10^{-5}
Sodium arsenite	3×10^{-5}
Mercuric chloride	3×10^{-6}

[a]From Bernheimer (1949).

f. Effect of Antimetabolites and Amino Acid Analogs. Younathan and Barkulis (1957), Ginsburg (1958), and Ginsburg and Grossowicz (1958) found that formation of RNA, albumin, and Tween hemolysin by resting streptococci was inhibited by β-phenylserine (10^{-3} M) and by β-3-DL-thienylalanine (10^{-2} M) in a system which contained maltose and Mg^{2+}. The effect of the analogs was completely reversed by equimolar concentrations of DL-phenylalanine.

Inhibition of SLS formation by phenylserine was not effective in the presence of sulfhydryl compounds (Ginsburg and Bentwich, 1964). As little as 0.005 M of cysteine completely reversed the inhibition caused by 0.1 M phenylserine. Both thioglycolic and thiomalic acids showed a similar effect, while ascorbic acid failed to affect the inhibition caused by phenylserine. These results explain the failure of phenylserine to inhibit the formation of SLS in the presence of cysteine. Phenylglycine and acetylproline strongly inhibited hemolysin formation. However, inhibition was also reversed by cysteine and other sulfhydryl compounds. This phenomenon of the reversal by sulfhydryl compounds of inhibition of SLS formation by phenylserine is not understood. Attempts to reverse the inhibition by phenylalanine, glycine, or proline failed. Moreover, as little as 0.002 M of these amino acids markedly inhibited hemolysin formation.

Younathan and Barkulis (1957) showed that DL-ethionine (2.5×10^{-2} M) and 5-methyl-DL-tryptophan (2.5×10^{-2} M) caused appreciable inhibition of RNA-hemolysin formation. The inhibition could not, however, be reversed by an equimolar concentration of the corresponding natural amino acid. The following amino acid analogs at 1×10^{-3} M were inactive in suppressing SLS formation: DL-ethionine; 5-methyl-DL-tryptophan, ω-trifluoro-DL-threonine, DL-proparglycine, *cis*-ω-chloro-DL-allylglycine, and γ-chloro-DL-allylglycine.

Although these results clearly suggest that the various analogs compete with the natural amino acid for metabolic processes leading to hemolysin formation, the exact mechanism of inhibition is still poorly understood.

g. Effect of Purine and Pyrimidine Analogs. Younathan and Barkulis (1957) and Ginsburg and Grossowicz (1958) showed that benzimidazole, a purine antagonist (Woolley, 1944) at a concentration of 10^{-2} M caused 85% inhibition of RNA and Tween hemolysin formation. However, the addition of an equimolar concentration of adenine or guanine failed to restore SLS production. Ginsburg (1958) showed that formation of CBH by resting streptococci was markedly inhibited by 2,6-diaminopurine sulfate, 5-methylthiouracil, diazouracil, and 8-chloroxanthine. No inhibition occurred with 2,4,6-triaminopyrimidine, 6-mercaptopurine, azaguanine, uracil, or guanine.

h. Effect of Derivatives of Dihydroxyazobenzene. R. Ito *et al.* (1948b) and Himeno (1955) showed that a number of structural relatives of the dihydroxyazobene series inhibited production of RNA hemolysin by resting cells. 6-(2'-hydroxy-3,5'-dinitrophenylazo)-4-hexylresorcinol and 6-(2'-hydroxy-3',5'-dichlorophenylazo)-4-ethylresorcinol are very potent inhibitors of the production of SLS. These two azo compounds were as potent inhibitors as 2,2'-dihydroxy-3,3',5,5'-tetrabromoazobenzene, studied by R. Ito *et al.* (1948b). However, no inhibition of SLS formation occurred with urethane, nitrogen mustard, nitromin, 3-hydroxyanthranilic acid, colchicine, nicotinic acid amide, *p*-aminobenzoic acid, L-methionine, or thiochrome.

i. Effect of Ultraviolet Irradiation. Washed streptococci irradiated with UV light for 1-10 minutes lost their capacity to form RNA, Tween, or cell-bound hemolysin (Ginsburg and Grossowicz, 1958; Ginsburg *et al.*, 1965). However, the rate of inactivation was much higher in the case of RNA hemolysin compared with Tween hemolysin or CBH. It is of interest that prolonged irradiation of the preformed hemolysins did not affect their hemolytic activities.

3. FORMATION BY PROTOPLASTS

Maruyama *et al.* (1959, 1960), Sugai and Egami (1960), and Maruyama and Sugai (1960) studied the production of SLS by streptococcal protoplasts, by subcellular fractions, and by "ghosts" derived from these organisms. The protoplasts were prepared by treating washed group A streptococci with bacteriophage lysates of group C streptococci. The optimal system for hemolysin production contained sodium succinate (0.5 M), magnesium sulfate (0.002 M), maltose (0.005 M), and an oligonucleotide fraction of the RNA core (200 μg/ml). The rate of hemolysin formation by the protoplasts was greater than that of intact streptococci. Succinate, which was required for the SLS formation by ghosts, inhibited SLS formation by intact streptococci. As in the case of intact streptococci (Ginsburg and Bentwich, 1964), sulfhydryl compounds were also found to enhance the formation of hemolysin by ghosts (Sugai and Egami, 1960).

Streptococcal ghosts obtained by lysing protoplasts in hypotonic media were shown to form streptolysin S if succinate was present in the incubation medium. Sulfhydryl compounds (thioglycolic acid, cysteine, or glutathione) stimulated streptolysin formation by ghosts. As in the case of intact streptococci, chloramphenicol (10^{-5} M) and β-DL-phenylserine (10^{-3} M) inhibited streptolysin formation by ghosts. Inhibition by the latter was reversed by phenylalanine (10^{-3} M).

Acid hydrolyzed casein or a mixture of 17 purified amino acids enhanced streptolysin formation by ghosts and by intact streptococci. On one hand, a very marked reduction of hemolysin production by ghosts was obtained, however, when proline and histidine were omitted from a mixture of 17 amino acids. On the other hand, omitting these two amino acids from a mixture of 17 amino acids markedly enhanced the production of SLS by intact streptococci.

4. Formation by Protoplast Membranes

More recently, Sokawa and Egami (1965) showed the release of a hemolytic component with properties similar to streptolysin S from a crude preparation of protoplast membrane fraction. The membranes were obtained from streptococci following treatment with group C phage lysin by a modified method described by Markowitz and Dorfman (1962). No data are given on the purity of such membranes and the degree of contamination with intact streptococci or with cell wall components. The reaction mixture was comprised of protoplast membrane fractions to which either oligonucleotide or Tween 40, sodium succinate, ATP, and Mg^{2+} were added. It was found that the release of hemolysin from these structures was not inhibited by chloramphenicol, puromycin, or streptomycin.

For the release of hemolytic components from the membrane fraction, ATP could be replaced by GTP, UTP, CTP, ADP, and by a mixture of creatine phosphate and creatine kinase. The fact that creatine phosphate was effective only in the presence of creatine kinase indicated that catalytic amounts of ADP were present in the membrane system. However, neither GDP, UDP, CDP, nor a mixture of four nucleoside monophosphates were effective. It is also of interest that glucose and maltose, which were required for the formation of SLS by resting streptococci, were not effective with the membrane fractions.

The release of the hemolytic component by ATP and Mg^{2+} was suppressed by trypsin, but not by pancreatic RNAses, RNAse T_1, RNAse T_2, chloramphenicol, puromycin, actinomycin D, sodium fluoride, PCMB, or DNP. Rabbit RBC were lysed directly by membranes in the presence of ATP and Mg^{2+} in the absence of oligonucleotide or Tween 40 and no free hemolysin was detected in supernatant fluids obtained from membrane suspensions (see also Ginsburg and Harris, 1965). Membranes derived from intact streptococci preincubated with chloramphenicol, puromycin, or streptomycin yielded much less hemolysin compared with controls.

5. Formation by Cell-Free System

A. Taketo and Taketo (1964a) studied the synthesis of SLS in a cell-free system. The streptococci were either ground from the frozen state with quartz or subjected to sonification with a 20 kc sonic disintegrator.

A crude extract obtained following centrifugation at 30,000 g was further centrifuged at 105,000 g and the supernatant fluid derived was precipitated with 60% saturated ammonium sulfate. When the crude extracts were incubated with RNA core in the presence of potassium chloride, Mg^{2+}, ATP, GTP, glutathione, maltose, and amino acids, the increase of hemolytic activity depended on the addition of oligonucleotides. The reaction was temperature dependent and maximal hemolytic activity was attained within 20 to 40 minutes. Further studies showed that an increase of hemolytic activity also occurred without the addition of ATP, GTP, reduced glutathione or amino acids mixtures. Chloramphenicol and 5-methyltryptophan, potassium cyanide, dinitrophenol, arsenite, and arsentate, which are inhibitors of the synthesis of high energy phosphate compounds, did not show significant inhibition. However, the increase of hemolytic activity was considerably reduced by EDTA. Also ultraviolet irradiation previously shown to inhibit RNA-hemolysin formation by intact streptococci (Ginsburg and Grossowicz, 1958) did not affect the increase of hemolytic activity by the cell-free polynucleotide-dependent reaction. The removal of the nucleic acid moiety from the crude extract by ultracentrifugation and streptomycin precipitation did not destroy the oligonucleotide-dependent increase in the hemolytic activity. These results further support the evidence for the synthesis of the hemolysin. The new hemolysin formed in the cell-free system was oxygen stable and unaffected by antistreptolysin O but was inhibited by trypan blue.

Ribonucleotide found associated with the hemolysin showed properties similar to that produced by intact cells. The cell-free reaction was insensitive to various agents known to inhibit protein synthesis. The increment of hemolytic activity was proportional to the amount of preformed intracellular hemolysin, and the inactivation of this hemolysin always resulted in loss of formation of RNA SLS. These data further support the hypothesis put forward by Ginsburg and Harris (1963) that RNA hemolysin is formed in the streptococci by transferring a hemolytic moiety, probably identical with the intracellular streptolysin or CBH, from a certain cellular carrier to oligonucleotide or other carrier moieties. This transfer may involve the release of the hemolytic moiety from certain masking substances associated with the cellular carrier with the simultaneous increase of hemolytic activity.

6. SYNTHESIS DE NOVO VERSUS EXTRACTION OF PREFORMED HEMOLYSIN

In any consideration of the mode of production of SLS by group A streptococci, it must be stressed that no appreciable amounts of pre-

formed hemolysin are found either inside or upon the streptococcal cells
(Bernheimer, 1949; Younathan and Barkulis, 1957; Ginsburg and Grossowicz, 1958), and that although these organisms cannot synthesize the
15 amino acids essential for growth (Slade et al., 1951; Ginsburg and
Grossowicz, 1957), no exogenous amino acid source except cysteine is
required for SLS formation by resting cells (Ginsburg and Bentwich,
1964). Since cysteine can be replaced by thioglycolic acid or by thiomalic
acid, cysteine probably acts as a donor of sulfhydryl groups rather than as
an essential amino acid (Ginsburg and Bentwich, 1964). To explain the
dispensability of amino acids in this reaction, it must be kept in mind that
streptococci, like other gram-positive organisms, possess a large intracellular pool of amino acids (Gale, 1951). Analysis of the endogenous pool
during SLS formation revealed that approximately half of the pool was
utilized during the incubation of resting streptococci in amino acid-free
medium for 2 hours whether or not oligonucleotide was present (Younathan and Barkulis, 1957). Thus, while the oligonucleotide caused a phe-
nomenal enhancement of the hemolysin production it did not bring about
an appreciable change in the overall rate of utilization of endogenous
amino acids. Streptococci starved for 2 hours in the absence of oligonucleotides produced 75% less hemolysin when transferred to oligonucleo-
tide-containing medium. This drop does not seem to be due solely to the
exhaustion of the intracellular amino acid supply, since the addition of a
mixture of 19 amino acids did not restore SLS formation (Younathan and
Barkulis, 1957; Ginsburg, 1958). However, a mixture of 17 amino acids
(Gly L-Pro, L-Glu, DL-Met, L-Lys, L-Leuc, DL-Val, DL-Ala, DL-Thz,
S-Scr, L-Tyz, L-His, L-Asp, L-Phe, L-Arg, DL-Try, and Cys) (Sugai,
1961) or 22 amino acids (the 17 mentioned plus L-Arg, Glyc, L-Val;
DL-Iso, L-Glu, DL-Asp, Ginsburg and Grossowicz, 1958) either replaced glucose as an energy source or enhanced hemolysin formation by
intact streptococci incubated with glucose (or maltose) and RNA. Also,
the balance among various amino acids was found to be important for
securing optimal formation of RNA hemolysin. It was thus shown that
omitting proline or histidine from a mixture of 17 amino acids caused a
four- to sixfold increase in hemolysin formation (Sugai, 1961). Also
phenylalanine, glycine and proline were found to inhibit SLS formation
when added to resting streptococci incubated with oligonucleotide, Mg^{2+},
and cysteine (Ginsburg and Bentwich, 1964). However, both glutamic
acid and serine shown by Koyama and Egami (1963) to be the major
components of the hemolytic moiety of SLS (Table III) markedly enhanced RNA hemolysin formation (Ginsburg and Bentwich, 1964).
Since there is evidence that net protein formation is accompanied by a
concomitant active nucleic acid synthesis and since nucleic acids and
some of their precursors were found to stimulate enzyme formation (Gale

and Folks, 1955; Gale, 1956), the effect of purines and pyrimidines on the SLS formation was examined (Younathan and Barkulis, 1957). It was found that a mixture containing equimolar amounts of uracil, thymine, cytosine, adenine sulfate, guanine HCl, xanthine, and hypoxanthine failed to enhance the formation of hemolysin in the absence or presence of oligonucleotide.

All the data presented (Bernheimer and Rodbardt, 1948; Bernheimer, 1949; Hayano, 1952; Younathan and Barkulis, 1957; Ginsburg, 1958; Ginsburg and Grossowicz, 1958; Sugai, 1961; Ginsburg et al., 1963, 1965; Ginsburg and Bentwich, 1964) leave very little doubt that the appearance of hemolysin in the suspension medium of resting streptococci depends upon an active metabolic process rather than on a physical extraction of a preformed intracellular hemolysin.

B. FORMATION in Vivo

The nonimmunogenicity of any of the forms of SLS has hampered any efforts to establish whether or not streptococci produce SLS in vivo. No detectable intravascular hemolysis accompanies streptococcal infections in humans, and no jaundice has been reported to develop following such infections. Also, no circulating SLS can be found in sera of patients suffering from streptococcal infections (Ginsburg, unpublished observations).

The fact, however, that serum is a potent inducer of SLS formation makes it highly probable that SLS is produced in inflammatory sites (e.g., tonsils) but because of its high affinity for cell membranes it is readily inactivated. Also, the inhibition of SLS activity by phospholipids and serum β-lipoprotein probably causes the immediate inactivation of any SLS formed.

Recently it has been reported (Snyder, 1960) that SLS could be isolated from kidneys and spleens of rabbits infected with group A streptococci. The hemolytic activity found in these organs 4 days following infection was neutralized by lecithin. No hemolysin was detected in the heart, liver, lungs, lymph nodes, brain, or skin. These results must, however, be regarded with some caution since the only evidence that the hemolysin is streptolysin S was its inhibition by lecithin, which is by no means a specific inhibitor of SLS. It is possible that other materials found in crushed organs are responsible for the hemolysis observed. If, however, the presence of SLS in active form in the circulation or in internal organs is confirmed, it would be of great importance, since it might thus reach other vital organs such as the heart via the circulation and cause cellular damage before it is either bound to red blood cells or leukocytes or neutralized by serum lipoproteins.

VIII. Inhibition of SLS Activity

Streptolysin S can be inactivated by agents which can destroy either the carrier molecule or the hemolytic moiety (peptide). Investigations concerning the inhibitors which affect the carrier molecule (e.g., *Aspergillus* RNAse; extreme pH values) has been fully described in Sections VI and IX. Of the inhibitors that affect the hemolytic moiety, diverse agents such as β-lipoproteins, aniline dyes, proteases, and inhibitors from higher fungi have been described.

A. ROLE OF PHOSPHOLIPIDS

The capacity of human sera to inhibit SLS was first studied extensively by Todd *et al.* (1939). The chemical basis for such an inhibition was found to be complex. Since ovolecithin was known to be a potent inhibitor, it would seem reasonable that serum lecithin alone could account for inhibition. However, it has been repeatedly observed, that lecithin loses its inhibitory power when diluted in serum, and the mere addition of ether to serum, without removal of serum components, results in a marked loss of inhibitory power (Humphrey, 1949b; Stollerman *et al.*, 1950).

Prolonged treatment with pepsin (Humphrey, 1949b) or trypsin (Stollerman *et al.*, 1950), long storage of serum at 4°C, heating serum to a temperature just below the coagulation point, and fractionation of serum with ammonium sulfate all markedly increased the inhibitory power of serum (Stollerman *et al.*, 1950). However, a major reduction of its inhibitory ability occurred when serum was treated with phospholipase C of *Clostridium welchii* (Stollerman *et al.*, 1950) or if extracted in the cold with an ether and alcohol mixture (Stollerman *et al.*, 1950; Humphrey, 1949a). The foregoing results, together with observations on serum fractions obtained by fractionation with cold methanol (e.g., Cohns fractions III and III-0) (Ginsburg *et al.*, 1963), show that the inhibition of streptolysin is not due to a specific antibody but to the normal components of serum. The serum components responsible for inhibition appear to be labile lipoprotein complexes (Stollerman *et al.*, 1950; Humphrey, 1949b; Ginsburg *et al.*, 1963).

Sera of patients having diseases associated with hyper- and hypolipemic states (Stollerman *et al.*, 1952) show a degree of inhibition which was related to the total phospholipid content of the sera. It was also demonstrated that a significant increase in inhibitory capacity of serum occurred when hyperphospholipemia was induced in rabbits by repeated intravenous injection of a neutral detergent, by ligation of the common bile duct, or by feeding cholesterol. The inhibitory capacity of sera having a very high cholesterol content was no greater than that of sera containing less cholesterol and the same amount of phospholipids. Since neither cholesterol nor neutral fat inhibits streptolysin S, it appears that phospholipids in the form of lipoprotein complexes plays a major role in streptolysin S inhibition.

Further studies (Elias *et al.*, 1966) have shown that SLS activity was inhibited by purified phospholipids (phosphatidylcholine, phosphatidylethanolamine, phosphatidylserine, phosphatidylinositol, phasphatidic acid, lysolecithin), by diglycerides derived from lecithin, by phospholipase C activity, and by sphingomyelin. It has also been shown that finely dispersed cholesterol which was subjected to sonic oscillation inhibited SLS activity. These results do not, however, agree with the findings of Humphrey (1949b) and Stollerman *et al.* (1952). This discrepancy cannot be explained at present unless we assume that the degree of dispersion of cholesterol is an important factor in the inhibition of SLS (Table VI).

The inhibitory power of sera taken from patients during the acute phase of rheumatic fever tended to be lower than that of sera from the same patients during periods of rheumatic inactivity. Humphrey (1949a) also found the inhibitory action of sera of patients having acute rheumatic fever to be lower than normal, but he also found decreased antistreptolysin S levels in streptococcal pharyngitis, scarlet fever, and rheumatoid arthritis. Stollerman and Bernheimer (1950) observed the antistreptolysin S titer to be lower than normal in 80% of patients having rheumatic activity, but to be normal in a series of patients having acute streptococcal pharyngitis. Abnormally low titers were occasionally observed in the sera of patients with other diseases, and it would appear that decrease in antistreptolysin S, although a common manifestation in rheumatic fever, is not specifically associated with this disease.

B. ROLE OF ANILINE DYES

R. Ito (1940a) has made an extensive study of the capacity of various dyes to inhibit SLS. The most potent *in vitro* inhibitors were trypan blue, dianyl blue, benzol blue, and Congo red. Trypan blue showed detectable inhibition of hemolysis in concentrations as low as 1:50,000,000 to 1:100,000,000.

Miyaji (1953) showed that the inhibition of RNA hemolysin activity by trypan blue could be reversed by dissociating the trypan blue following filtration through thick filter paper or through activated charcoal. Under such conditions, SLS activity could be totally regained. It was suggested that inhibition of SLS hemolysis by trypan blue or Congo red is neither

TABLE VI

EFFECT OF PURIFIED LIPIDS AND ISOLATED LIPID CONSTITUENTS OF RED BLOOD
CELL GHOSTS ON SLS ACTIVITY[a]

Compound tested	Concentration[b] (mg/ml)	Inhibition of SLS activity[c] (%)
Phosphatidylcholine	1.05	70
Phosphatidylcholine	4.00	100
Diglyceride (natural) (1:2)	4.00	65
Diglyceride (synthetic) (mainly 1:2)	4.00	65
Phosphatidylethanolamine	0.85	100
Phosphatidylserine	0.53	80
Phosphatidylinositol	0.14	75
Sphingomyelin (beef brain)	0.77	20
Cholesterol (synthetic)	1.37	70
Cerebroside (beef brain)	0.30	0
Ganglioside (beef brain)	0.50	0
Lysolecithin (egg lecithin)	0.09	90
Phosphatidic acid (egg lecithin)	0.09	90
Sialic acid	0.06	0
	(μmoles/ml)	
O-Phosphorylcholine	0.30	0
O-Phosphorylethanolamine	0.13	0
O-Phosphorylserine	0.17	0
Glycerophosphorylcholine	0.40	0
α-Glycerophosphate	0.19	0
Ethanolamine	0.06	0
Choline	0.12	0
Inositol	0.18	0
Serine	0.10	0
Sialic acid	0.30	0

[a]From Elias et al. (1966).

[b]Concentration of the various compounds given in mg/ml or μmoles are approximately equivalent to those found in 1 ml of packed red cells.

[c]2250 units/ml of SLS were incubated for 30 minutes at 37°C with the various compounds and the residual hemolytic activity was determined as described in the methods.

due to direct chemical reaction between SLS and the dye nor due to destruction of SLS in presence of dye. The author also emphasizes that the phenomenon of inhibition of SLS by this dye is due to competition for red blood cells.

Ginsburg et al. (1965) and Ginsburg and Harris (1965) showed that trypan blue inhibited the hemolytic activity of RNA, albumin, and Tween hemolysin as well as the transfer of hemolysin from washed streptococci (CBH) to red blood cells. However, trypan blue failed to affect hemolysis of red blood cells which have interacted with any of the hemolytic forms of SLS.

The inhibition of SLS was found to be dependent upon concentration of dye employed. When the hemolysin was incubated with 25 μg/ml of dye and then diluted serially, it was found that up to a dilution of 1:160 no trace of hemolysis occurred. Partial hemolysis, however, was found at dilution of 1:320 and 1:640, suggesting the dissociation of the SLS from trypan blue. Since it was shown that the hemolytic moiety of SLS can be transferred from one carrier to another (Ginsburg and Harris, 1963), it was suspected that trypan blue, although an inhibitor of SLS, can at low concentrations serve as a carrier of the hemolytic moiety. This assumption was fully established by showing that trypan blue (1–20 μg/ml) yielded a soluble hemolysin from washed streptococci incubated with glucose, Mg^{2+}, and cysteine. The hemolytic activity which was associated with trypan blue (trypan blue hemolysin) was inhibited by lecithin, papain and by excess of trypan blue (>30 μg/ml). Under similar conditions lecithin failed to induce extracellular hemolytic activity from washed streptococci.

C. ROLE OF PROTEOLYTIC ENZYMES

The hemolytic activity of RNA hemolysin is inactivated by chymotrypsin, papain, ficin, and cathepsin. The inhibition by the latter three enzymes depended on the presence of cysteine (Bernheimer, 1949). No inactivation of SLS occurred with trypsin, pepsin, lysozyme, hyaluronidase, lipase, or muramidase (Bernheimer, 1949; A. Taketo and Taketo, 1964a). Later on it was shown that similar patterns of inhibition occurred with cell-bound hemolysin as well as with albumin and detergent hemolysins (Ginsburg et al., 1965). Ishikura (1962) and Koyama and Egami (1963) demonstrated that in addition to the sulfhydryl-dependent proteases, both pronase (Streptomyces griseus proteinase) and nagarse (Bacillus subtilis proteinase) inactivated RNA hemolysin.

D. ROLE OF FUNGAL EXTRACTS

Bernheimer (1949) studied the inhibition of SLS by materials extracted from higher fungi (Basidiomycetes) and found that extracts of Lepiota procera and Clitocybe candicans inhibited SLS activity, but no data on the active principles in the extract were given.

E. ROLE OF OTHER FACTORS

Koyama and Egami (1963) showed that treatment of RNA hemolysin with phenol resulted in loss of hemolytic activity. Such treatment removed most of the polypeptide moiety from the oligonucleotide carrier.

The RNA hemolysin is inactivated by 8 M urea, but not by 6 M guanidine or 8 M sodium chloride (Koyama and Egami, 1963).

IX. The Purification of SLS

As has been stressed above, SLS of group A streptococci may exist as a complex between nonspecific carrier molecules (albumin, β-lipoprotein, detergents, RNA) and a specific hemolytic moiety, a peptide containing 12 amino acids. Most of the efforts to purify SLS were directed toward the isolation and characterization of the carrier molecules rather than toward the isolation of the hemolytic moiety.

Herbert and Todd (1944) were the first to describe a partial purification of the serum hemolysin. The most purified hemolysin preparation obtained by precipitation with carbon dioxide and saturation with ammonium sulfate was very opalescent, although no precipitate was obtained on centrifugation at 16,000 rpm for 3 hours. The preparation contained 12.1% nitrogen, 9.4% phosphorus, and 0.1% carbohydrates as glucose. The material gave a strong biuret reaction and had a lipid content of 20% as judged by extraction with alcohol-ether. The serum SLS could be completely destroyed by shaking with ethanol-ether (3:1), or with ethyl acetate. Also, serum thus treated failed to extract hemolysin from streptococci. The low nitrogen and high phosphorus content suggested that the serum hemolysin was associated with lipoprotein. Bernheimer (1954) however questioned this point on the basis of the relatively low specific activity of their purified preparations (52 units/mg). The most purified preparations of albumin hemolysin obtained yielded approximately 500-750 HU/mg albumin (Ginsburg, unpublished data). The hemolysin contained high amounts of lipid material.

The first report on the partial purification of RNA hemolysin was given by Bernheimer (1949). Employing resting streptococci (strain C203S) to which RNA-resistant core, and Mg^{2+} were added, he obtained a potent hemolytic product which, following lyophilization, yielded 30,000 HU/mg dry weight. This preparation although free of streptokinase, hyaluronidase, and proteinase was contaminated with appreciable amounts of a substance with deoxyribonuclease activity.

Cinader and Pillemer (1950) achieved considerable purification of RNA hemolysin by fractionation of crude streptococcal filtrate with methanol under controlled conditions of pH, ionic strength, and temperature. The best preparations of hemolysin were obtained by an initial precipitation with 25% methanol at 0°C followed by a second precipitation which occurred in the absence of methanol when the pH of the crude hemolysin was brought to 1.6 and the ionic strength adjusted to 0.165. This preparation contained 354,000 HU/mg nitrogen. Electrophoretically the material was separated into 2 peaks; the fast migrating component was found to contain SLS activity. With the development of ion-exchange chromatography, it was shown (Ishikura, 1961, 1962) that RNA hemolysin produced by group A streptococci strain S could be isolated in high yield following stepwise salt fractionation on Ecteola-cellulose. RNA core, digested with RNase T₁ was chromatographed on Ecteola-cellulose, and fractions eluted with salt concentrations higher than 0.3 M were used to produce hemolysin from resting streptococci.

The highest activity of hemolysis was eluted from the column at 0.75 M sodium chloride. The material was then subjected to gel filtration on Sephadex G-75 columns and the hemolysin was further purified by zone electrophoresis on starch. This method yielded 40,000 HU per optical density unit at 260 mμ. Koyama and Egami (1963) have purified RNA hemolysin by successive application of zone electrophoresis on starch and DEAE-cellulose column chromatography and obtained preparations containing 100,000 HU per optical density unit at 260 mμ, calculated to possess approximately 2,000,000 HU/mg dry weight. Y. Taketo (1963) employed methylated serum albumin-coated Kieselgur columns to purify RNA hemolysin. The RNA hemolysin applied to the column at 0.05 M phosphate was then eluted at 0.4–0.6 M sodium chloride.

Ginsburg and Bentwich (1964), employing strain S84 of group A streptococci, obtained high yields of purified SLS following chromatography of RNA hemolysin on DEAE-Sephadex. The starting material contained 10,000–30,000 HU/ml. Fractions eluted at 0.75 M potassium chloride were rechromatographed and the eluates were further concentrated by precipitation with 8 volumes of methanol at −20°C. Preparations containing 250,000 units/ml were obtained by this method. No data on the attempted isolation and purification of the hemolytic peptide are available.

X. Stability of SLS

A. EFFECT OF TEMPERATURE

Serum, albumin, detergent, and RNA hemolysins are very unstable in aqueous solutions and lose most of their activity on standing at 25°C for a few hours. However, SLS is much more stable in the dry state. Bernheimer (1950) found that potassium chloride at 0.5 M, potassium phosphate at 0.2 M, and ammonium chloride at 1 M prevented the inactivation of SLS heated to 50°C for 30 minutes. As little as 1/2000 M potassium afforded partial protection. However, lithium and calcium ions failed to protect while magnesium and barium ions gave partial protection. It was also found that in the absence of potassium over 90% inactivation of SLS occurred over a wide pH range. In the presence of potassium little or no in-activation occurred in solution over the range of pH of 3.0–9.0. Purified RNA hemolysin formed a soluble complex with silver salts (Shimitzu, 1956; Shoin, 1954; T. Ito, 1955). Such complexes did not lose their he-molytic power even after heating at 100°C for several hours. The hemo-lytic activity could be generated with vitamin C without appreciable loss in activity. Hydrogen sulfide was much less effective.

It was also reported that completely heat-inactivated SLS could be par-tially reactivated with absolute alcohol (Okamoto, 1962; Sugiyama, 1956). The mechanism of protection of SLS by cations is not under-stood.

B. EFFECT OF pH

The susceptibility of SLS to pH varies with the different forms of the hemolysins. Thus, it was shown (Ginsburg and Harris, 1963) that incu-bating the RNA hemolysin at pH 11.0 for 30 minutes results in its com-plete inactivation, while the albumin hemolysin was very stable at this pH. Similarly, albumin hemolysin was readily inactivated at pH 2 but was very stable at pH 11.0. Under similar experimental conditions, Tween or Triton hemolysins were not affected by such extreme pH values.

It was also shown that when the hemolytic moiety associated with the albumin hemolysin was transferred to RNA, the newly formed complex showed a pH susceptibility characteristic for the RNA hemolysin.

Since it is known that the albumin molecule is modified at pH 2 (Foster, 1960) and RNA is destroyed at pH 11, while Tween or Triton are stable at a wide range of pH values, it is reasonable to assume that the stability of the various forms of hemolysins depends solely on the stability of the car-rier molecules. No data on the optimal stability of the hemolytic moiety (the peptide) to temperature or pH values are available.

XI. The Role of SLS in the Virulence of Group A Streptococci

Stevens et al. (1921) reviewed the early literature on the relationship between the virulence of streptococci and their capacity to produce SLS. Although he believed that there was an intimate connection between hemolysin production and virulence, he considered that the data available were not sufficient to come to a conclusion on this matter. Stevens et al. (1921) showed that streptococcal strains whose virulence has been in-creased for any one species of animal did not produce greater concentra-tions of hemolysin than the original strain. More recently Stollerman and Bernheimer (1950) have shown that there was no difference in SLS production by strains of group A streptococci isolated from patients with streptococcal pharyngitis or with rheumatic fever. Leedom and Barkulis (1959) showed that the enhanced virulence of streptococci after mouse passage was associated with decreased SLS production. Snyder and Hamilton (1961) showed that group A streptococci produce more SLS than did streptococci group C or G and that the passage of streptococci in mice enhanced the production of SLS but did not enhance their virulence. The significance of SLS production by group A, C, or G streptococci is not understood. It has been suggested, however, that since group A streptococci produce larger amounts of hemolysin than do streptococci group C or G, this hemolysin may have a significant role in human infections (Snyder and Hamilton, 1961).

XII. Toxicity of SLS

Only a few reports in the literature deal with the toxic manifestation of different forms of SLS in laboratory animals. Although the toxicity of the hemolysins parallels the development of tissue alterations, the description of the two manifestations will be presented separately.

A. TOXICITY TO MICE

Weld (1934, 1935), Hare (1937), and Barnard and Todd (1940) studied the toxic effects of the serum-extracted hemolysin in the mouse following intervenous injections. The appearance of toxic manifestations depended on the amount of hemolysin injected. An injection of 15–30 HU resulted in death within 24 hours; larger amounts caused death within an hour. The animals dying after such short periods showed dyspnea, weakness, prostration, and intravascular hemolysis. The animals which survived 90 minutes showed hematuria and considerable enlargement of liver and spleen (see Section XIV). The toxic effects caused by these preparations could be prevented by heating to 50°C for 6 minutes. Since the preparations of hemolysin used in these studies were not purified, it is difficult to determine whether the effect described was actually caused by the hemolysin present in the preparation. It has been found (Ginsburg, et al. 1963) that similar serum filtrates prepared by the method of Weld (1934) contain a variety of streptococcal products (streptokinase, streptolysin O, RNase, etc.) which are also inactivated by heating to 50°C. However, in view of the more recent findings on the cytopathogenic effects of partially purified albumin hemolysin or RNA hemolysin on cells (see Section XIII), it may be assumed that at least part of the toxicity described was caused by the hemolysin.

Rosendall and Bernheimer (1952) found that the toxicity of mixtures containing Congo red (a potent inhibitor of SLS) and a lethal dose of SLS in mice was found to be a function of the amount of dye used. When the amount was small (of the order of 1 μg) the mixtures possessed little or no toxicity. However, when large amounts of dye were used (100 μg), which were far below the toxic dose of Congo red alone, the mixtures proved toxic. This paradoxical effect of Congo red could not be fully explained. It was also shown (Rosendall and Bernheimer, 1952) that no protection was afforded to mice by pretreatment with Congo red regardless of whether small or large doses were used. Binding of the Congo red by serum accounted for the failure of SLS to be inhibited *in vivo*. Ginsburg and Harris (1965) showed that trypan blue or Congo red at concentrations of 1–30 μg proved to be carriers capable of inducing soluble SLS from streptococci. At higher concentrations, trypan blue completely inhibited hemolytic and cytotoxic activity on mammalian cells (see Section X).

Sharpless and Schwab (1960) studied the toxicity of the intracellular hemolysin of group A streptococci in mice. The intracellular hemolysin was derived from a 1-liter culture of group A streptococci following 4 hours of sonic oscillation. The LD_{50} dose following intravenous injection was approximately 0.22 ml. Time of death depended on the dose and varied from less than 1 hour with very large volumes to as long as 5 days with the smallest lethal dose. Following inoculation, the animals were normally active for 10–15 minutes after which they became quiet and huddled together. Death typically occurred with violent convulsions. Autopsy consistently revealed hemoglobinuria, pulmonary hemorrhage, and edema. The lethal factor was heat labile, losing most of its activity after standing at 37°C for 30 minutes. Since the loss of lethal activity paralleled the loss of hemolytic activity, it was assumed that the intracellular hemolysin (IH) was responsible for toxicity. The relationship between IH and streptolysin S in not clear, however, since serum of rabbits immunized with the extract of sonically disrupted group A streptococci neutralized its hemolytic activity and since the fraction of the serum responsible for the neutralization was γ-globulin but not lipoprotein, it appears that IH is immunogenic and thus may be different from the classic SLS.

B. TOXICITY TO RABBITS

Ginsburg *et al.* (1968a) studied the toxic effects of purified streptolysin S in rabbits following intravenous injection. The LD_{50} of the hemolysin varied greatly in different experiments and in different animals. Approximately 6000 units of purified RNA hemolysin per kilogram of body weight will kill approximately 50% of the animals within 45-60 minutes. The rabbits employed were of a local stock and weighed 2-3 kg. A few rabbits appeared very refractory to SLS and were only killed by 10,000-25,000 units/kg. Approximately 15 minutes following the injection of a lethal dose the animals became restless. All animals injected showed electrocardiographic signs of tachicardia, ischemia, and arythmia which ended with a complete block. Twenty to thirty minutes following the injection of a lethal dose marked intravascular hemolysis was found which increased gradually and reached 30-35% a few minutes before the death of the animals. The animals had hemoperitoneum and passed bloody urine.

Rabbits appeared to be very refractory to intraperitoneal injections of the hemolysin. In this series of experiments rabbits tolerated up to 200,000 hemolytic units with the development of only small zones of parenchymal necrosis of the liver.

XIII. Effect of SLS on Cells and Tissues *in Vitro*

A. EFFECT ON NORMAL MAMMALIAN CELLS

1. RED BLOOD CELLS

Most of the studies on the activity of streptolysin S have been performed with red blood cells of various animal species. The use of red blood cells is very convenient since it is possible to measure quantitatively the hemoglobin released following hemolysis. Differences in susceptibility of red blood cells obtained from different animal species to bacterial and snake venom hemolysins have been described (Turner, 1957). The differences in susceptibility were attributed to the different phospholipids of the cell membrane. Thus, Bernheimer (1954) found that while mouse red blood cells are extremely resistant to SLO, they are very susceptible to SLS, and the difference in susceptibility was attributed to the high cholesterol contents of mouse red blood cells (Table VII).

Ginsburg *et al.* (1965) studied the relationship of the cell-bound hemolysin (CBH) to RNA hemolysin by comparing the susceptibility of red blood cells from various animal species to the hemolysins. The hemolytic effect in units per milliliter was determined for the erythrocytes of various animal species tested and these are shown (Table VII) as ratios to the hemolytic effect on human erythrocytes. In each case the ratio is greater than 1 but does not exceed 4. However, in the case of the two species with nucleated red blood cells (chicken and frog), the susceptibility to RNA hemolysin was much lower (6- to 20-fold) than to CBH. A similar

TABLE VII
RELATIVE SUSCEPTIBILITY OF RED BLOOD CELLS OF VARIOUS
ANIMAL SPECIES TO CBH AND RNA HEMOLYSIN[a]

Source of red blood cells	Ratio of hemolytic units for red blood cells of various species to that for human red blood cells	
	CBH	RNA hemolysin
Human	1.00	1.00
Rabbit	1.30	1.20
Chicken	1.66	0.25
Goat	1.80	1.20
Rat	2.20	2.90
Mouse	4.00	3.10
Cat	2.40	1.20
Sheep	1.00	1.10
Chicken	1.60	0.25
Frog[b]	0.30	0.015

[a]From Ginsburg et al. (1965, p. 647.)

[b]Similar results were obtained when frog Ringer solution was used instead of phosphate saline buffer.

observation of relatively lower susceptibility to RNA hemolysin than to CBH was also found in the case of Ehrlich ascites tumor cells. These experiments indicate that nucleated red blood cells behave differently from the mammalian red blood cells in their relative susceptibility to CBH and RNA hemolysin. Similar low susceptibility of avain red blood cells to IH was found by Schwab (1956b).

Red blood cells reacting with SLS undergo rapid swelling, and hemoglobin leaks out from the cells. Ghosts prepared by SLS contain much less hemoglobin than ghosts prepared with distilled water. No gross morphological changes can be detected in red blood cell ghosts following SLS action as seen by light microscope. (See Section XIV.)

2. LEUKOCYTES

Weld (1934) using serum hemolysin, Ginsburg and Grossowicz (1960) using albumin hemolysin and cell-bound hemolysin, and Bernheimer and Schwartz (1960) and Hirsch et al. (1963) using RNA hemolysin reported distinct cytopathogenic effects on mouse and rabbit leukocytes in vitro. However, Hare (1937) using serum hemolysin, Matsuda (1942), Snyder and Hamilton (1963), and Ginsburg and Grossowicz (1960) using similar amounts of RNA hemolysin failed to show cytopathic changes in mouse leukocytes. This apparent discrepancy has not been resolved. Usually leukocytes are 5-10 times more resistant to SLS than red blood cells.

The changes induced in the leukocytes appeared rapidly and were characterized by swelling, by the appearance of blebs, and by a decrease in the viability of the cells, indicating that the permeability and continuity of the cell membrane had been altered. Heating SLS to 100°C for 10 minutes or treatment of the hemolysin with trypan blue or lecithin (Ginsburg and Grossowicz, 1960) abolished the cytopathic effect on the cells. Hirsch *et al.* (1963) using rabbit peritoneal granulocytes and alveolar macrophages demonstrated that the initial toxic event observed following treatment with RNA hemolysin was lysis of the cytoplasmic granules into the cell sap rather than into vacuoles. Degranulation occurred 15–30 minutes following addition of 700 HU of SLS and was accompanied by formation of cytoplasmic granules which disappeared slowly. Also, filamentous changes in the cell membrane and nuclear fusion were sometimes seen, but these were in general less striking than those seen with streptolysin O.

The authors hypothesize that since SLS has been shown to release hydrolases from isolated liver lysosomes (see Section XV,B,1), it might also break lysosomes in intact leukocytes and thus release autolytic enzymes with a resulting general cell damage and death. The problem of whether death of leukocytes is associated with lysosomal rupture or is accompanied by such events remains to be established. Hirsch *et al.* (1963) also stressed the difference between degranulation during phagocytosis and that following SLS action. Whereas SLS degranulation is rapidly followed by severe cell damage, degranulation following phagocytosis shows no cytopathic changes, and the leukocyte continues to move about quite normally. It is also suggested, however, that the lysosomal theory is by no means proven and that SLS might damage multiple structures directly and also cause metabolic changes which may affect granules, cell membranes, and nuclei (see Section XIV). Hirschhorn, *et al.* (1966) studied the action of SLS on peripheral lymphocytes of normal people and patients with acute rheumatic fever. They showed that cultured lymphocytes show a nonspecific response to SLS similar to that found with phytohemagglutinin. This response is markedly and specifically diminished in cells obtained from patients with acute rheumatic fever not treated with penicillin. Such cells, however, retain their ability to respond to phytohemagglutinin and specific antigens. The authors suggest that since SLS is not immunogenic (see below), this phenomenon represents the counterpart of the *in vivo* neutralization of this substance, and that the diminution of this response in patients with acute rheumatic fever may represent a loss of the ability to neutralize SLS adequately during streptococcal infections. In view of the high familial incidence of this disease, it is possible that a genetic defect is responsible for the loss of the postulated defense mechanisms when the individual is subjected to stress by the presence of SLS in the body. Because of such a loss of neutralization, SLS may remain free in the organism to produce tissue damage associated with acute rheumatic fever. In order to accept such a hypothesis one must first demonstrate that the binding capacity of lymphocytes from rheumatics for SLS is indeed much lower than that from nonrheumatics. Another interpretation of the findings of Hirschhorn *et al.* (1966) is that lymphocytes of rheumatics may be more resistant to SLS action. This may be true if for genetic reasons such cells possess more binding sites for SLS on the cell membrane (e.g., higher levels of phospholipids). The authors also conclude that since cells obtained from patients with streptococcal infections in the absence of rheumatic fever responded normally to SLS, this relatively simple laboratory test may be helpful in the diagnosis of rheumatic fever (Hirschhorn *et al.*, 1966).

More recently Geri and Ben-Ezra (personal communications) have found that the diminished response of lymphocytes to SLS was not strictly specific for rheumatic fever, since lymphocytes obtained from four cases of juvenile rheumatoid arthritis also did not respond to SLS. The effect of penicillin treatment on the blast transformation by SLS as described by Hirschhorn *et al.* (1966) could not be fully corroborated. Lymphocytes taken from 27 cases of rheumatic fever patients who received penicillin prophylaxis all showed diminished response to SLS.

3. OTHER CELL TYPES

Snyder and Hamilton (1963) showed that RNA hemolysin inhibited the growth of McCoy cells, HeLa cells, KB cells, and heart cells (Giardi cells) grown in tissue cultures. The amounts of SLS needed to induce destruction of the cells varied from 25 units in the case of heart cells to 200 units in the case of HeLa cells. The cytotoxic effect of SLS was inhibited by lecithin. Oxygen uptake or glucose metabolism by rabbit spleen, heart, and kidney tissue slices was unaffected by 6000 HU of SLS/ml. The lack of effect is explained on the grounds that the hemolysin probably affected the permeability of the cells and that the enzymes released from such injured cells continued to metabolize glucose. Lawrence (1959) showed that preparations of serum hemolysin containing 2–10 HU/ml failed to affect the viability and integrity of human and guinea pig skin cells grown in tissue culture.

Marcus *et al.* (1966) studied the effect of washed streptococci possessing CBH and RNA hemolysin on tissue cultures of rat heart and kidney cells. Streptococci possessing approximately 1000 HU/ml of CBH and 1000 HU of RNA hemolysin exerted cytopathic changes on the cells as soon as 10 minutes following addition to the tissue cultures. The major changes seen were the appearance of large dense cytoplasmic granules (observable with a phase contrast microscope) of varying sizes. Some areas of cytoplasm contained several vacuoles which accumulated mostly around the swollen nuclei (Fig. 6A,B). By the end of 60 minutes, there was a complete disintegration of most of the heart cells though some nuclei were left intact. These effects were completely blocked by trypan blue. Strain C203U, shown to produce neither CBH nor RNA or albumin hemolysin, failed to induce any cytopathic changes in the cells. In other experiments, beating rat heart cells maintained in tissue culture were used as target cells. Five to ten minutes following the addition of RNA hemolysin, both the amplitude and the number of beats markedly decreased and by the end of 15 minutes no contractions were visible (Ginsburg, unpublished data). The heart cells then underwent cytopathic changes similar to those described above.

Lowry and Quinn (1964) and Quinn and Lowry (1967) showed that human cells obtained from tonsil, liver, conjunctiva, buccal carcinoma, intestine, and heart, as well as human monocytes and lymphocytes all grown in tissue cultures were destroyed when incubated with living strep-

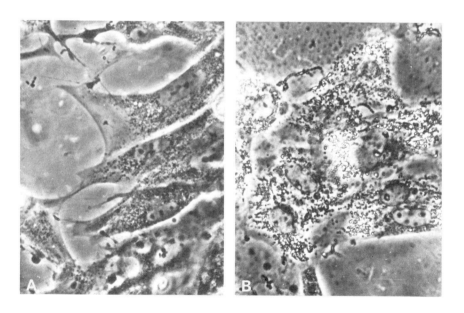

FIG. 6. (A) Four-day-old normal rat heart culture, zero time. Note a few streptococcal chains in the preparation (phase contrast, × 400). (B) The effect of CBH on rat heart cells after 10 minutes of incubation at 37°C (× 400). From Marcus *et al.* (1966).

tococci belonging to serological groups A, C, and G. No data as to the CBH content of these streptococci were given, however (see below). Medium in which streptococci and the tissue culture cells had grown had no observable effect on the cells. The cytopathic effect of the streptococci on the cells was prevented when the group A streptococci were separated from the cells by membrane filter diffusion chambers. (see Section XV). Attempts to duplicate the effect of the living streptococci with SLO, SLS (1400 HU per milliliter of medium) or by hyaluronidase failed.These results differ from those described by Bernheimer and Schwartz (1960), Ginsburg (1959), Ginsburg and Grossowicz (1960), and Snyder and Hamilton (1963).

4. EFFECT OF SLS ON PLATELETS

Rabbit blood platelets suspended in plasma were lysed by RNA hemolysin preparation containing as little as 60 HU/ml (Bernheimer and Schwartz, 1965a). In the absence of plasma, less than 0.1 unit of SLS was sufficient to cause 50% destruction of the platelet suspension (100,000/mm^3 within 45 minutes at 35°C. These concentrations of SLS were much less than those needed to lyse rabbit red blood cells. The authors suggest that, as in the case of red blood cells, SLS ruptures the membranes of platelets. It is also suggested that SLS might be responsible for the thrombocytopenia of rheumatic fever.

B. EFFECT ON TUMOR CELLS

The role of streptococcal infections (e.g., erysipelas) in tumor regression has been reported by several investigators (Fehleisen, 1882; Coley, 1893) and the early literature in this field has been reviewed by Nauts *et al.* (1953). More recent studies pointed to the possible role of SLS in the phenomenon of regression of experimental tumors in animals (Okamoto *et al.*, 1967).

Koshimura *et al.* (1955), Ohta (1957), and Havas *et al.* (1958) showed that Ehrlich ascites tumor cells incubated with certain group A streptococci lost their capacity to proliferate in mice. The cytotoxic effect on the cells was completely abolished by heating the streptococci to 50°C, but treatment of streptococci with penicillin not only did not prevent cytotoxicity, but markedly enhanced their effect on the tumor cells. Ginsburg (1959), Ginsburg and Grossowicz (1960), and Y. Taketo and Taketo (1967) showed that group A streptococci which possessed cell-bound hemolytic activity caused a distinct cytopathogenic effect on Ehrlich ascites tumor cells. This effect was characterized by marked swelling of the cells and by the development of blebs. The cells, which readily absorbed trypan blue, failed to proliferate in mice upon intraperitoneal injection. There was a direct correlation between the hemolytic and oncolytic properties of the streptococci; usually a few streptococcal chains adhered to the surface of damaged cells, but no invasion of streptococci into the tumor cells was apparent (Fig. 7A,B).

The cytopathic effect of the streptococci on red blood cells and tumor cells was completely abolished by SLS inhibitors, i.e., trypan blue, papain, and lecithin (Ginsburg and Grossowicz, 1958; Ginsburg, 1959; Ginsburg and Harris, 1965), and by metabolic poisons and antibiotics (Ginsburg and Grossowicz, 1958; Y. Taketo and Taketo, 1967), as well as by EDTA (Taketo and Taketo, 1967). Streptococcal mutants (strain C203U) which lacked CBH- or SLS-forming capacity failed to injure the tumor cells. Since the effect of CBH on the tumor cells could be duplicated by RNA, albumin, and Tween hemolysins (Ginsburg, 1959; Ginsburg and Grossowicz, 1960; Havas *et al.*, 1963; Y. Taketo and Taketo, 1966), it was assumed that SLS was responsible for cytotoxicity.

The synergistic effect of CBH or RNA hemolysin with proteolytic enzymes on Ehrlich ascites tumor cells was demonstrated by Ginsburg (1959). Tumor cells incubated with the various forms of the hemolysins underwent cytopathic changes. Various proteases (streptococcal proteinase, trypsin, papain), which caused no apparent injury to tumor cells, disintegrated the cells that had been damaged by the hemolysins. The lack of specificity of streptococcal proteinase in this effect suggests that other proteolytic enzymes of tissue or blood origin (cathepsin, plasmin) may act in a similar way, thus augmenting cellular damage induced by the rupture of subcellular organelles by SLS. Similarly, the synergistic effect of cytotoxic antibodies, complement, and plasmin or trypsin on Ehrlich ascites tumor cells has been described (Ginsburg and Ram, 1960; Hirata, 1963). Koshimura *et al.* (1955) who claimed that RNA hemolysin was not active against Ehrlich ascites tumor cells postulated a different mechanism of injury to tumor cells by streptococci. They showed that when living streptococci were incubated with Ehrlich ascites tumor cells, a significant amount of RNA hemolysin was produced by the streptococci. According to these authors, hemolysin was produced at the expense of the RNA of the tumor cells. (Koshimura *et al.*, 1958, 1960, 1961). To explain this phenomenon these authors postulated that the streptococci produced an enzyme which induces the RNA of the tumor cells to form SLS, and that the SLS thus formed may be injurious to the tumor cells. They further showed that following incubation of cell-free extracts (CPE) prepared from group A streptococci by grinding with alumina and precipitation with acetone with basal medium containing yeast RNA, high hemolytic activity was obtained. Also, tumor cells incubated with acetone lost their

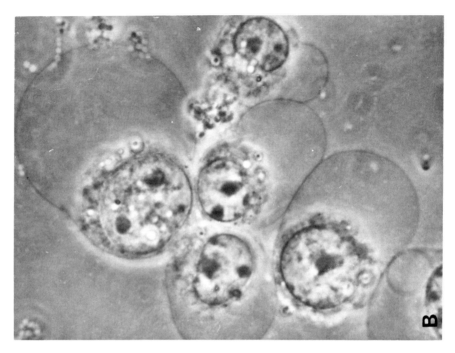

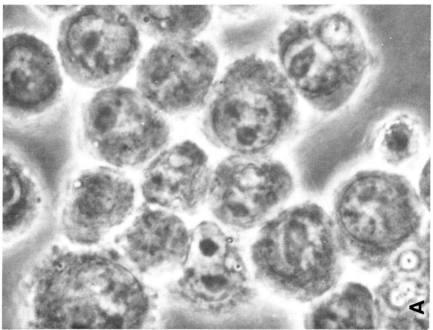

capacity to proliferate in mice. Both the anticancer activity and SLS syn-
thetizing activity were found in the same supernatant fluid derived from
CPE by centrifugation at 140,000 g for 120 minutes (Koshimura *et al.*,
1961; Okamoto *et al.*, 1967). Further studies by Okamoto *et al.* (1966a,b)
have shown that a potent antitumor activity was also obtained when
streptococci suspended in a basal medium (RNA, maltose Mg^{2+}) (Bernheimer, 1949) and penicillin (3 × 10⁴ units) were heated to 45°C for 20
minutes. This preparation was devoid of SLS-forming capacity; it was not
toxic for mice, but was pyrogenic for rabbits. The authors suggest that
SLS-producing streptococci contain two closely related factors, an SLS-
forming factor (or an SLS-synthesizing enzyme) and an antitumor factor.
Upon heating the streptococci to 45°C in the presence of the basal medium and penicillin, the SLS-forming factor is transformed to the antitumor factor. In the absence of more data on these apparently distinct factors and in view of the fact that both SLS and CBH have distinct
cytotoxic effects on tumor cells (Ginsburg and Harris, 1964; Y. Taketo
and Taketo, 1966) in the absence of penicillin or heating, it is not possible
at present to further evaluate the results of Okamoto *et al.* (1966a,b). This
is not intended, however, to rule out the possibility that as a result of heating, the streptococci release a factor toxic to the tumor cells. Further
studies are needed to elucidate this interesting problem.

In view of the complex nature of SLS (oligonucleotide–peptide) the following mechanisms of action of streptococci on tumor cells is suggested.
It may be postulated that several streptococcal chains possessing CBH
interact with the cell membrane of some tumor cells with the resulting
transfer of the hemolytic peptide on to the cell membrane. As a result
there is leakage out of ribonucleic acids (Y. Taketo and Taketo, 1966)
which now become recognized as carriers. The RNA interacts with CBH
(peptide) which is attached to its natural carrier in or upon the streptococcal cells, resulting in the release of RNA hemolysin into the surrounding
medium. By virtue of the high affinity of phospholipids of the cell membrane of neighboring tumor cells for the hemolytic moiety, the latter interacts with new sites on other tumor cell membranes causing leakage of
more RNA which in turn induces more synthesis of RNA hemolysin. At
the time of the injury to the outer cellular membrane, other membranous
structures (e.g., lysosomes) are also affected and this results in the release

---

Fig. 7. (A) Ehrlich ascites tumor cells at the beginning of incubation with streptococci
(× 1000). (B) Same as in (A) after 30 minutes of incubation at 37°C. Note the swollen cells
and the pseudopod-like structures. Few streptococcal chains adhere to the cell membrane
(phase contrast, × 1000). From Ginsburg and Harris (1965).

of hydrolytic enzymes (e.g., acid ribonucleases, acid phosphatase, etc.). The RNAse acts on the RNA released from the tumor cells to induce RNA core rich in guanylic acid (Section IV) with the formation of more RNA hemolysin.

An alternative theory is that small numbers of tumor cells die spontaneously and release sufficient RNA which in turn releases the hemolytic peptide from the streptococcal cells.

C. EFFECT ON BACTERIAL PROTOPLASTS AND MYCOPLASMA

1. EFFECT ON INTACT BACTERIA

Snyder (1961) and Bernheimer and Schwartz (1965a), employing a variety of gram-positive and gram-negative organisms have stressed that repeated attempts to demonstrate a significant effect of SLS (1000–6000 HU/ml) on the intact bacteria have been consistently negative. The explanation of the insensitivity of whole bacteria in contrast to wall-less bacteria (see below) is that the unaltered bacterial cell wall physically prevented access of toxin to the underlining membrane which is the site of action of SLS.

2. EFFECT ON BACTERIAL PROTOPLASTS, SPHEROPLASTS, AND L-FORMS

The data described in Sections VIIIA, XIIIAB, and XV suggest that SLS injures mammalian cells either by interacting with the phospholipids of the cell membrane or by affecting phospholipid membranes of subcellular organelles (i.e., lysosomes, mitochondria). Further insight into the mechanism of action of SLS on membranes came from a series of studies by Bernheimer and Schwartz (1965b), Davie and Brock (1966), and Bernheimer (1966) who have shown that protoplasts, spheroplasts, and L-forms derived from a variety of gram-positive organisms were lysed by RNA hemolysin (Table VIII). In the spectrum of its action SLS qualitatively resembled staphylococcal α-toxin. It is of interest, however, that protoplasts derived from several group A streptococcal strains, with the notable exception of one strain, were not lysed by SLS. It is also of interest that staphylococcal α-toxin lysed protoplasts of the (Wood 46) organism that made the α-toxin. It follows, therefore, that there must exist in the whole organism a protective mechanism against self destruction. It is also notable that all wall-less microorganisms whose membranes do not contain cholesterol, or are presumed not to, proved insensitive to streptolysin O. In this respect they differ from mammalian cells of various types and from parasitic strains of mycoplasma (See below) whose membranes do contain cholesterol. The lysis of wall-less bacteria by SLS is probably

TABLE VIII

SENSITIVITY OF VARIOUS WALL-LESS BACTERIA TO TOXINS[a]

Test organism	Preparation of test organism	α-toxin	Streptolysin S	Streptolysin O
Staphylococcus aureus (Wood 46) protoplasts	Lysostaphin	++	+++	0
Streptococcus pyogenes (GL8:A19) protoplasts	Phage-associated enzyme	++	0	0
Streptococcus pyogenes (C203S:A3) protoplasts[b]	Phage-associated enzyme	++	0	0
Streptococcus faecalis (ATCC 9790) protoplasts	Lysozyme	++	++	0
Micrococcus lysodeikticus (2665) protoplasts	Lysozyme	+	±	0
Sarcina lutea protoplasts[b]	Lysozyme	++	+	0
Bacillus megaterium (KM) protoplasts[b]	Lysozyme	++	+++	0
Escherichia coli (W) spheroplasts[b]	Lysozyme + EDTA	++	+	0
Escherichia coli (W) spheroplasts[b]	Penicillin	+	+	0
Pseudomonas aeruginosa (Toplin) spheroplasts	Lysozyme	0	0	0
Rhodospirillum rubrum spheroplasts	Lysozyme + EDTA	+	±	0
Vibrio metschnikovii spheroplasts[b]	Penicillin	0	0	0
Vibrio comma (Ogawa) spheroplasts[b]	Antibody + complement	0	0	0
Halobacterium halobium		0	0	0
Halobacterium cutrubrum (NRL-9)		0	0	0
S. pyogenes (AD-L:A12) L forms		++	0	0
S. pyogenes (GL8:A19) L forms		++	++	0
S. faecalis (F24L) L forms		++	0	0
Streptococcus zymogenes (Z30L) L forms		++	±	0
Proteus mirabilis (52) L forms		0	0	0

[a] From Bernheimer (1966). Symbols: 0 = no lysis observed; ± = barely significant lysis; + = significant lysis, but reduction in optical density less than 50% at 50 μg/ml; ++ = half maximal lysis caused by 20–50 μg/ml; +++ = half maximal lysis caused by 2–19 μg/ml; ++++ = half maximal lysis caused by 2 μg/ml.

[b] Data from Bernheimer and Schwartz (1965b).

due to its interaction with phospholipids of the membranes. The questions concerning the particular membrane phospholipids involved and whether enzymatic hydrolysis occurs remain unanswered (see also Bangham *et al.*, 1965; Elias *et al.*, 1966).

3. EFFECT ON MYCOPLASMA

Bernheimer and Davidson (1965) showed that of the six strains of mycoplasma (three parasitic and six saprophytic) examined for susceptibility to lysis by RNA hemolysin, streptolysin O, and staphylococcal α-toxin, only two of the parasitic strains (*M. gallisepticum* and *M. neurolyticum* A) were lysed by SLS, whereas all six strains were lysed by staphylococcal α-toxin. The authors suggest that the receptor for SLS in the membranes of the parasitic mycoplasma, probably phosphatidylethanoloamine, differ from those of α-toxin and are presumably missing from the membranes of the saprophytic PPLO. It is of interest that, like SLS, streptolysin O affects only the parasitic mycoplasma strains.

From all these studies it may be concluded that the inability of SLS to affect the viability of microorganisms possessing a rigid cell wall structure is probably due to its inability to penetrate through such a barrier to reach the protoplast membrane. Further studies on the phospholipid structure of the various wall-less bacterial forms will probably shed more light on the specific receptors or substrates in cell membranes susceptible to SLS and may also further explain the mode of action of SLS.

XIV. Pathogenicity of SLS

Because of the distinct hemolytic and cytotoxic properties exhibited by SLS, it was hoped that an understanding of its mode of action might explain, at least in part, the pathological manifestations which accompany group A streptococcal infections in humans.

A. SYSTEMIC EFFECTS

Barnard and Todd (1938) showed that mice injected intravenously with serum hemolysin that survived 2–8 hours had, in addition to hematuria, marked degenerative changes in the tubular epithelium of the kidney. The glomeruli revealed no histological changes. There was also marked necrosis of the lymphoid cells as well as the follicles of the spleen and small focal necrosis in the liver. In animals surviving more than 8 hours, there was almost always marked jaundice. Animals which survived 1 week showed very little pathological change in the liver, but renal hemorrhages were still found.

Ginsburg *et al.* (1968a) and Bentwich *et al.* (1968) showed that rabbits injected intravenously with amounts of RNA hemolysin smaller than a lethal dose and sacrificed 3 days following injection had mild proliferative glomerulitis. A few animals had foci of necrosis of the liver and hemorrhages in the omentun. A lipogranuloma with the appearance of giant cells developed 7 days following injection. No lesions in the heart were found in any of the animals injected with the hemolysin.

The intraperitoneal injection of large doses (10,000-20,000 units) which was usually nonlethal for the rabbit, caused liver necrosis. The necrotic areas were surrounded by granulation tissue containing foreign body giant cells abutting upon cellular debris. Zeiri *et al.* (1967) studied the effects of intratonsilar injection of RNA hemolysin in the rabbit. Animals which received 5000 units of SLS did not show any pathological alterations in any of the tissues examined. Also, SLS did not enhance the heart and liver lesions which were induced by streptococcal exo-products.

Tan *et al.* (1961) found that necrosis of renal tubules was produced in mice exposed to group A streptococci grown in intraperitoneal diffusion chambers. This was followed by rapid regeneration of the tubular epithelial cells. The renal lesions were accompanied by an increased proteinuria with many renal tubular cells and casts in the urine. Hematuria was observed rarely. These abnormal urinary findings correlated with the renal pathology and disappeared rapidly with regeneration of the renal tubules.

The renal lesions and abnormal urinary findings were not specific for nephritogenic type 12 streptococci but were also produced by two nonnephritogenic strains of types 12 and 14. Strains other than group A streptococci did not produce renal lesions or abnormal urine. SLS-deficient streptococcal mutants failed to induce lesions. In a study conducted to identify the streptococcal factor responsible for the renal tubular lesions, Tan and Kaplan (1962) showed that no streptococcal antigens could be demonstrated in the renal lesions by immunofluorescence techniques using human γ-globulin derived from humans and rabbits infected with group A streptococci (Kaplan, 1958). The failure to induce passive protection of mice with rabbit and human antisera suggested that the nephritogenic substance was nonimmunogenic. Highly purified preparations of SLS (3000-3500 units) injected intraperitoneally regularly caused tubular lesions and abnormal urine sediments similar to those induced in the diffusion chamber experiments. Such animals revealed only tiny areas of necrosis in the livers and hearts. Since SLS is nonimmunogenic but highly cytotoxic, the authors consider the possibility that SLS may be responsible for tubular disease which accompany human acute glomerulonephritis.

Tan and Kaplan (1963) further studied the alterations in the renal tubular basement membrane in mice injected intraperitoneally with a single
dose of RNA hemolysin (3000–5000 HU). In animals sacrificed 12–24
hours following injection, destruction of the tubular basement membrane
occurred as observed following staining with FITC-labeled rabbit anti-
mouse β-globulin fraction. The β-globulin fraction was found to share
common antigens with the tubular basement membranes. Staining of
glomerular basement membrane was, however, not noticeably diminished
or altered at this dose of hemolysin.

Formalin-fixed kidney stained with the periodic acid–Schiff (PAS)
method showed smudging and fragmentation of tubular basement membrane compared to the reaction of normal mouse kidney. PAS-stained
sections showed no alteration of glomerular basement membrane. Animals given similar doses of streptolysin S were killed at various intervals
after injection. It was observed that alteration of basement membrane
staining was not present at 6 hours, became apparent at 9 hours, and persisted for 36–48 hours after injection. After this period, staining of tubular
basement membrane was observed again. The return of basement membrane staining was seen in association with regeneration of damaged tubular segments.

A similar course of events was observed in mice with implanted intraperitoneal diffusion chambers containing group A streptococci. Tubular
basement membrane staining was observed to disappear during the period
of acute tubular necrosis and to return after tubular regeneration.

Although it was shown that a single injection of streptolysin S resulted
in altered staining reaction of tubular basement membrane with fluorescent conjugate, no alteration of staining in glomerular basement membrane was observed. The effect of a second injection was examined. Intraperitoneal injection of 5000 HU of streptolysin S was followed in 3 hours
by a similar injection of toxin, and the kidneys were examined 5 hours after the last injection. In sections of formalin-fixed kidney stained with
hematoxylin and eosin, the glomerular capillaries were seen to be filled
with homogeneous eosinophilic material which was PAS-positive. When
sections of frozen kidney were stained with fluorescent conjugate,
large accumulations of fluorescent material were present in the glo-
merulus together with a marked decrease in staining of glomerular
capillary loops. Tubular basement membrane staining was absent and
in certain areas focal aggregates of staining were present in the inter-
tubular spaces. The latter finding has been seen in some animals receiving single injections of streptolysin S but the glomerular changes have
not been observed except after a second injection.

B. LOCAL EFFECTS

1. EXPERIMENTAL ARTHRITIS

Weissmann *et al.* (1965) found that SLS injected into the knee joints of rabbits, regularly elicited an acute arthritis. Upon repeated injections, a chronic arthritis was induced which was characterized by hyperplasia of synovial lining cells, infiltration of synovium by lymphocytes and plasma cells, fibrinoid necrosis, and true pannus formation, with destruction of underlying articular cartilage (Figs. 8 and 9). No other streptococcal exoproduct induced such changes. Despite the nonantigenicity of the injected lysin, six of eight rabbits with chronic severe arthritis developed complement fixing antibody directed against subcellular particles (lysosomes) obtained from homologous liver homogenates. Sera from such animals had the capacity to stabilize isolated lysosomes against disruption by various agents. The data are compatible with the hypothesis that streptolysin S, an agent which has previously been shown capable of disrupting lysosomes *in vitro* and *in vivo* disrupts the lysosomes of synovial tissue, thereby releasing tissue-damaging substances.

Cook and Fincham (1966) have also reported on the induction of arthritis in rabbits and goats following the intraarticular injection of 2–9 doses (each of 1000–2000 HU) of RNA hemolysins. Aspirated synovial fluids showed an exudate comprising of polymorphs as soon as 24 hours following injections, followed by an exudate containing plasma cells and lymphocytes. Animals that received two injections showed only transitory infiltration with granulocytes. After nine injections pannus had replaced the articular cartilage and penetrated the bone. Rabbits that received chloroquine showed a more severe arthritis than untreated animals. These results confirmed those of Weissmann *et al.* (1965), but, contrary to the findings of these authors, Cook and Fincham could not find complement-fixing antibodies to rabbit liver lysosomes or to synovial homogenates. Also, they could not repeat the findings with respect to the inhibition of release of enzymes from lysosomes by the sera of the rabbits that have been injected with SLS. This apparent discrepancy remains to be elucidated.

More recently, Hollingsworth and Atkins (1966) have found that the development of arthritis in rabbits by SLS may not be due to the direct effect of the hemolysin on the synovial cells but to the effect of endotoxins which accidently contaminated the SLS preparation. Group A streptococci have been shown to possess an endotoxin-like material capable of causing a local and generalized Schwartzman phenomenon (Stetson, 1956). It may be considered that small amounts of such an endotoxin-like

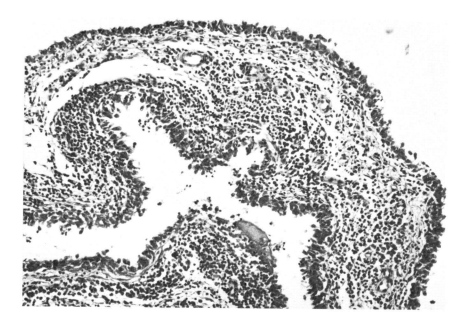

F1G. 8. Rabbit synovium 72 hours after the last of 5 injections of SLS into the knee joint. The synovium has become villous. The lining cell layer has become markedly thickened and the whole tissue has become infiltrated by small and large mononuclear cells. Fibroblast proliferation is evident; the joint has become the seat of a chronic inflammatory response. The joint was sterile. (×150) From Weissmann *et al.* (1965).

material may be released from the streptococci during the prolonged incubation with RNA. This may explain the findings of Hollingsworth and Atkins (1966). It is also of interest that Snyder (1961) obtained an endotoxin-like effect in rabbits injected with SLS preparation. Further studies employing endotoxin-free SLS will probably shed more light on this subject.

Ginsburg *et al.* (1968b) showed that acute and subacute arthritis was induced in rabbits following the intraarticular injection of a pool of extracellular antigens derived from streptococcal cultures grown in a chemostat. The antigen pool did not contain any SLS or SLO. In this respect, these results differ from those of Weissmann *et al.* (1965) who claimed that SLS was the only streptococcal exo-product capable of inducing arthritis.

2. EXPERIMENTAL MYOSITIS AND MYOCARDITIS

Ginsburg *et al.* (1968c) and Bentwich *et al.* (1968) showed that mice injected intramuscularly with 500 units of RNA hemolysin developed marked swelling and edema as soon as 12 hours following injection. Animals killed 16 hours following injection showed severe degenerative and necrotizing changes of the myofibers associated with inflammatory infiltration. Many of the damaged myofibers were invaded by granulocytes. Animals sacrificed on the third day showed rarified areas of muscle degeneration and subacute inflammation. Ninety-six hours following injection, most of the cellular debris had been removed and persisting myofibers as well as newly formed regenerating multinucleated myofiber buds remained. By the tenth day, fibroblastic proliferation was pronounced. The myofiber buds disappeared but granulocytic proliferation was still prominent. No pathological alterations were encountered in mice injected with heat-inactivated SLS. Similar results were obtained with saponin indicating that the toxic effect of SLS was probably related to its hemolytic capacity (see Section XIV). The cytopathological changes in the mouse muscle were completely inhibited by pretreating with cortisone.

Rabbits injected intramuscularly showed pathological alterations similar in some aspects to those encountered in mice. However regenerating fibers were not present. The inflammatory areas consisted of a multitude

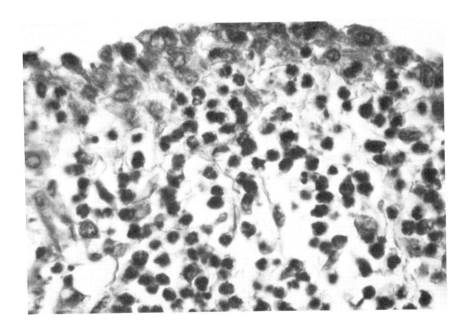

FIG. 9. Higher power view of rabbit synovium shown in Fig. 8. The synovial lining layer is swollen and hyperplastic lymphocytes and plasma cell infiltration is evident. (×500) From Weissmann *et al.* (1965).

of small, round, sharply outlined eosinophilic amorphous clumps surrounded by histiocytes and multinucleated giant cells (Fig. 9).

In rabbits injected intramyocardially with SLS, a large portion of the
injected site as well as adjacent areas underwent degeneration and necrosis. The areas of muscle damage were infiltrated with numerous mononuclear cells and histiocytes and many multinucleated giant cells were
found in the midst of necrotic fibers (Fig. 10).

Snyder (1960) showed that preparations of the RNA hemolysin were
pyrogenic in rabbits and that the pyrogenicity could be abolished by lecithin. The maximal temperature response was observed 4 hours after
injection. In the absence of data on the degree of purity of the hemolysin
employed, it is difficult to evaluate the results (see Holingsworth and Atkins, 1966). RNA hemolysin was also found to enhance the mortality of
rabbits challenged with *S. typhosa* endotoxin. These results were similar
to those obtained by preparing the animals with extracts of streptococcal
skin lesions and then challenging them with endotoxin (Schwab *et al.*,
1953). Examination of the animals revealed a Schwartzman-like lesion
affecting the heart and the kidneys.

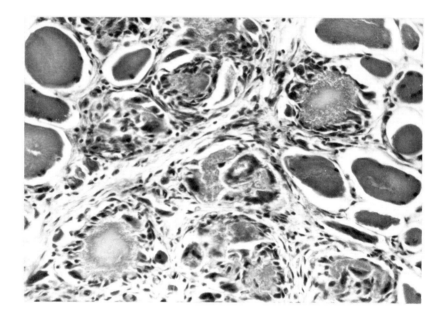

FIG. 10. Rabbit muscle 7 days following local injection of SLS. Subtotal replacement of
necrotic myofibers by granulation tissue. The latter contains several round to oval amorphous basophilic clumps, surrounded by reactive layer of histiocytic cells. (×240) From
Bentwich *et al.* (1968).

Snyder (1960) studied the effect of SLS on the isolated rabbit auricle and the isolated perfused heart of the frog and rabbit. Unlike SLO (Bernheimer and Cantoni, 1947), no effect on the rate and amplitude of contraction of the heart after additions of streptolysin S (2000 units/ml) was noted.

XV. Mode of Action of SLS

A. MOLECULAR LEVEL

1. LYSIS OF CELLS BY CELL-BOUND HEMOLYSIN

The phenomenon of lysis of red blood cells by washed streptococci is still intriguing (Weld, 1934; Smith, 1937; Hare, 1937; Ginsburg and Grossowicz, 1958). The relationship between the hemolytic effect of washed streptococci and the presence of CBH has been confirmed recently (Ginsburg and Harris, 1965; Y. Taketo and Taketo, 1967). Also, streptococcal mutants which lost their capacity to form CBH or SLS failed to show any cytotoxic effects. Neither in the studies of Weld (1934) and Smith (1937) nor in the studies by Ginsburg and Grossowicz (1958), and by Ginsburg and Harris (1965) was it possible to demonstrate any trace of hemolysin in the suspending medium derived from streptococci with considerable CBH activity. It was also shown that neither washings or hemolyzates of red blood cells, nor urea extracts of the streptococci contained any material capable of inducing the production of hemolysin by streptococci. It was postulated that lysis of red blood cells does not involve intermediary soluble hemolysin in detectable concentrations. Red blood cells separated from streptococci by means of a Millipore filter, which allows the free diffusion of RNA hemolysin, failed to become hemolyzed, indicating that close proximity of CBH-bearing streptococci with red blood cells is necessary for lysis (Ginsburg and Harris, 1965; Y. Taketo and Taketo, 1967; Quinn and Lowry, 1967). The direct evidence for the transfer of hemolytic material from streptococci to red cells was obtained in experiments showing that when streptococci possessing CBH activity were incubated with red blood cells for periods of time not sufficient to cause lysis, and then separated from each other by passage through cellulose columns. Under such conditions streptococci were completely trapped on the column, while red blood cells went through. Sufficient hemolytic material was transferred to red blood cells to cause subsequent lysis in the absence of streptococci (Ginsburg and Harris, 1965).

The transfer of hemolytic material from streptococci to red blood cells was temperature-dependent. It was possible to block the transfer of the hemolytic activity from streptococci to red cells by trypan blue (Fig. 11). These observations suggested that the hemolytic moiety of SLS transferred from streptococci to red blood cells has presumably such a high affinity for the sites on the surface of either of these cells that the concentration of hemolysin in free solution was below detectable levels, even in incubation mixtures in which hemolysis occurred. This hypothesis is consistent with observations described in Section VI in which the hemolytic moiety of SLS can be transferred among adequate carrier molecules.

2. Interaction of SLS with Cell Membranes

Very little is known about the mechanism by which SLS damages cells. Since the permeability of different cell membrane systems (erythrocytes, numerous nucleated mammalian cells and their subcellular organelles, bacterial spheroplasts, protoplasts, and mycoplasma) are altered by SLS (Section XIII) and since phospholipids present in cell membranes can block the cytotoxic effects of SLS (Section VIII), it may be assumed that the hemolysin interacts with and modifies cell membrane phospholipids.

Elias *et al.* (1966) showed that SLS is irreversibly bound to intact red

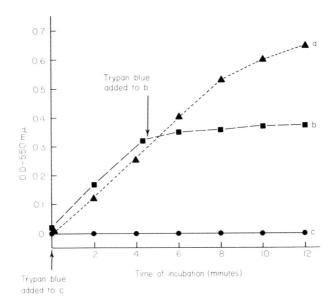

FIG. 11. The lysis of red blood cells separated from CBH-producing streptococci after various periods of time (a); (b) and (c) show the effects of interruption of the incubation. From Ginsburg and Harris (1965).

blood cells or to red blood cell ghosts. Treatment of such ghosts with phospholipase A and D, trypsin, lipase, or neuraminidase did not affect the degree of binding of SLS. However, treatment with phospholipase C from *Clostridium welchii*, which split the phospholipid to a diglyceride and phosphoryl base, reduced the binding capacity of SLS. Whereas 90% of the phospholipids of the ghosts were split by phospholipase C and the release of phosphorus was proportional to the decrease in binding, only about 40% of the capacity of the ghosts to bind SLS was lost. Also, purified lecithin split by phospholipase C lost about 40% of its capacity to inhibit SLS activity. Since sphingomyelin, ganglioside, sialic acid, and the various protein components of red blood cells did not inhibit SLS action, it was suggested that glycerol phosphatides constitute some of the binding sites for SLS in red blood cell membranes. Further indirect evidence that SLS interacts with cell membrane phospholipids came from the studies of Dishon *et al.* (1967), who showed that Streptolysin S blocked receptors in human red blood cells for a hemosensitizing factor (HF) produced by group A streptococci. Since the sensitization of the cells by HF was found to be completely blocked by lecithin, cephalin, as well as by *O*-phosphorylcholine and *O*-phosphorylethanolamine, it was assumed that both SLS and HF probably have common phospholipid receptors. It is of interest that phosphatidylserine, phosphatidylethanolamine, and phosphatidylinositol also inhibited lysis of red blood cells by rabbit antibodies and complement (Ginsburg, 1960). It seems, therefore, that phospholipids constitute substrates for the action of different hemolytic and cell-sensitizing factors (see below).

Further insight into the mode of action of RNA hemolysin was given by Bangham *et al.* (1965) who studied the interaction of SLS with artificial phospholipid structures. These consisted of concentric bimolecular lamellae composed of ovolecithin, cholesterol, and dicetyl phosphoric acid (in a ratio of 75:10:15), and resembled, in aqueous suspensions, such membrane-bounded biological bodies as mitochondria, red blood cells, or more closely, the myelin-figure form of lysosomes. Also, SLS treatment of the artificial structures caused a marked leakage of Na^+ and K^+. The effect of SLS was similar to that induced by diethylstilbestrol or deoxycholate. Similarly, SLS, like many other lysosome labilizers (Keiser *et al.*, 1964), released acid phosphatase from the large granule fractions of rabbit liver (see below). Electron micrographs showed that SLS treatment of the artificial membranes caused distinct alterations in their structure which consisted of segmentation of the membrane (Fig. 12). Although the membrane appeared to be intact, many new channels appeared between the inner aqueous compartments and the bulk aqueous medium. This effect is

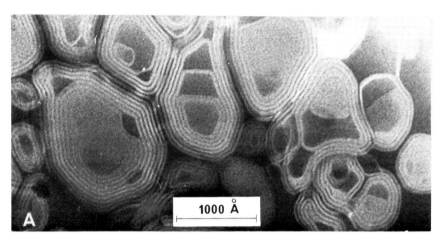

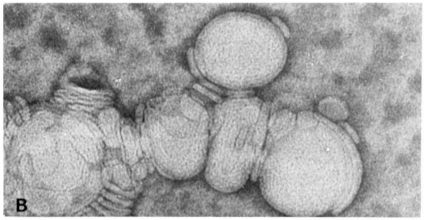

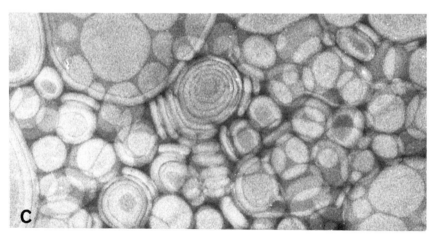

similar to that of lysolecithin on dispersions of lecithin-containing cholesterol (Bangham and Horne, 1964). Cortisone did not protect membranes against either lytic agent.

The inability of SLS to cause "holes" in the membranes and the fact that SLS probably does not possess phospholipase-like action on red blood cell ghosts as determined by thin layer chromatography (Elias *et al.*, 1966) suggest that SLS may alter the permeability of the cell membrane by mechanisms not yet known which may not necessarily involve degradation of cell membrane components. More recent electron micrographic studies by Humphrey and Durmashkin (1965) and by Durmashkin and Rosse (1966) have shown that the interaction of sensitized red blood cells with complement resulted in the formation of membrane holes. These appeared black in positive prints and therefore represented areas filled with negative stain. The holes were surrounded by a clear rim and the black portions measured 88Å in diameter. Other hemolytic agents such as streptolysin O and phospholipase C produced holes in the membranes of about 500 Å in diameter. However, interaction of SLS with red blood cell membranes did not result in the production of structural changes that were evident by negative staining of thin sections.

B. PHYSIOLOGICAL LEVEL

1. ACTION OF SLS ON SUBCELLULAR OGANELLES

The morphological changes in mammalian cells following interaction with SLS are usually characterized by swelling and by the development of pseudopod-like structures (Bernheimer, 1954; Ginsburg and Grossowicz, 1958; Ginsburg and Harris, 1965). There is leakage of macromolecules (i.e., RNA and proteins) and the cells readily take up vital dyes such as trypan blue and eosin. These results suggested that as in the case of the action of complement on sensitized cells (Goldberg and Green, 1959), SLS alters the permeability of cells and probably also damages other cell structures.

Treatment of rabbit polymorphonuclear leukocytes by SLS resulted in degranulation and cellular damage (Hirsch *et al.*, 1963). Keiser *et al.* (1964), Weissmann *et al.* (1964), and Bernheimer and Schwartz (1964) demonstrated that "granular" fractions of tissue homogenates prepared from liver, heart, spleen, and lymph nodes incubated with SLS and SLO

FIG. 12. Electron micrographs negatively stained with potassium phosphotungstate. (A) Control. Lecithin cholesterol dicetyl phosphoric acid. (B) Treated with streptolysin S. (C) Treated with lysolecithin. (× 240,000) From Bangham *et al.* (1965).

resulted in lysis and the release of β-glucuronidase and acid phosphatase from lysosomes and malic dehydrogenase from mitochondria (Table IX). Although the hemolytic action of each lysin paralleled the effect on lysosomes at equivalent levels of hemolytic activity, SLS was approximately 10 times more active on lysosomes than SLO. Pretreatment of animals with cortisone decreased the susceptibility of their isolated lysosomes to SLO but failed to prevent SLS action on lysosomes. No other streptococcal extracellular products were as active on lysosomes as the streptolysins, although activated streptococcal proteinase released some hydrolases from the granules. The similarity between the action of SLO and SLS on red cells and lysosomes suggested that the membranes bounding lysosomes and red cells have common properties. In further studies Keiser et al. (1964) showed that both SLO and SLS induced mitochondrial swelling and released malic dehydrogenase from mitochondria. This effect could be inhibited by Mg^{2+}, cyanide, dinitrophenol, bovine serum albumin, or antimycin. Only the latter two agents prevented release of malic dehydrogenase from the particles. Vitamin A induced swelling of mitochondria with release of malic dehydrogenase. In these effects, SLS and vitamin A resembled cysteine and ascorbate which induced swelling and lysis of mitochondria together with solubilization of enzymes. It was possible to dissociate the effects on mitochondria and lysosomes since less SLS was necessary to damage lysosomes than mitochondria. Injury to mitochondria resulted from the direct action of these agents, since the lysosomal enzymes released as a consequence of their action were not capable of inducing mitochondrial swelling or release of enzymes under the conditions studied.

Since streptolysins are capable of releasing hydrolases from lysosomes in vitro, they might also break lysosomes in intact leukocytes, thus releasing autolytic enzymes with resulting general cell damage and death. This assumption is strengthened by the findings that the initial morphological alterations in these cells is in fact degranulation. The granule content appeared to be discharged into the cytoplasm rather than into vacuoles. Subsequent changes such as cytoplasmic liquification and nuclear fusion are consistent with activation of autolytic enzymes. Hirsch et al. (1963) emphasize, however, that their observations only support, and by no means prove the postulated intracellular sequence of toxic events. One has to further postulate that in order to reach the subcellular organelles of the cell SLS must cross the cellular membranes. This can be achieved either by pinocytosis or by rupturing the cellular membrane. If the latter hypothesis is correct, irreversible permeability alterations will affect the integrity of the cell long before degranulation of lysosomes will occur. It is, therefore, possible that injury to subcellular organelles with all its implications may be only secondary to the intitial cell membrane damage.

XVI. Kinetics of SLS Action on Red Blood Cells

Bernheimer (1947), Cinader and Pillemer (1950) and Koyama (1965) studied the kinetics of action of RNA hemolysin on rabbit red blood cells. The initiation of the lysis of the cells was always preceded by a lag period. The rate of hemolysis then increased linearly and finally began to decline. The presence of a lag period distinguished SLS from SLO. Time curves of hemolysis were found to be of sigmoid shape, and semilogarithmic plots showed that the interaction of SLS with the red blood cells consisted of three phases, a lag period, a constant rate, and a decreasing rate. The lag phase was found to be inversely proportional to the concentration of the hemolysin. This phase was found to decrease with decreasing red blood cell concentrations. A large part of the hemolysin always remained in the supernatant fluid during the lag phase, but nevertheless, red blood cells obtained from this phase always underwent complete hemolysis. The lag period is the property SLS shares with *Clostridium septicum* hemolysin (Bernheimer, 1947). While there is little doubt that SLO combines irreversibly with the red blood cell membrane before hemolysis commences, this probably does not occur with SLS. Although detailed kinetic data on hemolysis by SLS are available (for the mathematical approach to this problem, see Koyama, 1965), the chemical reactions leading to the modification of the cell membrane and to the leakage out of hemoglobin are still poorly understood. Also, no indications exist that SLS is an enzyme (Elias *et al.*, 1966). The fact, however, that lecithin and cephalin prevent hemolysis by SLS indicate that membrane phospholipids may be the target for SLS action (see Sections VIII and XV).

XVII. Immunology and Immunochemistry

The question of whether any of the forms of SLS are immunogenic is still unanswered. It is agreed, however, by the majority of investigators (Bernheimer, 1949; Robinson, 1951) that no antibodies to SLS appear either in patients suffering from streptococcal infections or in animals immunized with partially purified SLS. Snyder (1960) injected rabbits with RNA hemolysin in Freund's adjuvant or following adsorption to kaolin particles. No antibodies could be detected in the animal sera capable of neutralizing SLS. In other studies he showed that kaolin particles adsorbed with either the active fraction of RNA core or with RNA hemolysin were agglutinated with sera obtained from animals inoculated with SLS-adsorbed kaolin particles. Such "immune" sera were found to be nonspecific. More recent studies by Getnick (1968) showed that RNA hemolysin complexed either with methylated bovine serum albumin (MBSA) or coupled to rabbit serum with carbodiimide failed to elicit anti-

TABLE IX

Release of Enzymes from a Granular Fraction of Rabbit Liver in 0.25 M Sucrose by Streptolysin S and Related Products[a]

Streptolysin preparation	Degree of granule suspension (μg/ml)	Hemolytic units per milliliter granule suspension	Number of experiments	Enzyme activity (%) released by controls[b]		
				β-Glucuronidase	Acid phosphatase	Malic dehydrogenase
Controls	—	—	24	100[c]	100[d]	100[e]
Streptolysin	130.0	1000	6	975 ± 92[f]	951 ± 102[f]	301 ± 103[f]
	65.0	500	6	874 ± 108[f]	812 ± 96[f]	297 ± 68[f]
	32.5	250	4	730	660	241
	26.0	200	4	710	400	192
	13.0	100	4	550	327	108
	6.5	50	4	331	199	112
	0.65	5	2	225	140	103
	0.65	5	2	225	140	103
	0.65	5	2	225	140	103
	0.13	1	2	102	98	107

Streptolysin S lacking mutant	130.0	< 10	2	110	97	98
	65.0	< 5	2	106	116	141
	32.5	< 2.5	1	108	106	87
RNA core used in SLS preparation	130.0	< 10	2	71	106	90
	65.0	< 5	1	95	105	96
	32.5	< 2.5	1	92	122	98
SLS heated at 100° C	32.5	–	1	111	126	35
SLS, granules at 4° C	32.5	250	1	104	85	115
SLS + cholesterol	130.0	1000	2	929	–	320
SLS + cortisol $(1.5 \times 10^{-4}\ M)$	130.0	1000	3	963	942	293

[a] From Weissmann et al. (1963).

[b] All experiments in the presence of 0.09% sodium chloride.

[c] Controls released $10.4 \pm 1.7\%$ of the "total" β-glucuronidase activity of the granules (17.5 ± 2.5 μg phenolphthalein/100 μg protein/hour).

[d] Controls released $11.3 \pm 1.2\%$ of the "total" acid phosphatase activity of the granules (5.91 ± 1.7 μg phenolphthalein/100 μg protein/hour).

[e] Controls released $24.2 \pm 6.8\%$ of the "total" malic dehydrogenase activity of the granules (250 ± 8.6 malic dehydrogenase units/μg protein).

[f] $p = <0.01$.

body formation to SLS in the rabbit. Also, SLS when bound to a Seitz filter was not immunogenic when implanted intraperitoneally. In some rabbits, however, a marked increase in the streptolysin inhibitor titer was observed following implantation. Such an increase in the nonspecific inhibitor was due to a transient hyperlipemia which developed in these rabbits. It is of interest that all rabbits injected with RNA hemolysin developed antibodies to ribonuclease used to prepare the RNA core employed for hemolysin production. Snyder (1960) studied the antibody response of rabbits following injections of rabbit heart modified by prior treatment with high amounts of SLS. No precipitins or complement-fixing antibodies to either SLS or heart were found. Todd (1938) and Hosoya et al. (1949b) are the only authors who claimed that that immunization of rabbits with living streptococci led to the production of neutralizing antibodies to SLS and these could be determined both in vitro and in vivo. Whether or not the neutralizing effect of these sera was due to the presence of antibodies or to nonspecific inhibitors remains to be established.

The controversy over the nonantigenicity of any of the forms of SLS may involve several hypotheses. It is possible that the amounts of hemolytic peptide associated with RNA or albumin which are injected into an animal or are formed in vivo during infections are too small to elicit antibody formation. The most purified preparations of SLS obtained (Koyama and Egami, 1963) contained 2×10^5 HU/mg dry weight. Thus, the amount of material associated with 1 HU is 5×10^{-5} mg or less. Since the amount of SLS used to immunize animals is usually in the range of 1000-2000 HU per rabbit per injection, the total amount of material injected is 5×10^{-3} mg. Of that small amount of complex, the carrier molecules (RNA and albumin) form the bulk of the dry weight employed. Thus, the absolute amount of peptide injected is even smaller, (see Section V). The recent findings of Bernheimer (1967) that the hemolytic peptide is of a very low molecular weight (approximately 2800) may conceivably account for its nonimmunogenicity. Another possibility is that the nonimmunogenicity of SLS is due to the absence of aromatic and sulfur-containing amino acids from the peptide (Koyama and Egami, 1963). Also, immunogenicity, if present at all, may depend on the arrival of the hemolytic peptide in active form at the antibody-producing cells. This is very unlikely since SLS is rapidly inactivated by interacting with the membranes of red blood cells and other cells (Elias et al., 1966).

Whatever may be the reason for the nonimmunogenicity of SLS, this hemolysin continues to interest and intrigue investigators, especially those interested in the role of streptococci in tissue damage. The fact, however, that lipoproteins of normal serum serve as natural inhibitors and the fact that these decrease during acute rheumatic fever further stresses the importance SLS may have in the pathogenesis of post-streptococcal sequelae.

REFERENCES

Albert, A. (1953). *Nature* **172**, 201.
Andrews, P. (1964). *Biochem. J.* **91**, 222.
Bangham, A. D., and Horne, R. W. (1964). *J. Mol. Biol.* **8**, 600.
Bangham, A. D., Standish, M. M., and Weissmann, G. (1965). *J. Mol. Biol.* **13**, 253.
Barnard, W. G., and Todd, E. W. (1938). *J. Pathol. Bacteriol.* **51**, 42.
Bentwich, Z., Boss, J. H., and Ginsburg, I. (1968). *Pathol. Microbiol.* **31**, 233.
Bernheimer, A. W. (1947). *J. Gen. Physiol.* **30**, 337.
Bernheimer, A. W. (1949). *J. Exptl. Med.* **90**, 373.
Bernheimer, A. W. (1950). *J. Exptl. Med.* **92**, 129.
Bernheimer, A. W. (1952). *Phosphorous Metab., Symp., Baltimore, 1951* Vol. 2, p. 358.
Bernheimer, A. W. (1954). *In* "Streptococcal Infections" (M. McCarty, ed.), p. 19. Columbia Univ. Press, New York.
Bernheimer, A. W. (1966). *J. Bacteriol.* **91**, 1677.
Bernheimer, A. W. (1967). *J. Bacteriol.* **93**, 2045.
Bernheimer, A. W., and Cantoni, G. L. (1947). *J. Exptl. Med.* **86**, 193.
Bernheimer, A. W., and Davidson, M. (1965). *Science* **148**, 1229.
Bernheimer, A. W., and Rotbart, M. (1948). *J. Exptl. Med.* **88**, 149.
Bernheimer, A. W., and Schwartz, L. L. (1960). *J. Pathol. Bacteriol.* **79**, 37.
Bernheimer, A. W., and Schwartz, L. L. (1964). *J. Bacteriol.* **87**, 1100.
Bernheimer, A. W., and Schwartz, L. L. (1965a). *J. Pathol. Bacteriol.* **89**, 209.
Bernheimer, A. W., and Schwartz, L. L. (1965b). *J. Bacteriol.* **89**, 1387.
Carlson, L. A. (1960). *Clin. Chim. Acta* **5**, 528.
Cinader, B., and Pillemer, L. (1950). *J. Exptl. Med.* **92**, 219.
Coley, W. B. (1893). *Am. J. Med. Sci.* **105**, 487.
Cook, J., and Fincham, W. J. (1966). *J. Pathol. Bacteriol.* **92**, 461.
Davie, J. M., and Brock, T. D. (1966). *J. Bacteriol.* **91**, 595.
Dishon, T., Finkel, R., Marcus, Z., and Ginsburg, I. (1967). *Immunology* **13**, 555.
Durmashkin, R. R., and Rosse, W. F. (1966). *Am. J. Med.* **41**, 699.
Egami, F., Shimamura, M., Yagi, Y., Hayashi, T., Mase, T., and Hosoya, S. T. (1950). *Japan. J. Exptl. Med.* **20**, 527.
Elias, N., Heller, M., and Ginsburg, I. (1966). *Israel J. Med. Sci.* **2**, 302.
Fehleisen, F. (1882). *Deut. Med. Wochschr.* **8**, 553.
Foster, J. F. (1960). *In* "The Plasma Proteins" (F. W. Putnam, ed.), p. 179. Academic Press, New York.
Gale, E. F. (1951). *Bacteriol. Rev.* **4**, 135.
Gale, E. F. (1956). *Biochem. J.* **62**, 40 P.
Gale, E. F., and Folks, J. P. (1955). *Biochem. J.* **59**, 675.
Getnick, R. (1968). Ph.D. Thesis, New York University School of Medicine.
Ginsburg, I. (1958). Ph.D. Thesis, Hebrew University, Jerusalem.
Ginsburg, I. (1959). *Brit. J. Exptl. Pathol.* **40**, 33.
Ginsburg, I. (1960). *Brit. J. Exptl. Pathol.* **41**, 648.
Ginsburg, I., and Bentwich, Z. (1964). *Proc. Soc. Exptl. Biol. Med.* **117**, 670.

Ginsburg, I., and Grossowicz, N. (1957). *Proc. Soc. Exptl. Biol. Med.* **96**, 108.

Ginsburg, I., and Grossowicz, N. (1958). *Bull. Res. Council Israel* **E7**, 237.

Ginsburg, I., and Grossowicz, N. (1960). *J. Pathol. Bacteriol.* **80**, 111.

Ginsburg, I., and Harris, T. N. (1963). *J. Exptl. Med.* **118**, 919.

Ginsburg, I., and Harris, T. N. (1964). *Ergeb. Mikrobiol., Immunitaetsforsch. Exptl. Therap.* **38**, 198.

Ginsburg, I., and Harris, T. N. (1965). *J. Exptl. Med.* **121**, 647.

Ginsburg, I., and Ram, M. (1960). *Nature* **185**, 328.

Ginsburg, I., Harris, T. N., and Grossowicz, N. (1963). *J. Exptl. Med.* **118**, 905.

Ginsburg, I., Bentwich, Z., and Harris, T. N. (1965). *J. Exptl. Med.* **121**, 633.

Ginsburg, I., Bentwich, Z., Zeiri, N., Silberstein, Z., and Lavi, S. (1968a). *In* "Current Research on Group A Streptococci" (R. Caravano, ed.), P. 239. Excerpta Med. Found. Amsterdam.

Ginsburg, I., Silberstein, Z., Spira, G., Bentwich, Z., and Boss, J. H. (1968b). *Experientia* **24**, 256.

Ginsburg, I., Zeiri, N., Bentwich, Z., Boss, J. H., and Harris, T. N. (1968c). *In* "Current Research on Group A Streptococci" (R. Caravano, ed.), p. 207. Excerpta Med. Found., Amsterdam.

Goldberg, B., and Green, H. J. (1959). *J. Exptl. Med.* **109**, 508.

Hare, R. (1937). *J. Pathol. Bacteriol.* **47**, 71.

Havas, H. F., Groesbeck, M. E., and Donelly, A. J. (1958). *Cancer Res.* **18**, 141.

Havas, H. F., Donnelly, A. J., and Porreca, A. V. (1963). *Cancer Res.* **23**, 700.

Hayano, S. (1952). *Japan. J. Exptl. Med.* **22**, 139.

Heppel, L. A., and Hilmoe, R. J. (1952). *Federation Proc.* **11**, 229.

Herbert, D., and Todd, E. W. (1944). *Brit. J. Exptl. Pathol.* **25**, 242.

Himeno, Y. (1955). *Ann. Rept. Res. Inst. Tuberc., Kanazawa Univ.* **12**, 111.

Hirata, A. (1963). *J. Immunol.* **91**, 625.

Hirsch, J. G., Bernheimer, A. W., and Weissmann, G. (1963). *J. Exptl. Med.* **118**, 223.

Hirschhorn, K., Schreibman, R. R., Verbo, S., and Gruskin, R. H. (1966). *Proc. Natl. Acad. Sci. U.S.* **52**, 1151.

Hollingsworth, J. W., and Atkins, E. S. (1966). *Arthritis Rheumat.* **9**, 513.

Hosoya, S. T., Hayashi, T., Mori, Y., Homma, Y., Egami, F., Shimamura, M., and Suzuki, Y. (1949a). *Japan. J. Exptl. Med.* **20**, 25.

Hosoya, S., Hayashi, T., Homma, Y., Egami, F., Shimamura, M., and Yagi, Y. (1949b). *Japan. J. Exptl. Med.* **20**, 27.

Humphrey, J. H. (1949a). *Brit. J. Exptl. Pathol.* **30**, 345.

Humphrey, J. H. (1949b). *Brit. J. Exptl. Pathol.* **30**, 365.

Humphrey, J. H., and Durmashkin, R. R. (1965). *Ciba Found. Sympo., Complement* p. 175.

Ishikura, H. (1961). *biochim. Biophys. Acta* **51**, 189.

Ishikura, H. (1962). *J. Biochem.* (Tokyo) **51**, 12.

Ito, R. (1940a). *Folia Pharmacol. Japon.* **28**, 41.

Ito, R. (1940b). *Japan. J. Med. Sci., IV. Pharmacol.* **13**, 23.

Ito, R. (1940c). *Folia Pharmacol. Japon.* **30**, 124.

Ito, R., Okami, T., and Yoshimura, M. (1948a). *Japan. Med. J.* **1**, 253.

Ito, R., Okami, T., Yoshimura, M., and Sagara, S. (1948b). *Japan. Med. J.* **1**, 260.

Ito, T. (1955). *Juzen Igakukai Zasshi* **57**, 1762.

Kabat, E. A., and Meyer, M. (1961). "Experimental Immunichemistry," 2nd ed. Thomas, Springfield, Illinois.

Kaplan, M. H. (1958) *J. Exptl. Med.* **107**, 341.

Keiser, H., Weissmann, G., and Bernheimer, A. W. (1964). *J. Cell Biol.* **22**, 101.

Klinge, K. (1962a). *Pathol. Microbiol.* **25**, 610.

Klinge, K. (1962b). *Z. Immunitaetsforsch.* **124**, 346.

Klinge, K. (1963). *Med. Welt* **42**, 3.

Koshimura, S., Murasawa, K., Nakagawa, E., Veda, M., Bando, Y., and Hirata, R. (1955). *Japan. J. Exptl. Med.* **25**, 93.

Koshimura, S., Shimizu, R., Masusaki, T., Ohta, T., and Kishi, G. (1958). *Japan. J. Microbiol.* **2**, 23.

Koshimura, S., Shimizu, R., Bando, Y., Hirata, R., and Shoin, S. (1960). *Japan. J. Microbiol.* **4**, 19.

Koshimura, S., Hirata, R., and Shoin, S. (1961). *Cancer Chemotherapy Rept.* **13**, 107.

Koyama, J. (1963). *J. Biochem. (Tokyo)* **54**, 146.

Koyama, J. (1964). *J. Biochem. (Tokyo)* **56**, 355.

Koyama, J. (1965). *J. Biochem. (Tokyo)* **57**, 103.

Koyama, J., and Egami, F. (1963). *J. Biochem. (Tokyo)* **53**, 147.

Koyama, J., and Egami, F. (1964). *J. Biochem. (Tokyo)* **55**, 629.

Koyama, J., Sokawa, Y., and Egami, F. (1963). *Biochem. Z.* **338**, 206.

Lawrence, J. C. (1959) *Brit. J. Exptl. Pathol.* **40**, 8.

Leedom, J. M., and Barkulis, S. S. (1959). *J. Bacteriol.* **78**, 687.

Lowry, P. N., and Quinn, R. W. (1964). *Proc. Soc. Exptl. Biol. Med.* **116**, 46.

Marcus, Z., Davis, A. M., and Ginsburg, I. (1966). *Exptl. Mol. Pathol.* **5**, 93.

Markowitz, A., and Dorfman, A. (1962). *J. Biol. Chem.* **237**, 273.

Marmorek, A. (1895). *Ann. Inst. Pasteur* **9**, 593.

Maruyama, Y., and Sugai, S. (1960). *Z. Allgem. Mikrobiol.* **1**, 19.

Maruyama, Y., Sugai, S., and Egami, F. (1959). *Nature* **184**, 832.

Maruyama, Y., Sugai, S., and Egami, F. (1960). *Z. Allgem. Mikrobiol.* **1**, 25.

Matsuda, K. (1942). *Folia Pharmacol. Japon.* **36**, 171.

Miyaji, Tm. (1953). *Ann. Rept. Res. Inst. Tuberc., Kanazawa Univ.* **10**, 237.

Nauts, H. C., Fowler, G. A., and Bogatko, F. H. (1953). *Acta Med. Scand.* Suppl. 276, 1.

Ohta, T. (1957). *Japan. J. Exptl. Med.* **27**, 107.

Okamoto, H. (1939). *Japan. J. Med. Sci., IV. Pharmacol.* **12**, 167.

Okamoto, H. (1962). *Ann. Rept. Res. Inst. Tuberc., Kanazawa Univ.* **19**, 165.

Okamoto, H. (1964). *Japan. J. Exptl. Med.* **34**, 109.

Okamoto, H., Kyoda, S., and Ito, R. (1941a). *Japan. J. Med. Sci., IV. Pharmacol.* **14**, 99.

Okamoto, H., Matsuda, K., and Kyoda, S. (1941b). *Folia Pharmacol. Japon.* **32**, 1.

Okamoto, H., Minami, M., Shoin, S., Koshimura, S., and Shimizu, R. (1966a). *Japan. J. Exptl. Med.* **36**, 175.

Okamoto, H., Shoin, S., Minami, M., Koshimura, S., and Shimizu, R. (1966b). *Japan. J. Exptl. Med.* **36**, 161.

Okamoto, H., Shoin, S., Koshimura, S., and Shimizu, R. (1967). *Japan. J. Microbiol.* **11**, 323.

Peterson, E. A., and Sober, H. A. (1960). *In* "The Plasma Proteins" (F. W. Putnam, ed.), p. 105. Academic Press, New York.

Quinn, R. W., and Lowry, P. N. (1967). *J. Bacteriol.* **93**, 1825.

Robinson, J. J. (1951). *J. Immunol.* **66**, 661.

Rosendal, K., and Bernheimer, A. W. (1952). *J. Immunol.* **68**, 53.

Sato, K., and Egami, F. (1957). *J. Biochem. (Tokyo)* **44**, 753.

Sato-Asano, K., Hayashi, K., and Egami, F. (1960). *J. Biochem. (Tokyo)* **48**, 292.

Schwab, J. H. (1956a). *J. Bacteriol.* **71**, 94.

Schwab, J. H. (1956b). *J. Bacteriol.* **71**, 100.

Schwab, J. H. (1960). *J. Bacteriol.* **79**, 488.

Schwab, J. H., Watson, D. S., and Cromartie, W. J. (1953). *Proc. Soc. Exptl. Biol. Men.* **82**, 754.

Sharpless, E. A., and Schwab, J. H. (1960). *J. Bacteriol.* **79**, 496.

Shimizu, R. (1956). *J. Pharm. Soc. Japan* **76**, 156.

Shoin, S. (1954). *Japan. J. Exptl. Med.* **24**, 13.

Shoin, S., Tokuda, T., Ito, T., Yamamoto, S., and Kitagawa, S. (1955). *Juzen Igakukai Zasshi* **57**, 1385.

Slade, H. D., and Knox, G. A. (1950). *J. Bacteriol.* **60**, 301.

Slade, H. D., Knox, G. A., and Slamp, W. C. (1951). *J. Bacteriol.* **62**, 669.

Smith, F. (1937). *J. Bacteriol.* **34**, 585.

Snyder, I. S. (1960). Ph.D. Thesis, University of Michigan, Ann Arbor, Michigan.

Snyder, I. S., and Hamilton, T. R. (1961). *Proc. Soc. Exptl. Biol. Med.* **106**, 836.

Snyder, I. S., and Hamilton, T. R. (1963). *J. Pathol. Bacteriol.* **86**, 242.

Sokawa Y., and Egami, F. (1965). *J. Biochem.* (*Tokyo*) **57**, 64.

Stetson, C. A. (1956). *J. Exptl. Med.* **104**, 921.

Stevens, F. A., Brady, J. W. S., and West, R. (1921). *J. Exptl. Med.* **33**, 223.

Stollerman, G. H., and Bernheimer, A. W. (1950). *J. Clin. Invest.* **29**, 1147.

Stollerman, G. H., Bernheimer, A. W., and MacLeod, C. M. (1950). *J. Clin. Invest.* **29**, 1636.

Stollerman, G. H., Brodie, B. B., and Steele, J. M. (1952). *J. Clin. Invest.* **31**, 180.

Strom, A. (1935). "Production of Diphtheria Toxin." A. S. Haakensen & Co., Oslo.

Sugai, S. (1961). *J. Biochem.* (*Tokyo*) **49**, 348.

Sugai, S., and Egami, F. (1960). *Proc. Japan. Acad.* **36**, 141.

Sugiyama, T. (1956). *Ann. Rept. Res. Inst. Tuberc., Kanazawa Univ.* **14**, 271.

Taketo, A., and Taketo, Y. (1964a). *J. Biochem.* (*Tokyo*) **56**, 552.

Taketo, A., and Taketo, Y. (1964b). *J. Biochem.* (*Tokyo*) **56**, 562.

Taketo, A., and Taketo, Y. (1965). *J. Biochem.* (*Tokyo*) **57**, 787.

Taketo, Y. (1963). *Ann. Rept. Res. Inst. Tuberc., Kanazawa Univ.* **21**, 97.

Taketo, Y., and Taketo, A. (1966). *J. Biochem.* (*Tokyo*) **60**, 357.

Taketo, Y., and Taketo, A. (1967). *J. Biochem.* (*Tokyo*) **61**, 450.

Tan, E. M., and Kaplan, M. H. (1962). *J. Infect. Diseases* **110**, 55.

Tan, E. M., and Kaplan, M. H. (1963). *Immunology* **6**, 331.

Tan, E. M., Hackel, D. B., and Kaplan, M. H. (1961). *J. Infect. Diseases* **108**, 107.

Tanaka, K. (1958). *J. Biochem.* (*Tokyo*) **45**, 109.

Tanaka, K., Maekawa, S., Hayashi, T., and Kuroiwa, Y. (1956a). *J. Biochem.* (*Tokyo*) **43**, 827.

Tanaka, K., Maekawa, S., and Hayashi, T. (1956b). *J. Biochem.* (*Tokyo*) **43**, 833.

Tanaka, K., Egami, F., Hayashi, T., Winter, J. E., Bernheimer, A. W., Mii, S., Ortiz, P., and Ochoa, S. (1957). *Biochim. Biophys. Acta* **25**, 663.

Tanaka, K., Hayashi, T., and Maekawa, S. (1958a). *J. Biochem.* (*Tokyo*) **45**, 97.

Tanaka, K., Egami, F., Hayashi, T., and Maekawa, S. (1958b). *J. Biochem.* (*Tokyo*) **45**, 593.

Todd, E. W. (1938). *J. Pathol. Bacteriol.* **47**, 423.

Todd, E. W. (1939). *J. Hyg.* **39**, 1.

Todd, E. W., Coburn, A. F., and Hill, A. B. (1939). *Lancet* **II**, 1213.

Turner, J. C. (1957). *J. Exptl. Med.* **105**, 189.

Weissmann, G., Keiser, H., and Bernheimer, A. W. (1963). *J. Exptl. Med.* **118**, 205.

Weissmann, G., Becher, B., and Thomas, L. (1964). *J. Cell Biol.* **22**, 115.

Weissmann, G., Becher, B., Widerman, G., and Bernheimer, A. W. (1965). *Am. J. Pathol.* **46**, 129.

Weld, J. T. (1934). *J. Exptl. Med.* **59**, 83.

Weld, J. T. (1935). *J. Exptl. Med.* **61**, 473.

Woolley, D. W. (1944). *J. Biol. Chem.* **152**, 225.

Younathan, E. S., and Barkulis, S. S. (1957). *J. Bacteriol.* **74**, 151.

Zeiri, N., Bentwich, Z., Boss, J. H., Ginsburg, I., and Harris, T. N. (1967). *Am. J. Pathol.* **51**, 351.

CHAPTER 4

Erythrogenic Toxins*

DENNIS W. WATSON AND YOON BERM KIM†

I. Introduction

The current dogma presented in modern textbooks relative to the nature and role of erythrogenic toxins in the pathogenesis of group A streptococcal infections can be stated briefly as follows: They are produced only by certain so-called scarlet fever strains and are responsible for the erythematous rash characteristic of clinical scarlet fever in man. Antitoxins are capable of neutralizing these toxins, which explains the immunological basis for a negative Dick test. Antitoxin injected into the rash may neutralize the toxin within the skin and cause a local blanching of the rash (Schultz-Charlton test). There is a possibility that more than one immunologically distinct toxin exists. These toxins are low molecular weight proteins. Individuals immune to these toxins are susceptible to group A streptococcal infections, and therefore, unlike diphtheria toxin in diphtheria, these toxins play an insignificant role in the pathogenesis of group A streptococcal infections and their sequelae.

A perusal of the literature reveals little interest in these toxins among most investigators interested in group A streptococcal diseases. In reviewing the literature on the importance of the various known extracellular factors of group A streptococci, one of us, in collaboration with Dr. W. J. Cromartie (Watson and Cromartie, 1951), stated, "The direct action of erythrogenic toxin explains only the toxic phenomena peculiar to

*Synonyms: Dick toxins, scarlet fever toxins, streptococcal exotoxins, streptococcal pyrogenic exotoxins.

†The work by the authors presented here was supported by USPHS Grants HE 5360 and AI 06487. Doctor Kim is a Research Career Development Awardee of the NIAID K3 AI 37,388.

scarlet fever. Therefore, most of the toxic reactions associated with these infections cannot be ascribed to a primary effect of this substance." We had assumed, as had others, that the erythematous reaction as claimed by Dick and Dick (1924) was the only toxic activity of these toxins. At this time, in collaboration with our students, we initiated an approach first proposed by Bail (1904) and later applied successfully to the anthrax bacillus (Cromartie et al., 1947; Watson et al., 1947). This concept is based on the fact that the complex environment within the tissues of the host may influence the metabolic activities of the group A streptococci so that these microorganisms produce materials not formed when they multiply in available culture media. At the time, we were optimistic for the success of this approach because of the highly significant and important observations of Murphy and Swift (1950), who had repeatedly produced rheumatic-like cardiac lesions in rabbits following repeated infections with various types of group A streptococci. These results are compatible with the concept that certain host factors are required for the production, by the group A streptococci, of unknown toxins capable of inducing these lesions.

As a result of these investigations, we found one primary group of substances that are readily produced when group A streptococci grow in the skin of rabbits (Schwab et al., 1953, 1955; Watson, 1954). These soluble factors in the streptococcal lesion extracts were characterized by their ability to enhance the lethal and cardiotoxic properties of gram-negative bacterial endotoxins and streptolysin O. They were labile when heated at 56°C for 30 minutes. They were immunogenic in rabbits and the activity did not appear to be related to any known group A streptococcal product. Further investigations revealed other properties such as pyrogenicity and at least three distinct immunological types. The failure of these toxins to induce an erythematous reaction in the skin of rabbits had eliminated any possible relationship to scarlet fever toxins. Later it was shown, however, that a highly purified erythrogenic toxin also failed to give an erythematous reaction in these animals, but manifested most of the properties of the toxins present within the skin-lesion extracts. Further studies revealed their relationship to the scarlet fever group of toxins (Watson, 1960).

In this chapter we will stress the fact that the ability of these toxins to produce erythema in the skin is only a secondary manifestation of a more important primary toxicity. A review of the literature reveals that this is not a new concept. The ability of all group A streptococci tested to produce these toxins in vivo and their profound and varied toxicities should create new interests in a possible role for these toxins in group A streptococcal infections, their nonsuppurative sequelae, and modification of the host response to other injuries such as endotoxin shock.

II. Early Literature

A. PRIMARY TOXICITY

When the Dicks (1924, 1938) described the so-called Dick test as a method for the detection of susceptible human beings to scarlet fever, the analogy with the Schick test and diphtheria was inevitable. The analogy has persisted to the present time. The neutralization by antitoxin and the classic flocculation observed in the toxin–antitoxin reactions were comparable to those observed with the diphtheria toxin–antitoxin system (Rane and Wyman, 1937; Hottle and Pappenheimer, 1941). From the beginning, however, there were many discrepancies. These have been reviewed by Hooker and Follensby (1934) who believed that most of these discrepancies could be explained by the presence of more than one immunological type of toxin.

B. ALLERGIC CONCEPT

The same year the Dicks (1924) described this toxin, Dochez (1924) independently discovered and reported the presence of skin-reacting substances from filtrates of streptococcal cultures. Unlike the Dicks, Dochez and Stevens (1927) emphasized the role of hypersensitivity in the pathogenesis of the Dick test. These results are well reviewed in a paper entitled, "Allergic View of the Dick Test" (1930). Of the earlier investigators, Cooke (1927, 1928a,b) added convincing evidence of the importance of hypersensitivity in the reaction to these toxins. It was recognized early that young children did not give positive reactions to the intradermal injection of Dick toxin. This was usually explained as being due to the presence of maternal antitoxin. Cooke (1927), however, showed that the serum of these negatively reacting infants had no neutralizing power. In addition, streptococci isolated from children without clinical scarlet fever were excellent toxin producers *in vitro*.

Zinsser (1931), in his excellent paper "Bacterial Hypersensitiveness," reviewed the evidence for primary toxicity versus the allergic concept. After a careful consideration of the evidence he made the following astute summary: "It is, therefore, at least important to consider the possibility that sensitization to an organism which so frequently invades the human throat may take place and thereby give rise to an allergic condition to which many of the manifestations of scarlet fever could be attributed . . . . Such a conception adds to, rather than detracts from, the importance of the observation made by the Dicks. For it would seem that, in the Dick toxin, we are confronted with an entirely new type of bacterial substance, one which injures the sensitized body, giving rise to symptoms not unlike those to be expected from a primary toxic action; and which, though heat stable and essentially an allergic antigen, is still neutralizable by an antiserum — a mechanism which adds a new and important chapter to the sum of immunological knowledge."

At about this time, Ando *et al.* (1930) showed that Dick filtrates contained both an allergic and a primary toxic constituent. This concept, however, was not pursued.

During World War II, Powers and Boisvert (1944) reviewed the concept of streptococcosis and the importance of age as a factor in the various clinical manifestations of streptococcal disease. As emphasized by the early investigators, scarlet fever is not seen in the infant and increases only after repeated streptococcal infections reaching a maximum incidence at the age of 6 years. At about the same time Rantz, Boisvert, and Spink (1946), after testing 1280 men of military age, concluded that positive Dick tests were infrequent in men whose premilitary residence had been in a geographical area in which hemolytic streptococcal disease is known to be low. With these data, they presented convincing evidence that previous exposure to hemolytic streptococci is essential for the establishment of a positive Dick reaction. They concluded, "The Dick reaction is probably the result of acquired hypersensitivity to the products of the streptococcus rather than of a natural susceptibility to a true toxin."

We have presented so far in this chapter good evidence for the two extreme points of view: (1) that they are true toxins, and (2) that they are simply a manifestation of a hypersensitivity reaction. We believe that our recent results can reconcile both concepts, and we shall give the evidence in a later section (Section III, B).

III. Production, Purification, and Characterization

A. PURIFICATION AND ERYTHROGENIC PROPERTIES OF THE STREPTOCOCCAL EXOTOXINS

After the Dicks (1924) described the presence of erythrogenic toxin in streptococcal culture filtrates, early attempts at purification and concentration were made by Hartley (1928) and Pulvertaft (1928). They were able to concentrate the toxin by alcohol precipitation and found the products lethal for rabbits. Veldee (1938) also produced an active toxin and precipitated it with tannic acid.

More recently, the most significant work on the purification of these toxins was accomplished by Stock (1939, 1942) and his associates, Krejci *et al.* (1942). Electrophoretically purified preparations had a molecular weight of 27,000. The toxin was precipitable by trichloroacetic acid and contained 15.2% nitrogen; it had the properties of a protein. This preparation was highly active [150×10^6 skin test doses (STD) per milligram]. Hottle and Pappenheimer (1941) also isolated a purified protein toxin. Their preparations contained 14 and 12.5% nitrogen and gave strong tests for protein. Like others, they found the preparations to be resistant to the proteolytic enzymes pepsin, trypsin, and papain. The flocculation reaction as measured quantitatively was found to be specific for scarlet fever toxin and antitoxin. This material contained 1.3×10^8 skin test doses per milligram of nitrogen.

The original preparation of Stock (1942) and Krejci et al. (1942) was heat coagulable and did not flocculate with antitoxin in contrast to the preparation of Hottle and Pappenheimer (1941). To determine if methodological differences could account for the variability in properties, Stock and Verney (1952) reinvestigated and purified toxins by different methods. These toxins were flocculated by most antitoxins, and they were more stable to heat, confirming the results of Hottle and Pappenheimer (1941).

Hooker and Follensby (1934) presented good evidence that more than one immunologically distinct toxin existed and described two types—A and B. They believed that more than two types could occur and that a single toxigenic strain could produce A or B or both. Stock and Lynn (1961) prepared concentrated type B and found it to be protein in nature, precipitable by trichloroacetic acid. In contrast to toxin A, it was inactivated by trypsin confirming the observations of Hooker and Follensby (1934). A and B toxins were immunologically distinct as determined by flocculation reactions with anti-A antitoxin and in agar gel diffusion methods. More recently, Mitrica et al. (1965) described a method for the crystallization of the toxin. Toxin recrystallized four times was electrophoretically homogeneous and contained 15.6% nitrogen. The activity was 1.04×10^9 STD/mg N as tested in New Zealand and chinchilla rabbits.

B. Purification and Biological Activity of the Streptococcal Exotoxins with Pyrogenic and Other Activities

1. Relationship of Erythrogenic and Pyrogenic Exotoxins

So far we have discussed these toxins only in terms of their erythrogenic activity as determined in the skin of rabbits or human beings. As pointed out earlier, Schwab et al. (1953) had demonstrated factors in streptococcal lesion extracts capable of enhancing the lethal and tissue-damaging properties of gram-negative bacterial endotoxins and streptolysin O. Later it was shown that pyrogenicity in rabbits was the most useful parameter of toxicity (Watson, 1960). With the aid of this method, it was possible to show that these toxins, produced *in vivo*, were associated with erythrogenic toxin. This was made possible by the availability of a highly purified preparation (1014C) obtained from Dr. Aaron Stock* and prepared as described by Stock and Verney (1952); this toxin had all of the biological activity of the *in vivo* preparations. This was confirmed by purified toxins made in our laboratory (Watson, 1960) and more recently by Kim and Watson (1967, 1970).

The pyrogenic assay is essentially that developed by Beeson (1947) for determining pyrogenic tolerance in rabbits against gram-negative bacterial endotoxins. In rabbits repeated intravenous injections given daily or every other day immunize specifically against the pyrogenic activity of erythrogenic toxin. An injection of 5 Lf intravenously gives a biphasic fever curve which reaches a maximum in approximately 3 hours. After a series of five IV injections the animals become immune to the pyrogenic activity of toxin as manifested by a change in temperature of less than 1°F at 3 hours. Such immunized animals were not immune to gram-negative bacterial endotoxins and commercial antitoxin neutralized the pyrogenic activity to the A toxin of Hooker and Follensby (1934).

By this pyrogenic assay, A toxin was found to be the most common toxin; it has been produced by types 28, 12, 17, and 10 (NY-5); B toxin was found in NY-5 [as reported by Hooker and Follensby (1934)] and type 19. A new toxin designated C was produced by a type 18 isolated at NMRU-4, Great Lakes, Illinois (Watson, 1960). As stated above, the type A toxin is neutralized by commercial antitoxin in contrast to the type C toxin which is not neutralized by this antiserum.

2. PURIFICATION

For the purpose of producing these exotoxins *in vitro*, a pyrogenic-free dialyzable medium was developed from that originally described by Stock (Watson, 1960). So far, Kim and Watson (1967, 1970) have prepared, in a highly purified form, both A and C toxins. The physicochemical and biological properties of A toxin have been determined. The NY-5 strain type 10 was used in this pyrogen-free dialyzable medium. Purification was accomplished by combined differential solubility and centrifugation in alcohol and acidic buffer. We have avoided the use of chromatographic methods and gel filtration because of the presence of gram-negative bacterial endotoxins within some of these material (Kim, Eng and Watson, unpublished). Purity was determined by homogeneity and symmetry of

*We are grateful to the late Dr. Aaron Stock whose interest and investigations contributed greatly to the defining of the chemical properties of these toxins.

the boundary in sedimentation velocity experiments and immunoelectro-phoretic analysis. The exotoxin A is an acidic protein as shown by amino acid composition. The average molecular weight was 27,000 as deter-mined by sedimentation equilibrium. This molecular weight is in good agreement with that given by Stock (1942). The highly purified exotoxin was free of streptolysins O and S, NADases, DNases, mucopeptides, and endotoxin as shown in Table I.

TABLE I
CHARACTERISTICS OF A PURIFIED
STREPTOCOCCAL PYROGENIC EXOTOXIN (NY-5)

Property	Results
Protein	80%
Hyaluronic acid	20%
Lipid	Trace
Heat stability of toxin (65° C at 30 minutes)	Labile
Sedimentation velocity ($s_{20,w}$)	1.8 S
Molecular weight (by sedimentation equilibrium)	27,000
Streptolysin O	Absent
Streptolysin S	Absent
NADases (DPNases)	Absent
DNases	Absent
Mucopeptides (cell wall)	Absent
Endotoxin	Absent

3. BIOLOGICAL ACTIVITY

The biological activities for this purified exotoxin A are summarized in Table II (Kim and Watson, 1967, 1970).

a. Pyrogenicity and Lethality. The purified exotoxin (type A) was highly active, giving a minimal pyrogenic dose at 3 hours (MPD-3) (Wat-son and Kim, 1964) of 0.07 μg/kg IV and LD$_{50}$ of 3500 μg/kg IV in young adult 3-month-old American Dutch rabbits. Both pyrogenic and lethal activities could be neutralized by specific immunization with the toxin. The pyrogenic activity of erythrogenic toxins and their specific neutrali-zation by antitoxin has been confirmed by Schuh (1965). He and his col-leagues have also demonstrated the liberation of so-called endogenous pyrogen from granulocytes incubated with exotoxin (Schuh and Hribalo-va, 1966). It is also of interest that glucocorticoids–hydrocortisone inhib-ited the pyrogenic and lethal activity.

b. Skin Reactivity. We have reviewed much of the convincing evidence for the role of hypersensitivity in one or more of the activities of erythro-genic toxins. Parish and Okell (1930) reported the relative insusceptibility

TABLE II

BIOLOGICAL ACTIVITIES OF PURIFIED STREPTOCOCCAL PYROGENIC EXOTOXIN (NY-5)

Activity	Animal[a]	Unit[b]	Results
Pyrogenicity	Rabbit	MPD-3	0.07 μg/kg IV
Lethality	Rabbit	LD_{50}	3,500 μg/kg IV
Skin reactivity	Rabbit (old or sensitized)	STD	1.0 μg ID
	Guinea pig (old or sensitized)	STD	0.1 μg ID
	Adult man	STD	< 0.000001 μg ID
Cytotoxicity	Rabbit spleen (macrophage)	CI (0.5)	10 μg/ml
Tissue damage	Rabbit	–	Cardiac muscle necrosis
Enhanced susceptibility to endotoxin shock	Rabbit	LD_{50}	> 100,000-fold
Reticuloendothelial function	Rabbit	PI (K)	Suppressed
Antibody synthesis	Rabbit	H_{50}, PFC	Suppressed
Antigenicity	Rabbit	–	Specific immunity (antitoxin)

[a]All animals used, except for skin reactivity determinations, were "normal" young adult American Dutch rabbits 3 months old.

[b]Unit: MPD-3 is a minimal pyrogenic dose (3 hours) which is defined as the smallest amount of toxin giving a mean rise of 1° F, 3 hours after IV injection; LD_{50} is a 50% lethal dose; STD is a skin test dose which is a dose giving a positive skin reaction greater than 6 × 6 mm at 24-48 hours; CI is a cytotoxic index (= average migration in millimeters of culture with toxin/average migration in millimeters controls); CI (0.5) represents 50% reduction of the migration; PI (K) is a phagocytic index: $K = (\log C_0 - \log C)/(t - t_0)$ where C_0 and C represent the concentration in blood at time t_0 and t in minutes; H_{50}, PFC are 50% hemolytic units and plaque-forming cells to sheep erythrocytes.

of young rabbits. This applies to both the skin reaction and lethality. Veldee (1932) gave a careful evaluation of animal variation and age of rabbits in the development of his method employing the ear of the white rabbit. He used old rabbits in excess of 4 pounds in weight because young rabbits did not respond to toxin as well as those fully matured, confirming the observations of Parish and Okell (1930) and Trask (1932). As stressed earlier, our failure to relate the pyrogenic toxins to erythrogenic toxin resulted from the failure of young American Dutch rabbits to give a skin reaction. We also found that older rabbits do give skin reactions, although results in these rabbits may vary. Veldee (1932) reported that in older rabbits within a single strain, only 74% were positive for one human skin test dose. He believed that susceptibility was an inherited characteristic. Hribalova and Schuh (1967) reported that steroids suppressed the skin reactivity of the toxins in rabbits which is more consistent with a hypersensitivity component. In guinea pigs we have confirmed the observations of Dochez and Sherman (1925). Young inbred guinea pigs of the N.I.H. strain 2 are not susceptible to the skin test, but the injection of small quantities of toxin sensitizes them so they become reactive. Dochez and Sherman (1925) were able to neutralize these acquired reactions by mixing the toxin with antitoxin. Kim and Watson (unpublished) sensitized the inbred guinea pigs with a single dose of purified type A toxin suspended in Freund's incomplete adjuvant and injected into the foot pads. Within 6 days these animals developed skin sensitivity which increased at 2-3 weeks. This acquired skin sensitivity to the toxin could be passively transferred by injecting spleen and lymph node cells from sensitized to nonsensitized animals. These results add evidence to the role of delayed type hypersensitivity in the pathogenesis of the skin reaction to these toxins.

All eight volunteers among laboratory personnel tested gave positive skin tests with 10^{-6} μg of the purified A toxin. This activity is greater than 10^9 skin test doses per milligram of protein, and therefore indicates a higher activity than previously described by Stock (1939, 1942) and Hottle and Pappenheimer (1941). However, it should be emphasized that our human volunteers had been working with group A streptococci and might have acquired a higher degree of hypersensitivity to the toxin than those subjects tested by others. For this reason, the skin test as an assay may not be quantitative for toxicity, because it will be influenced not only by true primary toxicity but also by the immunological state of the host, namely hypersensitivity and immunity.

c. *Cytotoxicity.* The tissue culture method of Heilman (1965) was used for measuring the cytotoxicity of the toxin. Young adult rabbit spleen macrophages gave a greater than 50% inhibition of macrophage migration at 96 hours giving a cytotoxic index of less than 0.5 with 10 μg of toxin per milliliter (Kim and Watson, 1967, 1970). This is consistent with the *in vivo* test of reticuloendothelial system suppression and the immunosuppressive effects of the toxin (Hanna and Watson, 1965, 1968).

d. *Enhancement of Susceptibility to Gram-Negative Bacterial Endotoxins and Other Injuries.* Perhaps the most dramatic biological activity of these streptococcal exotoxins is their ability to modify the susceptibility of animals to endotoxin shock (Schwab *et al.*, 1953, 1955; Watson, 1954, 1960). These studies have been confirmed and extended by Kim and Watson (1965, 1970). A quantitative analysis of this enhancement effect was made in three species of animals including American Dutch rabbits, cynomolgus monkeys, and Balb/Sy mice. The exotoxin used was the A type described in Table I and the endotoxin was from *Salmonella typhosa* 0901W. Animals highly resistant to endotoxin, when given as little as 0.1 μg/kg 3 hours prior to the injection of endotoxin, became highly susceptible to endotoxin shock. In American Dutch rabbits enhancement in excess of 100,000-fold was observed. Adult cynomolgus monkeys were highly resistant to endotoxin lethal shock. These animals were refractory to 2000 μg of streptococcal exotoxin and 8000 μg of endotoxin when these doses were given separately. When, however, these monkeys were pretreated with 500 μg of exotoxin and 3 hours later were given 2000 μg of endotoxin, all of the animals died within 24 hours.

Boroff (1951) reported an interesting observation which might be related to the enhancement phenomenon described above. If erythrogenic toxin is given intradermally at 24-hour intervals at different sites, the reaction to the second injection is more intense than that to the first. The author interpreted this as an allergenic property of the toxin because the reaction appeared specific for erythrogenic toxin and there was no enhancement of skin reactions to other antigens such as M-protein. It is not clear, however, whether the animals were sensitive to the skin-test materials used. In a preliminary report Kayute and Watson (1955) sensitized rabbits to bovine gamma globulin. The sensitized rabbits were divided into two groups; one group received streptococcal lesion extract containing A toxin. Four hours later both groups were given an intravenous injection of the sensitizing antigen, bovine γ-globulin. There was no manifest distress in the control group, but rabbits receiving streptococcal toxin gave intense anaphylactic reactions and five animals within this group died. No deaths were recorded in control groups which received only the γ-globulin. Those surviving were killed on the fourteenth day, and a consistent type of myocardial pathology was found. Lesions were more severe in those animals given the streptococcal toxin prior to the sensitizing antigen. It is obvious, therefore, that the enhancement of susceptibility as first shown for gram-negative bacterial endotoxin and streptolysin O (Schwab et al., 1955) is not specific for any one toxic reaction but rather creates a state of hypersusceptibility to a wide variety of stressful events.

e. Inhibition of Reticuloendothelial Function. Streptococcal lesion extract containing C toxin when injected intravenously into American Dutch rabbits depressed reticuloendothelial function for a least 24 hours. In contrast, the intravenous injection of an equivalent pyrogenic dose of gram-negative bacterial endotoxin (COO8) caused an early depression of reticuloendothelial function, but, after 24 hours, a stimulation occurred which doubled in 48 hours. The prolonged depression of the reticuloendothelial system brought about in these animals by these pyrogenic exotoxins could explain at least partially the mechanism by which these toxins potentiate lethality and tissue damage by toxins such as streptolysin O and endotoxins of gram-negative bacteria (Hanna and Watson, 1965).

f. Immunosuppression. Hanna and Watson (1968) predicted on the basis of reticuloendothelial inhibition that these pyrogenic exotoxins might have immune suppressive activity. If antigens, especially particulate antigens, must be processed by the reticuloendothelial system (Harris and Ehrich, 1946; Fishman, 1961), a reticuloendothelial inhibitor could inhibit or at least suppress antibody formation. The highly purified A type toxin (Kim and Watson, 1967, 1970) as described in Table I was used. When given to American Dutch rabbits the purified exotoxin at 0.002 of the LD_{50} dose suppressed the antibody response to injected sheep erythrocytes. A control experiment using gram-negative bacterial endotoxin at comparable pyrogenic levels did not induce antibody suppression, but did induce the well-known adjuvant effect. It is obvious from our knowledge of antibody-forming spleen cells in the so-called "normal" animal that, with this antigen–antibody system, the inhibition involves the secondary rather than the primary response. Thus these exotoxins are capable of blocking the anamnestic response, certainly an important defensive mechanism of the host.

g. Antigenicity. These low molecular weight toxins do not appear to be highly antigenic. It follows that if they are immunosuppressive to other antigens they would also be immunosuppressive to themselves. Although Halbert (1958) found measurable anti-erythrogenic toxin antibodies in pooled human serum, Hanson and Holm (1961), comparing frequency of antibodies in human sera to various streptococcal extracellular antigens, found antistreptolysin O in almost all sera from adults, whereas antibodies to erythrogenic toxin were found in only a few. It should be pointed out that both groups of investigators were measuring only the anti-A antibody. These observations do not preclude the importance of erythrogenic toxins in human infections. Indeed it might be expected that the most effective toxins or factors involved in pathogenicity would be the least antigenic.

There has been no effective method of toxoiding these toxins and also maintaining their immunogenicity. The most effective antigen was developed by Veldee (1938). After some purification, the toxins were precipitated by tannic acid and used as a tannic acid–toxin complex suspended in a protective colloid, acacia. This preparation given intradermally in three doses was effective in converting children from Dick-positive to Dick-negative reactions (Veldee *et al.*, 1941). Preparations of a similar type were used by Wasson and Brown (1942) in a controlled immunization study on ambulatory patients suffering from rheumatic heart disease. There was a reduction in the number of attacks of acute rheumatic fever and a general improvement in health. Because of the various generalized toxicities associated with these toxins, it would not seem advisable to continue such tests in human subjects, especially those highly sensitized, until a method is found to detoxify the preparations. Indeed, it is conceivable, as suggested by Rantz (1952) that immunization procedures could induce resistance within human tissues to the development of the rheumatic process even though group A streptococcal infection should occur.

IV. Proposed Mechanism of Activity of Exotoxins

The two widely divergent concepts given in this chapter are both well supported by reliable experimental observations. We believe the two extreme concepts—the primary toxicity versus the allergic concept—are reconcilable into a single mechanism which has common features with the proposed mechanism for activity of gram-negative bacterial endotoxins reported by Watson and Kim (1964). As given in Fig. 1, the toxin is produced within the host or *in vitro*, in a complex form closely associated with hyaluronic acid. The hyaluronic acid is not necessary for the primary toxicity but acts as a carrier. The primary toxicity, which can act either independently or interdependently of acquired hypersensitivity, is associated with the heat-labile portion of the low molecular weight protein. This portion of the molecule exists in more than one antigenic form and accounts for the immunological specificity; at least three toxins can be identified, A, B, and C. There are probably additional types. Manifestations of the primary toxicity are pyrogenicity, lethality, cytotoxicity, reticuloendothelial suppression, immunosuppression, and perhaps the most significant, the modification or enhancement of the host response to in-

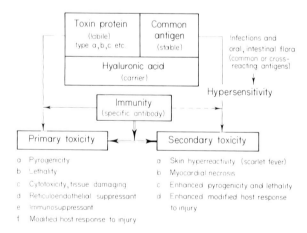

Fig. 1. Proposed mechanisms for activity of group A streptococcal exotoxin.

jury. For example, these toxins are capable of enhancing the susceptibility of American Dutch rabbits 100,000 times to gram-negative bacterial endotoxins. Associated with the toxin is a heat-stable portion which is antigenically common to all of the toxins and accounts for the secondary toxicity. As a result of repeated streptococcal infections, the host develops an allergy to infection by this component. In the absence of specific neutralizing antibody, the labile active portion of the toxin makes the tissues hyperreactive so that they manifest a hypersensitivity reaction to an extremely small amount of the common antigen. Neutralization of the toxin with antiserum or destruction of the primary toxic portion by heat, eliminates or reduces the hyperactivity and a reduced reaction results because the primary and secondary toxicities are mutually interdependent. Thus, the rash in the Dick test and scarlet fever results from the combination of a primary toxicity and a delayed type of acquired hypersensitivity to a portion of the toxin. This enhancement or hyperreactivity of the host induced by the primary toxicity can also bring about other secondary toxicities as a result of hypersensitiveness brought about by other infections, intestinal flora, and cross-reacting antigens. Antibodies specific for the toxins protect against secondary toxicities by blocking the primary toxicity. In defining the biological activity of these toxins one must take into consideration the immunological state of the host — relative immunity and hypersensitivity. Thus, two individuals of the same species could be negative to the Dick test for different reasons. The young child may not have acquired the hypersensitivity; the adult may have hypersensitivity but high neutralizing antibody blocks the primary toxicity. Thus, the great number of variables within the host and the fact that more than one immunological type of toxin exists could account for all the discrepancies associated with the nature of the biological activity within this group of exotoxins.

It seems unfortunate to us that the rash, which is the result of a secondary toxicity (probably the least significant toxic property of these toxins), has done so much to obscure the importance of this group of toxins in the pathogenesis of group A streptococcal infections and their late sequelae.

REFERENCES

"Allergic View of the Dick Test." (1930). *Ann. Pickett-Thomson Res. Lab.* 6, 123.
Ando, K., Kurauchi, K., and Nishimura, H. (1930). *J. Immunol.* 18, 223.
Bail, O. (1904). *Centr. Bakteriol., Abt I. Orig.* 37, 270.
Beeson, P. B. (1947). *J. Exptl. Med.* 86, 29.
Boroff, D. A. (1951). *J. Bacteriol.* 62, 627.
Cooke, J. V. (1927). *Proc. Soc. Exptl. Biol. Med.* 24, 314.

Cooke, J. V. (1928a). *Am. J. Diseases Children* **35**, 762.

Cooke, J. V. (1928b). *Am. J. Diseases Children* **35**, 784.

Cromartie, W. J., Watson, D. W., Bloom, W. L., and Heckly, R. J. (1947). *J. Infect. Diseases* **80**, 14.

Dick, G. F., and Dick, G. H. (1924). *J. Am. Med. Assoc.* **82**, 265.

Dick, G. F., and Dick, G. H. (1938). "Scarlet Fever." Year Book Publ., Chicago, Illinois.

Dochez, A. R. (1924). *J. Am. Med. Assoc.* **82**, 542.

Dochez, A. R., and Sherman, L. (1925). *Proc. Soc. Exptl. Biol. Med.* **22**, 282.

Dochez, A. R., and Stevens, F. A. (1927). *J. Exptl. Med.* **46**, 487.

Fishman, M. (1961). *J. Exptl. Med.* **114**, 837.

Halbert, S. P. (1958). *J. Exptl. Med.* **108**, 385.

Hanna, E. E., and Watson, D. W. (1965). *J. Bacteriol.* **89**, 154.

Hanna, E. E., and Watson, D. W. (1968). *J. Bacteriol.* **95**, 14.

Hanson, L. A., and Holm, S. E. (1961). *Acta Pathol. Microbiol. Scand.* **52**, 59.

Harris, T. N., and Ehrich, W. E. (1946). *J. Exptl. Med.* **84**, 157.

Hartley, P. (1928). *Brit. J. Exptl. Pathol.* **9**, 259.

Heilman, D. H. (1965). *Intern. Arch. Allergy Appl. Immunol.* **26**, 63.

Hooker, S. B., and Follensby, E. M. (1934). *J. Immunol.* **27**, 177.

Hottle, G. A., and Pappenheimer, A. M., Jr. (1941). *J. Exptl. Med.* **74**, 545.

Hribalova, V., and Schuh, V. (1967). *Folia Microbiol. (Prague)* **12**, 477.

Kayute, S. W., and Watson, D. W. (1955). *Bacteriol. Proc.* p. 94.

Kim, Y. B., and Watson, D. W. (1965). *Bacteriol. Proc.* p. 45.

Kim, Y. B., and Watson, D. W. (1967). *Bacteriol. Proc.* p. 87.

Kim, Y. B., and Watson, D. W. (1970). *J. Exptl. Med.* **131**, 611.

Krejci, L. E., Stock, A. H., Sanigar, E. B., and Kraemer, E. O. (1942). *J. Biol. Chem.* **142**, 785.

Mitrica, N., Pleceas, P., and Mesrobeanu, L. (1965). *Z. Immunitaets- Allergieforsch.* **129**, 78.

Murphy, G. E., and Swift, H. F. (1950). *J. Exptl. Med.* **91**, 485.

Parish, H. J., and Okell, C. C. (1930). *J. Pathol. Bacteriol.* **33**, 527.

Powers, G. F., and Boisvert, P. L. (1944). *J. Pediat.* **25**, 481.

Pulvertaft, R. J. V. (1928). *Brit. J. Exptl. Pathol.* **9**, 276.

Rane, L., and Wyman, L. (1937). *J. Immunol.* **32**, 321.

Rantz, L. A. (1952). "The Prevention of Rheumatic Fever." Thomas, Springfield, Illinois.

Rantz, L. A., Boisvert, P. L., and Spink, W. W. (1946). *New Engl. J. Med.* **235**, 39.

Schuh, V. (1965). *Folia Microbiol. (Prague)* **10**, 156.

Schuh, V., and Hribalova, V. (1966). *Folia Microbiol. (Prague)* **11**, 112.

Schwab, J. H., Watson, D. W., and Cromartie, W. J. (1953). *Proc. Soc. Exptl. Biol. Med.* **82**, 754.

Schwab, J. H., Watson, D. W., and Cromartie, W. J. (1955). *J. Infect. Diseases* **96**, 14.

Stock, A. H. (1939). *J. Immunol.* **36**, 489.

Stock, A. H. (1942). *J. Biol. Chem.* **142**, 777.

Stock, A. H., and Lynn, R. J. (1961). *J. Immunol.* **86**, 561.

Stock, A. H., and Verney, E. (1952). *J. Immunol.* **69**, 373.

Trask, J. D. (1932). *J. Immunol.* **22**, 41.

Veldee, M. V. (1932). *Public Health Rept. (U.S.)* **47**, 1043.

Veldee, M. V. (1938). *Public Health Rept. (U.S.)* **53**, 909.

Veldee, M. V., Peck, E. C., Franklin, J. P., and DuPuy, H. R. (1941). *Public Health Rept. (U.S.)* **56**, 957.

Wasson, V. P., and Brown, E. E. (1942). *Am. Heart J.* **23**, 291.

Watson, D. W. (1954). *In* "Streptococcal Infections" (M. McCarty, ed.), pp. 92–108. Columbia Univ. Press, New York.

Watson, D. W. (1960). *J. Exptl. Med.* **111**, 255.

Watson, D. W., and Cromartie, W. J. (1951). *Bull. Univ. Minn. Hosp.* **22**, 188.

Watson, D. W., and Kim, Y. B. (1964). *In* "Bacterial Endotoxins" (M. Landy and W. Braun, eds.), pp. 522–536. Rutgers Univ. Press, New Brunswick, New Jersey.

Watson, D. W., Cromartie, W. J., Bloom, W. L., Kegeles, G., and Heckly, R. J. (1947). *J. Infect. Diseases* **80**, 28.

Zinsser, H. (1931). "Resistance to Infectious Diseases," 4th ed., Chapter XXII, pp. 452–469. Macmillan, New York.

Staphylococcal α-Toxin*

John P. Arbuthnott

I. Introduction

A. General Remarks

Of the several toxic and potentially toxic products of pathogenic staphylococci, the most potent is the α-toxin. The relative ease with which it can be produced and its striking biological effects have served to attract many investigators. Despite recent advances in our knowledge of this intriguing toxin, much remains to be elucidated; in particular, we still do not know the nature of its substrate or receptor site in cell membranes or its true role in the pathogenesis of human disease.

Three phases seem to emerge in the development of knowledge of staphylococcal toxins. An initial period of activity between 1870 and 1920 comprised the discovery of a "toxin," antitoxin, and the first descriptions of its toxic activities. The second phase, between 1928 and 1940, saw the emergence of α-toxin as a distinct entity. This was initiated by the tragedy in the small Australian town of Bundaberg in which 12 of

*The material for this chapter was compiled in June 1968.

21 children died in the course of immunization against diphtheria. The vaccine was contaminated with a staphylococcus and the Royal Commission (1928) set up to investigate the cause of the fatalities concluded that ". . . death resulted from an overwhelming toxaemia at the early stage of the invasion of the organism." As a result of this, many workers, notably Burnet (1929, 1930, 1931) turned their attention to staphylococcal toxins in general, their multiplicity, production, properties, and their possible roles in pathogenicity and immunization.

The emergence of a potent exotoxin, α-toxin, which was lethal for laboratory animals and which was produced by the vast majority of pathogenic staphylococci led almost logically to the belief that staphylococcal disease was analogous to monotoxic diseases such as diphtheria, and that neutralization of the toxin by its antitoxin would alleviate the symptoms of infection. Both passive immunization with hyperimmune sera and active immunization with toxoid were employed. Many conflicting and contradictory reports were published on the effectiveness of such therapy. At first, results were encouraging, but later reappraisal and use of more rigorous controls indicated that, at best, experimental animals could be protected only for a few days. The general opinion around 1940 was of failure and with the tremendous initial success of antibiotics, interest in staphylococcal toxins fell off markedly. The background to this failure of antitoxic therapy is admirably discussed in the review of Elek (1959).

Two reasons have led to the recent revival of interest in staphylococcal toxins. First, is the realization that staphylococcal infections due to antibiotic resistant strains are a matter of growing concern. Thus, a greater knowledge of the exotoxins of staphylococci and their role in pathogenesis may provide information of direct medical importance. Second, recent interest has focused on the nature and mode of action of cytolytic bacterial toxins from a broader biological viewpoint. They may provide useful tools in the study of the structure and function of membranes and pose interesting questions as to their possible enzymatic nature. The field is now dominated by contemporary biochemical and biophysical techniques. Despite recent advances which have led to a partial understanding of the physical and chemical properties of α-toxin and its site and mechanism of action, it must be emphasized that it is still a relatively "young" toxin; preparations of satisfactory purity (noncrystalline) have been obtained only in the past 5 or 6 years, whereas the classic toxins such as diphtheria, tetanus, and botulinum were all crystallized more than 14 years ago. As will become apparent, fundamental gaps in our knowledge still exist, and the present chapter can at best be considered as a progress report.

B. DISCOVERY OF α-TOXIN

In a consideration of all the qualifications and restrictions of interpreting pioneer work carried out more than 60 years ago, it is clear that the four main properties now associated with staphylococcal α-toxin, lethal action, dermonecrosis, hemolysis, and damage to rabbit leukocytes, had been described by the early 1900's. The first experimental demonstration of a staphylococcal toxin was probably brought by von Leber (1888); the active principle (phlogozin) when precipitated by alcohol and injected into the anterior chamber of the eye of rabbits, caused inflammation. In the same year, De Christmas (1888) reported that culture filtrates and their alcohol precipitates caused inflammation of the skin of the conjunctiva of rabbits. Two years later Breiger and Fraenkel (1890) showed that "toxalbumins" obtained by salting out or alcohol precipitation of culture fluids killed guinea pigs and rabbits: the formation of sterile pus and intense inflammatory reaction with necrosis at the site of injection was also observed. Confirmations of the lethal property of staphylococcal toxin were soon forthcoming from Rodet and Courmont (1892), von Lingelsheim (1900), and Kraus and Pribram (1906). A fundamental contribution was made by van de Velde (1894), who showed that leukocytes in the pleural effusion of rabbits infected with a virulent strain of staphylococcus were badly damaged. The active principle, termed "leukocidin," could be obtained *in vitro*. Van de Velde also noted that both his strains hemolyzed rabbit blood. Neisser and Wechsberg (1901) obtained cell-free hemolysin, confirmed the leukocidic action on rabbit leukocytes, and standardized the technique of assessing hemolysis around colonies of staphylococci on blood agar plates. Antiserum to many of these early preparations neutralized the various toxic activities.

By the early 1900's, then, it was clearly established that cell-free products of the staphylococcus were toxic both *in vivo* and *in vitro*. Certain inconsistences and discrepancies in the results (e.g., heat sensitivity, lethal activity, and hemolytic activity) slowly attracted the attention of some workers but it was only some 20 years later that these led finally to the suspicion that more than one toxin was present in staphylococcal filtrates. Gradually there emerged a differentiation of hemolysins according to the species of erythrocyte on which they acted.

In 1921 Walbum described a hemolysin which did not lyse goat erythrocytes at 37°C but caused rapid lysis on cooling to 0°C. This so-called hot–cold hemolysin was subsequently reinvestigated by Biggar, Boland, and O'Meara (1927) and found to be active on sheep erythrocytes. Moreover, Glenny and Stevens (1935) showed that this second hemolysin was immunologically distinct from the rabbit lysin; they designated the rabbit hemolysin (α-) and the sheep hemolysin (β-), a terminology which has survived to the present time. Several authors suggested that there are at least two serologically distinct rabbit hemolysins (Morgan and Graydon 1936; M. L. Smith and Price, 1938; D. D. Smith, 1956) and the designations α_2- and γ-toxin were introduced. In spite of considerable evidence in favor of the existence of such a lysin, the term γ-toxin has not been generally accepted in the literature.

Williams and Harper (1947) reported the existence of yet another hemolysin, termed δ-hemolysin. This hemolysin was further investigated by Marks and Vaughan (1950) and Marks (1951). Its solubility in organic solvents suggested that it may be lipid in nature but the work of Yoshida (1963) clearly indicates the existence of a proteinaceous toxin of low hemolytic activity, acting nonspecifically on erythrocytes of different species. This toxin together with β-toxin will be reviewed in Chapter 6.

The existence of several serologically distinct hemolysins may well explain the discrepancies and confusion in early work and clearly indicates the care required in designating which particular toxin is being investigated. Preferably three criteria should be used to define a hemolytic staphylococcal toxin — (1) hemolysis (taking into account species sensitivity and potency), (2) animal toxicity, and (3) specific neutralization with antitoxin.

In addition to the hemolytic exotoxins, staphylococci produce a large number of potentially toxic factors and enzymes, including leukocidin, enterotoxin, lipase, phospholipase, protease, phosphatase, hyaluronidase, staphylokinase, and coagulase. Indeed, the greatest difficulty in formulating a working hypothesis for the mechanism of pathogenicity of staphylococci is the evaluation of the relative importance of this plurality of toxic products.

C. Unitarian Hypothesis

Much of the work on α-toxin from 1930 onward was devoted to proving or disproving the "unitarian hypothesis" first put forward by Burnet (1930) that the main activities of α-toxin were manifestations of a single toxic protein. By 1940, the bulk of the available evidence was in favor of the unitarian point of view. Despite a few exceptions, the activities paralleled one another in culture filtrates, their properties were similar, and they could be neutralized in parallel by α-antitoxin. The results of studies employing purified preparations of α-toxin from several different laboratories leave little doubt that the main properties of α-toxin are due to a single toxic substance; highly purified preparations of the toxin judged to be pure by a variety of criteria possessed all the activities attributed to crude α-toxin. Two recent reports lend further support to this view. Manohar *et al.* (1966) showed that heat reactivated α-toxin (Section III, C, 2b) was hemolytic, lethal, and dermonecrotic. Also, the interesting genetic experiments of McLatchey and Rosenblum (1966a), who investigated the properties of α-toxin mutants obtained by ultraviolet irradiation, showed that the majority of mutants lost all three toxic activities, presumably as a result of a single mutational event. However there were isolated a few mutants which were deficient in hemolytic activity but retained, to a varying degree, the lethal and dermonecrotic activities and produced a protein which cross reacted with α-toxin in gel diffusion tests. This suggests either that the α-toxin molecule possesses two or more active sites or that those mutants retaining lethal and dermonecrotic activity but not hemolytic activity produce an α-toxin molecule having an altered primary structure which in turn affects the specificity of a single active site.

II. Toxicity of α-Toxin

A. HEMOLYTIC ACTIVITY

By far the most convenient and sensitive method of assaying staphylococcal α-toxin is by measurement of its hemolytic activity; rabbit erythrocytes are the most sensitive and are most commonly used. Thus, hemolysis presents a rapid method for the determination of specific activity during purification procedures, the specific activity being taken as the number of hemolytic units per milligram of protein. As can be seen in Table I, the sensitivity of the erythrocytes of different species differs widely. Notably, human erythrocytes are particularly resistant to α-toxin. Moreover, it is well known that the erythrocytes of different individuals belonging to the same species vary in sensitivity; for instance, erythrocytes from different rabbits may vary by up to fivefold with the same batch of toxin (Cooper *et al.*, 1966). Such variability has presented problems in the standardization of the hemolytic assay for α-toxin and as yet there is no internationally accepted hemolytic unit. Moreover, the hemolytic assays of different workers involve the use of different times of incubation, different methods of dilution, diluents of different composition, and erythrocyte suspensions of differing concentration. Such factors probably explain the range of values obtained for the hemolytic unit of α-toxin in terms of micrograms of protein. Published results for this value vary between 0.008 μg (Lominski *et al.*, 1963) and 0.6 μg (Robinson and Thatcher, 1963). A detailed comparison of hemolytic units is shown in

TABLE I

RELATIVE SENSITIVITY OF ERYTHROCYTES OF DIFFERENT SPECIES TO α-TOXIN[a]

Species	Sensitivity as compared with the rabbit
Rabbit	100
Wallaby	20
Hamster	11–27
Dog	10–25
Rat	10
Mouse	9
Cat	9
Deer	5
Wood duck	4
Bear	1
Sheep	0.6–1.0
Human	0–0.8
Chicken	0–0.5
Guinea pig	0–0.1
Horse	0–0.06
Monkey	0

[a]From Bernheimer (1968).

Table IV. Some degree of standardization is desirable, and it seems that a procedure such as that adopted by Bernheimer and Schwartz (1963) which can be adapted either for qualitative or quantitative determinations presents a satisfactory, rapid, and reproducible method. When testing an unknown preparation of toxin, reference should be made to a standard preparation of toxin (for instance a crude precipitate of toxin maintained under ammonium sulfate or lyophilized crude toxin) having an arbitrary assigned hemolytic activity (that determined on the first day of testing). Assuming that the standard toxin does not spontaneously lose activity, this procedure circumvents difficulties arising from day to day variation of the erythrocyte suspension. It is interesting to note that a direct comparison of the hemolytic assay of Lominski and Arbuthnott (1962) with that of Bernheimer and Schwartz (1963) revealed a fivefold difference in sensitivity of the assays. Thus, different techniques largely explain the difference in published values for the hemolytic unit. The adoption of an internationally accepted hemolytic unit would greatly facilitate the evaluation of work in different laboratories. These considerations apart, it is clear that a fraction of a microgram of α-toxin is sufficient to cause hemolysis of rabbit erythrocytes, although streptolysin S, cereolysin, and staphylococcal β-toxin, which are hemolytic down to approximately 0.001 μg are weight for weight considerably more hemolytic than staphylococcal α-toxin. The kinetics and mechanism of the hemolytic reaction will be discussed later (Section IV A).

B. LETHAL EFFECT

All species of experimental animals tested thus far have been found to be susceptible to staphylococcal α-toxin. However, there are wide differences in species sensitivity (Table II). When compared on the basis of LD_{50} in micrograms of toxin protein per kilogram of body weight, the rabbit is by far the most sensitive test species and the frog the most resistant. The rapid lethal effect of large doses of α-toxin is striking (Table III). There seems to be a threshold dose below which death is slow and above which it is extremely rapid.

TABLE II
COMPARATIVE TOXICITY OF α-TOXIN FOR EXPERIMENTAL ANIMALS[a]

Species	LD_{50} (μg)	LD_{50} (μg toxin/kg body weight)
Mouse	1	40
Rabbit	5	2
Frog	10	400
Chicken	80	60

[a]Calculated from data of Arbuthnott (1964).

TABLE III
RELATIONSHIP BETWEEN DOSE OF α-TOXIN AND TIME TO DEATH IN MICE[a]

Dose (HU)	Time to death						Mortality (%)
	Minimum		Maximum		Mean		
32,000	11	seconds	32 seconds	17	seconds		100
4,000	20	seconds	40 seconds	36	seconds		100
1,000	1.5	minutes	2 minutes	2	minutes		100
500	4	minutes	6 minutes	5	minutes		100
250	5	minutes	3 hours	1.25	hours		100
128	3	hours	4 days	—			50

[a]From Arbuthnott (1964).

It is customary, but to a large extent meaningless, to calculate the presumed lethal dose of bacterial toxins for man on the basis of the sensitivity of the most sensitive species. When this is done for staphylococcal α-toxin, the presumed lethal dose for man becomes 0.14 mg. Reference to the table of comparative toxicities of a variety of toxins (van Heyningen, 1970) places staphylococcal α-toxin close to *Clostridium welchii* α-toxin. It is therefore comparatively much less toxic than diphtheria, tetanus, and botulinum toxins. The use of data obtained with rabbits to calculate the toxicity for man is misleading, especially since human erythrocytes are known to be many times more resistant than those of the rabbit. It is perhaps more realistic to base an estimate of the lethal dose for man on the toxicity for a species having erythrocytes of comparable sensitivity. When the chicken is used for such a comparison, a value of 4.2 mg is obtained for the presumed toxicity in man. This too may be a fallacious estimate, since the membranes of certain vital cell types may be more or less sensitive than the erythrocyte membrane.

For routine laboratory toxicity tests, rabbits are not suitable on the criteria of size and expense. Thus, the mouse, though less sensitive, is the most commonly used laboratory animal. The results of Bernheimer and Schwartz (1963) and Lominski *et al.* (1963) for the LD_{50} in mice are in good agreement; both reported values of 1.0 μg. However, Goshi *et al.* (1963a) found that the LD_{50} for mice was 12 μg. It is notable that the latter did not use the Wood 46 strain for toxin production and a comparative study of the toxicity of α-toxin preparations from different strains would be useful.

C. ADDITIONAL TOXIC EFFECTS OF α-TOXIN

1. DERMONECROSIS

The injection of small amounts of α-toxin into the skin of experimental animals causes extensive necrosis. The published values of the smallest dose of purified α-toxin causing dermonecrosis in rabbits are in reasonably good agreement. In four independent studies, this value varies between 0.5 and 2.4 μg. of purified toxin. Dermonecrosis, although presenting further evidence of the cytotoxic action of α-toxin, is not entirely suitable for quantitative assay of toxic activity because it is often difficult to measure the extent of the lesion accurately. It is interesting to note that Goshi *et al.* (1963a) observed that the injection of small amounts (1–6 hemolytic units) of purified α-toxin into human skin produced a large inflammatory lesion in 6–24 hours without visible necrosis. The mechanism of the dermonecrotic reaction is probably complex. According to Thal and Egner (1961), dermonecrosis, like other necrotizing effects of α-toxin is due primarily to a selective action of the toxin on the smooth muscle of the blood vessels of the skin, in turn causing anemic infarction of the skin following prolonged local ischemia. However, the well-known cytotoxic effect of α-toxin for a variety of cells in tissue culture raises the possibility that necrosis may result from the direct action of the toxin on skin tissues without necessarily involving vascular effects.

2. EFFECTS ON MUSCLE

Considerable attention has been focused on the myotoxic action of staphylococcal α-toxin, particularly its effect on smooth muscle preparations. That α-toxin causes a contraction and subsequent paralysis of several smooth muscle preparations is now clearly established (Brown et al., 1959; Thal and Egner, 1961; Wiegershausen and Rašková, 1961; Wiegershausen, 1962, 1965; Brown et al., 1965). The effect can be achieved with purified α-toxin and contraction can be prevented by the addition of antitoxin (Wurzel et al., 1966). The contraction proceeds even after the removal of the toxin from the suspending fluid and is accompanied by a loss of sensitivity of the muscle tissue to stimulant drugs such as norepinephrine (Brown and Quilliam, 1965; Wurzel et al., 1966). This contractile effect of α-toxin on smooth muscle appears to be relatively specific, since Wurzel et al. (1966) showed that certain other bacterial toxins, including endotoxin, streptolysin S, streptolysin O, tetanus toxin, and diphtheria toxin did not cause contraction. Wiegershausen considered that the action of α-toxin on smooth muscle results in the release of a contracting substance such as serotonin. However, Brown and Quilliam (1965) neither detected the release of such a substance from guinea pig ileum segments nor succeeded in demonstrating modification of the toxic response by specific antagonists of known spasmogenic agents. These results together with those of Wurzel et al. (1966) suggest a direct action of the toxin on smooth muscle rather than an indirect action mediated by the release of pharmacologically active substances.

Lominski et al. (1962b) reported an action of staphylococcal α-toxin on voluntary muscle of mice in vivo and in vitro. Subcutaneous injection of toxin resulted in flaccid paralysis of the muscles nearest to the site of injection. When large doses of α-toxin were employed, paralysis preceded the appearance of histological lesions. Isolated mouse skeletal muscle treated with α-toxin progressively lost the ability to react to electrical stimulation. Moreover, the fact that isolated muscle preparations from mice previously paralyzed with tubocurarine (known to block nerve endings and the neuromuscular junction) behaved in the same way suggested that the paralysis was due to direct action of the toxin on muscle rather than on nerve. These effects were shown to be specific for α-toxin. Thal and Egner (1961) reported that rabbit skeletal muscle is resistant to α-toxin. However, Gulda (1965) observed that close intraarterial injection of crude α-toxin into denervated rabbit gastrocnemius muscle produced a contraction similar to that induced by acetylcholine. Toxin, however, depressed the normal acetylcholine contraction. Much of the above-mentioned work has been carried out using crude toxin preparations and certain aspects should be reinvestigated employing highly purified α-toxin. The mechanism of action of α-toxin on skeletal muscle is not understood but may involve loss of the normal permeability properties of the muscle cells.

3. Effects on Cells and Subcellular Organelles

a. Cells in Tissue Culture. Damage or destruction of a variety of iso-lated cells and cells in tissue culture by α-toxin has been demonstrated by many workers including Nogrady and Burton (1961), Thal and Egner (1961), Gabliks and Solotorovsky (1962), Felton and Pomerat (1962), Artenstein *et al.* (1963), Madoff *et al.* (1963), Korbecki and Jeljaszewicz (1965), and Jeljaszewicz *et al.* (1965). Among the cell types sensitive to α-toxin are human esophageal epithelium and rabbit fibroblasts, rabbit kid-ney cells, human amnion cells, Krebs 2 ascites tumor cells, K.B. cells, L and monkey kidney cells. Initially, studies of the cytopathic effect of α-toxin on cells in tissue culture involved the use of crude preparations of toxin, yielding results of limited significance. However, the more recent investigations of Madoff *et al.* (1963) and Jeljazewicz *et al.* (1965) were carried out using purified toxin. The former examined the liberation of methionine-^{35}S-labeled protein from toxin-treated cells and found that 68% of labeled protein was released by rabbit kidney cells in tissue cul-ture after a 30-minute contact with 600 hemolytic units of α-toxin. By contrast, human amnion cells were much more resistant. The latter group investigated effects of α-toxin on the enzymatic activities of K.B. cells in culture; loss of 5'-nucleosidase activity, decrease in glucose utilization and lactic acid production, and disappearance of dehydrogenases were the most striking effects. Recently, inhibition of the ability of washed sus-pensions of Krebs 2 ascites tumor cells to oxidize glucose has been noted (Symington and Arbuthnott, 1969) together with a striking stimulation of succinate oxidation (Fig. 1). Marked morphological changes in Krebs 2 ascites tumor cells, detected using phase contrast microscopy, have been reported (Madoff *et al.,* 1963), Toner *et al.* (1969) have reinvestigated these morphological effects using electron microscopy. Preliminary results indicate that the main changes include loss of normal mem-brane convolutions and loss of electron density of the cytoplasm fol-lowing treatment with α-toxin (Fig. 2). All the cytopathic effects of α-toxin so far described can be explained by an action of the toxin on the cell membrane, resulting in disorganization of the membrane and loss of the cell's normal permeability properties. In some cases, the end result of such a functional impairment is lysis of the cell.

The introduction of an assay system for α-toxin based on its cytopathic action may be useful for some purposes. Recently, Felsenfeld and Felsen-feld (1966) have employed a method for the estimation of both α-toxin and α-antitoxin based on the titration of the cytopathogenic effect in human embryonic kidney cell cultures.

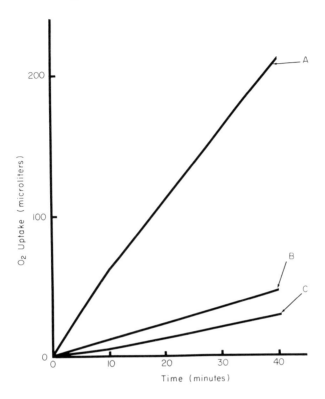

FIG. 1. Effect of purified α-toxin on succinate oxidation by washed suspensions of Krebs 2 ascites tumor cells. A=cell treated with 430 HU α-toxin per milliliter for 30 minutes; B=control suspension; C=endogenous respiration. (Symington and Arbuthnott, 1969).

b. Polymorphonuclear Leukocytes and Platelets. As indicated by Gladstone (1966), the existence of at least three staphylococcal extracellular products (α-toxin, Penton Valentine leukocidin, and δ-toxin) each capable of killing leukocytes led to confusion in early work. Again, the availability of purified preparations has clarified the position to some extent and the comparative activities of the three factors have been described by Gladstone (1966). Although α-toxin is well known to be toxic for rabbit leukocytes, there is conflicting evidence regarding its effect on human leukocytes. Goshi *et al.* (1963a) claimed that α-toxin affected both human and rabbit leukocytes, whereas Gladstone (1966) confirmed the early work of Wright (1936), finding that human leukocytes were resistant to large doses of α-toxin (up to 350 μg). Toxin-treated polymorphs appeared microscopically normal and retained their ability to move across glass. By

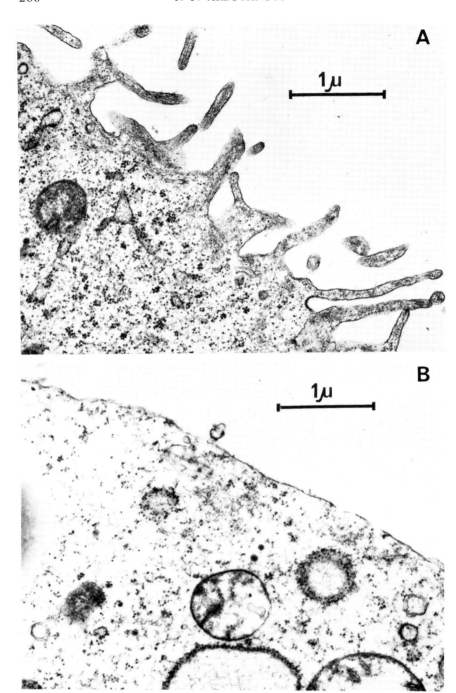

contrast, Gladstone (1966) also found human monocytes to be sensitive to α-toxin. A possible reason for the conflicting reports of Goshi *et al.* (1963a) and Gladstone (1966) may lie in the fact that different strains were employed for toxin production, emphasizing the need for comparative study of α-toxin preparations from different strains.

The ability of staphylococci to destroy platelets was first described by Gengou (1935a,b) who rightly attributed the effect to the action of α-toxin. This effect was not reinvestigated until 1964 when Siegel and Cohen (1964) reported that staphylococcal α-toxin caused loss of structural and functional integrity of platelets. Bernheimer and Schwartz (1965a) using purified toxin then carried out a comprehensive study of the action of staphylococcal α-toxin and several other bacterial toxins on rabbit platelets. α-Toxin caused a rapid reduction in the optical density of platelet suspensions and loss of contents into the suspending medium; phase contrast microscopy revealed gross structural damage. The amount of toxin required to cause half-maximum reduction in optical density was 0.5 μg. Other hemolytic bacterial toxins shared the capacity to affect platelets in this way, while nonhemolytic toxins did not. Jeljaszewicz *et al.* (1966) have suggested that the lysis of platelets by α-toxin is preceded by aggregation. More recently, Manohar *et al.* (1967) have confirmed the platelet-damaging activity of α-toxin, and their finding that heat-reactivated α-toxin is platelet-damaging leaves little doubt that the effect is another manifestation of the toxicity of the α-toxin moiety. Electron microscopy of toxin-treated platelets (Manohar *et al.*, 1967) revealed loss of cell contents and irregularities in the outline of the cell membrane. The final magnification (× 30,000) was probably too low to reveal further details of membrane damage.

c. Wall-less bacteria. It is well known that intact bacteria are resistant to α-toxin. However, in an interesting series of papers, Bernheimer and his co-workers (Bernheimer and Schwartz, 1965b; Bernheimer and Davidson, 1965; Bernheimer, 1966) showed that protoplasts and L forms derived from a number of gram-positive species were lysed by small amounts of 70% pure α-toxin. By contrast, spheroplasts and L forms from a selection of gram-negative bacteria were either considerably more resistant to or unaffected by the toxin. These experiments suggested that a systematic analysis of cell membranes from resistant and sensitive species might reveal the nature of the substrate or receptor for α-toxin. How-

---

FIG. 2. Fine structural changes in Krebs 2 ascites tumor cells following treatment with 800 HU purified α-toxin: (A) surface of an untreated cell showing normal surface projections; (B) surface of a toxin treated cell showing loss of electron density and loss of surface projections (Toner *et al.*, 1969).

ever, the most recent work of Bernheimer *et al.* (1968a), has shown that the lytic action of α-toxin preparations on protoplasts and spheroplasts may be due to the presence of small contaminating amounts of δ-toxin. α-Toxin purified by careful density gradient ultracentrifugation did not lyse protoplasts and spheroplasts in amounts of 50 μg. It seems, therefore, that certain toxic activities previously attributed to α-toxin must be reinvestigated. Toxin neutralized by α-antitoxin and by heating must be included in such investigations. Indeed a convenient method for the preparation of monospecific α-antitoxin would be of considerable value in this respect (Section V,A). Also, comparative studies of the actions of highly purified staphylococcal α- and δ-toxins in a number of systems are required.

  d. Subcellular organelles. Bernheimer and Schwartz (1964) investigated the disruption of leukocyte lysosomes by a number of bacterial toxins. Again the known cytolytic toxins, including purified α-toxin and δ-toxin had striking lytic effects; that of staphylococcal α-toxin was neutralized by antitoxin. It was also notable that, whereas α-toxin both lysed leukocyte lysosomes and caused the release of marker enzymes from liver lysosome preparations, δ-toxin acted only on the leukocyte lysosomes. There is evidence, however, that α-toxin does not affect all intracellular organelles. For instance, Lominski *et al.* (1964) found that purified α-toxin did not impair succinic oxidase activity of mouse liver mitochondria. Moreover, Gemmell (1968) has found that α-toxin, unlike succinic oxidase factor, does not induce mitochondrial swelling as judged by decrease in optical density at 540 mμ. This substantiates the observation of Paradisi (1967) that even tissue culture cells showing marked cytopathic effect due to α-toxin contained normal mitochondria. We can speculate, therefore, that whereas the lysosomal membrane is susceptible to the action of α-toxin, the outer mitochondrial membrane is resistant.

  e. Artificial models. Although it is doubtful whether one can refer properly to the action of bacterial toxins on artificial systems in terms of "toxicity," it is interesting to note at this point that purified preparations of α-toxin caused leakage of trapped ions from artificial phospholipid membranes (Weissmann *et al.*, 1966). Also, Freer *et al.* (1968) have shown that highly purified α-toxin caused extensive morphological changes in these artificial membranes (Section IV,A).

  From the above summary of the diverse toxic activities of staphylococcal α-toxin, it is clear that this toxin is a cytolytic toxin having a broad spectrum of activity. The term "catholic cytotoxin" introduced by Elek (1959) is appropriately descriptive. However, many studies have not involved the use of toxin of the highest purity and even purified preparations may contain traces of contaminating toxic proteins. Thus, it is still uncertain whether all of the cytotoxic properties attributed to α-toxin are due solely to the action of α-toxin. Nevertheless, if investigators had awaited the availability of absolutely pure toxin, the experiments would not have been carried out and much invaluable information missed. A more definitive evaluation of the toxicity of α-toxin, especially at the cellular and subcellular level, must await future experimentation.

III. Production and Nature of α-Toxin

A. PRODUCTION

There is little detailed knowledge of the factors which affect the production of α-toxin. Certain empirical rules exist, which, if followed, will ensure good yields. This situation is not surprising, since the main aim of most workers has been the study of the nature and mode of action of the toxin rather than its production and biosynthesis.

1. TEST ORGANISM

Although α-toxin is produced by the vast majority of coagulase-positive staphylococci, one particular strain, Wood 46, has been employed since the time of Burnet. In the author's opinion, Wood 46 is not outstanding in toxigenicity; some strains routinely isolated from human infections show comparable toxin production. As is the case with many other toxins, the organism tends to lose toxigenicity on repeated subculturing. Elek (1959) holds the view that the level of toxin production in a culture reflects a balance between α-toxin positive and α-toxin negative variants present in the population, and in order to obtain high levels of toxin, the environmental conditions must favor the predominance of the α-toxin positive variant. That conditions *in vivo* favor such selection was supported by the finding that passage in rabbits yielded organisms of high toxigenicity (Mercier and Richou, 1944). Moreover, W. D. Foster (1963) has shown that even strains which are α-toxin negative *in vitro* produce toxin *in vivo*. As with diphtheria toxin and other bacterial toxins, there appears to be a relationship between toxigenicity and lysogeny. In 1961, Blair and Carr showed that toxigenicity could be conferred on nontoxigenic strains by lysogenization with phages from toxigenic strains.

2. CULTURAL CONDITIONS

The first effort to standardize production of staphylococcal toxin was made by Neisser and Wechsberg (1901); the basis of their media was meat infusion broth. Such media, however, did not yield high titers of

α-toxin. Walbum (1909) and Russ (1916) introduced the technique of extracting cultures of staphylococci grown on solid media. This procedure resulted in fluids rich in hemolysin. The next major advance was made by Parker, Hopkins, and Gunther (1926) who achieved a marked increase in toxic activity by incubating cultures in 10% carbon dioxide, 90% air. Soon after this, Burnet (1930) combined the use of agar and carbon dioxide to obtain high titers of α-toxin. Using a semisolid nutrient medium and an atmosphere of 20% carbon dioxide, 80% air, he achieved good toxin production. This method proved reliable and variations of it have been employed in several recent studies (Kumar and Lindorfer, 1962; Robinson and Thatcher, 1963; Lominski et al., 1963). The main disadvantage of this method is the technical inconvenience in preparing large quantities of crude toxin for purification.

The beneficial effect of carbon dioxide has not yet been fully explained. That it acts as a buffer preventing an excessive rise in pH (to pH > 7.5) is certain, and this may largely explain its activity (Elek, 1959). However, attempts to replace carbon dioxide by buffering the medium have not proved entirely successful. Moreover, Burnet (1930) described mutants which produced high yields of α-toxin in the absence of carbon dioxide. The work of Ganczarski (1962), who demonstrated the incorporation of $^{14}CO_2$ into staphylococcal proteins, including the α-toxin moiety, suggested the possibility that carbon dioxide fixation reactions may play a role in the formation of one of the amino acids essential for toxin production. If this is so, it should be possible to replace the requirement for carbon dioxide by the addition of the products of carbon dioxide fixation (e.g., oxaloacetic acid). Such experiments have not, to the author's knowledge, been reported. It would also be of interest to compare the rate of incorporation of labeled carbon dioxide or amino acids into α-toxin and total cellular protein.

The enhancement of toxin production by small amounts of agar is easier to explain. McLean (1937) suggested that agar acts by absorbing some unidentified component of the metabolism or product of the staphylococcus inhibitory to toxin production. Its action can be simulated by other absorbent materials. Seiffert (1935) and McLean (1937) showed that cellophane, kieselguhr, kaolin, and even pieces of filter paper acted in the same way. The polysaccharide portion of agar was found to remove inhibitory material, while the calcium portion was inhibitory by itself (McIlwain, 1938). The use of solid or semisolid media is, however, inconvenient and alternative methods employing shaken liquid cultures proved more useful. Initially, such shaken culture methods were unreliable. The rate and direction of shaking proved to be critical —

e.g., Favorite and Hammon (1941) found horizontal shaking gave good toxin production, while end over end shaking yielded almost no toxin. Also, overvigorous shaking gave low yields presumably because of inactivation of the toxin due to denaturation (Gladstone, 1938; Rud, 1955). These difficulties have since been largely overcome. Madoff and Weinstein (1962) successfully employed a casein hydrolyzate medium using an atmosphere of 30% carbon dioxide, 70% oxygen. Subsequently, Bernheimer and Schwartz (1963) introduced a method based on the use of liquid media comprising casein hydrolyzate and yeast diffusate. The presence of yeast diffusate removed the requirement for the addition of carbon dioxide to the atmosphere. Such methods regularly yield crude toxin of high titer and are suitable for production of large volumes of crude toxin for purification. Coulter (1966) also employed a liquid medium aerated with 70% oxygen, 30% carbon dioxide.

Extremely little is known about the specific nutrient requirements for α-toxin production. Following the work of Knight and his co-workers (Knight, 1935, 1937a,b,c; Knight and McIlwain, 1938), who showed that nicotinic acid, nicotinamide, and thiamine were required for good growth of staphylococci in a basal medium of amino acids, these compounds and crude preparations of yeast extract have regularly been incorporated into media for toxin production (Favorite and Hammon, 1941; Bramann and Norlin, 1951; Bernheimer and Schwartz, 1963).

Few attempts have been made to produce α-toxin in chemically defined media. However, in 1938, Gladstone carried out a comprehensive study of the amino acids required for toxin production. In a complete medium containing 16 amino acids, thiamine, nicotinamide, glucose, and inorganic salts which supported the growth of staphylococci, only traces of toxin were formed. However, working on the basis that the further addition of selected amino acids, especially arginine, stimulated toxin production (Gengou, 1935b), Gladstone (1938) succeeded in producing increased yields of toxin in fully synthetic media. Not only the individual amino acids but also their relative concentrations were important. The basic requirement was for arginine, glycine, alanine, proline, valine, phenylalanine, lysine, tryptophan, and methionine. Under these conditions, the presence of oxygen was essential for production and carbon dioxide enhanced the yield. Perhaps the relatively low yields of toxin obtained using this defined medium discouraged further attempts to employ fully synthetic media. It seems likely that the interrelationships of individual amino acids is extremely complex. Nevertheless, an extension of these early findings may throw light on the mechanism of biosynthesis of α-toxin. The production of α-toxin *in vivo* will be discussed in Section VI.

3. BIOSYNTHESIS OF α-TOXIN *in Vitro*

Since staphylococcal α-toxin is a typical protein (Section III, C), it is presumed that its biosynthesis is by reactions typical of general protein synthesis. However, toxin biosynthesis is not simply related to the formation of cellular protein, since it is possible to obtain good growth of toxigenic staphylococci without toxin production. Environmental factors play an important role, and the mechanism of control of α-toxin synthesis is not understood. The work of de Repentigny and his co-workers (Sonea *et al.*, 1965; Turgeon *et al.*, 1966) has shown that the purine and pyrimidine antagonists, 8-azaguanine and 5-fluorouracil cause reduced growth and virulence of strain Wood 46 and also a reduction in the number of antigenic components of crude toxin. More recently, this group (Leboeuf-Trudeau *et al.*, 1967) reported that the tryptophan analogs 4- and 5-methyltryptophans and 7-azatryptophan caused loss of the hemolytic and lethal activities of strain Wood 46 which could be reversed by the addition of L-tryptophan, anthranilic acid, or indole. Thus, impairment of normal nucleic acid and protein synthesis appears to result in impaired toxin production.

The interesting transductional analysis of recombination between α-toxin mutants (McClatchey and Rosenblum, 1966b) suggested that at least two genetic loci are involved in toxin synthesis. They also suggest the existence of a regulatory gene controlling both α-toxin and fibrinolysin production. The extension of this genetic approach should be most fruitful.

There are conflicting views on the mechanism of release of α-toxin during growth. Raynaud *et al.* (1955), who carried out a comprehensive study of the secretion of a number of bacterial toxins, observed that α-toxin was liberated into the culture fluid during the logarithmic phase of growth after a lag of approximately 1 hour. Figure 3 shows the time course of α-toxin production in a complex shaken liquid medium (McNiven and Arbuthnott, unpublished) aerated with 70% oxygen, 30% carbon dioxide. Such a pattern of events suggested that α-toxin is a true extracellular toxin (Pollock, 1962), the toxin being released without apparent autolysis. However, Bernheimer and Schwartz (1961) observed that culture filtrates from 24-hour cultures contained fairly large amounts of nucleic acid, which they considered as resulting from autolysis during growth. Thus, the evidence at present is not conclusive.

If α-toxin and other cytolytic toxins are indeed released without autolysis, then the mechanism of their release presents an interesting biological problem. It has been shown (Bernheimer and Schwartz, 1965b) that protoplasts and spheroplasts from a variety of bacteria were lysed by

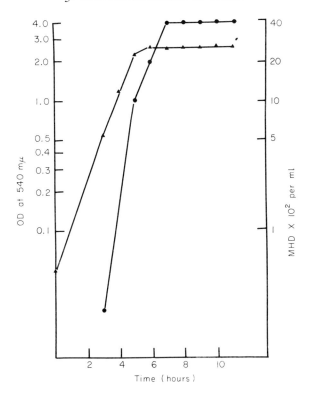

FIG. 3. Production of α-toxin by strain Wood 46 in a shaken culture in nutrient broth at a temperature of 37°C in an atmosphere of 70% oxygen, 30% carbon dioxide. ▲ = growth as measured by OD at 540 mμ; ● = hemolytic titer (McNiven and Arbuthnott, 1968).

cytolytic toxins. Even protoplasts prepared from the parent strain Wood 46 were lysed. Thus, cytolytic toxins are capable of damaging the membranes of bacterial cells. How then are such membrane-damaging toxins released from the bacterial cell without causing irreversible damage to the parent cell? Three possibilities appear likely. (1) potentially self-damaging cytolytic toxins may be secreted as inactive precursors or protoxins which subsequently become activated extracellularly; (2) the interior surface of the bacterial cell membrane may be inherently resistant to the action of such toxins; (3) such toxins are synthesized or activated between the outer surface of the cell membrane and the cell wall (Pollock, 1962). An investigation, similar to that of Gerwing *et al.* (1968), of the cytoplasmic contents of staphylococci at different times during growth may throw light on this problem.

In summary, it can be said that although relatively little is known about the factors controlling toxin production or the mechanism of its secretion from the staphylococcus, methods have been developed which yield high titer toxin suitable for purification.

B. PURIFICATION

Within the past 5 years staphylococcal α-toxin has been purified to a high degree in a number of laboratories (Madoff and Weinstein, 1962; Kumar and Lindorfer, 1962; Goshi *et al.,* 1963a; Robinson and Thatcher, 1963; Jackson, 1963; Bernheimer and Schwartz, 1963; Lominski *et al.,* 1963; Cooper *et al.,* 1966; Coulter, 1966; Arbuthnott *et al.,* 1967). The properties of these preparations are summarized in Table IV. Although highly purified toxin has been obtained, which by a number of criteria behaved as a single protein, none of the methods has resulted thus far in crystallization. In summarizing factors affecting purification we must bear in mind the possibility that the purification procedures may to some extent alter the toxin molecule. Indeed, Haque (1967) considers that results obtained with highly purified toxin may be misleading.

Early attempts to fractionate α-toxin were concerned with the production of potent toxoid for therapeutic use (Holt, 1936; Boivin and Izard, 1937; Kodama and Nishiyama, 1938) and of toxin for investigating the toxoiding reaction mechanism (Burnet and Freeman, 1932). After a lapse of some 10 years, the problem was reexamined with the sole aim of purification (Wittler and Pillemer, 1948). These investigators devised a method involving strict control of pH, temperature, ionic strength, protein concentration, and methanol concentration. This yielded a potent preparation of toxin, subsequently shown to be impure. Nevertheless, the first stages of the method of Wittler and Pillemer (1948) are suitable for concentrating crude toxin and have been retained by some workers (Lominski *et al.,* 1963; Coulter, 1966). In 1954 Turpin *et al.* developed a complex procedure combining many of the previous methods. The product was potent but again impure. The method of Butler (1959) yielded neither potent nor serologically pure toxin. By contrast with these early partially purified preparations which were concentrated but impure, the first reports of the production of toxin judged to be pure, on the basis of immunological tests (Madoff and Weinstein, 1962; Kumar and Lindorfer, 1962; Goshi *et al.,* 1963a), suffered from a major limitation; the final preparations contained very small amounts of toxic protein which was often highly unstable. An important contribution was made by Bernheimer and Schwartz (1963). Their method of purification, which combined the use of fractional precipitation with ammonium sulfate, continuous paper curtain electrophoresis, density gradient ultracentrifugation, and electrophoresis in sucrose gradients yielded potent toxin of high purity. Much of the subsequent work on the effects of α-toxin on various membrane-bound systems was done using this material. In the same year, Lominski *et al.* (1963) described a method which combined gel filtration on G75 and DEAE-A50 Sephadexes with methanol fractionation under carefully controlled conditions. Yields of toxin were low but the material, by different criteria, behaved in a similar manner to that of Bernheimer and Schwartz (1963). This method has recently been employed successfully by Felsenfeld and Felsenfeld (1966). Coulter (1966) reinvestigated the purification of α-toxin, using partial purification by the method of Wittler and Pillemer (1948) followed by gel filtration on Sephadex G100 and subsequent electrophoresis on columns of Sephadex G100. Again the product appeared to be pure by several criteria. Coulter's preparations however were highly unstable, having a half-life of only 3 days when stored at 0°C. More recently in the course of work on the study of the physical properties of α-toxin, Arbuthnott *et al.* (1967) showed that heat aggregated α-toxin could be disaggregated and reactivated by treatment with 8 *M* urea. Reactivated toxin after the removal of urea possessed similar physical chemical and biological properties to native α-toxin and the method also resulted in substantial purification. At present the possibility that heat purified α-toxin suffers from some degree of irreversible alteration in tertiary structure cannot be excluded (Arbuthnott *et al.*, 1967).

No generally accepted purification procedure has yet been adopted for staphylococcal α-toxin. Recent methods vary considerably in details of methodology, presumably largely as a result of the differing facilities available in different laboratories. Nevertheless, a few general points have emerged concerning factors influencing purification. It is desirable to start with large volumes of crude toxin having high titer; the use of nonproteinaceous culture media for toxin production probably simplifies the task of isolating purified toxin. The first stages of purification must involve concentration of the toxic protein. This can be achieved conveniently by salting out with ammonium sulfate or precipitation with methanol at pH 4.0 at temperatures below −5°C. Subsequent purification can be achieved by a variety of procedures. However, the high isoelectric point of *a*-toxin (pI 8.6) (Wadstrom, 1968) probably explains the success of preparative electrophoretic methods (paper curtain, density gradient, gel, isoelectric focusing) and of ion exchange chromatography (DEAE-Sephadex, DEAE-cellulose, carboxymethylcellulose). Further purification and concentration can be achieved by fractional precipitation with ammonium sulfate. Organic solvents, e.g., methanol, if used at this stage of purification, must be employed under extremely carefully controlled conditions of temperature. Moreover, it is now clear that highly purified staphylococcal α-toxin

TABLE IV

COMPARISON OF PURIFICATION PROCEDURES AND PROPERTIES OF α-TOXIN[a]

Authors	Strain	Purification procedure	Hemolytic unit (μg)	Mouse LD$_{50}$ (μg)	Specific activity	Precipitation lines—Ouchterlony or immunoelectrophoresis	Chemical nature	Physical properties
Kumar et al. (1962)	Wood 46	(1) Continuous curtain electrophoresis; pH 5.6 (2) Refractionation; pH 8.6	?	?	800 HU/ml[b]	1	Protein carbohydrate	M.W. = 10,000–15,000; 1.4 S
Bernheimer and Schwartz (1963)	Wood 46	(1) Fractional precipitation with ammonium sulfate (2) Curtain electrophoresis (3) Zone electrophoresis in sucrose density gradient (4) Ultracentrifugation in sucrose density gradient	0.05	1	19,000 HU/mg	1	Protein	M.W. = 44,000: 90% 3 S, 10% 12 S: 4 components in electrophoresis (all active)
Goshi et al. (1963a)	Local strain phage type 80/81/42B/52	(1) Precipitation with acetic acid and TCA; 4° C (2) Methanol 15%; 4° C (3) DEAE-cellulose column (4) Hydroxyapatite column	0.012	12	80,000 HU/mg[c]	1	90% protein, 10% carbohydrate	No data
Lominski et al. (1963)	Wood 46	(1) Acetic acid–methanol precipitation; −5° C (2) Sephadex G 75 column (3) Sephadex DEAE A50 column, pH 6.5 (4) Methanol fractionation (5) DEAE A50 Sephadex column, pH 5.8	0.008	1	119,000 HU/mg	1	Protein	90% 3.1 S, 10% 16 S
Jackson (1963)	(1) Wood 46 (2) "209-60"	(1) Zinc acetate precipitation (2) Ethanol; −10° to −20° C (3) Hydroxyapatite column	0.2	3.9	?	?	Protein	No data

	Local strain phage type	Purification		?		?	Protein	
Robinson and Thatcher (1963)	80/81	(1) Zinc acetate precipitation (2) Ethanol −10°C (3) Carboxymethyl cellulose, column (4) Starch gel electrophoresis	0.6	?	?	?	Protein	No data
Cooper et al.[a] (1966)	Wood 46	(1) Zinc acetate precipitation (2) Sephadex G25 (3) Curtain electrophoresis (4) DEAE-cellulose column (5) Carboxymethyl cellulose column	0.21	?	1,200,000 HU/ml	1	Protein	2.8 S
Coulter (1966)	Wood 46	(1) Acetic acid-methanol precipitation (2) Acetate extraction (3) Sephadex G100 column (4) Electrophoresis on Sephadex G100	?	?	10,000 HU/mg	1	Protein	2.8 S; M.W. = 29,600 and 21,200; spontaneous aggregation to insoluble precipitate
Arbuthnott et al. (1967)	Wood 46	(1) Partial purification by method of Bernheimer and Schwartz (1963) (2) Heated 1 minute at 60°C (3) 8 M urea; pH 8.3 (4) Dialysis 0.03 M borate; pH 8.3	0.05	1	20,400 HU/mg	1	Protein	90% 3 S, 10% 12 S; S value in urea = 1.9S

[a] Modified from Gladstone (1966).
[b] Cited by Manohar et al. (1966).
[c] Calculated from data of Goshi et al. (1963a).
[d] Modification of the original method of Madoff and Weinstein (1962).

may undergo spontaneous aggregation to high molecular weight polymers of low biological activity (Section III, C, 2a). Although the conditions governing aggregation are still poorly understood, it is advisable not to maintain pure toxin in solution under conditions of low ionic strength. Also, unnecessary freezing and thawing and lyophilization should be avoided. Different workers are not in total agreement about the stability of α-toxin, but storage of purified preparations under 70-90% ammonium sulfate at 0-4°C is probably the best storage method.

Multiple criteria should be employed to assess purity. Analytical centrifugation, Ouchterlony double diffusion tests, and immunoelectrophoresis are convenient and sensitive indicators of purity. Disk gel electrophoresis may be valuable but, caution must be exercised in analyzing spontaneously aggregating proteins such as staphylococcal α-toxin by this method. Moreover, it has recently been shown that small amounts of a second hemolysin, probably δ-toxin, may be present even in highly purified preparations of α-toxin (Freer et al., 1968; Bernheimer et al., 1968a). As yet, a simple method for total removal of δ-toxin does not exist, but Bernheimer et al. (1968a) have successfully removed δ-toxin by carefully controlled density gradient ultracentrifugation. Since many of these factors have only recently been determined, results pertaining to the mode of action of α-toxin obtained employing impure toxin preparations may require reinvestigation.

C. Chemical and Physical Nature

1. Chemical Nature

Purified α-toxin consists almost entirely of protein and its activity is destroyed by proteolytic enzymes (Lominski and Arbuthnott, 1962; Bernheimer and Schwartz, 1963; Coulter, 1966). The presence of up to 10% of carbohydrate has been recorded by Goshi et al. (1963a), who found that treatment with both α- and β-amylase destroyed the toxic activity of their preparations. The effects of amylases, particularly β-amylase, could not be explained by the presence of contaminating proteolytic enzymes. On the basis of these findings, Goshi et al. proposed that α-toxin was a protein-polysaccharide complex. By contrast, Bernheimer and Schwartz (1963) found less than 1% carbohydrate measured as glucose and Felsenfeld and Felsenfeld (1966) reported only 1.3% carbohydrate. This discrepancy has not yet been satisfactorily explained, although it may be significant that Bernheimer and Schwartz (1963) employed strain Wood 46 while Goshi et al. (1963a) used a locally isolated phage type 80/81 strain.

Amino acid analyses have been carried out independently by Bernheimer and Schwartz (1963) and Coulter (1966) (Table V). These findings are in fair agreement, despite minor discrepancies, and indicate that α-toxin contains no unusual amino acids. It is notable that both groups of workers reported the absence of cysteine, indicating that α-toxin contains no disulfide bridges or free sulfhydryl groups. Coulter (1966) suggested that the high positive charge carried by α-toxin may be explained if most of the glutamic and aspartic acid residues are present as glutamine and asparagine. The high concentration of ammonia in the hydrolyzate supports this suggestion. In addition the N-terminal amino acids, as determined by Coulter (1966), were arginine and histidine. Neither is commonly present in the N-terminal position of proteins (Noll, 1966), although *Clostridium botulinum* type B toxin has arginine as N-terminal amino acid (Gerwing *et al.*, 1966).

TABLE V

AMINO ACID COMPOSITION OF α-TOXIN

Constituent	Residues calculated on a M.W. = 44,000 (Bernheimer and Schwartz, 1963)	Residues calculated on a M.W. = 21,000 (Coulter, 1966)[a]
Lysine	23	13 (26)
Histidine	4	2 (4)
Ammonia	71	52 (104)
Arginine	10	4 (8)
Aspartic acid	44	25 (50)
Threonine	23	12 (24)
Serine	22	10 (20)
Glutamic acid	21	11 (22)
Proline	7	5 (10)
Glycine	23	12 (24)
Alanine	12	7 (14)
Valine	12	8 (16)
Methionine	10	2[b] (4)
Isoleucine	13	8 (16)
Leucine	15	7 (14)
Tyrosine	9	5 (10)
Phenylalanine	10	5 (10)
Cysteic acid	0	?
Cystine	0	—
Tryptophan	?	?

[a]Figures in parentheses represent Coulter's data calculated on a M.W. = 42,000 for direct comparison with Bernheimer's data.
[b]Total of methionine + methionine sulfoxide + methionine sulfone.

2. PHYSICAL PROPERTIES OF α-TOXIN

a. Molecular aggregation. Highly purified preparations of α-toxin characteristically show the presence of a slow-moving peak in the ultracentrifuge, having a sedimentation coefficient of 2.8–3.1 S (Bernheimer and Schwartz, 1963; Lominski *et al.*, 1963; Cooper *et al.*, 1966; Coulter, 1966). The presence of an additional small fast-moving peak (accounting for 10–15 % of the total protein) with a sedimentation coefficient of 12–16 S was reported independently by Bernheimer and Schwartz (1963) and Lominski *et al.* (1963). The significance of the 12 S component, which possesses little or no lethal and hemolytic activity and can be separated from the 3 S component by density gradient ultracentrifugation, has been reinvestigated recently (Arbuthnott *et al.*, 1967). Three pieces of evidence suggested that the 12 S component is a molecular aggregate of α-toxin: (1) purified 12 S material was disaggregated by urea to yield biologically active toxin; (2) the 12 S component spontaneously reformed when urea solutions of heat aggregated α-toxin were dialyzed against 0.03 M borate buffer pH 8.3; the amount of 12 S component in such preparations was similar to that observed in unheated partially purified toxin; (3) in Ouchterlony double diffusion tests, purified 12 S material gave a line of partial identity with the main α-toxin line of precipitation. Thus, the heavy component was termed α_{12S}-toxin. Purified α_{12S}-toxin also had a strikingly uniform appearance when examined by negative staining in the electron microscope (Fig. 5a). It consisted of small rings having an outside diameter of approximately 90 Å which appeared to consist of a hexagonal arrangement of six subunits each measuring 20–25 Å in diameter. It has since been shown to have a molecular wight of 250,000–300,000 (Forlani, unpublished). As yet, little is known about the conditions which lead to the formation of α_{12S}. However, the constancy of the ratio between α_{12S} and α_{3S} in purified preparations suggests an equilibrium between the two forms. More recently, Freer *et al.* (1968) observed that α_{12S} formation was induced by artificial phospholipid spherules (Section IV, A).

The existence of even larger aggregates of α-toxin was first suggested by Coulter (1966) who observed the formation of an insoluble precipitate in purified α-toxin preparations after standing at 0°C. This nontoxic insoluble material, when injected into rabbits gave rise to toxin-neutralizing antibody. The recent work of Arbuthnott *et al.* (1967) supports Coulter's hypothesis. They obtained an insoluble precipitate, which had no biological activity, by brief heating at 60°C. This material could be disaggregated by 8 M urea to yield biologically active toxin (Table VI). Subsequent removal of urea by dialysis yielded a product which closely resembled native α-toxin in its physical properties and biological activity. The possi-

TABLE VI
HEAT AGGREGATION AND UREA DISAGGREGATION OF α TOXIN[a]

Sample	Protein (mg/ml)	HU/ml	Initial protein (%)	Initial hemolytic activity (%)	Specific activity
Stage 5 toxin	6.5	50,000	100	100	7,700
Supernatant fluid after heating	3.5	2,400	67	6	685
Precipitate in PBS	—	<20	—	<0.05	—
Precipitate dissolved in 8 M urea	7.3	80,000	30	44	11,000
Supernatant fluid from dialysis	2.6	53,000	12	32	20,400
Precipitate from dialysis	—	85	—	0.05	—
Precipitate from dialysis dissolved in 8 M urea	6.12	26,000	13	6.7	4,320

[a] From Arbuthnott et al. (1967).

ble significance of such aggregation reactions in the explanation of the "Arrhenius effect" will be referred to in Section III, C, 2b. The degree and nature of aggregation probably depends on a number of factors including purity, ionic strength, protein concentration, pH, and temperature. The possibility that high molecular weight aggregates of α-toxin do not consist exclusively of α-toxin molecules cannot be completely excluded at present (Bernheimer, 1968).

There is increasing evidence that the characteristic biologically active form of staphylococcal α-toxin (α_{3S}) is itself not molecularly homogeneous (Bernheimer, 1968). Sucrose density gradient electrophoresis of purified α-toxin revealed the presence of three or four distinct peaks having different electrophoretic mobilities but similar biological activities (Bernheimer and Schwartz, 1963). Moreover, recent data for highly purified α-toxin examined by ultracentrifugation (Forlani, unpublished) and by isoelectric focusing (Wadstrom, 1968) have shown that the α_{3S} component is not homogeneous. Molecular weight determinations by a variety of methods (Bernheimer and Schwartz, 1963; Coulter, 1966) support this conclusion; α_{3S}-toxin appears to consist of a mixture of molecules having molecular weights between 21,000 and 50,000. There is also some evidence that α_{3S}-toxin can be disaggregated to a 1.9 S component in urea (Arbuthnott et al., 1967). Current work, therefore, suggests that α-toxin exists in varying degrees of molecular association and in this respect resembles a number of other bacterial toxins.

b. Heat Stability—the "Arrhenius Effect." Most proteins are denatured on heating, although a few, notably ribonuclease, are relatively heat stable. There have been numerous conflicting reports on the heat sensitivity of staphylococcal α-toxin. As early as 1900, it was apparent that different preparations of staphylococcal toxin differed in heat stability. In 1907, Arrhenius observed the paradoxical effect toward heat now known as the "Arrhenius effect." He showed that crude toxin, when heated to 70°C lost almost all of its hemolytic activity, but that reheating of the inactive mixture to 100°C resulted in the reappearance of a substantial portion of hemolytic activity. This unusual property has since attracted the attention of numerous investigators. A possible explanation was first put forward by Landsteiner and von Rauchenbichler (1909) who suggested that the inactivation at low temperature was due to the formation of an inactive complex consisting of toxin and a component of the culture filtrate; subsequently reheating to a higher temperature was said to dissociate the complex with the release of active toxin. Such an explanation assumes that α-toxin is intrinsically heat stable.

The Arrhenius effect was not, however, easily repeatable and the work of Landsteiner and von Rauchenbichler (1909) was ignored for some years. Conflicting reports on the heat stability of α-toxin continued to appear throughout the 1930's. This led Tager (1941) to undertake a comprehensive study of the inactivation at 60°C. He demonstrated that a variety of autolytic products of bacteria and other substances, including pepsin and lecithin, combined with the toxin at 60° but not at 80°C. In 1959, Elek concluded that "all this evidence suggests that α-lysin itself is highly thermostable and the apparent inactivation is due to another mechanism."

Reinvestigation of the effect of heat awaited the preparation of highly purified α-toxin. The studies of Manohar *et al.* (1966) and Cooper *et al.* (1966) were at first sight contradictory, although each provided valuable information. The former demonstrated reappearance of hemolytic, lethal, and dermonecrotic activities on reheating 60°-inactivated crude α-toxin to 100°C. Thus, heat-reactivated toxin had the same biological activities as native unheated toxin. On one hand, Manohar *et al.* (1966) reported that purified α-toxin could not be reactivated at 100°C after prior inactivation at 60°C. On the other hand, Cooper *et al.* (1966), who used more concentrated preparations of toxin, found an appreciable reactivation when 60°-inactivated, purified toxin was reheated at 80°C. Cooper *et al.* (1966) also observed that heating to 60°C resulted in the formation of an insoluble precipitate which, when harvested and reheated to 80°C, liberated detectable amounts of active toxin. Cooper *et al.* (1966) interpreted these results in terms of denaturation of toxin at 60°C with formation of insoluble denatured protein containing some trapped soluble toxin which was released on further heating to 80°C. They suggested that much of the controversy surrounding the Arrhenius effect was due to the use of toxin preparations of differing potency and purity, prolonged heating periods, and different temperatures. Subsequently, Arbuthnott *et al.* (1967) demonstrated that the insoluble precipitate obtained at 60°C could be reversibly disaggregated by treatment with 8 *M* urea. It seems likely, therefore, that heating for short periods at 60°C induces aggregation of active α-toxin to an insoluble, nontoxic form, and that reheating to higher temperatures results in a partial reversal of this reaction with the release of soluble active toxin. This soluble toxin itself is probably destroyed if the reheating period is prolonged or if the temperature is raised to 100°C. Such an explanation differs from that of Cooper *et al.* (1966) mainly in terminology; the term "denaturation" implies irreversible alteration of the toxic protein. In 1907, therefore, Arrhenius posed an intriguing problem which has remained a topic of controversy until the present day.

IV. Mechanism of Action

A. *In Vitro* MEMBRANE INTERACTIONS

From studies of the cytotoxicity of staphylococcal α-toxin (Section II, C), it became clear that the toxin had a direct action on cells, probably due to its effect on the cell membrane. The exact nature of the reaction between α-toxin and cell membranes is not yet fully understood. Despite an intensive search in a number of laboratories, no substrate or receptor substance has been demonstrated unequivocally. The lack of a known substrate has presented difficulties in investigating the mode of action of α-toxin. Most work has been carried out using hemolysis of rabbit erythrocytes as a quantitative method of assay. This system suffers from the inherent limitation that hemolysis represents the end result of a series of events and is thus an indirect assay. Recently, artificial phospholipid membrane systems known as spherules or liposomes have been employed. These also suffer from a major limitation in that they cannot be considered as being necessarily identical to natural membranes.

A further understanding of the mode of action of many cytolytic toxins awaits the elucidation of the physicochemical structure of membranes, which is a subject of intense current interest. Indeed, cytolytic toxins may present the biochemist with valuable tools for the investigation of membrane structure. The recent work of Lenard and Singer (1968) using *Clostridium welchii* α-toxin supports this view.

1. KINETICS OF HEMOLYSIS

Most work on the kinetics of hemolysis of staphylococcal α-toxin has centered around the possibility that the toxin is an enzyme. In the early 1930's, Forssman (1933, 1934a,b,c) first postulated that staphylococcal hemolysin was enzymatic. He suggested this on the grounds that the reaction between the hemolysin and erythrocytes of rabbit and sheep was characterized by a weak, irregular, and easily reversible adsorption. However, Levine (1938, 1939) observed that the hemolytic, dermonecrotic, and lethal effects of the toxin were strongly adsorbed by concentrated suspensions of erythrocytes. From this, he concluded that the reaction obeyed the Freundlich adsorption isotherm, implying that the reaction between toxin and erythrocytes was stoichiometric. This dialogue continued with the statement of Forssman (1939) that "to embody these phenomena in a mathematical formula is not an easy task. At any rate they cannot be classed under the formula employed by Levine."

The quantitative kinetics of hemolysis of a number of bacterial toxins other than those of *Staphylococcus aureus* were first investigated by Bernheimer (1944, 1947). He compared these agents with some known surface active agents such as saponin. Bernheimer concluded at that time that "in view of the fact that all the lytic agents showing the direct proportionality appear to be proteins, it seems not improbable that some or all of the lysins of this class are enzymes." A turbidimetric assay of the kinetics of hemolysis of staphylococcal α-toxin was introduced by Mangalo and Raynaud (1959) who determined a mathematical relationship between the time to reach 50% hemolysis and the concentration of α-toxin; no conclusion was reached as to the enzymatic nature of the toxin. Lominski and Arbuthnott (1962) reinvestigated the kinetics of hemolysis. The S-shaped curves typical of hemolysis by α-toxin can be seen in Fig. 4. There is a characteristic prelytic lag phase, followed by a period of rapid hemolysis, and finally, a tailing off. Taking the slopes of the curves at the time of maximum rate of hemolysis as an index of the velocity of the reaction, they observed that the rate of hemolysis was directly proportional to the concentration of toxin at low α-toxin concentrations. Split titration experiments indicated little or no loss of toxin in the course of hemolysis. These findings were not inconsistent with the toxin being enzymatic. A more detailed investigation of the kinetics of hemolysis was carried out independently by Marucci (1963a,b) and Madoff and his co-workers (1964; Cooper *et al.*, 1964a, b); both groups obtained evidence in favor of the enzymatic hypothesis. The primary interaction between α-toxin and the erythrocytes, which occurred in the prelytic phase, resulted in the loss of the selective permeability of the erythrocyte membrane as evidenced by

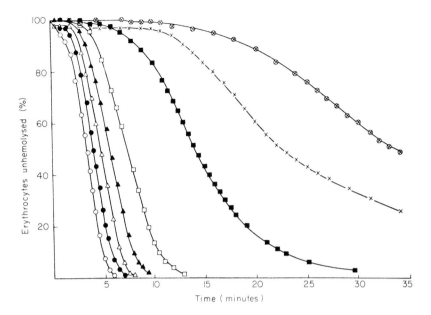

FIG. 4. Kinetics of hemolysis of rabbit erythrocytes by different concentrations of α-toxin: ○ = 160 MHD/ml; ● = 80 MHD/ml; △ = 40 MHD/ml; ▲ = 30 MHD/ml; □ = 20 MHD/ml; ■ = 10 MHD/ml; × = 5 MHD/ml; ⊕ = 2.5 MHD/ml. (Lominski and Arbuthnott, 1962).

leakage of potassium ions. Subsequent lysis of the damaged erythrocytes was independent of the continued presence of toxin. During the prelytic phase toxin became rapidly adsorbed on the erythrocyte surface and could be visualized by fluorescent antibody (Klainer et al., 1964). The addition of antitoxin very early in the prelytic phase prevented lysis and the release of potassium ions. However, if the addition of antitoxin was delayed, then hemolysis could not be inhibited. Certain osmotic stabilizers — e.g., sucrose and polyethylene glycol — prevented hemolysis, probably due to protection of the irreversibly damaged erythrocyte membrane from osmotic shock (Cooper et al., 1964b). Unlike Lominski and Arbuthnott (1962), Madoff et al. (1964) observed that α-toxin was used up in the hemolytic reaction. This difference may reflect a difference in the purity of the preparations used; the former used only partially purified toxin, whereas the latter employed highly purified toxin.

Although these studies of the kinetics of hemolysis suggested an enzymatic action of α-toxin during the prelytic phase on a substrate present in the erythrocyte membrane, the substrate has not yet been identified. Moreover, there has been no unequivocal demonstration of a correlation between α-toxin activity and any known enzyme present in staphylococcal culture filtrates (see reviews of Bernheimer, 1965; Gladstone, 1966). At present, evidence in favor of the enzymatic mode of action of α-toxin cannot be considered conclusive.

2. ARTIFICIAL MEMBRANES

The artificial phospholipid model membranes characterized by Bangham and his co-workers (Bangham and Horne, 1964; Bangham et al., 1965a,b), known as spherules or liposomes, possess selective permeability properties having many features in common with natural membranes. In addition, their lamellar structure, as revealed in the electron microscope, is characteristically myelinic (Fig. 5b). The physical and biological properties of spherules have been reviewed in detail by Sessa and Weissmann (1968).

When prepared in salt solutions, spherules trap ions between the constituent bilayers and the subsequent release of trapped ions has been used as a model system to study the activity of a number of surface-active agents including steroids, drugs, detergents, and polyene antibiotics. Thus, Weissmann et al. (1966) studied the effects of staphylococcal α-toxin on spherules of varying lipid composition. Like streptolysin S, α-toxin caused rapid release of cations, anions, and other marker molecules from the spherules; prior incubation with α-antitoxin neutralized the lytic effect. The spherulytic action of α-toxin was independent of the net surface charge, since spherules containing dicetyl phosphate were as sensitive as those containing stearylamine. Moreover, both staphylococcal α-toxin and streptolysin S induced the release of trapped ions independent of the presence of cholesterol in the artificial membrane. These findings indicated that staphylococcal α-toxin acted on the phospholipid component of spherules and that the interaction may involve hydrophobic portions of the toxic protein.

This aspect has recently been extended by Freer et al. (1968) who reinvestigated the action of highly purified α-toxin on spherules composed of lecithin, cholesterol, and dicetyl phosphate (70:10:20) and carried out a comparative study of morphological changes caused by α-toxin in both artificial and natural membranes. Employing highly purified α-toxin, they confirmed the lytic effect on spherules and isolated a second lytic factor

---

FIG. 5. Interaction of α-toxin with spherules (lecithin-cholesterol-dicetyl phosphate; 70:10:20). (A) Purified α_{12S}-toxin showing hexagonal packing of molecules (arrows). (B) Preparation of lipid spherules showing concentric lipid bilayers. (C) Lipid spherules after treatment with heat purified α-toxin: rings can be seen on the surface of lipid sheets. All preparations were examined by negative staining (Freer et al., 1968).

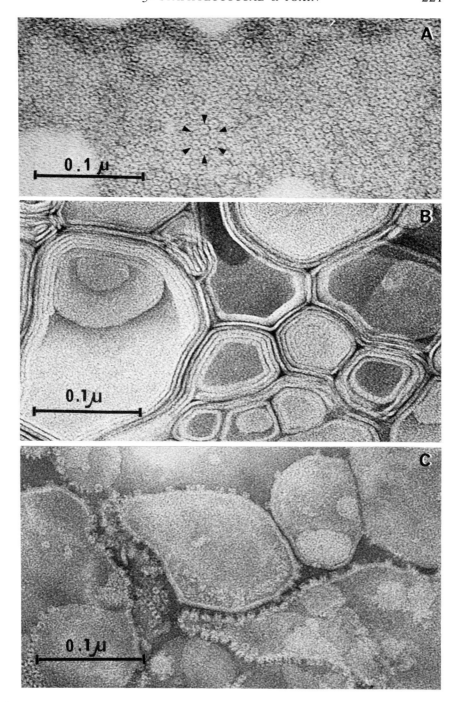

(release factor) from partially pure toxin. Purified α_{12S}-toxin which was only weakly hemolytic for rabbit erythrocytes had a marked lytic effect on spherules. The disruption of spherules was accompanied by the appearance of ring structures (Fig. 5c), having similar dimensions to α_{12S}-toxin, and adsorption of toxic protein. The morphological changes differed considerably from those produced by streptolysin S (Bangham et al., 1965b). A detailed study of ring formation suggested that α-toxin polymerized on the surface of the lipid membranes to form aggregates closely resembling α_{12S}-toxin. Experiments carried out on lipid monolayers having the same molar ratio of lipids as the spherules revealed changes in the surface pressure and surface potential consistent with a penetration of the monolayers by α-toxin due to a hydrophobic interaction.

That the effects of α-toxin on artificial membranes bore some relationship to its action on natural membranes was shown by the fact that ring structures appeared on α-toxin-treated erythrocyte ghosts (Figs. 6a and b); both rabbit and human ghosts induced ring formation. While rings appeared randomly distributed on rabbit ghosts, the distribution was often rectilinear on human ghosts. It must be stressed however that no rings were observed on erythrocytes harvested prior to hemolysis. Thus, ring formation on ghosts may represent a secondary interaction between α-toxin and an already partially disorganized membrane.

The work of Woodin and Wieneke (1966a,b) indicated that staphylococcal leukocidin also undergoes polymerization on cell membranes and dispersed phospholipids. In addition, Kapral (1967) has reported the inactivation of staphylococcal δ-toxin by phospholipids.

Three possible hypotheses could account for the mechanism of action of α-toxin at the molecular level: (1) α-toxin may interact reversibly, but not necessarily enzymatically, with a phospholipid component of cell membranes causing disorganization of the membrane, loss of selective permeability, and subsequent lysis; (2) α-toxin may become adsorbed on cell membranes by hydrophobic interaction, and once specifically orientated, may become enzymatically active, causing hydrolytic cleavage of an as yet unidentified substrate and subsequent lysis; (3) α-toxin may be a mutant or incomplete enzyme capable of interacting with its substrate but unable to hydrolyze it; such an interaction may result in disorganization of the cell membrane. Two experimental approaches may throw light on this obviously complex interaction. A detailed comparison of the compo-

Fig. 6.   Interaction of α-toxin with erythrocyte ghosts.(A) Membrane fragment from α-toxin-lysed rabbit erythrocyte ghost. (B) Fragment of osmotically lysed human erythrocyte ghost after treatment with α-toxin. Note random arrangement of rings on rabbit ghost and rectilinear arrays on human ghost. (Freer et al., 1968).

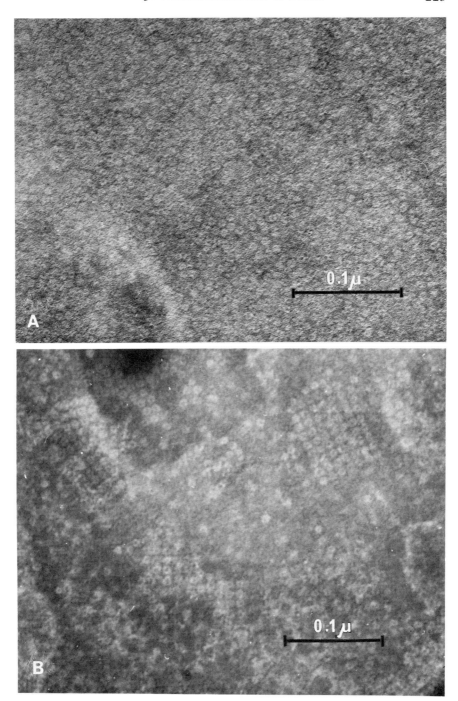

sition and structure of sensitive and resistant membranes (both the lipid and protein components), together with a study of the physicochemical conditions governing the action of α-toxin on artificial membranes of varying composition may yield further information on the nature of the α-toxin–membrane interaction. Moreover, the use of aromatic polysulfonic acid inhibitors of α-toxin may provide a clue to the nature of the active site on the toxin molecule (Robson Wright *et al.*, 1968; Arbuthnott *et al.*, 1968).

B. MECHANISM OF ACTION *in Vivo*

The many toxic effects of staphylococcal α-toxin observed *in vitro* serve only to underline the problem of explaining the mode of action of this toxin *in vivo*; it is extremely difficult to evaluate which *in vitro* effect, if any, predominates *in vivo*. It is also clear that α-toxin acts on the membranes of different cell types, and therefore, that it does not possess the strikingly specific *in vivo* action typical of certain other bacterial exotoxins. Moreover, workers in different disciplines have approached the problem from different standpoints. Microbiologists and biochemists have concentrated their efforts on the purification, the chemical and physical nature, and the mechanism of action of the toxin in relatively simple *in vitro* systems with the hope that a uniform working hypothesis of the mode of action would emerge. By contrast, physiologists and pharmacologists have been concerned with evaluating the dominant physiological changes in the whole animal brought about by crude preparations of staphylococcal α-toxin. This latter approach is entirely justifiable, since α-toxin itself is probably not the sole determining factor in staphylococcal disease. Thus, a study of the whole crude toxic complex containing in addition to α-toxin, leukocidin, δ-toxin, and other factors can be judged to be of greater value. Nevertheless, in considering the mode of action of α-toxin itself, the latter approach is necessarily of limited value. At this time, little can be said of the pharmacological action of highly purified preparations of α-toxin *in vivo*. Also the preceding discussion of the mechanism of action of α-toxin *in vitro* emphasized the complexity of the problem. When one considers all the possible interactions involved in the whole animal, the situation becomes even more complex. It therefore must be emphasised that the combined efforts of workers in several disciplines will be required to determine the main effects of α-toxin *in vivo*. Such studies must involve the use of highly purified α-toxin. They may well yield findings of intrinsic and fundamental interest to physiologists and pharmacologists.

Certain general points can be made, which apply to both crude and purified α-toxin. For instance, the time to death is dose-dependent; large doses kill extremely rapidly, whereas small doses kill only over a prolonged period (1–4 days). The causes of death in rapid and slow death are probably quite different. This is emphasized by the fact that rapid death is characterized by few distinctive histological changes whereas slow death is accompanied by severe kidney necrosis. Also, the symptoms of death are similar for crude and purified α-toxin. With large doses, animals show unsteadiness, irregularity in the breathing and death occurs after intermittent tetanic spasms although at death the body and limbs are completely flaccid. With intermediate doses, the animal remains normal for a period of time, then becomes progressively weaker, shows staring of the coat, a drop in body temperature, and reduced respiration; the animal may remain comatose for periods up to an hour or even longer. Such symptoms by themselves reveal little about the mode of action of the toxin, but do suggest a basic similarity between crude and purified α-toxin.

Early work on the physiological and pharmacological effects of α-toxin *in vivo* have been admirably reviewed by Elek (1959). It is merely intended at this point to summarize the main findings. The action of crude staphylococcal toxin on blood pressure, on the heart, on the small vessels, and on the nervous system were all recorded prior to 1920 (van de Velde and Denys, 1895; Neisser and Levaditi, 1901; Kraus and Pribram, 1906; Russ, 1916; Le Fèvre de Aric, 1919). Kelloway *et al.* (1930) carried out a detailed study of the effect of crude toxin on the blood pressure of rabbits and cats. Intravenous injection of toxin caused an initial fall in blood pressure, then an "excessive recovery" followed by a rapid terminal drop. The initial fall was shown to be due to pharmacologically active constituents of the medium and the recovery to the release of adrenaline. The terminal fall was considered to result from the obstruction of the pulmonary circulation. In addition, toxin was found to have an effect on the heart itself, and death of experimental animals was considered to result from the combined effects of these actions. However, Rigdon (1935) found no obstruction of the pulmonary circulation. In addition to finding a progressive fall in blood pressure, Nélis *et al.* (1934) described the appearance of cardiac irregularities on electrocardiograms; the work of Dingle *et al.* (1937), however, did not confirm these findings. The necrotic action of staphylococcal α-toxin on skin and kidney has been long known (Neisser and Levaditi, 1901). On injection of sublethal doses of α-toxin, De Navasquez (1938) observed typical symmetrical cortical necrosis of the kidney and suggested paralysis of the interlobal arteries and efferent arterioles resulting in stasis and necrosis. Distension of the glomerular capillaries with leakage of toxin and subsequent damage of the cells of the epithelium was the suggested mechanism of von Glahn and Weld (1935) and this was supported by the work of Simmonds *et al.* (1946). The possibility that the ischemic effect was due entirely to vasospasm of the small vessels has been argued by Thal (1951) and Thal and Egner (1954, 1961). Similarly, Thal and Molestina (1955) found that direct introduction of toxin into the pancreatic duct caused a highly fatal hemorrhagic pancreatic necrosis due to suppression of the pancreatic blood flow. Spasm of the smooth muscle of the blood vessels could explain the fatal drop in blood pressure.

The action of crude staphylococcal α-toxin on the central nervous system was described by Travassos (1933a,b). Intracerebral injection of the toxin caused spasm, rapid respiration, and finally Cheyne–Stokes breathing. Also, direct injection into the lumbar region of the spinal chord resulted in paralysis of the hind legs and spreading of the symptoms to the cerebral region. A direct action of the toxin on the respiratory center was suggested by Nélis (1935) and Nélis and Bonnet (1935). Although many other effects were noted, the above-mentioned are the best documented and most significant. Therefore, by 1960 it was clear that crude preparations of staphylococcal toxin acted on the peripheral circulation, on the heart, and on the central nervous system. It is interesting to note that despite its powerful hemolytic activity staphylococcal α-toxin is not considered to act *in vivo* primarily by causing intravascular hemolysis. Intravascular hemolysis does occur but to a highly variable extent and the degree of hemolysis is insufficient to explain rapid death even in the rabbit, which is the most sensitive species. Since 1960, most work on the effects of α-toxin has been carried out on isolated organs and tissues *in vitro*. The striking paralysis of smooth muscle preparations has already been referred to. Wiegershausen (1960, 1962) also examined the action of crude toxin on perfused isolated heart muscle from a number of species. The rabbit, fowl, and cat were found to be sensitive while the common snail, and to a lesser extent, the guinea pig, were resistant. Together with the systolic arrest, toxin caused constriction of the coronary arteries. It is difficult to conclude from Wiegershausen's experiments whether cardiac arrest resulted from restricted flow of nutrient through constricted coronary arteries, whether the effect was direct on muscle, or whether both contributed. Since cardiac arrest *in vitro* is preceded by a long time lag of up to 20 minutes, it is doubtful whether such an effect can by itself explain rapid death which occurs in a considerably shorter time. This serves to emphasize the difficulty of transposing results obtained *in vitro* to observations made *in vivo*. The work of Wurzel *et al.* (1966) also underlines this point; they concluded that the amount of purified toxin required to cause paralysis of smooth muscle *in vitro* was some ten times greater than the lethal dose in rabbits.

Lominski *et al.* (1965) examined the lethal effect of crude and purified toxin in cold-blooded animals. They observed that death, as judged by a number of criteria, preceded cardiac arrest and concluded that, in cold-blooded animals at least, the predominant effect of toxin may be on the central nervous system.

The possibility that the release of pharmacologically active substances plays a role *in vivo* is also a subject of controversy. On the one hand, the work of Wiegershausen supports such a hypothesis, while the investigations of Brown and his co-workers suggest that the release of such substances *in vivo* does not play a dominant role.

Two Czechoslovakian groups (Šamánek and Zajíc, 1965; Švihovec *et al.*, 1965), carried out detailed investigations of pharmacological effects of crude toxin *in vivo*. The former concluded that the most striking finding was the gradual decline in cardiac output and the increase of the peripheral resistance, the main carotid artery pressure rising in the initial phase and falling rapidly in the terminal phase. Small decreases in the respiratory and pulse rates were recorded with a definite fall in the preterminal phase. The latter group emphasized the role of blood pressure changes, possibly resulting from an effect on smooth muscle of the blood vessels. Thus, at the present time, no unified concept of the mode of action of α-toxin *in vivo* exists. We must await further work with highly purified preparations.

V. Immunology

A. Toxoid and Antitoxin

Staphylococcal α-toxin and its toxoid are antigenic in most experimental animals. Subcutaneous or intramuscular injection of toxoid alone or with adjuvant elicits the formation of circulating antibody which neutralizes the several toxic activities of α-toxin and precipitates the antigen *in vitro*. Limited available evidence (Felsenfeld and Felsenfeld, 1966) indicates that the toxin neutralizing antibody belongs to the IgG class of immunoglobulins; IgM and IgA did not neutralize the toxin. This study, however, was based on neutralization of the cytopathic effect of purified α-toxin in tissue cultures and the immunoglobulin fractions were obtained from pooled sera of humans suffering from chronic staphylococcal infection. A further detailed study of the nature of the immunoglobulins produced in experimental immunization with α-toxoid would seem to be required.

Antitoxic levels in serum can be accurately determined using neuralization of the hemolytic effect as indicator. A standard international unit (IU) of antitoxin was introduced in 1938 by M. L. Smith and Ipsen and is still in use. Limitations affecting the determination of the hemolytic unit of α-toxin (Section II, A) also apply to the neutralization test. However, the circular definition of a hemolytic unit (Lh) based on the use of standard antiserum presents an alternative to the direct hemolytic assay. The use of antitoxin strips to differentiate hemolysin patterns on rabbit and sheep blood agar (Elek and Levy, 1950) presents a suitable method for the rapid screening of strains for toxin production.

The toxoiding of α-toxin with formaldehyde was investigated by Burnet and Freeman (1932). The rate of toxoiding was found to be dependent on the concentration of formaldehyde and to be proportional to the square root of the hydroxyl ion concentration; the reaction had a high temperature coefficient. Crude α-toxin, therefore, can be readily toxoided by overnight incubation at 37°C at a slightly alkaline pH, in the presence of 0.4% formaldehyde. Such treatment results in almost complete inactivation of hemolytic activity, and this rapid toxoiding reaction contrasts with the long incubation periods required for other bacterial toxins. Recently, Bernheimer et al. (1968b) have shown that highly purified α-toxin could be toxoided at low concentrations of formaldehyde. The product, by gel filtration on Sephadex, had a similar molecular weight to α_{3S}-toxin. This contrasts with the findings of Murphy (1967) (for tetanus toxin) who reported the formation of high molecular weight polymers during the toxoiding reaction. A detailed study of the influence of different concentrations of formaldehyde and different concentrations of toxic protein should be undertaken since high concentrations of formaldehyde may well induce aggregation of α-toxin.

That nontoxic aggregates of α-toxin elicited the formation of toxin-neutralizing antibody was shown by Coulter (1966). Insoluble aggregate, spontaneously formed in the cold, induced antitoxin production in rabbits. Moreover, the α_{12S}-aggregate gave a reaction of partial identity with the α-toxin line of precipitation in Ouchterlony double diffusion tests (Arbuthnott et al., 1967). Such aggregates may be of value in the preparation of monospecific antisera. A useful method for the production of monospecific antibody has been described by Goudie et al. (1966). The α-toxin precipitin line from gel diffusion tests was cut out, washed, and the antigen–antibody complex was emulsified in the complete Freund's adjuvant and injected into the popliteal lymph nodes of the rabbit. The use of such specific antitoxin should be of great value in elucidating further the biological activity of α-toxin.

Crude α-toxin itself has been reported to have adjuvant activity. In 1936, Swift and Schultz observed that "staphylotoxin" enhanced the immune response to beef lens protein. This adjuvant effect may reflect the action of α-toxin on the membranes of antibody-forming cells (Munoz, 1964). A detailed study of the adjuvant activity of purified α-toxin may prove rewarding. Another interesting immunological effect of α-toxin and α-toxoid has been investigated by Goshi and his co-workers (1963b; E. W. Smith *et al.*, 1963). Intracutaneous injection of α-toxin or toxoid in humans and experimental animals having raised serum levels of antitoxin causes a hypersensitivity reaction. In man the reaction is biphasic. The initial phase is characterized by a wheal and flare response and by cellular changes indistinguishable from the immediate reactions of ragweed and timothy antigens. The second phase consisted of the formation of an indurated area of erythema, the dimensions of which could be correlated with the serum antitoxin level.

B. Immunity

Immunity to staphylococcal infection has been the subject of much recent discussion and speculation (Rodgers and Melly, 1965; Ekstedt, 1965). The detailed critical review of Elek (1959) emphasized the lack of convincing evidence that acquired or passive immunity to α-toxin protected against staphylococcal infection in man and animals. At best, an increased survival time in lethal infections, or reduction in size of local lesions could be achieved.

In certain types of experimental infection, however, the protective role of α-antitoxin can be demonstrated. For instance, Kapral (1965) studying experimental staphylococcal peritonitis in mice found that a conventional, noncapsulated strain of staphylococcus (18Z) killed 60% of the mice in 15 hours; administration of antitoxin 2 hours prior to challenge, greatly reduced mortality. However, injection of antitoxin prior to infection with the capsulated "diffuse type" Smith strain, although resulting in an increased survival time, did not significantly reduce mortality. Also, antitoxin has been shown to protect against staphylococcal rabbit-burn infections (Johnson, 1966). These models, however, represent only two of the numerous ways of studying staphylococcal infection and the current view remains that, in general, α-antitoxic immunity by itself is not protective. Unlike monotoxic diseases such as diphtheria, no single staphylococcal product has been shown to play a dominant role, and staphylococcal infection can best be described as multifactorial (Rodgers and Melly, 1965). Many different vaccines — e.g. those incorporating whole cells, and cell fractions (Stamp, 1961), coagulase (Lominski *et al.*, 1962a), surface polysaccharide (Fisher *et al.*, 1963), and leukocidin toxoid (Mudd *et al.*, 1965) — have been tested with varying degrees of success. Assessment of the relative value of these vaccines is difficult because different experimental models were employed. Also, there is evidence that different strains of staphylococci may produce different types of infection. For instance, a vaccine rich in coagulase protected rabbits against phage group III staphylococci but not against phage group I organisms (Lominski *et al.*, 1962a). In addition, the capsulated "diffuse type" Smith strains show markedly increased virulence in mice as compared with "compact" or wild type strains (Koenig and Melly, 1965). Immunization with heat-killed Smith "diffuse type" cells or capsular material will confer a high degree of protection against such strains. Thus, any generalization about staphylococcal immunity at this time is of doubtful value. However, Rodgers (1966) has expressed the interesting, if pessimistic, view that clinical staphylococcal disease observed in experimental animals and adult humans probably represents an infection superimposed on a high degree of natural humoral immunity. Active immunization is therefore unlikely to prove successful. In his view, attention should be focused now on methods of stimulating nonspecific mechanisms of immunity.

VI. Role in Pathogenicity

It is accepted that the mechanism of staphylococcal pathogenicity is extremely complex. "It is generally held that none of the extracellular products that are characteristic of pathogenic staphylococci has thus far been shown unequivocally to be a major determinant of infection and disease" (Blair, 1965). Indeed, the extracellular armory of the pathogenic staphylococcus is impressive. It includes α-toxin, β-toxin, δ-toxin, enterotoxin, leukocidin, coagulase, hyaluronidase, nuclease, lecithinase, lipase, and protease. Moreover, the great importance of surface components such as bound coagulase and capsular material is now realized. Therefore, it is impossible to view the role of α-toxin in isolation. However, dismissal of α-toxin as a contributory factor is equally untenable.

For α-toxin to exert its effect *in vivo* it must be produced in sufficient quantity. There is now direct evidence that hemolysin is formed in detectable amounts *in vivo* (Cohn, 1963a; W. D. Foster, 1963; E. A. Foster, 1965, 1967). The elegant demonstration by E. A. Foster (1965, 1967) of hemolysin production in the rabbit kidney is particularly noteworthy. Foster's studies suggested that both α- and δ-toxin were produced *in vivo*. In addition, Kapral (1965) has extended the earlier work of Gladstone and Glencross (1959) who showed the formation of α-toxin by cultures of staphylococci grown in dialysis sacs implanted in the peritoneal cavity. Both capsulated and noncapsulated strains yielded considerable amounts of toxin when grown under these conditions (Kapral, 1965). Moreover, the kinetics of α-toxin production *in vivo* and *in vitro* were not dissimilar. Toxin was produced only during active cell division, the amount remaining constant when the stationary phase was reached. Kapral's data also suggested that toxin production *in vivo* was adaptive and that fully induced organisms showed a tenfold increase in the virulence for mice by the intraperitoneal route in comparison with noninduced organisms. Staphylococci, therefore, can produce substantial amounts of α-toxin *in vivo*. Also as mentioned previously, the prior injection of α-antitoxin substantially reduced the mortality of mice challenged with staphylococci by the intraperitoneal route.

A working hypothesis has been proposed by Kapral (1965) for the role of α-toxin in the mouse intraperitoneal model. Using this system, Cohn (1963a,b,c) showed that the primary host defence mechanism was phagocytosis by peritoneal mononuclear cells and invading granulocytes. Subsequently, Kapral (1965) suggested that conventional noncapsulated staphylococci rapidly formed large aggregates in the peritoneum due to the action of bound coagulase. He suggested that the organisms at the center of such clumps were protected from phagocytosis, could multiply, and produce a lethal amount of α-toxin. By contrast, the more virulent capsulated strains do not clump and are resistant to phagocytosis by virtue of their capsules; again, death is thought to result from the elaboration of α-toxin. A similar role for bound coagulase in mouse kidney infections has been suggested by Gorrill *et al.* (1966). Such model systems, although providing useful information, are necessarily artificial, and conclusions based on such results do not hold for all types of staphylococcal infection. Challenge by the intraperitoneal route, for instance, cannot be compared directly with other routes of injection. Moreover, observations made in mice and rabbits cannot be directly extrapolated to humans. Human polymorphonuclear leukocytes are resistant to α-toxin, while those of the mouse and rabbit are sensitive (Gladstone, 1966). Thus, in human infections, δ-toxin and leukocidin, which are leukocidic for human leukocytes, probably play an important role in the spread of infection by neutralizing the protective effect of phagocytosis.

It seems likely that the role of α-toxin in pathogenicity depends on the type of lesion produced. In a localized lesion such as a skin or kidney abscess, the necrotic effect of α-toxin will contribute to tissue damage. In septicemia, lethal amounts of α-toxin may be produced, and similarities have been noted between the symptoms of α-toxin death in experimental animals and certain symptoms seen in staphylococcal septicemia. It also seems likely that α-toxin may act synergistically with other extracellular products of the staphylococcus. For instance, α-toxin may destroy the normal permeability properties of cells, allowing the entry of agents capable of disrupting normal cellular metabolism such as succinic oxidase factor (Lominski *et al.*, 1968), nuclease, and lipases. The development of more sensitive methods for determining the amounts of α-toxin and other staphylococcal products present in the tissues and the blood stream during experimental infections together with a detailed study of the time sequence of the elaboration of these products in disease may allow a new experimental approach to a study of the mechanism of pathogenicity.

ACKNOWLEDGMENTS

The author thanks the late Professor Iwo Lominski for facilities, Dr. C. G. Gemmell for reading the manuscript, and Mrs. M. G. Marshall for secretarial assistance.

REFERENCES

Arbuthnott, J. P. (1964). Ph.D. Thesis, University of Glasgow.
Arbuthnott, J. P., Freer, J. H., and Bernheimer, A. W. (1967). *J. Bacteriol.* **94**, 1170.
Arbuthnott, J. P., Lominski, I. R. W., and Robson Wright, M. (1968). *Biochem. J.* **108**, 49.
Arrhenius, S. (1907). "Immunochemistry." Macmillan, New York.
Artenstein, M. S., Madoff, M. A., and Weinstein, L. (1963). *Yale J. Biol. Med.* **35**, 373.
Bangham, A. D., and Horne, R. W. (1964). *J. Mol. Biol.* **8**, 660.
Bangham, A. D., Standish, M. M., and Watkins, J. C. (1965a). *J. Mol. Biol.* **13**, 238.
Bangham, A. D., Standish, M. M., and Weissmann, G. (1965b). *J. Mol. Biol.* **13**, 253.
Bernheimer, A. W. (1944). *J. Exptl. Med.* **80**, 333.
Bernheimer, A. W. (1947). *J. Gen. Physiol.* **30**, 337.
Bernheimer, A. W. (1965). *Ann. N.Y. Acad. Sci.* **128**, 112.
Bernheimer, A. W. (1966). *J. Bacteriol.* **91**, 1677.
Bernheimer, A. W. (1968). *Science* **159**, 847.
Bernheimer, A. W., and Davidson, M. (1965). *Science* **148**, 1229.
Bernheimer, A. W., and Schwartz, L. L. (1961). *Proc. Soc. Exptl. Biol. Med.* **106**, 776.
Bernheimer, A. W., and Schwartz, L. L. (1963). *J. Gen. Microbiol.* **30**, 455.
Bernheimer, A. W., and Schwartz, L. L. (1964). *J. Bacteriol.* **87**, 1100.
Bernheimer, A. W., and Schwartz, L. L. (1965a). *J. Pathol. Bacteriol.* **89**, 209.
Bernheimer, A. W., and Schwartz, L. L. (1965b). *J. Bacteriol.* **89**, 1387.
Bernheimer, A. W., Avigad, L. S., and Grushoff, P. (1968a). *J. Bacteriol.* **96**, 487.
Bernheimer, A. W., Freer, J. H., Lominski, I., and Sessa, G. (1968b). *J. Bacteriol.* **96**, 1429.
Bigger, J. W., Boland, C. R., and O'Meara, R. A. Q. (1927). *J. Pathol. Bacteriol.* **30**, 271.
Blair, J. E. (1965). *Ann. N.Y. Acad. Sci.* **128**, 451.
Blair, J. E., and Carr, M. (1961). *J. Bacteriol.* **82**, 984.
Boivin, A., and Izard, Y. (1937). *Compt. Rend. Soc. Biol.* **124**, 25.
Bramann, J., and Norlin, G. (1951). *Acta Pathol. Microbiol. Scand.* **29**, 127.
Breiger, L., and Fraenkel, C. (1890). *Berlin Klin. Wochschr.* **27**, 241.

Brown, D. A., and Quilliam, J. P. (1965). *Brit. J. Pharmacol.* **25**, 781.

Brown, D. A., Prichard, B. N. C., and Quilliam, J. P. (1959). *Brit. J. Pharmacol.* **14**, 59.

Brown, D. A., Casewell, M. C., and Quilliam, J. P. (1965). *Proc. 2nd Intern. Pharmacol. Meeting, Prague, 1963* Vol. 9, p. 207. Pergamon Press, Oxford.

Burnet, F. M. (1929). *J. Pathol. Bacteriol.* **32**, 717.

Burnet, F. M. (1930). *J. Pathol. Bacteriol.* **33**, 1.

Burnet, F. M. (1931). *J. Pathol. Bacteriol.* **34**, 471.

Burnet, F. M., and Freeman, M. (1932). *J. Pathol. Bacteriol.* **35**, 477.

Butler, L. O. (1959). *Biochem. J.* **71**, 67.

Cohn, Z. A. (1963a). *Yale J. Biol. Med.* **35**, 12.

Cohn, Z. A. (1963b). *Yale J. Biol. Med.* **35**, 29.

Cohn, Z. A. (1963c). *Yale J. Biol. Med.* **35**, 48.

Cooper, L. Z., Madoff, M. A., and Weinstein, L. (1964a). *J. Bacteriol.* **87**, 127.

Cooper, L. Z., Madoff, M. A., and Weinstein, L. (1964b). *J. Bacteriol.* **87**, 136.

Cooper, L. Z., Madoff, M. A., and Weinstein, L. (1966). *J. Bacteriol.* **91**, 1686.

Coulter, J. R. (1966). *J. Bacteriol.* **92**, 1655.

De Christmas, M. J. (1888). *Ann. Inst. Pasteur.* **2**, 469.

De Navasquez, S. (1938). *J. Pathol. Bacteriol.* **46**, 47.

Dingle, J. H., Hoff, H. E., Nahum, L. H., and Carey, B. W. (1937). *J. Pharmacol.* **61**, 121.

Ekstedt, R. D. (1965). *Ann. N.Y. Acad. Sci.* **128**, 301.

Elek, S. D. (1959). "Staphylococcus Pyrogenes and Its Relation to Disease." Livingstone, Edinburgh and London.

Elek, S. D., and Levy, E. (1950). *J. Pathol. Bacteriol.* **62**, 541.

Favorite, G. D., and Hammon, W. McD. (1941). *J. Bacteriol.* **41**, 305.

Felsenfeld, O., and Felsenfeld, A. D. (1966). *Proc. Soc. Exptl. Biol. Med.* **122**, 442.

Felton, H. M., and Pomerat, C. M. (1962). *Exptl. Cell Res.* **27**, 280.

Fisher, M. W., Devlin, H. B., and Erlandson, A. L. (1963). *Nature* **199**, 1074.

Forlani, L. Unpublished data cited by Bernheimer (1968).

Forssman, J. (1933). *Biochem. Z.* **265**, 291.

Forssman, J. (1934a). *Acta Pathol. Microbiol. Scand.* **11**, 214.

Forssman, J. (1934b). *Acta Pathol. Microbiol. Scand.* **11**, 452.

Forssman, J. (1934c). *Compt. Rend. Soc. Biol.* **117**, 639.

Forssman, J. (1939). *Acta Pathol. Microbiol. Scand.* **16**, 335.

Foster, E. A. (1965). *Science* **149**, 1395.

Foster, E. A. (1967). *Am. J. Pathol.* **51**, 913.

Foster, W. D. (1963). *J. Pathol. Bacteriol.* **86**, 535.

Freer, J. H., Arbuthnott, J. P., and Bernheimer, A. W. (1968). *J. Bacteriol.* **95**, 1153.

Gabliks, J., and Solotorovsky, M. (1962). *J. Immunol.* **88**, 505.

Ganczarski, A. (1962). *Lodz. Towarz. Nauk. Wydzial IV*, Nr. 44, 1–84.

Gemmell, C. G. (1968). Ph.D. Thesis, University of Glasgow.

Gengou, O. (1935a). *Ann. Inst. Pasteur* **54**, 428.

Gengou, O. (1935b). *Ann. Inst. Pasteur* **55**, 129.

Gerwing, J., Dolman, C. E., Kason, D. V., and Tremaine, J. H. (1966). *J. Bacteriol.* **91**, 484.

Gerwing, J., Morrell, R. W., and Nitz, R. H. (1968). *J. Bacteriol.* **95**, 22.

Gladstone, G. P. (1938). *Brit. J. Exptl. Pathol.* **19**, 208.

Gladstone, G. P. (1966). *Postepy Mikrobiol.* **5**, 145.

Gladstone, G. P., and Glencross, E. J. G. (1959). *Brit. J. Exptl. Pathol.* **41**, 313.

Glenny, A. T., and Stevens, M. F. (1935). J. Pathol. Bacteriol. **40**, 201.

Gorrill, R. H., Klyhn, K. M., and McNeil, E. M. (1966). *J. Pathol. Bacteriol.* **91**, 157.

Goshi, K., Cluff, L. E., and Norman, P. S. (1963a). *Bull. Johns Hopkins Hosp.* **112**, 15.

234   J. P. ARBUTHNOTT

Goshi, K., Smith, E. W., Cluff, L. K., and Norman, P. S. (1963b). *Bull. Johns Hopkins Hosp.* **113**, 183.
Goudie, R. B., Horne, C. H. W., and Wilkinson, P. C. (1966). *Lancet* **II**, 1224.
Gulda, O. (1965). *Proc. 2nd Intern. Pharmacol. Meeting, Prague, 1963* Vol. 9, p. 207. Pergamon Press, Oxford.
Haque, R. (1967). *J. Bacteriol.* **93**, 525.
Holt, L. B. (1936). *Brit. J. Exptl. Pathol.* **17**, 318.
Jackson, A. W. (1963). *Can. J. Biochem. Physiol.* **41**, 219.
Jeljaszewicz, J., Szmigielski, S., Korbecki, M., and Zak, C. (1965). *J. Infect. Diseases* **115**, 421.
Jeljaszewicz, J., Niewiarowski, S., and Poplawski, A. (1966). *Postepy Microbiol.* **5**, 203.
Johnson, J. E. (1966). *Proc. Soc. Exptl. Biol. Med.* **122**, 584.
Kapral, F. A. (1965). *Ann. N.Y. Acad. Sci.* **128**, 259.
Kapral, F. A. (1967). *Bacteriol. Proc.* p. 64.
Kelloway, C. H., Burnet, F. M., and Williams, F. E. (1930). *J. Pathol. Bacteriol.* **33**, 889.
Klainer, A. S., Madoff, M. A., Cooper, L. Z., and Weinstein, L. (1964). *Science* **145**, 714.
Knight, B. C. J. G. (1935). *Brit. J. Exptl. Pathol.* **16**, 315.
Knight, B. C. J. G. (1937a). *Nature* **139**, 628.
Knight, B. C. J. G. (1937b). *Biochem. J.* **31**, 731.
Knight, B. C. J. G. (1937c). *Biochem. J.* **31**, 996.
Knight, B. C. J. G., and McIlwain, H. (1938). *Biochem. J.* **32**, 1241.
Kodama, T., and Nishiyama, S. (1938). *Kitasato Arch. Exptl. Med.* **15**, 247.
Koenig, M. G., and Melly, M. A. (1965). *Ann. N.Y. Acad. Sci.* **128**, 231.
Korbecki, M., and Jeljaszewicz, J. (1965). *J. Infect. Diseases* **115**, 205.
Kraus, R., and Pribram, E. (1906). *Wien. Klin. Wochschr.* **19**, 493.
Kumar, S., and Lindorfer, R. K. (1962). *J. Exptl. Med.* **115**, 1095.
Kumar, S., Locken, K. I., Kenyon, A. J., and Lindorfer, R. K. (1962). *J. Exptl. Med.* **115**, 1107.
Landsteiner, K., and von Rauchenbichler, R. (1909). *Z. Immunitaetsforsh.* **1**, 439.
Leboeuf-Trudeau, T., de Repentigny, J., Frenette, R. M., and Sonea, S. (1967). *Bacteriol. Proc.* p. 64.
Le Fèvre de Aric. (1919). *Compt. Rend. Soc. Biol.* **82**, 1313.
Lenard, J., and Singer, S. J. (1968). *Science* **159**, 738.
Levine, B. S. (1938). *J. Immunol.* **35**, 131.
Levine, B. S. (1939). *J. Pathol. Bacteriol.* **48**, 291.
Lominski, I., and Arbuthnott, J. P. (1962). *J. Pathol. Bacteriol.* **83**, 515.
Lominski, I., Smith, D. D., Scott, A. C., Arbuthnott, J. P., Gray, S., Muir, D., Turner, G. H., and Hedges, C. K. (1962a). *Lancet* **I**, 1315.
Lominski, I., Arbuthnott, J. P., Scott, A. C., and McCallum, H. M. (1962b). *Lancet* **II**, 590.
Lominski, I., Arbuthnott, J. P., and Spence, J. B. (1963). *J. Pathol. Bacteriol.* **86**, 258.
Lominski, I., Arbuthnott, J. P., Gemmell, C. G., Gray, S., and Marshall, W. A. (1964). *Lancet* **II**, 503.
Lominski, I., Arbuthnott, J. P., and Gemmell, C. G. (1965). *J. Pathol. Bacteriol.* **89**, 387.
Lominski, I., Gemmell, C. G., and Arbuthnott, J. P. (1968). *J. Gen. Microbiol.* **52**, 107.
McIlwain, H. (1938). *Brit. J. Exptl. Pathol.* **19**, 411.
McLatchey, J. K., and Rosenblum, E. D. (1966a). *J. Bacteriol.* **92**, 575.
McLatchey, J. K., and Rosenblum, E. D. (1966b). *J. Bacteriol.* **92**, 580.
McLean, D. (1937). *J. Pathol. Bacteriol.* **44**, 47.
McNiven, A. C., and Arbuthnott, J. P. (1968). Unpublished observations.
Madoff, M. A., and Weinstein, L. (1962). *J. Bacteriol.* **83**, 914.

Madoff, M. A., Artenstein, M. S., and Weinstein, L. (1963). *Yale J. Biol. Med.* **35**, 382.

Madoff, M. A., Cooper, L. Z., and Weinstein, L. (1964). *J. Bacteriol.* **87**, 145.

Mangalo, R., and Raynaud, M. (1959). *Ann. Inst. Pasteur* **97**, 188.

Manohar, M., Kumar, S., and Lindorfer, R. K. (1966). *J. Bacteriol.* **91**, 1681.

Manohar, M., Maheswaran, S. K., Frommes, S. P., and Lindorfer, R. K. (1967). *J. Bacteriol.* **94**, 224.

Marks, J. (1951). *J. Hyg.* **49**, 52.

Marks, J., and Vaughan, A. C. T. (1950). *J. Pathol. Bacteriol.* **62**, 597.

Marucci, A. A. (1963a). *J. Bacteriol.* **86**, 1182.

Marucci, A. A. (1963b). *J. Bacteriol.* **86**, 1189.

Mercier, P., and Richou, R. (1944). *Compt. Rend. Soc. Biol.* **138**, 834.

Morgan, F. G., and Graydon, J. J. (1936). *J. Pathol. Bacteriol.* **43**, 383.

Mudd, S., Gladstone, G. P., and Lenhart, N. A. (1965). *Brit. J. Exptl. Pathol.* **66**, 455.

Munoz, J. (1964). *Advan. Immunol.* **4**, 397.

Murphy, S. C. (1967). *J. Bacteriol.* **94**, 586.

Neisser, M., and Levaditi, C. (1901). *Compt. Rend. 13th Cong. Intern. Méd., Paris. 1900., Sect Pathol. Gén.* 475.

Neisser, M., and Wechsberg, F. (1901). *Z. Hyg. Infektionskrankh.* **34**, 299.

Nélis, P. (1935). *Bull. Acad. Med. Belg.* **15**, 539.

Nélis, P., and Bonnet, H. (1935). *Compt. Rend. Soc. Biol.* **118**, 136.

Nélis, P., Bouckaert, J. J., and Picard, E. (1934). *Ann. Inst. Pasteur* **52**, 597.

Nogrady, G., and Burton, A. L. (1961). *Pathol. Biol.* **9**, 831.

Noll, H. (1966). *Science* **151**, 1241.

Paradisi, F. (1967). *Experientia* **23**, 1045.

Parker, J. T., Hopkins, J. G., and Gunther, A. (1926). *Proc. Soc. Exptl. Biol. Med.* **23**, 344.

Pollock, M. R. (1962). *In* "The Bacteria" (I. C. Gunsalus and R. Y. Stanier, eds.), Vol. 4, pp. 121–178. Academic Press, New York.

Raynaud, M., Bizzini, B., Fischer, G., and Prévot, A. R. (1955). *Ann. Inst. Pasteur* **88**, 454.

Rigdon, R. H. (1935). *A.M.A. Arch. Pathol.* **20**, 201.

Robinson, J., and Thatcher, F. S. (1963). *Can. J. Microbiol.* **9**, 697.

Robson Wright, M., Arbuthnott, J. P., and Lominski, I. R. W. (1968). *Biochem. J.* **108**, 41.

Rodet, A., and Courmont, J. (1892). *Semaine Med.* **12**, 32.

Rodgers, D. E. (1966). *Postepy Mikrobiol.* **5**, 279.

Rodgers, D. E., and Melly, M. A. (1965). *Ann. N.Y. Acad. Sci.* **128**, 274.

Royal Commission. (1928). *Med. J. Australia* **2**, 2.

Rud, E. (1955). *Acta Pathol. Microbiol. Scand.* **36**, 441.

Russ, V. K. (1916). *Z. Exptl. Pathol. Therap.* **18**, 220.

Šamánek, M., and Zajík, F. (1965). *Proc. 2nd Intern. Pharmacol. Meeting, Prague, 1963* Vol. 9, p. 199. Pergamon Press, Oxford.

Seiffert, W. (1935). *Zent. Bakteriol., Parasitenk., Abt. I. Orig.* **135**, 100.

Sessa, G., and Weissmann, G. (1968). *J. Lipid Res.* **9**, 310.

Siegel, I., and Cohen, S. (1964). *J. Infect. Diseases,* **114**, 488.

Simmonds, J. P., Linn, H. J., and Lange, J. (1946). *A.M.A. Arch. Pathol.* **41**, 185.

Smith, D. D. (1956). *Nature* **178**, 1060.

Smith, E. W., Goshi, K., Norman, P. S., and Cluff, L. E. (1963). *Bull. Johns Hopkins Hosp.* **113**, 247.

Smith, M. L., and Ipsen, J. (1938). *Quart. Bull. Health Organ. League of Nations* **7**, 845 (cited by Elek, 1959).

Smith, M. L., and Price, S. A. (1938). *J. Pathol. Bacteriol.* **47**, 379.

Sonea, S., de Repentigny, J., and Frappier, A. (1965). *Can. J. Microbiol.* **11**, 383.

Stamp, Lord. (1961). *Brit. J. Exptl. Pathol.* **42**, 30.

Švihovec, J., Mašek, K., and Jiřička, Z. (1965). *Proc. 2nd Intern. Pharmacol. Meeting, Prague, 1963* Vol. 9, p. 193. Pergamon Press, Oxford.

Swift, H. F., and Schultz, M. P. (1936). *J. Exptl. Med.* **63**, 703.

Symington, D. A., and Arbuthnott, J. P. (1969). *J. Med. Microbiol.* **2**, 495.

Tager, H. (1941). *Yale J. Biol. Med.* **14**, 68.

Thal, A. P. (1951). *Federation Proc.* **10**, 372.

Thal, A. P., and Egner, W. (1954). *A.M.A. Arch. Pathol.* **57**, 392.

Thal, A. P., and Egner, W. (1961). *J. Exptl. Med.* **113**, 67.

Thal, A. P., and Molestina, J. E. (1955). *A.M.A. Arch. Pathol.* **60**, 212.

Toner, P. G., Arbuthnott, J. P., Carr, K. E., Symington, D., and Gemmell, C. G. (1969). In preparation.

Travassos, J. (1933a). *Compt. Rend. Soc. Biol.* **114**, 369.

Travassos, J. (1933b). *Compt. Rend. Soc. Biol.* **114**, 371.

Turgeon, P., Grimard, S., and de Repentigny, J. (1966). *Can. J. Microbiol.* **12**, 588.

Turpin, A., Relyfeldt, E. H., Pillet, J., and Raynaud, H. (1954). *Ann. Inst. Pasteur* **87**, 185.

van de Velde, H. (1894). *Cellule* **10**, 401.

van de Velde, H., and Denys, J. (1895). *Cellule* **11**, 358.

van Heyningen, W. E. (1970). *In* "Microbial Toxins" (S. J. Ajl, T. C. Montie, and S. Kadis, eds.), Vol. I, 1-28.

von Glahn, W. C., and Weld, J. T. (1935). *J. Exptl. Med.* **61**, 1.

von Leber, T. (1888). *Forsch. Med.* **6**, 460.

von Lingelsheim, W. (1900). "Aetiologie und Therapie der Staphylokokken Infectionen." Urban, Berlin.

Wadstrom, T. (1968). *Biochim. Biophys. Acta* **168**, 228.

Walbum, L. E. (1909). *Z. Immunitaets forsch.* **3**, 70.

Walbum, L. E. (1921). *Compt. Rend. Soc. Biol.* **85**, 1205.

Weissmann, G., Sessa, G., and Bernheimer, A. W. (1966). *Science* **154**, 772.

Wiegershausen, B. (1960). *Arch. Exptl. Pathol. Pharmakol.* **238**, 144.

Wiegershausen, B. (1962). *Acta Biol. Med. Ger.* **9**, 517.

Wiegershausen, B. (1965). *Proc. 2nd Intern. Pharmacol. Meeting, Prague, 1963* Vol. 9, p. 183. Pergamon Press, Oxford.

Wiegershausen, B., and Rašková, H. (1961). *Biochem. Pharmacol.* **8**, 75.

Williams, R. E. O., and Harper, J. G. (1947). *J. Pathol. Bacteriol.* **59**, 69.

Wiseman, G. M. (1970). *In* "Microbiol Toxins" (S. J. Ajl, T. C. Montie, and S. Kadis, eds.), Vol. III, pp. 237-263.

Wittler, R. G., and Pillemer, L. (1948). *J. Biol. Chem.* **174**, 23.

Woodin, A. M., and Wieneke, A. A. (1966a). *Biochem. J.* **99**, 469.

Woodin, A. M., and Wieneke, A. A. (1966b). *Biochem. J.* **99**, 479.

Wright, J. (1936). *Lancet* **I**, 1002.

Wurzel, M., Bernheimer, A. W., and Zweifach, B. W. (1966). *Am. J. Physiol.* **210**, 360.

Yoshida, A. (1963). *Biochim. Biophys. Acta* **71**, 544.

CHAPTER 6

The Beta- and Delta-Toxins of *Staphylococcus aureus*

GORDON M. WISEMAN

I. Beta-Toxin

Glenny and Stevens (1935), investigating two preparations of α-toxin, observed that with the first, dermonecrotic and hemolytic activities were neutralized by equal amounts of antiserum as expected. For the second toxin, ten times as much antiserum was required for neutralization of its dermonecrotic activity. They further observed that following incubation at 37°C, the hemolytic effect of this second toxin was greatly intensified on standing for a period at room temperature or at 4°C. This "hot–cold" hemolysin, antigenically distinct from the α-toxin, was referred to by Glenny and Stevens as the β-toxin.

Bryce and Rountree (1936) found that the β-toxin was produced largely by *Staphylococcus aureus* strains of animal origin. According to their investigations, the erythrocytes of sheep and the ox were susceptible to its action while those of the ferret, rabbit, rat, guinea pig, and koala bear were resistant. The toxin had slight activity in the presence of human erythrocytes.

A. TOXICITY

1. EFFECT ON WHOLE ANIMALS

Early work on the toxicity of the β-toxin was limited to the observation of Glenny and Stevens that their preparation was lethal for rabbits but not mice. The toxin also caused no necrosis when injected subcutaneously into rabbits but did give rise to a mild erythema. Bryce and Rountree confirmed its toxicity for rabbits.

Thatcher and Matheson (1955), in a study of the kitten test for staphylococcal enterotoxin, made the claim that β-toxin, like enterotoxin, could cause emesis in cats. In contrast with enterotoxin, it could be inactivated by boiling with subsequent incubation in the presence of ascorbic acid.

Following the discovery by Jackson and Mayman (1958) that the hemolytic activity of the β-toxin is activated by Mg^{2+}, Heydrick and Chesbro (1962) claimed that intraperitoneal injection of the toxin was lethal for guinea pigs only in the presence of these ions. The work of Wiseman (1965a), who used a partially purified preparation of β-toxin from the R-1 and 252F strains of *S. aureus*, was at variance with earlier work which claimed that the toxin was lethal for rabbits. He found that mice and guinea pigs were insusceptible to the toxin whether or not it was injected intravenously in the presence and absence of Mg^{2+}. Subcutaneous inoculation of rabbits caused only a mild erythema. Maheswaran *et al.* (1967) were unable to demonstrate necrosis in the skin of rabbits when a highly purified preparation was injected with Mg^{2+}. Although hemolytic activity of β-toxin is enhanced in the presence of Mg^{2+}, there is, however, no evidence that parallel results are obtained *in vivo*.

2. Effect on Mammalian Cells in Culture

Much of the more recent work concerning toxicity has utilized tissue culture and suspensions of nucleated mammalian cells. Chesbro *et al.* (1965) have shown that β-toxin produced by the UNH-Donita strain of *S. aureus* has a leukocidal effect on suspensions of guinea pig macrophages. The cells' ability to reduce phenolindo-2,6-dichlorophenol (PIP) to a colorless compound was lost in the presence of toxin, and Giemsa-stained smears of such preparations revealed that the leukocytes were either disintegrated or swollen and distorted. Wiseman (1968) has also observed that β-toxin derived from *S. aureus* R-1 is toxic to suspensions of human amnion, KB, and monkey kidney cells on the basis of trypan blue uptake, absence of acid production in the medium, and inability to attach to glass surfaces. In addition, rabbit and sheep leukocytes were unable to reduce PIP in the presence of the toxin, but their ability to take up *Staphylococcus epidermidis* cells seemed unimpaired. Bernheimer and Schwartz (1964) were unable to disrupt rabbit leukocyte lysosomes or rabbit liver lysosomes as indicated by failure of β-toxin to reduce turbidity of a suspension or release lysosomal enzymes. In a later publication (1965), these authors found that the β-toxin attacked rabbit blood platelets. Korbecki and Jeljaszewicz (1965) observed that β-toxin prepared by fractional precipitation of culture supernates of *S. aureus* Wood 46 exerted a toxic effect on KB and monkey kidney cells. According to their report, two he molytic units of β-toxin per milliliter added to the medium caused detachment of KB cells from glass after 24 hours of incubation, along with the appearance of vacuolation and some disintegration. Monkey kidney cells treated with the toxin were granular in appearance, but the number of intact cells remaining was greater than was the case with KB cells. Histochemical studies of KB cells incubated with β-toxin (Jeljaszewicz et al., 1965) revealed no alteration in their alkaline phosphatase and 5′-nucleotidase activity, but the number of cells hydrolyzing β-naphthyl acetate and 5-bromoindoxyl acetate decreased significantly. The toxin also increased the number of cells containing lipids staining with Sudan B and markedly reduced the proportion showing acid phosphatase activity.

According to Gladstone and Yoshida (1967), the addition of crude β-toxin to HeLa, L, HL, FL, HeP, chick fibroblasts, and rat heart connective tissue cells had no effect after 2 hours. After incubating β-toxin with human, bovine, and monkey kidney cells, Hallander and Bengtsson (1967) were unable to show uptake of neutral red by the cells after 6 hours, indicating that the toxin was without effect.

3. CURRENT STATUS OF TOXICITY

In summary, early work with β-toxin cannot be relied upon to give an accurate picture of its toxicity for laboratory animals, since results were obtained with crude material. The presence of δ-toxin in these preparations could not be ruled out, as its presence in staphylococcal culture filtrates was undetected before 1947. Points upon which there is agreement at present are that the β-toxin is not lethal for mice and is not necrotic when injected subcutaneously into rabbits, but rather produces an erythematous flush. All of the early crude preparations killed rabbits, but partially purified material free of α- and δ-toxins did not (Wiseman, 1965a). It is difficult to compare the effects of the toxin upon laboratory animals with work done using cultures of mammalian cells, since the dose per cell is enormous in these tissue culture systems compared to that in whole animals. Studies of various investigators concerned with the effect of β-toxin on tissue culture cells are also not easily compared owing to the fact that observations on the cells were made at different times after addition of the toxin. Furthermore, toxin concentration and purity were not uniform.

B. PRODUCTION AND PURIFICATION

1. PRODUCTION

In a study of four strains of S. aureus, Wiseman (1963) found that β-toxin titers were higher on media containing 1.5% agar if the plates were incubated in a mixture of 25% carbon dioxide in air rather than 25% car-

TABLE I
EFFECT OF GASEOUS ENVIRONMENT ON β-TOXIN PRODUCTION[a]

Strain	Gas mixture	Growth (O.D. 650 mμ)	Sheep red cell titer (HU/ml)[b]
252F	Air	0.84	1,016
	CO_2-oxygen	0.76	1,280
	CO_2-air	0.91	2,560
R-1	Air	0.58	2,560
	CO_2-oxygen	0.43	20,480
	CO_2-air	0.59	32,510
P-92	Air	0.58	5,120
	CO_2-oxygen	0.51	16,260
	CO_2-air	0.54	65,010
G-128	Air	0.62	20,480
	CO_2-oxygen	0.48	16,260
	CO_2-air	0.64	130,100

[a] After Wiseman (1963).

[b] Values are the mean of two experiments. Plates were layered with cellophane, inoculated, and incubated for 24 hours. Two milliliters of 0.01 M phosphate–saline buffer were added to each plate and the growth was removed. Hemolysin titrations were carried out on the supernatant fluid after centrifugation and in the presence of 0.001 M Mg^{2+}.

bon dioxide in oxygen or air alone as shown in Table I. Growth was depressed slightly in the carbon dioxide and oxygen mixtures. Haque and Baldwin (1964) have also investigated the effect of various mixtures of carbon dioxide in air and oxygen on β-toxin formation. Carbon dioxide concentrations of 10, 20, 40, and 80% in air were of equal value in increasing titers in heart infusion broth to which 0.3% agar was added. In contrast with Wiseman's data, they found that 20% carbon dioxide in oxygen was as effective in increasing titers as mixtures of carbon dioxide in air. Haque and Baldwin also found that aeration of broth cultures by agitation or sparging was ineffective in improving yields.

A neutral pH favors growth with production of highest titers of toxin (Wiseman, 1963) as shown in Table II. Haque and Baldwin also studied the influence of pH and the addition of fermentable carbohydrates upon growth and toxin production, finding that best yields were obtained when pH was initially adjusted to 5.2–5.8. The pH rose to 8.5 after 48 hours of incubation, indicating absence of strong buffering action in the media, making these results difficult to compare with Wiseman's data. The addition of carbohydrates to the basal medium did not improve yields.

Chesbro et al. (1965) used a completely dialyzable medium for β-toxin production, stating that the addition of 0.5% L-arginine enhanced its formation. They employed 20% carbon dioxide in oxygen and incubated their cultures at 35°C for 24 hours with shaking, replenishing the gases

TABLE II
EFFECT OF pH ON PRODUCTION OF β-TOXIN ON SOLID MEDIUM

Buffer	pH	Growth (O.D. 650 mμ)	Sheep red cell titer (HU/ml)[a]
Acetate	5.0	0	<20
Phosphate	6.0	0.75	81,920
Phosphate	7.0	0.87	130,000
Borate	8.0	0.36	10,240
Borate	9.0	0	<20

[a] Values are the mean of two experiments. Buffers were 0.01 M with respect to Dolman–Wilson (1940) medium containing 1.5% agar. The pH did not change by more than 0.3 units after 24 hours of growth. The buffer salts themselves were not responsible for the effects upon growth and toxin production. After Wiseman (1963).

after 6 and 12 hours. Maheswaran *et al.* (1967) extracted toxin from medium containing 1.5% agar after incubation in an atmosphere of 50% carbon dioxide in oxygen.

Wiseman (1963) found that the rate of toxin production was maximal in strains R-1 and 252F during the early logarithmic growth phase (Fig. 1). Highest titers were reached after 24 hours of incubation with little or no decline detectable after 48 hours, which supports the observations of Haque and Baldwin (1964) based on work with semisolid media. As part

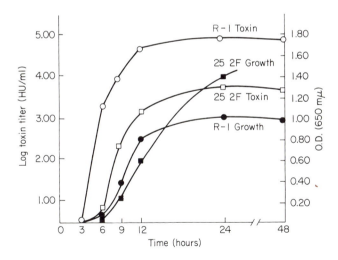

FIG. 1. Rate of β-toxin formation with respect to growth of strains R-1 and 252F. The toxins were produced on solid media and titrated in the presence of sheep erythrocytes and 0.001 M Mg^{2+}. The gaseous environment was 25% carbon dioxide in air. (Redrawn from Wiseman, 1963.)

of the same study, Wiseman also investigated amino acid requirements of growth and β-toxin production in the R-1 strain (Table III). He used the basal medium of Gladstone (1938) to which various amino acids and growth factors were added. For this strain, an absolute requirement for arginine, proline, and glycine was observed, growth and toxin formation being negligible if these three amino acids were omitted when compared to complete medium. Toxin titers were reduced if valine alone or aspartic and glutamic acids or cystine and methionine in combination were omit-

TABLE III

NUTRITIONAL REQUIREMENTS OF *Staphylococcus aureus* STRAIN R-1

Omissions from complete medium	Growth (O.D. 650 mμ)[a]	Sheep red cell titer (HU/ml)
Alanine, valine, leucine, glycine	0.47	80
Alanine	1.71	640
Leucine	1.37	640
Valine	0.59	160
Glycine	0.26	40
Proline, hydroxyproline, tryptophan, histidine	0.10	<20
Hydroxyproline	1.66	640
Tryptophan	1.53	320
Histidine	1.57	320
Proline	0.22	<20
Aspartic acid, glutamic acid	1.43	40
Aspartic acid	1.54	320
Glutamic acid	1.69	320
Cystine, methionine	0.35	<20
Cystine	1.14	160
Methionine	1.60	640
Phenylalanine, tyrosine	1.68	640
Lysine, arginine	0.13	<20
Lysine	1.74	640
Arginine	0.30	<20
Thiamine, nicotinamide	0.53	<20
Thiamine	0.67	<20
Nicotinamide	0.85	20
Complete medium	1.62	640

[a]Optical density (O.D.) measurements were made on suspensions diluted 1:20. The value obtained was multiplied by 20 to give the figures in the table.

ted. Aspartic and glutamic acids were interchangeable, but full growth and toxin production were not restored when cystine was substituted for methionine. The growth factors thiamine and nicotinamide were indispensable. In this study there was no clear distinction between amino acid requirements for growth and toxin production except possibly in the omission of both aspartic and glutamic acids. Growth, but not toxin production, in their absence nearly equaled that in the complete medium.

2. PURIFICATION

In an early attempt to free β-toxin from other exocellular products, Bryce and Rountree (1936) inactivated α- but not β-toxin in their preparations by heating at 60°C for 15 minutes. Kodama and Kojima (1939) were able to precipitate the active β-toxin by treatment with ethanol, methanol, or acetone. The feasibility of acetone as a precipitating agent was confirmed by Fulton (1943), who obtained maximum recovery if precipitation was carried out at pH 9.0.

The application of recent advances in methods of separation of proteins has facilitated recovery of highly purified β-toxin (Table IV). Robinson *et al.* (1958) combined ethanol precipitation with adsorption to calcium phosphate gel and subsequent electrophoresis, obtaining a 670-fold increase in specific activity. Yields were not reported, and tests of homogeneity were not carried out. The highest yields of any procedure to date have been achieved by Jackson (1963) using ethanol precipitation and complexing with Zn^{2+} followed by adsorption to hydroxyapatite. Recovery was about 50–60% with an overall 255-fold increase in specific activity. Chesbro *et al.* (1965) purified β-toxin from their UNH-Donita strain of *S. aureus* about 150-fold in a single step on cellulose phosphate, eluting the toxin by application of a buffer concentration gradient. They reported the presence of two antigens in their purified preparations. Doery *et al.* (1965) employed ammonium sulfate precipitation of β-toxin from strain 1062-17 followed by fractionation on hydroxyapatite. Like Chesbro *et al.*, they found two antigenic components in their best preparations. Wiseman and Caird (1967) achieved a 70-fold increase in specific activity by adsorption of crude β-toxin of the R-1 strain to hydroxyapatite and precipitation of impurities from the eluate at pH 4.0. Passage of the supernatant fluid through Sephadex G-100 resulted in a β-toxin preparation containing two antigens, with overall recovery of about 20–25%. Maheswaran *et al.* (1967) twice precipitated β-toxin with ammonium sulfate, obtaining a 23-fold purification. A further twofold increase was effected on Sephadex G-100. The active effluent was then passed through carboxymethyl-cellulose equilibrated with 0.005 *M* phosphate buffer at pH 7.0. β-Toxin was retained on the column and eluted with a phosphate buffer gra-

TABLE IV

COMPARISON OF METHODS FOR PURIFICATION OF β-TOXIN

Robinson et al. (1958)		Jackson (1963)		Wiseman and Caird (1967)		Maheswaran et al. (1967)	
Step	Specific activity	Step	Specific activity	Step	Specific activity	Step	Specific activity
Crude	1	Crude	1	Crude	1	Crude	1
Ethanol precipitation	15	Zinc–ethanol precipitated	3	Hydroxyapatite	20	Ammonium sulfate precipitated	23
Calcium phosphate treatment	30	Zinc–mercuric acetate precipitated	10	Acetate precipitated	35	Sephadex G-100	46
Starch electrophoresis	670	Hydroxyapatite	255	Sephadex G-100	70	Carboxymethylcellulose	245

dient containing 3% sodium chloride. They did not specify the concentration of buffer–sodium chloride which removed the toxin. Maheswaran's group reported an overall 245-fold increase in specific activity for the three-step procedure, but percentage recovery was not reported. Agar gel diffusion, immunoelectrophoresis and disk electrophoresis on polyacrylamide gel indicated the presence of one antigen in their purified toxin preparation. It is of interest to note that Sephadex G-100 in their investigations also resulted in an active effluent consisting of two antigenic components as observed by Wiseman and Caird.

In spite of the fact that several of the methods of purification reported have permitted recovery of highly purified β-toxin containing only one or two antigens, the application of rigorous criteria of homogeneity to high toxin concentrations has not been carried out. Criteria presently available include immunodiffusion, immunoelectrophoresis, disk electrophoresis, analytical ultracentrifugation, and N-terminal analysis. Recycling on an ion exchanger or Sephadex would also give some indication of purity, but these procedures have not as yet all been applied to a single toxin preparation.

Purified β-toxin was reported to be stable for as long as 4 months if freeze-dried (Maheswaran et al., 1967), but activity was lost rapidly if kept as a solution at 4°C. Chesbro et al. (1965) also noted marked instability of toxin in solution or if filtered or shaken. Jackson's toxin (1963) when freeze-dried lost no activity over a 6-month period, nor did that of Wiseman and Caird (1967).

C. CHARACTERISTICS

1. THE "HOT-COLD" REACTION

The property which first drew attention to the β-toxin was the classic "hot–cold" hemolytic phenomenon characteristic of the toxin (Bigger *et al.*, 1927). Hemolysis is incomplete at the lowest dilutions of toxin or is absent at 37°C and only becomes evident when the titration is further incubated at a lower temperature, hence the application of the term "hot–cold." If colonies of *S. aureus* producing β-toxin are incubated on sheep blood agar at 37°C, a zone of darkening is apparent which progresses to hemolysis if the plates are cooled. Concentric ring effects are frequently noticed surrounding the colony before the zone of red cells affected by the β-toxin begins to lyse. Flamm (1957) attributed this to the Liesegang phenomenon, which is a complex relationship between the growing colony producing the exocellular agent, its diffusion through the supporting gel, and its reaction with other microorganisms or with erythrocytes (Pulvertaft *et al.*, 1947).

The nature of the hot-cold effect has been the subject of some speculation as reflected in the work of Pulsford (1954) and Wiseman (1965b). Pulsford dealt with this phenomenon as it appeared on sheep blood agar, finding that the red cells incubated with β-toxin could be lysed at 37°C by rapid alteration of the pH or sodium chloride concentration above or below 0.85%. Wiseman confirmed Pulsford's findings for concentrations of sodium chloride below 0.80% in a fluid system, but above this level no lysis occurred. He furthermore observed that rapid adjustment of the pH from 6.9 downward resulted in increasing lysis of sensitized cells. Changes in pH from 6.9 to 9.8 did not cause hemolysis. It was also shown that glucose (0.5–3.0%) and sodium chloride (1.0–2.5%) inhibited lysis of sensitized sheep cells. The explanation of these findings may depend upon an increase in the cell volume under such conditions (Ponder, 1948), and inhibition of the lytic reaction by glucose and hypertonic sodium chloride tends to support this view. Since it is not known whether lysis of erythrocytes brought about by β-toxin is the result of membrane perforations or its disintegration, it could also be argued that hemolysis at 37°C caused by rapid pH changes or hypotonic sodium chloride concentrations is effected through enlargement of the perforations. Similarly, the explanation of the hot-cold phenomenon may be that sudden contraction of the red cell membrane as a result of lowered temperature has the effect of increasing the circumference of the perforations, allowing hemoglobin to leak out at some critical point.

2. THE ERYTHROCYTE SPECTRUM

There is some agreement that staphylococcal β-toxin lyses erythrocytes of the ox, sheep, and goat, while those of the rabbit, ferret, guinea pig, monkey, horse, rat, and mouse are quite resistant (Elek, 1959). Reports of the sensitivity of human erythrocytes are variable. The early investigations were, however, carried out with crude toxin and in ignorance of the effect of metal ions upon hemolysis of red cells in the presence of β-toxin. Wiseman (1965a) has tested the sensitivity of 13 species of erythrocytes to beta toxin from the R-1 and 252F strains of *S. aureus* (Table V) in the presence of Mg^{2+}. The highest titers in both cases were with sheep, ox, and human erythrocytes, while those of the horse, guinea pig, dog, frog, mouse, rat, and fowl were quite resistant. Pig, rabbit, and cat red cells occupied an intermediate position. In other work done some time later, Wiseman also found that monkey erythrocytes were resistant to the R-1 toxin, while goat red cells were about as sensitive as those of the rabbit.

Haque and Baldwin (1964) were unable to detect lysis of human, rabbit, or horse erythrocytes in the presence of purified β-toxin derived from their Parisi strain. There was some difference in their method of titration

TABLE V

SPECTRUM OF ERYTHROCYTE SENSITIVITY TO PARTIALLY PURIFIED
β-TOXINS OF STRAINS R-1 AND 252F

Erythrocyte species	Hemolytic titers (HU/ml) of β-toxins from strains	
	R-1	252F
Horse	<4	<4
Guinea pig	<4	<4
Dog	<4[a]	<4
Frog	<4[a]	<4[a]
Mouse	<4[a]	<4[a]
Rat	<4[a]	<4[a]
Fowl	<4[a]	<4[a]
Pig	32	32
Rabbit	64	32
Cat	64	64
Man	256	128
Ox	512	512
Sheep	2048	512

[a] Slight hemolysis, less than 50%, was observed at these dilutions. Titrations were performed in the presence of 0.001 M Mg^{2+} in 0.01 M phosphate–saline buffer at pH 7.0. All species showed the classic hot–cold effect after incubation for 1 hour at 37°C followed by standing overnight at 4°C.

TABLE VI

INFLUENCE OF ADDITION OF 0.001 M Mg^{2+} ON HEMOLYTIC TITERS OF
β-TOXINS FROM DIFFERENT STRAINS OF *Staphylococcus aureus*

Strains[a]	Mg^{2+} added	Hemolytic Titers (HU/ml) with cells of		
		Rabbit	Man	Sheep
P-92	−	<20	<20	20
	+	20	160	1,280
G-128	−	<20	<20	80
	+	40	640	2,560
R-1	−	20	40	160
	+	160	320	10,240
252F	−	<20	20	40
	+	20	80	320

[a] Partially purified β-toxin from these strains was tested.

from that of Wiseman, however. Tests were incubated for 80 minutes at 37°C followed by refrigeration for 30 minutes, when readings were taken.

The effect of Mg^{2+} on β-toxin titers with rabbit, human, and sheep red cells is observed in Table VI (Wiseman, 1965a). In the absence of Mg^{2+}, rabbit and human red cells are relatively insensitive to β-toxin, but lysis is greatly enhanced if these ions are present at 0.001 M concentrations, although lysis is still greater in sheep red cells. Roy (1937) and Kodama and Kojima (1939) also found that β-toxin lysed human red cells.

3. EFFECT OF METAL IONS

Jackson and Mayman (1958) showed that inactivation was the result of dialysis of β-toxin but that its hemolytic activity was restored in the presence of 0.01 M Mg^{2+} or Mn^{2+}. Calcium ions had no effect. The addition of citrate or EDTA to the toxin had the same effect as dialysis; that is, hemolytic activity was lost.

Robinson *et al.* (1958) reported that hemolytic activity of their β-toxin preparation in the presence of sheep erythrocytes was enhanced by Co^{2+}, Mg^{2+}, Mn^{2+}, Ni^{2+}, and Fe^{2+}, but not by Zn^{2+} or Ca^{2+} (Table VII). They have further reported that hemolysis of sheep cells in the presence of β-toxin is optimal at 0.00025 M concentrations of Mg^{2+} and Co^{2+}. Wiseman (1965a) confirmed this for Co^{2+}, Mg^{2+}, Mn^{2+}, and Ca^{2+} but noted that Ni^{2+} had no effect on R-1 and 252F toxins. Zinc ions at 0.001 M concentrations inhibited hemolysis. He also found that the activity optimum was in the range of 0.01–0.001 M Mg^{2+} and Co^{2+} in contrast with Robinson's data.

Other investigators have all noted increased hemolytic activity with Mg^{2+} (Haque and Baldwin, 1964; Chesbro *et al.*, 1965). The former au-

TABLE VII

EFFECT OF METAL CATIONS ON HEMOLYTIC ACTIVITY OF β-TOXIN

Cations added	Robinson et al.[a] (0.0005 M)	Wiseman[b] (0.001 M)	Haque and Baldwin[c] (0.001 M)
Co^{2+}	40	20,480	—
Ni^{2+}	24.5	640	—
Fe^{2+}	20.0	—	640
Mg^{2+}	18.7	20,480	2,560
Mn^{2+}	20.0	10,240	—
Ca^{2+}	0	320	40
Zn^{2+}	0	20	—
No additions	0	640	160

[a] Robinson et al. (1958). Activity was expressed as hemin (μg)/protein (μg).

[b] Wiseman (1965a). Activity was expressed as hemolytic units per milliliter, which were defined as the highest dilutions of toxin lysing 50% of red cells.

[c] Haque and Baldwin (1964). Their hemolytic units were similar to those of Wiseman.

thors confirmed the absence of increased hemolytic activity in the presence of Ca^{2+}. The effect of all these ions cannot be explained by their position in the periodic table, as would be expected from the relationships of nickel to cobalt and calcium to magnesium. Activation by a metal cation was the first evidence that the β-toxin was an enzyme. There is no record in the literature of anions enhancing hemolytic activity of the β-toxin.

D. MODE OF ACTION

1. In Vitro MODE OF ACTION

a. Analysis of End Products. In a study of ten strains of S. aureus producing α- and β-toxins, Doery et al. (1963) found that all hydrolyzed sphingomyelin, a common constituent of cell membranes. Ten strains producing only α-toxin had no effect on this phospholipid. Furthermore, the distribution of curtain electrophoretic fractions corresponded with those containing β-toxin. They also demonstrated that when phospholipid extracts of erythrocytes were chromatographed, sphingomyelin disappeared if the cells had been treated with the toxin before the extract was made.

The mode of action was determined by Doery's group using sphingomyelin prepared from ox brain as substrate. Their partially purified β-toxin was added to an emulsion of sphingomyelin at pH 7.5 and incubated at 37°C for 2.5 hours. Trichloroacetic acid was added to stop the reaction. The supernatant fluid was subjected to electrophoresis on paper at pH 6.5, pyridine–acetic acid–water (25:1:225) being used as solvent. It was noted that a spot staining with reagent specific for phosphorus had the same Rf value as an authentic sample of phosphorycholine chromatographed simultaneously. This led them to suggest the following reaction:

$$\text{Sphingomyelin} + \text{water} \xrightarrow{\beta\text{-toxin}} N\text{-acylsphingosine} + \text{phosphorylcholine}$$

Wiseman and Caird (1966, 1967) and Maheswaran and Lindorfer (1966, 1967) were able to confirm Doery's results. The data of Wiseman and Caird (Table VIII) show that phosphorus and nitrogen were recovered quantitatively in the chloroform extract of samples initially collected in the presence and absence of toxin. Since sphingomyelin is insoluble in water and soluble in chloroform, it is evident that no hydrolysis products could be detected in unincubated reaction mixtures. After 20 hours of incubation with toxin, nearly all of the phosphorus was recovered from the aqueous rather than the chloroform extract.With regard to nitrogen, 52% was found in the aqueous and 65% in the chloroform extracts. Thus, the presence of phosphorylcholine in the aqueous extract is confirmed. These data also support the suggestion of the formation of chloroform-soluble N-acylsphingosine as the other product of hydrolysis. The chloroform solution of this compound, unlike its parent compound sphingomyelin, gave a color with ninhydrin. Wiseman and Caird (1967) also showed that the occurrence of greater amounts of sphingomyelin in various species of erythrocytes was correlated with increased hemolysis in the presence of β-toxin.

b. Specificity of the reaction. Doery *et al.* (1965) studied the action of β-toxin only on one phospholipid other than spingomyelin, noting that the toxin also hydrolyzed lysophosphatidylcholine with the liberation of phosphorylcholine and a monoglyceride. Wiseman and Caird (1967) found that phosphatidylethanolamine, phosphatidylcholine, ribonucleic acid, sodium β-glycerophosphate, and disodium phenylphosphate were resistant to attack. It appears that the toxin is a quite specific enzyme, attacking, so far as is known, only sphingomyelin and lysophosphatidyl-

TABLE VIII

END PRODUCT ANALYSIS OF THE REACTION OF β-TOXIN WITH SPHINGOMYELIN[a]

Test	Incubation time (hours)	Phosphorus (%)		Nitrogen (%)	
		Aqueous extract	Chloroform extract	Aqueous extract	Chloroform extract
Sphingomyelin control	0	0	94	0	98
	20	5	87	0	100
Sphingomyelin + β-toxin	0	0	95	0	98
	20	93	0	52	65

[a] After Wiseman and Caird (1967).

choline. The mode of action of the β-toxin strongly suggests that it is similar to phospholipase C. *Clostridium perfringens* α-toxin, which is a phospholipase C, preferentially hydrolyzes phosphatidylcholine, resulting in the release of phosphorylcholine and a diglyceride, but it does not attack phenylphosphate, β-glycerophosphate, or nucleic acid. It has been reported to hydrolyze sphingomyelin slowly (van Heyningen, 1950), an observation which has been confirmed by Wiseman and Caird (unpublished data).

   c. Effect of Inhibitors and Activators. A study of the effect of inhibitors and activators on systems in which sphingomyelin is incubated with purified β-toxin has in general confirmed data obtained when erythrocyte stromata were used as substrate. Doery *et al.* (1965) showed that the hydrolysis of sphingomyelin by β-toxin is activated by Co^{2+} and Mg^{2+}, Co^{2+} being more effective than Mg^{2+}. Calcium ions inhibited the reaction. Using sphingomyelin as substrate in the presence of toxin, Maheswaran and Lindorfer (1967) confirmed that Mg^{2+} activated hydrolysis of the phospholipid. Furthermore, the addition of EDTA prevented release of aqueous organic phosphorus from this substrate, an observation also made by Jackson and Mayman (1958), Robinson *et al.* (1958), and Wiseman (1965a) on the toxin's hemolytic activity. These authors also found that citrate would inhibit the reaction, not an unexpected result in view of the demonstrated activation of β-toxin by cations. Chesbro *et al.* (1965) found that the thiol-inactivating agents *p*-chloromercuribenzoate and iodoacetate inhibited hemolytic activity of the toxin. Maheswaran and Lindorfer (1967) observed that these reagents prevented hydrolysis of sphingomyelin by the toxin.

2. *In Vivo* MODE OF ACTION

   There is no evidence at present that β-toxin attacks sphingomyelin *in vivo*. Normal rabbit serum *in vitro* does not inhibit lysis of sheep erythrocytes, but rather enhances it slightly at a concentration of 0.05–1.0%. Bovine serum albumin (0.05–0.1%) also increases hemolysis, but inhibition rather than enhancement is observed with similar concentrations of fibrinogen (Wiseman, 1965a).

   Working with rabbits, Corkill (1955) showed that injection of β-toxin increased blood sugar levels. Toxoided material when injected did not give rise to an elevated blood sugar. In connection with this observation it is interesting to note that Smith (1965) found that blood glucose in human patients dying of staphylococcal infections was significantly elevated the day before death. However, carcass analysis of mice dead of staphylococcal infection showed a decrease of total glucose. Bergman *et al.* (1965) reported that intravenous injection of rabbits and cats produced instantaneous biphasic changes of blood pressure followed by a slow decline to zero level. Their β-toxin killed both species of animal and stimulated respiration just before death. Both Bergmann *et al.* and Corkill used a β-toxin preparation of undefined purity, and the presence of other toxic products causing these effects cannot be ruled out. The relationship of their observations to phospholipase activity of the β-toxin is obscure. There is some evidence (Edwards and Ball, 1954) that phospholipases A, C, and D inhibit electron transport in mammalian cells. It has been shown recently by Wiseman (1968) that β-toxin destroys the ability of leukocytes to reduce the dye dichlorophenol–indophenol, but a specific study of inhibition in cell-free systems has not been made.

E. Antigenicity

Bryce and Rountree (1936) reported that in their experience the α- and β-toxins were antigenically distinct. Williams and Harper (1947) observed that δ-toxin could not be neutralized on sheep blood agar plates by antiserum to β-toxin. Thaysen (1948), using culture filtrates of *S. aureus* isolated from cases of furunculosis in dogs, differentiated on serological grounds a toxin which he referred to as β_2. He claimed that the β_2-toxin differed from the classic β-toxin in its antigenic properties and characteristic dose–time curve. Thaysen also stated that both toxins occur together in ordinary filtrates and that normal dog serum contains relatively large amounts of β_2-antitoxin. Although his observations were never confirmed, support for the existence of two toxins with similar characteristics comes from the work of Maheswaran *et al.* (1967) and Haque and Baldwin (1963) who reported separation of "anionic" and "cationic" β-toxins on DEAE-cellulose. Although Wiseman (1965a) found that β-toxins derived from the R-1 and 252F strains of *S. aureus* manifested slight differences in several properties, he noted that antiserum to 252F toxin would neutralize the R-1 toxin. Further work in this area is required before the concept of multiple forms of the toxin can be supported.

F. Relationship of Beta-Toxin to Pathogenicity of *S. aureus*

There is general agreement that β-toxin is produced only by strains which are coagulase positive, or rather, it has never been reported in coagulase-negative strains of *S. aureus*. Since coagulase is closely associated with pathogenicity, by implication β-toxin must also play a role in the disease process or its initiation. Of course, this has not been proved, nor has it been for any other toxin of *S. aureus* for that matter.

Although β-toxin production is associated with coagulase-positive strains, it is uncommon in strains isolated from lesions in man (Elek, 1959). Microorganisms taken from animals, however, generally produce it (Stamatin *et al.*, 1949; Burns and Holtman, 1960). In particular, β-toxin production is characteristic of *S. aureus* isolated from bovine mastitis (Slanetz and Bartley, 1953). Elek and Levy (1950) in a study of 59 coagulase-positive animal strains, noted that 88% produced detectable quantities of β-toxin on sheep blood agar (Table IX) in contrast with 74% and 86% for α- and δ-toxins, respectively. In the same study, they found that 59% of animal pathogens tested produced all three hemolysins. Only 7% of strains produced β-toxin alone.

Marandon and Oeding (1966) confirmed the results of Rountree (1947), which showed that strains of *S. aureus* producing β-toxin do not generally form staphylokinase and are most commonly isolated from animals. The reverse was also true. Marandon and Oeding further noted that strains producing β-toxin in the absence of staphylokinase were susceptible to phage 42D. Thus, staphylokinase-negative, β-toxin-positive staphylococci are characteristic of strains from animal sources (particularly bovine mastitis) and staphylokinase-positive, β-toxin-negative organisms are chiefly associated with disease in man. The significance of these findings in reference to the question of pathogenicity and virulence of staphylococci has not as yet been appreciated. Winkler *et al.* (1965) have shown that lysogenization of strains of *S. aureus* producing β-toxin by certain serological group F phages has resulted in loss of β-toxin production and gain in staphylokinase production. This appears to be a true lysogenic conversion of the type controlling toxigenicity in *Corynebacterium diphtheriae* and

TABLE IX
INCIDENCE OF HEMOLYSINS IN 359 STRAINS OF STAPHYLOCOCCI[a]

Group	Number of strains examined	Occurrence of hemolysin (%)				
		α	β	δ	ε	nil
I. Coagulase-positive human pathogens	200	96	11	97	0	0
II. Coagulase-positive animal strains	59	74	88	86	0	2
III. Coagulase-negative skin strains	77	0	0	0	95	5

[a] After Elek and Levy (1950).

Streptococcus pyogenes. The study of mutants of this type might shed light on the role of β-toxin in infection.

It is to be expected that possession of enzymes hydrolyzing components of the cell membrane would offer an advantage to staphylococci. However, in the case of β-toxin, *in vivo* sphingomyelinase activity has not yet been demonstrated. It is true that mammalian cell membranes generally contain sphingomyelin in varying concentrations and that certain tissues, notably brain, are rich in this phospholipid, but there is no evidence that such tissues are targets for β-toxigenic *S. aureus*.

II. Delta-Toxin

Twenty years after the discovery of the β-toxin, Williams and Harper (1947) observed that with various strains of *S. aureus* grown on sheep blood agar in the presence of α- and β-antitoxins, hemolysis was not suppressed. The substance responsible for this hemolytic activity was called δ-toxin. The δ-toxin was shown to have a wider spectrum of hemolysis than α- and β-toxins, acting on erythrocytes of rabbit, sheep, man, monkey, horse, rat, mouse, and guinea pig. Marks and Vaughan (1950), who confirmed the existence of δ-toxin, added that it acted synergistically with β-toxin on human and sheep erythrocytes.

A. TOXICITY

Until recently, little definite knowledge was available regarding the toxicity of δ-toxin. Jackson and Little (1956, 1957), working with crude toxin, thought that it might be identical with the leukocidin that acts on human leukocytes. They compared leukocidal activity of α-toxin with that of δ-toxin which had been freed of the former by filtration. In contrast with α-toxin, which caused swelling of the leukocytes, δ-toxin was lytic. Gladstone and van Heyningen (1957) noted that the leukolytic action of the δ-toxin ran parallel with its hemolytic action on human and horse red cells and, like hemolysis, was inhibited by cholesterol. In their experience, the δ-toxin affected the leukocytes of man, rabbit, guinea pig, and mouse. Gladstone and Yoshida (1967) found that polymorphonuclear leukocytes, lymphocytes, and blood macrophages of the rabbit, man, mouse, rat, guinea pig, pigeon, and fowl were all susceptible to the action of crystalline δ-toxin. HeLa, L, HLM, FL, and HEp cells, including chick fibroblasts and rat heart connective tissue cells, all showed essentially similar cytopathic changes in the presence of the toxin according to these authors. The δ-toxin also liberated aldolase and β-glucuronidase from HeLa cells, indicating that the toxin acted on both the cell membrane and on lysosomes. Unfortunately, after the work was completed, Gladstone and Yoshida found that their δ-toxin preparation was contaminated with β-toxin and ribonuclease. Their results, therefore, await confirmation with the use of toxin of demonstrated purity. Bernheimer and Schwartz (1964), using the same toxin preparation employed by Gladstone and Yoshida, found that it did not release significant amounts of β-glucuronidase and acid phosphatase from a large granule fraction of rabbit liver.

Data regarding toxicity of δ-toxin for laboratory animals are scant. Marks and Vaughan (1950) reported that it was dermonecrotic when injected into the skin of rabbits; this was confirmed by Gladstone (1966). Gladstone further observed that intravenous injection of mice with a 55% purified preparation was without visible effect.

B. Production and Purification

1. Production

Williams and Harper (1947) reported that δ-toxin production was not possible in a fluid medium and that carbon dioxide is not essential for its formation on solid media. This was confirmed by Marks and Vaughan (1950). Wiseman (1963) found that on solid media, carbon dioxide concentrations varying from 25 to 75% in air had little effect on growth and toxin production. α-Toxin titers were increased 13-fold in the same strain at 50% concentrations of carbon dioxide in air. Mixtures of carbon dioxide and oxygen also had only a slight effect on δ-toxin titers (Table X). In contrast with these data, Murphy and Haque (1967) found that production of δ-toxin on heart infusion agar plates was optimal at a concentration of 10% carbon dioxide in air. Differences between hemolytic titers in air alone and in the optimal carbon dioxide–air mixture were not large, however.

Yoshida (1963) achieved satisfactory production of δ-toxin in the dialyzable CCY medium of Gladstone and van Heyningen (1957). One liter of CCY medium was placed in a 3-liter conical flask and mechanically gyrated at 37°C for 18–24 hours. Aeration had to be carefully controlled if optimal titers were to be obtained. The inability of earlier investigators to produce the toxin in fluid media was probably due to their failure to appreciate the necessity for adequate aeration of the broth cultures. According to Yoshida, formation of δ-toxin in CCY medium proceeded without lag in association with bacterial growth, reaching a plateau after 18–24 hours. Using strain 146P, Murphy and Haque (1967) obtained similar results on heart infusion agar plates with the cultivation technique of Birch-Hirschfeld (1933). Toxin production reached a maximum after incubation for 20 hours.

TABLE X

EFFECT OF CARBON DIOXIDE CONCENTRATION IN AIR OR OXYGEN UPON PRODUCTION
OF δ-TOXIN BY THE E-DELTA STRAIN OF S. *aureus*[a]

Carbon dioxide concentration (%)	Air			Oxygen		
	Growth (O.D. 650 mμ)	Hemolytic titer (HU/ml)		Growth (O.D. 650 mμ)	Hemolytic titer (HU/ml)	
		α	δ		α	δ
0	0.50	100	50	—	—	—
25	0.49	200	40	0.41	160	40
35	0.51	400	40	0.32	200	40
50	0.67	2560	80	0.42	400	50
75	0.54	1590	40	0.53	640	80

[a] Figures are the means of three experiments. α-Toxin titers were obtained with rabbit erythrocytes and those of δ-toxin with human erythrocytes. After Wiseman (1963).

2. PURIFICATION

Several investigators have attempted to isolate the δ-toxin. Marks and Vaughan (1950) employed overnight extraction of cultures with ethanol at −4°C. After centrifugation, the ethanol was evaporated in a stream of air. Further overnight extraction with diethyl ether left a residue which contained the δ-toxin with an average yield of about 25%. The partially purified preparation was nondialyzable, could not be Seitz filtered without loss of activity, and suffered no change of titer after heating at 65° or 100°C up to 2 hours. In those strains of *S. aureus* producing both β- and δ-toxins, Marks and Vaughan also reported that the two could be separated by adsorption of the δ-toxin onto alumina at pH 8.0.

Jackson and Little (1958b) claimed that δ-toxin could be separated from α-toxin by heating at 60°C for 10–15 minutes. This treatment led to a sharp drop in δ-toxin hemolytic activity, which suggested the existence of two toxins, one heat labile and the other heat stable. Recovery of heat-stable δ-toxin was effected by precipitation of freeze-dried crude material with ethanol at pH 4.0 and at a temperature of −5° to −20°C. The precipitated toxin was further extracted with 75% ethanol in water resulting in a yield of 40% of the original toxin. Traces of α-toxin still remained, however.

Yoshida (1963) developed a procedure for the crystallization of α-toxin which satisfied two criteria of homogeneity — one peak was observed in the ultracentrifuge and one line of precipitation was obtained in Ouchterlony plates in the presence of antiserum. Nevertheless, the crystalline toxin was later shown to be contaminated with ribonuclease and β-toxin (Gladstone and Yoshida, 1967). As a result, one cannot accept their molecular weight and amino acid determinations.

The method of Wiseman and Caird (1968) results in a 30-fold increase in specific activity when crude δ-toxin is compared to purified material. Culture supernatant fluid was dialyzed against acetate buffer at pH 4.0. The active substance found in the precipitate after centrifugation was redissolved and treated with hydroxyapatite at pH 7.0 with elution of toxin being accomplished by addition of 2 M sodium chloride. Further purification was achieved on a column of diethylaminoethyl (DEAE) cellulose at pH 7.0. The hemolytic activity was not retained in the column under these conditions and appeared in the first of several protein peaks eluted in presence of a 0-0.5 M sodium chloride gradient. Although the toxin appeared to be pure when examined in agar gel diffusion plates using an antiserum to crude material prepared in rabbits, other tests of homogeneity were not carried out. Since this report was published, prolonged incubation has revealed the presence of an additional precipitation line. The purification procedure has therefore been modified to include precipitation with 30-45% saturated ammonium sulfate followed by chromatography on DEAE-cellulose. The active effluent was recycled once through the DEAE column in contrast with a single passage in the earlier procedure. Toxin (at a concentration of 6 mg/ml) obtained with the modified method gives one line of precipitation when examined by immunoelectrophoresis and agar gel diffusion techniques. One N-terminal amino acid residue is seen when an acid hydrolyzate of dinitrophenyl-toxin is chromatographed. Tentatively we have assigned the N-terminal position in δ-toxin to proline; its occurrence in this position is perhaps unusual. Disk electrophoresis preparations of the toxin also revealed only one strong stained band of protein.

C. CHARACTERISTICS

1. HEMOLYTIC SPECTRUM

Williams and Harper (1947) observed that the δ-toxin possessed a wider hemolytic spectrum than α- or β-toxins, being lytic for erythrocytes of rabbit, sheep, man, monkey, horse, rat, mouse, and guinea pig. Marks and Vaughan (1950) claimed that the toxin could be recognized by its lysis of human and horse red cells at 37°C and noted that it potentiated lysis of human and sheep erythrocytes by β-toxin. Gladstone (1966) stated that all erythrocyte species that have been tested are susceptible in varying degree to the action of the toxin, though the differential susceptibility is not as apparent as with α- and β-toxins. This is clear from Table XI in which Wiseman (unpublished data) has compared the sensitivities of β- and δ-toxins to various erythrocyte species. Thus, δ-toxin lyses all spe-

TABLE XI

HEMOLYTIC SPECTRUM OF STAPHYLOCOCCAL TOXINS[a]

| | Sensitivity of red cells (HU/ml) to | | | |
| | β-Toxin | | δ-Toxin | |
Red cells	R-1	252F	Newman	E-delta
Man	512	128	512	512
Monkey	< 16	—	—	256
Rabbit	64	32	128	128
Sheep	2048	512	128	64
Ox	512	512	64	64
Guinea pig	< 4	< 4	32	64
Horse	< 4	< 4	8	16

[a] Figures are the means of two determinations. Titrations of the two toxins were not carried out simultaneously, but erythrocyte sensitivity spectra for each toxin are reproducible. After Wiseman (unpublished data).

cies, whereas monkey, ox, and guinea pig cells are resistant to β-toxin. However, there has never been any clear agreement among investigators regarding the hemolytic spectra of staphylococcal toxins, a fact mediated by (1) variability of erythrocyte sensitivity to the toxins in a single animal, (2) differences in toxin concentration and technique of titration used in various laboratories, and (3) the use of impure preparations.

2. EFFECT OF INHIBITORS AND ACTIVATORS

Jackson and Little (1958a) found that a variety of substances would inhibit the hemolytic activity of δ-toxin. On the one hand, erythrocyte ghosts and hemoglobin reduced activity, and on the other, various proteins were inhibitory. Rabbit and human serums, globulins, albumin, and gelatin were all capable of reducing hemolytic activity; γ-globulin at a concentration of 1% was the most effective. Gladstone and Yoshida (1967) found that fibrinogen, α- and β-globulins, and mucoproteins markedly inhibited action of the toxin, while partial inhibition was achieved with γ-globulin and albumin (Table XII).

Wiseman and Caird (1968) also noted that δ-toxin of strains Newman and E-delta was strongly inhibited by 0.1% rabbit and human serums and to a lesser extent by 0.1% human γ-globulin, bovine albumin, and gelatin. They found that there was some inhibition by cholesterol at a concentration of 2 mg/ml, an observation in keeping with that of Gladstone and van Heyningen (1957) but which Gladstone and Yoshida (1967) were not able to confirm at a concentration of 10 mg/ml.

In contrast with β-toxin, metal cations have not been shown to enhance the activity of δ-toxin, nor was EDTA or citrate found to inhibit hemo-

TABLE XII

EFFECT OF VARIOUS PLASMA PROTEIN FRACTIONS AND LECITHIN ON
HEMOLYSIS BY PURIFIED δ-TOXIN[a]

Fraction	Final concentration (%)	Hemolysis (%)	Inhibition (%)
Fraction I (fibrinogen)	0.1	0	100
	0.01	25	65
Fraction II (γ-globulin)	0.5	31	55
Fraction III (β-globulin,			
lipoprotein)	0.1	0	100
	0.01	20	71
Fraction IV (α-globulin,			
lipoprotein)	0.1	0	100
	0.01	17	75
Fraction V (albumin)	0.5	62	10
Fraction VI (mucoprotein)	0.1	0	100
	0.01	60	15
Human serum	0.2	5	93
	0.1	24	65
	0.05	60	15
Rabbit serum (normal)	0.2	9	87
	0.1	18	75
Lecithin (animal)	0.2	72	0
	0.1	65	7
Control	—	70	—

[a] After Gladstone and Yoshida (1967).

lytic activity (Jackson and Little, 1958a). These observations were confirmed by Wiseman and Caird (unpublished data) who were unable to
enhance δ-toxin hemolytic titers over a range of 10^{-2}–10^{-6} M Mg^{2+} and
Ca^{2+}.

D. MODE OF ACTION OF DELTA-TOXIN AND ITS RELATIONSHIP
TO PATHOGENICITY OF *S. aureus*

1. IS THE TOXIN AN ENZYME?

Until recently, nothing was known of the chemical nature and mode of
action of the δ-toxin. Several investigators (Jackson and Little, 1958a;
Marks and Vaughan, 1950) have reported that δ-toxin was stable to heating, although Yoshida (1963) and Wiseman and Caird (unpublished) have
found that highly purified preparations are thermolabile and have noted
that such preparations are sensitive to the action of trypsin and chymotrypsin. That the toxin has a high molecular weight is indicated by the fact
that it is nondialyzable and will pass out in the void volume of a column of
Sephadex G-200 according to Hallander (1963) and to Wiseman and
Caird.

Kapral (1967) reported that the hemolytic activity of δ-toxin was "neutralized" by phospholipids. The activity appeared to be adsorbed to the phospholipids from which it could be recovered by removal of the phosphate radical by nonhemolytic *Bacillus cereus* phospholipase. The nature of the reaction between δ-toxin and phospholipids was not ascertained. Wiseman and Caird (1968), using a highly purified preparation, have shown that δ-toxin releases acid-soluble phosphorus from erythrocytes in direct proportion to their hemolytic sensitivity (Fig. 2). Thus, the evidence is strong that hemolytic and phosphorus-liberating activity are identical. They further showed that the toxin attacks phosphatidylinositol, releasing 19.5 μg phosphorus after 60 minutes of incubation (Table XIII). About 2 μg of phosphorus was released from phosphatidylserine and a trace from phosphatidyl-choline. Sphingomyelin was not hydrolyzed by δ-toxin in contrast with its susceptibility to β-toxin. It was also noted that the rate of release of acid-soluble phosphorus from phosphatidylinositol was linear with respect to time, indicating that the reaction follows first-order kinetics. The reaction rate of δ-toxin is directly propor-

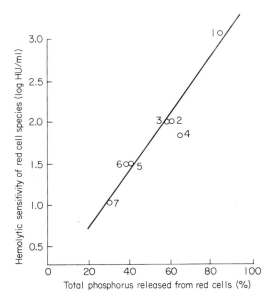

FIG. 2. The hemolytic sensitivity in hemolytic units per milliliter of all red cell species tested was plotted against the amount of acid-soluble phosphorus released from these species in the presence of δ-toxin. The linear correlation between the two phenomena is strong evidence that hemolysis is due to release of the organic phosphorus from a substrate containing it. Key: 1 = human; 2 = guinea pig; 3 = rabbit; 4 = bovine; 5 = goat; 6 = sheep; 7 = horse.

TABLE XIII

SPECIFICITY OF THE ACTION OF δ-TOXIN ON PHOSPHOLIPIDS

Substrate	Incubation time (minutes)	Phosphorus released[a] (μg)
Sphingomyelin	60	0
Phosphatidylcholine	30	0.5
	60	0.7
Phosphatidylserine	30	0.9
	60	2.3
Phosphatidylinositol	30	3.0
	60	19.5
Toxin control	60	0

[a] Figures are the differences between phosphorus released in the presence and absence of toxin. Toxin control is toxin without phospholipids.

tional to temperature between 20 and 56°C, whereas Doery *et al.* (1965) and Maheswaran and Lindorfer (1967) both found that maximum activity of β-toxin was in the region of 40°C.

2. WHAT KIND OF ENZYME IS THE DELTA-TOXIN?

Judging from the fact that the phosphorus released by δ-toxin from phosphatidylinositol is acid soluble, it is suggested without further proof that the enzyme is a phospholipase C-like β-toxin. The reaction may be as follows:

$$\text{Phosphatidylinositol} \longrightarrow \text{inositol phosphate} + \text{diglyceride}$$

It is not yet known whether the presence of a second or third atom of phosphorus on the inositol moiety would change the specificity of the δ-toxin. Furthermore, this work requires confirmation with highly purified substrate.

3. ANTIGENICITY AND *in Vivo* MODE OF ACTION — RELATIONSHIP OF DELTA-TOXIN TO PATHOGENICITY

It has not been possible to demonstrate conclusively the antigenicity of δ-toxin preparations in view of the fact that all normal serums and serum components so far tested have inhibited activity at relatively low concentrations (Table XII; Section C,2). Gladstone and Yoshida (1967), furthermore, noted that the zone of hemolysis did not correspond with the line of precipitation when δ-toxin was incubated with commercial α-antitoxin in a blood agar plate. Wiseman and Caird (1968) have observed that highly purified δ-toxin, when incubated with a rabbit-produced antiserum to crude δ-toxin, gives one strong line of precipitation in a double diffusion plate. Although prolonged incubation did yield an additional line, modification of the purification procedure (Section B,2) yielded a preparation considered to be homogeneous on the basis of several criteria. This material consistently gave one line of precipitation in double diffusion plates and in immunoelectrophoresis and disk electrophoresis experiments. In their opinion, then, it is very unlikely that the δ-toxin is not antigenic.

Nothing is known of the *in vivo* activity of δ-toxin. It has been suggested by various authors that δ-toxin is of no consequence in the pathogenesis of staphylococcal disease since its action is inhibited *in vitro* by normal serum components. Gladstone (1966) has however shown that the toxin is necrotic when injected intracutaneously into rabbits in large doses, but is not lethal for laboratory mice.

Elek and Levy (Table XI; Section I,F) have shown that in *S. aureus* strains from human sources, the association of δ-toxin production with disease is very nearly as high as that of coagulase. In addition, about 86% of coagulase-positive strains from animal sources produced δ-toxin. Joiris (1952) has also noted the close association of δ-toxin production with strains isolated from lesions in man. As with other staphylococcal toxins, it is nevertheless hard to ascribe a particular role to δ-toxin in the pathogenesis of staphylococcal disease.

Recently, Hoffmann and Streitfeld (1965) found that partially purified preparations of δ-toxin inhibited growth of several species of gram-positive bacteria including *S. aureus*; this suggests that the toxin might function as a selective growth agent for the strains producing it. In view of the widespread prevalence of antibacterial agents, this observation awaits confirmation with highly purified material.

REFERENCES

Bergmann, F., Gutman, J., and Chaimovitz, M. (1965). *Proc. 2nd Intern. Pharmacol. Meeting, Prague, 1963* Vol. 9, p. 221. Pergamon Press, Oxford.
Bernheimer, A. W., and Schwartz, L. L. (1964). *J. Bacteriol.* 87, 1100.
Bernheimer, A. W., and Schwartz, L. L. (1965). *J. Pathol. Bacteriol.* 89, 209.
Bigger, J. W., Boland, C. R., and O'Meara, R. A. Q. (1927). *J. Pathol. Bacteriol.* 30, 271.
Birch-Hirschfeld, L. (1933). *Z. Immunitaetsforsch.* 81, 260.
Bryce, L. M., and Rountree, P. M. (1936). *J. Pathol. Bacteriol.* 43, 173.
Burns, J., and Holtman, D. F. (1960). *Ann. N.Y. Acad. Sci.* 88, 1115.
Chesbro, W. R., Heydrick, F. P., Martineau, R., and Perkins, G. N. (1965). *J. Bacteriol.* 89, 378.
Corkill, J. M. B. (1955). *Can. J. Public Health* 46, 243.
Doery, H. M., Magnusson, B. J., Cheyne, I. M., and Gulasekharam, J. (1963). *Nature* 198, 1091.
Doery, H. M., Magnusson, B. J., Gulasekharam, J., and Pearson, J. E. (1965). *J. Gen. Microbiol.* 40, 283.
Dolman, C. E., and Wilson, R. J. (1940). *Can J. Public Health* 31, 68.
Edwards, S. W., and Ball, E. G. (1954). *J. Biol. Chem.* 209, 619.

Elek, S. D. (1959). *"Staphylococcus pyogenes* and its Relation to Disease." Livingstone, Edinburgh and London.

Elek, S. D., and Levy, E. (1950). *J. Pathol. Bacteriol.* **62**, 541.

Flamm, H. (1957). *Schweiz, Z. Allgem. Pathol. Bakteriol.* **20**, 358.

Fulton, F. (1943). *Brit. J. Exptl. Pathol.* **24**, 65.

Gladstone, G. P. (1938). *Brit. J. Exptl. Pathol.* **19**, 208.

Gladstone, G. P. (1966). *Postepy Mikrobiol.* **5**, 145.

Gladstone, G. P., and van Heyningen, W. E. (1957). *Brit. J. Exptl. Pathol.* **38**, 123.

Gladstone, G. P., and Yoshida, A. (1967). *Brit. J. Exptl. Pathol.* **48**, 11.

Glenny, A. T., and Stevens, M. F. (1935). *J. Pathol. Bacteriol.* **40**, 201.

Hallander, H. O. (1963). *Acta Pathol. Microbiol. Scand.* **59**, 543.

Hallander, H. O., and Bengtsson, S. (1967). *Acta Pathol. Microbiol. Scand.* **70**, 107.

Haque, R., and Baldwin, J. N. (1963). *Bacteriol. Proc.* p. 78.

Haque, R., and Baldwin, J. N. (1964). *J. Bacteriol.* **88**, 1304.

Heydrick, F. P., and Chesbro, W. R. (1962). *Bacteriol. Proc.* p. 63.

Hoffmann, F. M., and Streitfeld, M. M. (1965). *Can. J. Microbiol.* **11**, 203.

Jackson, A. W. (1963). *Can. J. Biochem. Physiol.* **41**, 755.

Jackson, A. W., and Little, R. M. (1956). *Bacteriol. Proc.* p. 88.

Jackson, A. W., and Little, R. M. (1957). *Can. J. Microbiol.* **3**, 101.

Jackson, A. W., and Little, R. M. (1958a). *Can. J. Microbiol.* **4**, 435.

Jackson, A. W., and Little, R. M. (1958b). *Can. J. Microbiol.* **4**, 453.

Jackson, A. W., and Mayman, D. (1958). *Can. J. Microbiol.* **4**, 477.

Jeljaszewicz, J., Szmigielski, S., Korbecki, M., and Zak, C. (1965). *J. Infect. Diseases* **115**, 421.

Joiris, E. (1952). *Rev. Belge Pathol.* **22**, 185.

Kapral, F. A. (1967). *Bacteriol. Proc.* p. 64.

Kodama, T., and Kojima, T. (1939). *Kitasato Arch. Exptl. Med.* **16**, 36.

Korbecki, M., and Jeljaszewicz, J. (1965). *J. Infect. Diseases* **115**, 205.

Maheswaran, S. K., and Lindorfer, R. K. (1966). *Bacteriol. Proc.* p. 44.

Maheswaran, S. K., and Lindorfer, R. K. (1967). *J. Bacteriol.* **94**, 1313.

Maheswaran, S. K., Smith, K. L., and Lindorfer, R. K. (1967). *J. Bacteriol.* **94**, 300.

Marandon, J., and Oeding, P. (1966). *Acta Pathol. Microbiol. Scand.* **67**, 149.

Marks, J., and Vaughan, A. C. T. (1950). *J. Pathol. Bacteriol.* **62**, 597.

Murphy, R. A., and Haque, R. (1967). *J. Bacteriol.* **94**, 1327.

Ponder, E. H. (1948). "Hemolysis and Related Phenomena." Grune & Stratton, New York.

Pulsford, M. F. (1954). *Australian J. Exptl. Biol. Med. Sci.* **32**, 347.

Pulvertaft, R. J. V., Greening, J. R., and Haynes, J. A. (1947). *J. Pathol. Bacteriol.* **59**, 293.

Robinson, J., Thatcher, F. S., and Gagnon, J. (1958). *Can. J. Microbiol.* **4**, 345.

Rountree, P. M. (1947). *Australian J. Exptl. Biol. Med. Sci.* **25**, 359.

Roy, T. E. (1937). *J. Immunol.* **33**, 437.

Slanetz, L. W., and Bartley, C. H. (1953). *J. Infect. Diseases* **92**, 139.

Smith, I. M. (1965). *Ann. N.Y. Acad. Sci.* **128**, 334.

Stamatin, N., Tacu, A., and Marica, D. (1949). *Ann. Inst. Pasteur* **76**, 178.

Thatcher, F. S., and Matheson, B. H. (1955). *Can. J. Microbiol.* **1**, 382.

Thaysen, E. H. (1948). *Acta Pathol. Microbiol. Scand.* **25**, 529.

van Heyningen, W. E. (1950). "Bacterial Toxins." Blackwell, Oxford.

Williams, R. E. O., and Harper, G. J. (1947). *J. Pathol. Bacteriol.* **59**, 69.

Winkler, K. C., de Waart, J., Grootsen, C., Zegers, B. J., Tellier, N. F., and Vertregt, C. D. (1965). *J. Gen. Microbiol.* **39**, 321.

Wiseman, G. M. (1963). Ph.D. Thesis, University of Edinburgh.

Wiseman, G. M. (1965a). *J. Pathol. Bacteriol.* **89**, 187.
Wiseman, G. M. (1965b). *Can. J. Microbiol.* **11**, 463.
Wiseman, G. M. (1968). *Can. J. Microbiol.* **14**, 179.
Wiseman, G. M., and Caird, J. D. (1966). *Can. Soc. Microbiol. Abstracts,* p. 16.
Wiseman, G. M., and Caird, J. D. (1967). *Can. J. Microbiol.* **13**, 369.
Wiseman, G. M., and Caird, J. D. (1968). *Proc. Soc. Exptl. Biol. Med.* **128**, 428.
Yoshida, A. (1963). *Biochim. Biophys. Acta* **71**, 544.

CHAPTER 7

Enterotoxins

MERLIN S. BERGDOLL

I. Introduction

The staphylococcal enterotoxins cause food poisoning common in many countries of the world. The ingestion of these substances results in a variety of symptoms, the most common being vomiting and diarrhea 2–6 hours after eating the food containing enterotoxin.

The purification of a protein (enterotoxin) that caused emesis in monkeys led to the discovery that the staphylococci produce more than one enterotoxin (Bergdoll *et al.*, 1959b), the basis for differentiation being their reactions with specific antibodies. It was suggested by Casman (1960) that the first two enterotoxins identified (Bergdoll *et al.*, 1959b; Casman, 1960) be called E and F, since staphylococcal strains isolated from foods implicated in food poisoning outbreaks appeared to produce only enterotoxin F, and many of the strains isolated from patients suffering from enteritis following antibiotic therapy (Surgalla and Dack, 1955) produced enterotoxin E.

In 1962 Bergdoll suggested, through correspondence to other investigators in the field, that a permanent nomenclature for the enterotoxins be established so that new enterotoxins could be named in an orderly manner as they were identified. As a result of this suggestion an open meeting was held on May 9, 1962, at the Sixty-second Annual Meeting of the American Society for Microbiology (Kansas City, Missouri) to establish a system of nomenclature for the enterotoxins. As a result of this meeting the enterotoxins are now designated as enterotoxins A, B, C, etc. (Casman *et al.*, 1963) using reactions with specific antibodies as the basis for differentiation. To date, enterotoxins A (Casman, 1960), B (Bergdoll *et al.*, 1959b), C (Bergdoll *et al.*, 1965a), and D (Casman *et al.*, 1967) have been identified, and E has been tentatively identified (Bergdoll *et al.*, 1968a).

II. Toxicity

A. In Humans

The availability of information about the toxicity of the enterotoxins in humans is almost nonexistent. Although the causative agent was originally determined through the use of human volunteers by Dack *et al.* (1930) to be a substance produced by the staphylococci, no means of determining the toxin content of the materials consumed by the volunteers was available. Two known attempts have been made to test the potency of purified or partially purified enterotoxin B in human volunteers *per os*. An experiment at the Food Research Institute with two individuals gave negative results with pure toxin (enterotoxin B), first with 1 μg and then with as much as 10 μg. In another laboratory, 50 μg of enterotoxin B of an estimated 50% purity was tested on three volunteers and all showed typical food poisoning symptoms within 2-4 hours after ingestion of the toxin (Raj and Bergdoll, 1969). The only other information available concerning humans susceptible to the enterotoxins is from careless handling of the enterotoxins in the laboratory or from volunteers eating food suspected of causing a food poisoning outbreak. Although people working in the laboratory have become ill after working with the enterotoxin and consuming food without washing of the hands, it was not possible from this type of contamination to conclude anything about dosage except that very small amounts were involved. Some information was obtained about the possible potency of enterotoxin A when the content of this toxin was estimated in cheese that had been consumed by human volunteers. The estimate indicated that the human that became ill after eating the smallest amount of cheese (20 gm) had received less than 1 μg. This finding is of greater significance than the results obtained with enterotoxin B, since A is the toxin most frequently encountered in food poisoning outbreaks. Determination of the minimum amount required to cause illness in humans is highly desirable in order to indicate when any given food is safe for human consumption.

B. In Monkeys

1. Per Os

The enterotoxins are toxic to a number of species of animals, particularly when injected intraperitoneally or intravenously. The primates are the only order that is relatively sensitive to the enterotoxins *per os*. The only member of this order other than man that has been used as test animals to any extent is the rhesus monkey (*Macacca mulatta*) (Surgalla *et al.*, 1953) although a few experiments were conducted with cynamologous monkeys and chimpanzees (*Pan*) (Wilson, 1959). This very limited study with five chimpanzees showed them to be about ten times more sensitive to enterotoxin than rhesus monkeys when the dosage is calculated on the basis of kilogram body weight. Much more information is available about the toxicity of enterotoxin B than the other enterotoxins in rhesus monkeys. In one study with about 100 animals (2.5-3 kg) the ED_{50} by the oral route was determined to be 0.9 μg per kilogram body weight (Schantz *et al.*, 1965). Biological activity was characterized by emesis or diarrhea within 5 hours after administration of the toxin through an infant feeding tube that was inserted through the nasal passage to the stomach. Many observations in the Food Research Institute laboratories indicate a dosage of approximately 5 μg per animal (2-3 kg) when emesis only was observed. In these laboratories the toxin is administered directly into the stomach by catheter tube in 50-ml amounts. Limited observations with enterotoxins A and C show them to cause emesis in monkeys in dosages of 5 μg per animal (Chu *et al.*, 1966; Borja and Bergdoll, 1967).

2. Intravenous

The effect of the enterotoxin by routes of administration other than oral (intraperitoneal or intravenous) has been studied. The use of these routes are subject to misinterpretation since products of the staphylococci other than the enterotoxins can cause symptoms similar to those of enterotoxin. Even when the enterotoxin-containing materials are treated with trypsin (Denny and Bohrer, 1963) or pancreatin (Casman and Bennett, 1963) to destroy the interfering substances, one is never sure that these materials have been completely inactivated in every instance. The intravenous injections of enterotoxins has proved very useful in studies where the purified enterotoxins can be used. In one study with enterotoxin B, over 200 rhesus monkeys were injected in the saphenous vein with purified enterotoxin in 0.02 M sodium phosphate buffer containing 0.85% sodium chloride. Illness characterized by vomiting or diarrhea was observed in 50% of the animals at 0.1 μg per kilogram body weight (Schantz *et al.*, 1965). Results of a study with purified enterotoxin A employing 30 monkeys and observing only emesis are given in Table I (Chu *et al.*, 1966). These results show that enterotoxin A injected intravenously is more reactive in the monkey than enterotoxin B.

III. Analysis

A. Introduction

A major problem that has confronted investigators in the enterotoxin field is the lack of practical sensitive methods for the detection and assay of the enterotoxins. The fact that the enterotoxins are proteins eliminates the possibility of developing chemical methods for their detection in that any method developed for one protein would not be specific for that protein alone. The method used must be specific for the biological activity of the enterotoxins or take advantage of some specific characteristic of the enterotoxin molecule.

Naturally, the best test animal for enterotoxin activity would be the human; however, humans are not readily available for experimentation. Many other types of animals have been tested in hopes that an inexpensive specific test could be found. Some animals that react to the entero-

TABLE I

EMESIS IN RHESUS MONKEYS BY ENTEROTOXIN A[a]

Route of administration	Dose	Result[b]
	(μg/animal)	
Intragastric	5	4/10
	10	16/30
	20	9/12
	(μg/kg)	
Intravenous	0.017	2/6
	0.035	2/9
	0.070	4/9
	0.140	5/6

[a] Chu et al., 1966.
[b] Number vomiting versus number challenged.

toxins are pigs (Hopkins and Poland, 1942), dogs (Minett, 1938; Sugiyama et al., 1960, Nikodemusz et al., 1963), cats and kittens (Dolman et al., 1936; Minett, 1938; Davison et al., 1938; Dolman and Wilson, 1940; Hammon, 1941; Matheson and Thatcher, 1955; Casman, 1958), and monkeys (Jordan and McBroom, 1931; Woolpert and Dack, 1933; Surgalla et al., 1953; Schantz et al., 1965). All of these animals with the exception of the monkey are relatively insensitive to the enterotoxins unless they are injected intraperitoneally or intravenously. A number of other animals, such as frogs (Robinton, 1949, 1950; Eddy, 1951), tropical fish (Raj and Liston, 1962), pigeons, nematodes (DeValle, 1960; Chang and Hall, 1963), and various protozoa (McIntosh and Duggan, 1965) did not respond to enterotoxin. Because emesis is the most readily observable reaction to enterotoxin, animals without a vomiting mechanism (e.g., rodents) have been of little value as test animals. In one instance, mice and rabbits pretreated by a parenteral injection of staphylococcal enterotoxin became more susceptible to the lethal action of bacterial endotoxins (Sugiyama et al., 1964a). The disadvantage here was that it was necessary to use partially purified enterotoxins and the injection solutions had to be pyrogen-free.

B. BIOLOGICAL METHODS

The methods most frequently employed are intraperitoneal or intravenous injections of cats and kittens (Dolman and Wilson, 1940; Hammon, 1941) and feeding of young rhesus monkeys (Surgalla et al., 1953). The cat method requires the inactivation of substances that may provoke symptoms similar to those caused by enterotoxin when administered by parenteral routes. Heating at 100°C for 20–30 minutes (Davison et al.,

1938; Dolman and Wilson, 1940) has been used to inactivate other biologically active substances such as the hemolysins; however, not all of the β-hemolysin may be destroyed (Thatcher and Matheson, 1955), and apparently, some strains of staphylococci produce other interfering substances that are not completely destroyed by heat. Although the enterotoxins once were considered to be quite heat stable, studies with the purified enterotoxins show that under some conditions they are readily destroyed by heating. Since α- and β-hemolysin are the primary interfering substances, specific antisera (Dolman, 1943) to these two substances have been used to inactivate them before injection of enterotoxin preparations. This method has limited value since there may be other biologically active substances that could interfere. Since the enterotoxins are resistant to proteolytic enzymes, digestion of crude enterotoxin preparations with trypsin (Denny and Bohrer, 1963) or pancreatin (Casman and Bennett, 1963) have been resorted to to destroy other proteinaceous biologically active substances. Next to the monkey, cats are the most reliable animal, although they are subject to nonspecific reactions. One disadvantage of cats is that they are relatively insensitive to enterotoxin C since 50 times as much of this enterotoxin as enterotoxins A or B is required to produce emesis in these animals. Cats are relatively cheap and could be raised in the laboratory if facilities were available.

The most reliable bioassay for the enterotoxins is the feeding of young rhesus monkeys (Surgalla et al., 1953). Of the toxic moieties produced by the staphylococci, only the enterotoxins cause emesis in these animals. Assays are made by administering the enterotoxins in solutions (usually 50 ml) to young monkeys (2–3 kg) by catheter. The animals are observed for 5 hours after feeding, and vomiting is accepted as a positive reaction for enterotoxin. To determine the presence of enterotoxin in a given sample, six monkeys are used and emesis in at least two animals is considered a positive reaction. The original cost of the animals and the expense of their upkeep limit their availability for routine testing. The cost is increased because the animals become resistant to the enterotoxin after several injections. Since other methods are now available for analyzing known enterotoxins, the use of monkeys is generally restricted to testing for new enterotoxins.

A number of studies have been undertaken to identify enterotoxin with biologic activities other than its emetic action on animals. Its effect on microorganisms, on isolated enzyme systems, etc., have been investigated with negative results. Negative results were obtained with tissue cultures (Milone, 1962) and monkey kidney cells (Kienitz and Schmelter, 1964), while Schaeffer et al. (1966) reported positive results with human embryonic intestinal cells, although relatively large amounts of enterotoxin

(40-60 μg/ml) were required. A study with chicken embryos (Kienitz and Preuner, 1959; Kicnitz, 1962) showed that enterotoxin did have a lethal effect, but there was interference from the hemolysins. Frequently, some type of effect is demonstrated with crude enterotoxin preparations, but not with the purified enterotoxin. Sometimes investigators are misled to believe that the particular activity under investigation is due to enterotoxin either because controls are inadequate or because purified enterotoxin is not used for test purposes.

C. SPECIFIC ANTIBODIES

One property of proteins, the eliciting of specific antibodies when injected into animals, has been taken advantage of in the development of specific assay methods. The fact that a precipitate is formed when antigens are mixed with their specific antibodies has been used as the basis of a number of methods for detecting enterotoxins. Although the antigen–antibody reaction may not necessarily indicate biological activity, in most instances, however, correlation between the two is adequate to justify using the immunological reaction in assaying for enterotoxin. Among the methods that have been proposed are the Oudin single gel diffusion tube test (Surgalla *et al.,* 1952), the Oakley double gel diffusion tube test (Bergdoll *et al.,* 1959a, 1961; Hall *et al.,* 1965), the comparator cell (Surgalla *et al.,* 1952; Bergdoll *et al.,* 1959b), Ouchterlony plates (Casman, 1958; Bergdoll *et al.,* 1959b, 1965a), the Wadsworth microslide (Casman and Bennett, 1963; Hall *et al.,* 1965), quantitative precipitin test (Silverman, 1963), hemagglutination inhibition (Morse and Mah, 1967; Johnson *et al.,* 1967), reversed passive hemagglutination (Silverman *et al.,* 1968), and immunofluorescence (Friedman and White, 1965; Genigeorgis and Sadler, 1966a). All of these methods have been used for the detection of the enterotoxins, with the single diffusion tube method (Bergdoll, 1962; Hall *et al.,* 1963; Read *et al.,* 1965b; Weirether *et al.,* 1966) and the quantitative precipitin test (Silverman, 1963) the only ones adapted for quantitative determination of the enterotoxins. The type of method employing the specific antigen–antibody reaction depends on the type of experiment being conducted. Each of the various methods has been found to be useful in certain instances.

1. SINGLE GEL DIFFUSION TUBE

The single gel diffusion tube test is most useful in production and purification work because the enterotoxin can be determined quantitatively (Bergdoll, 1962). In this method, an agar column (4 mm diameter) containing the enterotoxin antiserum is layered with the enterotoxin solution

(5-200 μg/ml). The front of the precipitate band formed by the interaction of the enterotoxin with its antibody moves down the agar column at a rate corresponding to the concentration of the enterotoxin and the concentration of the antibody. The distance the band moves within a given time is measured and the enterotoxin concentration calculated from a standard curve. The standard curve is obtained by plotting the log of known enterotoxin concentrations (μg/ml) against the distance that the precipitate band moves in millimeters into the agar column in a given time. Incubation for 7 days at 25°C is the standard procedure at the Food Research Institute; however, other investigators incubate for shorter periods of time at higher temperatures (Weirether et al., 1966). Because the movement of the precipitate band is affected by pH and salt concentration, the enterotoxin samples to be analyzed are either dialyzed against the standard gel diffusion buffer (0.02 M sodium phosphate buffer, pH 7.4 containing 0.85% sodium chloride and 1 : 10,000 merthiolate), or the enterotoxin used in preparing the standard curve is dissolved in the solution employed in the experiments (Kato et al., 1966). The limits of sensitivity of this method is 1-2 μg/ml of enterotoxin, which restricts its use when one is trying to detect very small amounts of enterotoxin, for example, in foods. It is not recommended as a method for the identification of enterotoxin since one cannot compare the unknown directly with a known enterotoxin.

2. DOUBLE GEL DIFFUSION TUBE

The double gel diffusion tube method is used to detect impurities in enterotoxin fractions obtained in purification procedures and in the purified enterotoxins (Bergdoll et al., 1959a). It also has been used to detect very small amounts of enterotoxin in toxin preparations (Hall et al., 1965). This method involves the placing of a layer of agar between the antibody-agar and antigen layers. A line of precipitate forms in the agar layer for each antigen-antibody system (providing the concentration of the reactants are not too unbalanced) with the position of the line being dependent on the relative concentrations of the two reactants. The length of the agar layer and the concentration of the antigen and antibody determine the time required for a line to appear. Lines will develop within 2 or 3 days if the agar layer is only a few millimeters thick and the antigen concentration is of the order of 10-20 μg/ml. It has been reported that as little as 0.05 μg/ml of enterotoxin can be detected by this method (Hall et al., 1965); however, the time required to detect a line with this small amount is up to 21 days. One disadvantage of this method is that the sample to be tested cannot be compared directly with a known enterotoxin. The double gel diffusion comparator cell technique is one attempt to overcome this problem (Surgalla *et al.*, 1952; Bergdoll *et al.*, 1959b). The comparator cell can be described as two to four single tubes combined with the agar-containing portions as one wide tube and the antigen-containing part as individual tubes. The unknown is placed in one tube and the known in another tube. When the lines develop in the agar, the line formed with the unknown will join with the line of the known enterotoxin if the unknown contains the reference enterotoxin.

3. OUCHTERLONY PLATE

The Ouchterlony plate technique is used for the detection of enterotoxins in unknown materials (Bergdoll *et al.*, 1965a). There are many modifications of the original method, involving primarily the shape and placement of the antigen and antibody wells in the agar. The wells are usually round and normally are in a circle around a center well with the edges of the outer wells 2–4 mm from the edge of the center well. The farther apart the wells are, the longer the time for development and the more concentrated the reagents need to be. Usually, good lines can be obtained overnight (25°C) with 5–20 μg enterotoxin/ml when the wells are 2–3 mm apart. To obtain lines with smaller amounts of toxin requires 2–3 days, but frequently the reagents disappear from the wells before the lines develop adequately. Normally, the antibody is placed in the center well and control toxin and unknown materials are alternated in the outer wells. This method is not as sensitive as the microslide technique, but it is adequate for detecting enterotoxin in concentrated supernates and is much easier for inexperienced personnel to use. Attempts are being made to modify this method to make it as sensitive as the microslide method.

4. MICROSLIDE

The microslide technique is used for the detection of very small amounts of enterotoxin in concentrated food extracts and in bacterial culture filtrates produced with staphylococci of unknown enterotoxigenicity (Casman and Bennett, 1963; Hall *et al.*, 1965). In this method an ordinary microscope slide is cleaned and plastic electrician's tape (two layers thick) is placed near each end of the slide leaving a space between of 2 cm. The space between the taped areas is coated with agar and dried. Hot buffered agar is placed between the taped areas and immediately covered with a template made of Plexiglas. The antiserum is placed in the center hole and the control enterotoxin and unknowns are placed in the outer holes. The slides are incubated at room temperature in a petri dish containing moist cotton for 1–3 days. After incubation, the template is removed and the lines of precipitate are observed under oblique lighting with the aid of a magnifying glass. As little as 0.1 μg/ml of enterotoxin has been detected by this method; however, in order to achieve this sensitivity a great deal of experience is necessary. This method appears to be the most difficult of the various gel diffusion methods for the uninitiated to obtain satisfactory results. The ratio of antigen to antibody must be very carefully controlled for the most sensitive operation. At the present time this method is the one of choice to detect the small amounts of enterotoxin present in concentrated food extracts. It is possible to concentrate food extracts to 0.1 ml for analysis by this method since very small amounts of solution are required.

5. QUANTITATIVE PRECIPITIN TEST

The quantitative precipitin test of Heidelberger and Kendall (1929) has been applied to the determination of enterotoxin B by Silverman (1963). In these tests 0.5 ml of antigen solution was mixed with 0.5 ml of antitoxin and incubated at 37°C for 4 hours and then at 4°C for 4 days. Washed precipitates were analyzed for total nitrogen by the micro-Kjeldahl technique. The enterotoxin content was calculated from a standard curve prepared with the purified toxin and antitoxin. This investigator reported that no significant difference in results between the gel diffusion and quantitative precipitin test was obtained.

6. HEMAGGLUTINATION INHIBITION

Two procedures employing hemagglutination inhibition for the detection of enterotoxins have been reported (Morse and Mah, 1967; Johnson *et al.,* 1967). So far, however, they have been used only for detection of enterotoxin B primarily in bacterial culture supernates. In one procedure, formalinized sheep erythrocytes were treated with tannic acid before sensitization with enterotoxin (Morse and Mah, 1967); in the other procedure the enterotoxin was coupled to the formalinized erythrocytes with bis-diazatized benzidine (Johnson *et al.,* 1967). The sensitized erythrocytes were added to various combinations of enterotoxin–antienterotoxin and only if insufficient enterotoxin was present did hemagglutination occur. This method is as sensitive or more sensitive than gel diffusion tests and it can be completed in several hours even with low concentrations of enterotoxin; however, experience is needed in interpretation of the results. One problem with this method is that some staphylococcal cultures contain hemagglutinins that are difficult to adsorb by sensitized erythrocytes or to destroy by heating (Johnson *et al.,* 1967).

7. REVERSED PASSIVE HEMAGGLUTINATION

In the reversed passive hemagglutination (Silverman *et al.,* 1968), formalin-preserved sheep erythrocytes were treated with tannic acid before sensitization with enterotoxin antibodies. The sensitized cells were preserved with either formalin or pyruvic aldehyde. In the test, enterotoxin solutions were treated with the sensitized erythrocytes and allowed to stand for 2 hours before the degree of agglutination was determined. With the antiserum used in the experiments reported by these investigators 0.0015 μg of enterotoxin/ml was the smallest amount that resulted in distinct hemagglutination. No particular difficulties were encountered with this method, although antiserum containing only antibodies to enterotoxin is essential. This method might become the one of choice where a very high degree of sensitivity is required.

8. FLUORESCENT ANTIBODY

Another method that has been proposed for the detection of enterotoxin is the use of fluorescent antibodies (Genigeorgis and Sadler, 1966a). Specific antibodies to the enterotoxins were conjugated with fluorescein isothiocyanate and used to stain fixed smears or to precipitate the enterotoxin in fluids containing living cells and enterotoxin or enterotoxin alone. After incubation the precipitates were caught on Millipore filter membranes and washed, and impression smears were made on slides. Enterotoxin produced in foods in the laboratory has been detected by this method, although the amount of enterotoxin present was relatively large, that is, several micrograms per milliliter of food slurry. The authors state that less than 0.05 μg/ml of enterotoxin can be detected by their method (Genigeorgis and Sadler, 1966b). This is misleading, however, since the enterotoxin was detected directly on the food where there was a relatively high local concentration of enterotoxin around the microorganisms, probably much greater than 0.05 μg/ml. The sensitivity of this method appears to be about 1 μg/ml.

D. DETECTION IN FOODS

The amount of enterotoxin required to cause illness in humans is not known, although a rough estimate for enterotoxin A (the enterotoxin most frequently involved in food poisoning outbreaks) has been made from a food poisoning outbreak involving cheese. An analysis of the cheese for its enterotoxin content along with some human volunteer studies indicated a dosage of around 1 μg. Since the amount of food consumed by an individual may be 50-100 gm, it is not possible to detect 1 μg in this amount of food by the methods currently being used for this purpose without some means of concentrating the enterotoxin. The degree to which a food extract must be concentrated depends on the sensitivity of the method used to detect the enterotoxin in the extract. Only two methods, double gel diffusion tube and microslide, have actually been used to detect the enterotoxin in concentrated food extracts, although reversed passive hemagglutination, immunofluorescence, and hemagglutination inhibition have been suggested. At present, immunofluorescence appears to be less sensitive than the other methods, and hemagglutination inhibition, even though it can detect as little as 0.04 μg/ml, may suffer from interference by impurities present in crude extracts. The most recent information concerning the double diffusion tube and microslide tests is that they are about equal in sensitivity on a toxin concentration basis (0.05-0.1 μg/ml); however, the double diffusion method requires a greater volume of solution than the microslide method (0.2 ml and 0.02 ml, respectively, per single analysis) and it is not possible to compare the unknown with a control. The current method of choice, therefore, is the microslide technique. Whether this method is adequate to detect the enterotoxin in concentrated extracts from foods containing the minimum amount of enterotoxin required to make a very sensitive individual ill is not known. It is adequate to detect the enterotoxin in most foods implicated in food poisoning outbreaks, although it may not be sensitive enough to establish the safety of a food under all circumstances.

The most recent method that has been proposed for detection of enterotoxins in foods is reversed passive hemagglutination (Silverman *et al.*, 1968). Since as little as 0.0015 μg of enterotoxin/ml can be detected by this method, it should be possible to detect 0.3 μg enterotoxin in 100 gm of food without concentration of the food extract. In tests with several foods to which 1 μg of enterotoxin B was added to 100 gm of food, the enterotoxin was detected without difficulty. This method has not been tested adequately on foods from food poisoning outbreaks or with enterotoxins other than B. It is not possible with this method to compare an unknown directly with a known enterotoxin as in the microslide technique; however, this method may become the method of choice for detecting very small amounts of enterotoxin in food extracts.

The efforts to detect enterotoxin in foods has been concentrated primarily on procedures for extracting and concentrating the enterotoxin from foods. The methods proposed include froth flotation with rhodamine B-labeled antibodies followed by gel filtration through Sephadex (Hopper, 1963), acid precipitation and chloroform extraction of milk and cheese extracts (Read *et al.*, 1965a,b), chromatography with the ion exchange resin Amberlite CG50 (Hall *et al.*, 1965), and chromatography with carboxymethylcellulose (Casman and Bennett, 1965). The latter three methods involve additional concentration of the extracts with polyethylene glycol 20,000.

In the froth flotation method the enterotoxin was determined in the concentrated extract by clumping the rhodamine B antibody-enterotoxin complex with latex polystyrene. Problems may be encountered from extraneous material in the food extracts which can complicate determination of a positive reaction. The limits of sensitivity of this method is about 1 μg/ml of concentrated extract.

The methods developed for milk and cheese by Read *et al.* (1965a, b) involve a series of precipitations and chloroform extractions. The authors reported that levels of 0.02–0.05 μg of enterotoxin/gm of cheese could be detected by their method using the double gel diffusion tube test. They were unable, however, to detect enterotoxin in the extract from cheese which had made human volunteers ill. Kollias (1967) used the first step of Read's procedure (acidification, centrifugation, and filtration) to detect enterotoxin B (2 μg/ml) added to milk by hemagglutination inhibition. This method is inadequate, however, for detection of the small amounts of enterotoxin (0.004 μg/ml) sometimes present in foods involved in food poisoning outbreaks, since the minimum amount that can be detected by hemagglutination inhibition is 0.04 μg/ml.

Hall *et al.* (1965) employed as the primary step for concentration and partial purification of the enterotoxin in food extracts chromatography using the ion exchange resin Amberlite CG-50. The enterotoxin in the concentrated extract was detected by either the double gel diffusion tube or microslide techniques. The authors reported that 0.05 μg of enterotoxin/gm of food could be detected by their method. It is currently in use by the authors to examine foods implicated in food poisoning outbreaks, but it has not been adequately tested by other workers in the field.

The method developed by Casman and Bennett (1965) also employed chromatography (carboxymethylcellulose) as the primary step for concentration of food extracts. For some foods such as cheese it has been necessary to use chloroform extractions to remove some of the interfering contaminants that are not removed by the carboxymethylcellulose. The extracts were concentrated to 0.1–0.2 ml and the enterotoxin detected by the microslide technique. As little as 0.25–0.5 μg of enterotoxin in 100 gm of food has been detected by this method. It has been used more widely than any other method and recently was used to examine over 4 million pounds of cheese for possible enterotoxin contamination (Zehren and Zehren, 1968). The limitation of this method as well as all the methods employing specific antibodies for the detection of the enterotoxin is governed by the availability of antiserum specific for the enterotoxins. Only those enterotoxins that have been identified with specific antibodies can be detected. This means that it is not always possible to detect the enterotoxin in foods implicated in food poisoning outbreaks, even though it may be present.

IV. Production

A. MEDIA

1. COMPOSITION – MAIN INGREDIENTS

The methods for the production of the enterotoxins has changed markedly since Dack *et al.* (1930) first produced enterotoxin in veal infusion broth. The choice of media is an important consideration in the production of enterotoxin and is governed to a large degree by the purpose of the production. For example, it is desirable to select the simplest medium possible when the enterotoxin is to be used in purification studies in order to avoid complicating the purification. The use of completely dialyzable media makes it possible to avoid substances such as other proteins that might be difficult to separate from the enterotoxin. If the purpose is merely detection or identification of the enterotoxin, then it is desirable to use the medium which will result in the greatest concentration.

Meat infusion broths such as veal (Woolpert and Dack, 1933; Segalove, 1947; Surgalla *et al.*, 1951), beef heart (Burnet, 1930; Hallander, 1965), beef (Dolman, 1934), and brain heart (Casman and Bennett, 1963; D'Arca Simonetti, 1965; McLean *et al.*, 1968) were and are still being used for the production of enterotoxin. Usually the meat infusion broths are supplemented with a small amount of peptone and in some cases glucose. One investigator reported that supplementation of brain heart infusion with 1% maltose resulted in better enterotoxin B production than any other medium used (D'Arca Simonetti, 1965). Casman and Bennett (1963) found that brain heart infusion broth was consistently superior to other media for the production of enterotoxin A, and these investigators have used it for the production of all enterotoxins (for identification purposes), even though Mullet and Friedman (1961) reported that this was a poor medium for production of enterotoxin B. Hallander (1965) obtained only one-thirtieth as much enterotoxin B in heart infusion as in a medium containing hydrolyzed casein. Genigeorgis and Sadler (1966c), however, obtained yields of enterotoxin B up to 188 μg/ml in brain heart infusion which is adequate for many types of experiments. Such yields of enterotoxin B are possible even in a poorer medium, since, in general, B-producing strains are higher yielders than strains that produce other enterotoxins. Yields of at least 900 μg/ml have been obtained with the B producing strain S-6 in media considered optimum for large-scale production of this enterotoxin. Much higher yields than this have been obtained by methods specifically designed for producing small volumes of very potent toxin (Casman and Bennett, 1963). The meat infusion broths have been and are used primarily for production of smaller volumes of relatively potent enterotoxin for detection and identification purposes.

The trend to simpler media began when Dolman and Wilson (1938) replaced beef infusion broth in their media with Difco Proteose peptone and Favorite and Hammon (1941) used casein hydrolyzed with hydrochloric acid as the main ingredient in their medium. Segalove (1947) was the first to employ pancreatic digests of casein for the production of enterotoxin. He used a product called Amigen (Mead Johnson and Co.) which later became the preferred main ingredient of the media used by the investigators at the Food Research Institute (Surgalla *et al.*, 1951; Kato *et al.*, 1966). This material made possible the use of a very simple media for production of the toxin for purification.

After Amigen was used for many years, it became temporarily unavailable — (it is now available as Protein Hydrolysate Powder (PHP), Mead Johnson International, Evansville, Indiana) — and it was necessary to investigate other pancreatic digests. A series of these are produced by Sheffield Chemical Co., Norwich, New York, and some of them have proved to be useful in the production of enterotoxins, especially when substituted with other materials (Table II). N-Z Amine A has been used in equal amounts with PHP for production of large volumes of enterotoxin (1000–2000 gallons) and N-Z Amine NAK (NAK) has been used in equal quantities with PHP for the production of enterotoxin B in high yields and as the main ingredient in the medium for production of enterotoxin A and C in large quantities in the laboratory (Kato *et al.*, 1966). N-Z

TABLE II

PANCREATIC DIGESTS OF CASEIN AS A MEDIUM FOR
PRODUCTION OF ENTEROTOXIN B [a]

Digest[b]	Final pH	Optical density[c]	Amount of enterotoxin[d] (μg/ml)
2% PHP	8.4	3.10	200
2% N-Z Amine A	8.4	1.20	40
4% N-Z Amine A	8.2	2.10	110
3% N-Z Amine A + 0.1% K_2HPO_4	8.3	2.60	210
1% PHP + 1% N-Z Amine A	8.3	2.30	190
3% PHP + 3% N-Z Amine NAK	8.2	9.60	480

[a] Kato *et al.*, 1966.

[b] Supplemented with 0.001% niacin and 0.00005% thiamin and adjusted to pH 6.5; incubation at 37°C for 18 hours on a gyrotory shaker (280 rpm).

[c] Optical density determined at 1:10 or 1:20 dilution at 655 mμ in a Coleman spectrophotometer and the result multiplied by the appropriate factor.

[d] Enterotoxin quantity determined by gel diffusion.

Amine A has been used for the production of enterotoxin D (Casman *et al.*, 1967) and for certain experiments with enterotoxin B (Rosenwald and Lincoln, 1966).

2. COMPOSITION – SUPPLEMENTS

Supplementation of most media used in the production of enterotoxin, particularly the casein hydrolyzates, is necessary for optimum growth of the staphylococci. Favorite and Hammon (1941) added thiamin, nicotinic acid, and glucose to their medium containing acid hydrolyzed casein. Casman (1958) found it necessary to supplement acid hydrolyzed casein with calcium pantothenate, thiamin, nicotinic acid, ferric citrate, potassium hydrogen phosphate, potassium dihydrogen phosphate, magnesium sulfate, sodium acetate (in place of the glucose in Favorite and Hammon's medium) L-cystine and L-tryptophan in order to obtain consistently good growth and enterotoxin production. Casman explained this difference by the fact that it was necessary for Favorite and Hammon to use a heavy inoculum prepared in meat infusion peptone broth to obtain good growth, thus supplying additional growth factors.

Segalove (1947) supplemented his pancreatic digest of casein medium, Amigen, with thiamin, nicotinic acid, calcium pantothenate, magnesium sulfate, potassium dihydrogen phosphate, ferrous ammonium sulfate, and glucose. Later experiments in the Food Research Institute laboratories with Amigen indicated that supplementation with thiamin and nicotinic acid only was sufficient for enterotoxin production (demonstrated by the monkey feeding test), although in most cases glucose was added.

Unfortunately, all of these studies were reported before a method for the quantitative measurement of enterotoxin was available (Bergdoll, 1962), and it is impossible to determine their relative value in enterotoxin production. Data obtained in the Food Research Institute laboratories since that time, however, show that supplementation of PHP with anything other than niacin and thiamin hydrochloride is unnecessary and almost as much enterotoxin B is produced when thiamin is left out (Table III). The use of PHP in Casman's medium (Casman, 1958) in place of Casamino acids yielded less enterotoxin than the same amount of PHP supplemented with niacin (Table III). Attempts to substitute N-Z Amine A for PHP indicated that equivalent results could be obtained when only part of the PHP was replaced or when larger amounts were used and the medium supplemented with a potassium salt in addition to the thiamin hydrochloride and niacin (Table II). Haynes *et al.* (1954) showed that potassium was required for optimum growth of staphylococci, and from the studies with N-Z Amine A it is apparent that this product lacks the amount of potassium required for optimum growth of these organisms.

TABLE III

SUPPLEMENTATION OF PROTEIN HYDROLYZATE POWDER (PHP)
FOR ENTEROTOXIN B PRODUCTION[a]

2% PHP supplement	Starting pH	Final pH	Optical density[b]	Amount of enterotoxin (μg/ml)
None	6.5	7.3	0.30	0
Thiamin[c]	6.5	7.5	0.40	15
Niacin[c]	6.5	8.5	2.70	210
Niacin + thiamin[c]	6.5	8.5	2.90	245
Niacin + thiamin[c]	7.6	8.4	3.10	200
Casman[d]	7.6	8.3	3.20	180

[a]Bergdoll, 1961.

[b]Optical density determined at 1:10 or 1:20 dilution at 655 mμ in a Coleman spectrophotometer and the result multiplied by the appropriate factor.

[c]Supplemented with 0.00005% thiamin and 0.001% niacin; incubation at 37°C for 18 hours on a gyrotory shaker (280 rpm).

[d]Casman, 1958.

Less work has been done in recent years on exploring media for the maximum yield of enterotoxin B since there is less need for producing it in quantity as large amounts of the purified toxin have already been prepared (Schantz et al., 1965). Media that is useful in the production of one enterotoxin may give different results with another, such as the results obtained with brain heart infusion broth for enterotoxins A and B as mentioned previously and with NAK for the same two enterotoxins (Kato et al., 1966). Even though 4% NAK gives somewhat higher yields of enterotoxin A and C than does 3% NAK plus 3% PHP, the fact that much higher yields of enterotoxin B are obtained in the latter medium recommends it as the medium of choice for producing volumes of any as yet unidentified enterotoxins for purification.

3. pH

The selection of the pH to which the medium should be adjusted is also of concern, although enterotoxin has been produced over a pH range. It should be pointed out that in most attempts to produce enterotoxin, only occasionally has an effort been made to maintain the pH of the medium constant throughout the incubation, since a buffer of high ionic strength would be required to counteract the pH effect of the metabolic products produced during the incubation. An attempt in the Food Research Institute laboratories to maintain a constant pH with phosphate buffers did indicate that at pH 7.5 the most enterotoxin was produced; however, the concentration of phosphate required to hold the pH within 0.2 of a pH unit inhibited the growth of the staphylococci and less total enterotoxin was produced than when no attempt was made to maintain a constant pH. The only other way to control pH is by automatically adding acid or base. Laboratory fermenters are available which incorporate pH control of the medium during incubation, although no reports have been made of their use in studying enterotoxin production.

Woolpert and Dack (1933) adjusted their medium to pH 6 in their early experiments on enterotoxin production. Dolman (1943) reported adjusting his medium to pH 7.2, and for many years nearly all investigators adjusted their media to pH 7.2-7.6. The latter pH was the one used in the Food Research Institute laboratories for over 15 years before meaningful experiments could be conducted on the effect of pH on enterotoxin production.

Studies on the effect of pH are complicated by the fact that the results obtained are dependent on the composition of the media and the manner in which the incubation is carried out. For example, when 15 liters of Amigen medium (pH 7.6) containing glucose was incubated in 5-gallon Pyrex bottles with sparging the pH after incubation was above 8 (Surgalla *et al.*, 1951). Incubation of Amigen medium (pH 7.6) with glucose in turning bottles (10 liters of medium in 12-gallon bottles, rotating on the side at a rate of 3 times per hour for 3 days) resulted in a pH of about 5.5, while incubation of 200 ml of medium in Roux bottles for 3 days resulted in a pH of about 6.5. When the medium was made semisolid with agar and incubated in Roux bottles, the final pH was over 7.

No studies similar to the ones described above have been conducted with enterotoxin B-producing strains since methods for quantitative measurement of enterotoxin were developed. Casman and Bennett (1963) have reported on the production of enterotoxin A by using different methods and media, but the results are less conclusive for A since the amounts of this enterotoxin produced are relatively small except in the cellophane sac method. These investigators recommend adjusting the pH to 5.3-5.5 when semisolid brain heart infusion agar is used, to pH 6.5-7.0 for the cellophane sac procedure, and to pH 5.5 for media rotated in 8-ounce nursing bottles. The investigations of Kato *et al.* (1966) with enterotoxin A indicate the best results were obtained with PHP and NAK media when they were adjusted to pH 6.0. The only method of incubation used in these experiments was rotation of the medium in Erlenmeyer flasks on a gyrotory shaker at 280 rpm for 24 hours at 37°C. Results of experiments with enterotoxin B indicated adjustment of the medium to pH 6 resulted in somewhat more toxin than at other pH's tested (Table IV). The pH of the media after incubation may be important as an indication of good growth and enterotoxin production. Under the conditions used in the

TABLE IV

EFFECT OF pH ADJUSTMENT OF MEDIA
ON ENTEROTOXIN B PRODUCTION[a]

Starting pH	Final pH	Optical density[b]	Amount of enterotoxin (μg/ml)
5.0	8.1	2.50	200
5.5	8.3	2.40	270
6.0	8.3	2.40	290
6.5	8.3	2.50	260
7.0	8.3	2.60	260
7.5	8.4	2.40	230
8.0	8.4	2.60	200

[a]Bergdoll, 1961; 2% PHP supplemented with 0.001% niacin and 0.00005% thiamin; incubation at 37°C for 18 hours on a gyrotory shaker (280 rpm).

[b]Optical density determined at 1:10 or 1:20 dilution at 655 mμ in a Coleman spectrophotometer and the result multiplied by the appropriate factor.

Food Research Institute laboratories, a rise during incubation to above pH 8 seems desirable. There is need for further information about the effect of pH with different media incubated under different conditions.

B. METHODS

1. SEMISOLID MEDIA

Several different methods of incubation have been used in the production of enterotoxin. Again, the choice of method depends a great deal on the purpose of the production. One of the early methods (Woolpert and Dack, 1933) involved the incubation of semisolid media (1% agar) in Kolle flasks under 20% carbon dioxide at 37°C for 48-72 hours. This method was developed in an attempt to produce a potent toxin before any means was available for determination of the enterotoxin content. This method has been used by other investigators and has proved useful for the preparation of small volumes of potent toxin, but it is too cumbersome for production of the volumes needed for purification studies. Semisolid and solid media are still in use today for the preparation of small volumes of concentrated enterotoxin. Casman and Bennett (1963) incubated 25 ml quantities of semisolid brain heart infusion media (0.6-0.7% agar) in standard petri dishes in air for 48-72 hours at 35-37°C. Semisolid media in petri dishes had been used by both Burnet (1931) and Dolman (1934) in the early days of enterotoxin production; however, in both cases, incubation was carried out in McIntosh-Fildes jars under a carbon dioxide-oxygen gas mixture. Inoculation (Casman and Bennett, 1963) was accomplished by spreading four drops of an aqueous suspension of the organisms over the surface. Enterotoxigenicity of strains producing less than 2.5–5.0 cat-vomiting doses of toxin A cannot be determined by this method without concentration of the toxin solution when the micro-slide technique is used for detection of the enterotoxin. Hallander (1965) used petri dishes (14 cm) containing solid media (1.5% agar) covered with autoclaved cellophane. The inoculum in 5 ml of phosphate buffered saline was poured onto the cellophane and incubation was carried out at 37°C for 24–72 hours. It is not possible to evaluate Hallander's method with other methods because the enterotoxin was not determined quantitatively.

2. DEEP CULTURE AERATION

Surgalla *et al.* (1951) used deep culture aeration, incubating 15 liters of medium in 5-gallon bottles by passing up to 30 liters of air per hour through sintered glass spargers placed near the bottom of the bottle. This method has been used only occasionally for production of enterotoxin in the laboratory, but has been adapted for use on a large scale in pilot plant operations (1000–2000 gallons). This is the only method usable for pilot plant production and has been used successfully for production of enterotoxins A, B, and C. The main problem with production of this scale is the recovery of the enterotoxins from such large volumes.

The deep culture aeration method has been used in other laboratories for enterotoxin production, but studies in the Food Research Institute using a small scale device (capacity of 1.5 liters of medium) designed to duplicate the results obtained in large tanks showed that with enterotoxin B less enterotoxin was produced by this method than by shaking. No direct comparison of the two methods have been made for enterotoxin A, but results obtained in another laboratory using large bottles similar to those used by Surgalla *et al.* (1951) indicated more A was produced than is currently obtained by shaking in the Food Research Insitute. One problem in aeration methods that must be dealt with is the necessity for use of antifoams. Many different materials have been tried, but the one that appears to give the best results is GE-silicone. Unless a device is available for automatically adding antifoam, the problem is to add sufficient amounts to the medium to control the foaming throughout the incubation. This is sometimes difficult since the staphylococci vary widely in their production of materials which cause foaming.

3. ROTATION

Several different methods involving rotation or movement of the medium containers during incubation have been reported. Favorite and Hammon (1941) carried out their incubations in 250-ml, narrow-necked

Pyrex nursing bottles with the medium in a carbon dioxide-oxygen atmosphere 48-96 hours at 37°C. Some were rotated on their horizontal axes and some, containing glass marbles, were turned end over end, both at 20 rph. Others were placed in a shaking machine. Casman and Bennett (1963) have also employed the horizontal rotation procedure using 8-ounce nursing bottles (25-ml medium in air atmosphere) but rotating at 20 rpm at 35-37°C for 18-24 hours. Surgalla *et al.* (1951) incubated 10 liters of medium in 12-gallon bottles under 20% carbon dioxide while rotating the bottles on their sides at the rate of 3 times per hour.

Investigators in the Food Research Institute have used gyrotory shakers for the past several years for production of quantities of enterotoxin for purification as well as small quantities for identification purposes. The procedure found best is to incubate 400-600 ml of media in 2-liter Erlenmeyer flasks for 18-24 hours at 37°C on a gyrotory shaker at 280 rpm (Kato *et al.*, 1966). For small quantities of more potent toxin the best procedure is to incubate 15 ml of media in 250-ml Erlenmeyer flasks under the same conditions. This method has been used by other investigators upon recommendation of the Food Research Institute workers.

4. DIALYSIS MEMBRANES

A method employing differential dialysis with three chambers and two membranes of different porosity has been used to effect the separation and concentration of enterotoxin B (Herold *et al.*, 1967). The culture was placed in the top chamber containing water which was separated by a 200-mμ pore diameter membrane filter from the middle chamber which also contained water. The middle chamber was separated by a 5-mμ pore diameter filter from the lower chamber which contained the medium. Teflon-coated steel balls were placed in the middle and bottom chambers and a perforated baffle in the top chamber for mixing. The medium was equilibrated throughout the chambers by shaking for 12 hours before inoculation. The maximum time incubation could be carried out was about 50 hours before staphylococci began appearing in the central chamber. Although a good portion of the toxin appeared in the central chamber, more than one-third remained in the top chamber. The total amount of toxin produced in this system was less than was produced in a two-chamber system with an ordinary dialysis membrane separating them. In this system, enterotoxin at a concentration of 1.1 mg/ml was obtained in the culture chamber.

The method which apparently gives the highest yield of enterotoxin per milliliter is the cellophane sac culture technique (Casman and Bennett, 1963). In this method, toxin production is confined to the interior of a cellophane sac lying on the surface of fluid medium in Roux bottles. An aqueous suspension (0.5 ml) of the organism is placed on the interior surface of the sac and incubated for 72 hours at 35–37°C in a horizontal position. Usually, it is necessary to add a little water or saline to aid in removing the growth from the sac, the total volume being kept at about 1 ml. For some strains, 100 times as much enterotoxin per milliliter was produced with the sac method as with the semisolid media in petri dishes. Even though more enterotoxin is produced with the sac method, Casman is promoting the semisolid media-plate method for general use, probably because it is much simpler to perform. According to the results reported by Hallander (1965) it would appear that his cellophane covered solid media-plate method is superior to Casman's plate method and might be the one of choice for production of small quantities of concentrated enterotoxin. Even if methods which result in larger volumes of less concentrated enterotoxin are chosen because of ease of performing them, it is relatively simple to concentrate the solutions to very small volumes by dialysis against Carbowax 20 M.

5. Temperature

Nearly all of the incubations for enterotoxin production have been carried out at 35–37°C. Little information is available about enterotoxin production at other temperatures and all that can be said is that from experiments that have been conducted in the Food Research Institute laboratories, enterotoxin can be produced at 25° and 30°C, but in lesser amounts than at 37°C. Some experiments by McLean et al. (1968) show that very small amounts of enterotoxin B are produced at both 16° and 20°C (10–20 µg/ml versus 340 µg/ml at 37°C), even though growth was about equivalent to that at 37°C. Until definitive experiments are conducted at various temperatures, 35–37°C should be used for enterotoxin production.

C. Enterotoxin-Producing Staphylococci

1. Percentage of Strains that are Producers

It is recognized that not all strains of staphylococci produce enterotoxin, but it has been impossible to determine what percentage are enterotoxigenic. The difficulty in obtaining such data is due to inadequacy of the enterotoxin detection methods. The enterotoxigenicity of strains that produce identified enterotoxins can be established by antigen–antibody techniques, although many strains produce as yet unidentified toxins. While there is no method that can be considered infallible, reasonably satisfactory results have been obtained by the monkey feeding test. One problem with this method is that the minimum amount of enterotoxin detectable is 5-10 μg in 50-70 ml of liquid, the maximum volumes that can be administered to a 2-3 kg animal. This is inadequate for detection of the small amounts that are produced by some strains (0.005 μg/ml of bacterial culture supernate), and to detect them a 20-fold concentration of the enterotoxin-containing fluids is necessary. This is the current procedure that is being followed in the Food Research Institute (Bergdoll, 1968) and several strains that by previous methods were classed as nonenterotoxigenic have been found to be enterotoxigenic. The number of strains that can be examined by this method is limited because of the cost involved, but results obtained so far indicate that the percentage that are enterotoxigenic is much higher than the 50% estimated from the results obtained by a combination of the antigen-antibody and cat methods (Casman et al., 1967). Hopefully, the task will become easier as additional enterotoxins are identified and their specific antibodies become available.

2. RELATIONSHIP OF ENTEROTOXIN PRODUCTION TO OTHER STAPHYLOCOCCAL PRODUCTS

Many attempts have been made to relate enterotoxin production to some other product of the staphylococci, for example, coagulase. It has been generally accepted that enterotoxin production is confined to coagulase-positive staphylococci (*Staphylococcus aureus*) (Evans et al., 1950), although the isolation of enterotoxigenic coagulase-negative strains have been reported (Thatcher and Simon, 1956; Omori and Kato, 1959; Bergdoll et al., 1967). Due to the divergence of coagulase tests used it is difficult to agree on when a strain is coagulase negative. Exhaustive studies of what appears to be a coagulase-negative strain may show it to be coagulase positive. The main concern, however, is that routine examination shows it to be coagulase negative, hence, nonenterotoxigenic by current practices. Work is being conducted in the Food Research Institute in an attempt to resolve this problem.

The relationship of enterotoxin to other products produced by the staphylococci such as hemolysins (Surgalla and Hite, 1945; Thatcher and Simon, 1956; Ritzerfeld et al., 1960), phosphatase (Thatcher and Simon, 1956), penicillinase (Parker and Lapage, 1957), and nuclease (Chesbro and Auborn, 1967) have been studied, but no consistent correlations are apparent. It is possible that 99% of enterotoxigenic strains may produce a given substance (e.g., coagulase), but to use this as a guide for eliminating strains as nonenterotoxigenic is questionable. If a food containing a coagulase-negative strain that happened to be enterotoxigenic were mishandled a food poisoning outbreak could result.

3. PHAGE TYPING

Phage typing of staphylococcal strains is done in a number of laboratories and an attempt to relate a particular pattern to the source of the organisms has been made by many investigators (Munch-Peterson, 1963; Wentworth, 1963; Hurst, 1965), apparently with some success. Enterotoxin production, however, cannot be correlated to any phage pattern or group, although many enterotoxigenic strains are lysed by group III phages. Phage typing of all strains isolated in connection with food poisoning outbreaks should be done since this is the only reliable method of tracing the source of contamination (Munch-Peterson, 1963).

At least two attempts have been made to convert nonenterotoxigenic strains to enterotoxin producers by the use of temperate phages. Read and Pritchard (1963) showed that for strain S-6 (primarily enterotoxin B producer with small amount of A) there was no correlation between the presence of prophage and enterotoxin production when they were able to isolate from this strain nonlysogenic cells that were enterotoxigenic. These investigators found that the temperate phages of the enterotoxin A-producing cultures were heterogeneous which suggested that a connection between the presence of a specific prophage and the ability to produce enterotoxin A does not exist.

Casman (1965) reported the conversion of 31 nonenterotoxigenic strains to enterotoxin producers when they were lysogenized with a purified temperate phage from an enterotoxin A producer. He was unsuccessful in attempts to confer enterotoxigenicity by temperate phages from two strains that were both A and B producers. Since this was a preliminary report and no further information has been published, the question of conversion of nonenterotoxigenic strains to enterotoxin producers remains open.

V. Purification

A. INTRODUCTION

Several early attempts were made to purify enterotoxin with little success (Jordan and Burrows, 1933; Davison and Dack, 1939; Hammon, 1941). Initial studies in the Food Research Institute laboratories made use of such methods as precipitation with ammonium sulfate, hydrochloric acid, and ethanol and methanol at subzero temperatures which resulted in partial purification of the toxin (Bergdoll et al., 1951). The fact that preparations of higher purity were obtained by chromatography with diatomaceous silica (Hyflo Super Cel) (Bergdoll et al., 1952) led to the use of other adsorbents such as alumina and the ion exchange resin Amberlite IRC 50 (XE-64) (Bergdoll et al., 1959a). With the advent of carboxymethylcellulose and the Sephadexes, purification can be accomplished without employing the more cumbersome precipitation techniques.

B. RECOVERY FROM SUPERNATES

One of the major concerns in the purification of the enterotoxins is the recovery of the toxin from the bacterial culture supernates. Since large volumes of supernates are required to provide sufficient toxin for the purification various precipitation techniques were tried. The one found initially to be most useful was adjustment of the supernates to pH 3.5 with phosphoric acid followed by filtration with the use of filter-aid (Bergdoll et al., 1959a). Handling of the precipitates was cumbersome and recovery of the toxin was in general rather poor. This method was abandoned for enterotoxin B when it was discovered that the enterotoxin could be adsorbed directly from the supernates by Amberlite IRC-50 (XE-64) (Bergdoll et al., 1961). For enterotoxins A and C recovery from the supernates was initially accomplished by adjustment of the supernates to pH 2.9 with trichloroacetic acid (Chu et al., 1966). Much better recovery was obtained by this method than with phosphoric acid precipitation; however, apparent partial denaturation of the toxins by the trichloroacetic acid made this procedure undesirable. In order to accomplish the purification of these enterotoxins, it was necessary to resort to smaller scale production and dialyze the supernate for 24-48 hours against an equal volume of 50% aqueous Carbowax 20 M (Union Carbide Corp., New York, N.Y.) for initial concentration. The crude enterotoxin (10-20 fold concentration) is used for purification either before or after freeze drying (Chu et al., 1966; Frea et al., 1963). This method is still being used in the Food Research Institute, although attempts are being made in this and other laboratories to adapt the ion exchange resin adsorption procedure for initial concentration of the various enterotoxins.

C. ENTEROTOXIN B

Purification of the first enterotoxin (enterotoxin B) was reported by Bergdoll et al. (1959a). The toxin was obtained in a high state of purity by the following steps: (1) precipitation at pH 3.5 with phosphoric acid; (2) adsorption on alumina from 0.03 M sodium phosphate at pH 6.3 and subsequent elution with 0.2 M disodium phosphate; (3) precipitation from 40% ethanol at $-7°C$; (4) adsorption on Amberlite IRC-50 (XE-64) (equilibrated with 0.05 M sodium phosphate at pH 6.8) from 0.02 M sodium phosphate at pH 6.2 and subsequent elution with 0.05 M sodium phosphate at pH 6.8; (5) precipitation from 25% ethanol at $-13°C$; (6) electrophoresis in 0.05 M sodium phosphate at pH 6 with starch as the supporting medium; (7) precipitation from 30% ethanol at $-13°C$; and (8) freeze drying. Since this method was lengthy and not readily adaptable for preparation of large quantities of the enterotoxin, it was modified for purification of enterotoxin B in multiple gram lots by Schantz *et al.* (1965) as follows: (1) adsorption on the ion exchange resin CG-50 from the culture supernate diluted with two volumes of water and adjusted to pH 6.4 and subsequent elution with 0.5 M sodium phosphate at pH 6.8 in 0.25 M sodium chloride; (2) adsorption on CG-50 (equilibrated with 0.05 M sodium phosphate at pH 6.8) from the dialyzed eluate from step 1 (to reduce salts to less than 0.01 M) and subsequent elution with 0.15 M disodium phosphate; (3) adsorption on carboxymethylcellulose (equilibrated with 0.01 M sodium phosphate at pH 6.2) from the dialyzed eluate from step 2 (to reduce salts to less than 0.01 M) and subsequent elution with a linear-gradient phosphate buffer from 0.02 M at pH 6.2 to 0.07 M at pH 6.8; and (4) dialysis to reduce the buffer salts to 2-3% of the protein concentration, centrifuged to remove any insoluble material, and freeze dried. The overall yield of purified toxin usually amounted to 50-60% based on gel diffusion tests on the original culture supernate.

D. OTHER ENTEROTOXINS

Enterotoxins A (Chu *et al.*, 1966), C_1 (Borja and Bergdoll, 1967), and C_2 (Avena and Bergdoll, 1967) have been purified by somewhat different procedures than those used for enterotoxin B. The procedures outlined below for the purification of enterotoxin A illustrate those used in the Food Research Institute laboratories for these and any as yet unidentified enterotoxins. The procedures are as follows: (1) concentration of the culture supernate 10-20-fold with Carbowax 20 M followed by dialysis against deionized water; (2) adsorption on carboxymethylcellulose (equilibrated with 0.01 M sodium phosphate at pH 5.7) and subsequent elution with 0.02 M disodium phosphate; (3) adsorption on carboxymethylcellulose (equilibrated with 0.01 M sodium phosphate at pH 6.0) from the dialyzed eluate (from step 2) adjusted to pH 6.0 and subsequent elution with a gradient phosphate buffer from 0.01 M at pH 6.0 to 0.05 M at pH 6.6; (4) gel filtration of the dialyzed lyophilized eluate (from step 3) dissolved in 5 ml of 0.05 M sodium phosphate at pH 6.8 with Sephadex G-100; (5) gel filtration of the lyophilized enterotoxin (from step 4) dissolved in 5 ml distilled water with Sephadex G-75 equilibrated and developed with 0.005 M sodium phosphate, pH 6.85; and (6) dialysis and freeze drying. The overall yield of purified enterotoxin A is usually 30-35% based on gel diffusion tests on the original culture supernates.

There is some variation in the procedures used for the different enterotoxins since the methods were worked out by different investigators. It is probable that the enterotoxins can be purified by the same methods, although some modifications would be necessary which take into account the differences in isoelectric points and the different impurities in the crude toxins.

Casman *et al.* (1967), has attempted to purify enterotoxin D by the procedures used for enterotoxin B by Schantz *et al.* (1965). No reliable tests for purity were made on their product and the tests that were made indicated the enterotoxin content of the product may be as low as 10%. Work is in progress in the Food Research Institute laboratories on the purification of enterotoxin D and E using methods similar to those employed for A and C.

An alternate procedure for the purification of enterotoxin A was reported by Denny *et al.* (1966a). The main procedure in the purification was the use of polyacrylamide gel electrophoresis. However, sufficient material was not obtained to determine purity of the final product. Attempts to adapt this method to larger scale use have been unsuccessful.

E. HOMOGENEITY

Each of the purified enterotoxins was tested for homogeneity by velocity ultracentrifugation, paper electrophoresis, and the double gel diffusion tube test. In the last method, antiserum prepared by using partially purified enterotoxin was used at varying concentrations with varying concentrations of the enterotoxins, usually 2 mg to 1 μg/ml. As little as 0.1% of an impurity can be detected by this method (Bergdoll *et al.,* 1959a, 1965a). Results indicated the purified toxins contained less than 5% impurities.

Electrophoresis in starch gel at pH 8.5 and 8.68 separated enterotoxin B into two components (Baird-Parker and Joseph, 1964). Both components reacted with the specific antibody to enterotoxin B, although initial experiments with piglets indicated only one component to be biologically active. Schantz *et al.* (1965) showed that electrophoresis of enterotoxin B in starch gel gave two major components in 0.02 M borate buffer at pH 8.6, but gave a single component in borate or Veronal buffer at pH 8.6 and in 0.02 M phosphate buffer at pH 7.0 when the ionic strength was raised to 0.1 with sodium chloride. Both components obtained in the borate buffer showed toxicity in monkeys and gel diffusion values equal to that of the original toxin. Joseph and Baird-Parker (1965) later found that both components were toxic and suggested that changes in the secondary or tertiary protein configuration may have caused the formation of the two bands. Separation into two bands in starch gel electrophoresis has been reported also for enterotoxin A (Chu *et al.*, 1966) and C_1 (Borja and Bergdoll, 1967).

VI. Nature

A. GENERAL PROPERTIES

The purified enterotoxins are fluffy, snow-white materials that are hygroscopic and readily soluble in water and salt solutions (Avena and Bergdoll, 1967; Bergdoll *et al.*, 1959a; Borja and Bergdoll, 1967; Chu *et al.*, 1966; Schantz *et al.*, 1965). Tests with the purified enterotoxins for carbohydrate, lipid, nucleic acids, α- and β-lysins, apyrase, coagulase, fibrinolysin, and proteolytic enzymes were negative. Some of the chemical and physical properties are given in Table V.

The diffusion coefficient value reported for enterotoxin B was obtained by the agar gel method of Schantz and Lauffer (1962) and is higher than the value (7.72) obtained by Schantz *et al.* (1965) with the synthetic boundary cell method. A valve-type synthetic boundary cell was used in the Food Research Institute for obtaining the diffusion coefficients of the other enterotoxins.

TABLE V

SOME PROPERTIES OF THE ENTEROTOXINS

	Enterotoxin			
	A^a	B^b	$C_1{}^c$	$C_2{}^d$
Emetic dose (ED_{50}) (μg/monkey)	5	5	5	5–10
Nitrogen content (%)	16.5	16.1	16.2	16.0
Sedimentation coefficient ($s_{20,w}$) (S)	3.04	2.78	3.00	2.90
Diffusion coefficient				
($D_{20,w}$) ($\times$ 10^{-7} cm^{2}sec^{-1})	7.94	8.22	8.10	8.10
Reduced viscosity (ml/gm)	4.07	3.81	3.4	3.7
Molecular weight	34,700	30,000	34,100	34,000
Partial specific volume	0.726	0.726	0.728	0.725
Isoelectric point	6.8	8.6	8.6	7.0
Maximum absorption (mμ)	277	277	277	277
Extinction ($E_{1\,cm}^{1\%}$)	14.3	14.4	12.1	12.1

[a] Chu *et al.*, 1966.
[b] Bergdoll *et al.*, 1965a.
[c] Borja and Bergdoll, 1967.
[d] Avena and Bergdoll, 1967.

The partial specific volumes for the enterotoxins given in Table V were determined from the amino acid compositions according to the method of Schachman (1957). The values obtained by pycnometry for enterotoxin B (0.743) by Wagman *et al.* (1965) and for enterotoxin C_2 (0.742) by Avena and Bergdoll (1967) are not in good agreement with the values obtained from the amino acid composition. The value for enterotoxin C_1 (0.732) obtained by pycnometry (Borja and Bergdoll, 1967) is in good agreement with the amino acid composition value and so is the value for enterotoxin B (0.730) found by Schantz (1966).

The molecular weight of 30,000 reported by Bergdoll *et al.* (1965b) for enterotoxin B does not agree with the molecular weight of 35,300 for this toxin reported by Wagman *et al.* (1965). The value reported by Bergdoll *et al.* (1965b) was an average between the value of 30,800 calculated from the Svedberg equation using the sedimentation coefficient, the diffusion coefficient, and the partial specific volume given in Table V and the molecular weight of 29,000 obtained from the half-cystine content of the toxin. Wagman *et al.* (1965) calculated the molecular weight by the Archibald Method (Ehrenberg, 1957), by use of the Svedberg equation, and from the amino acid composition (Spero *et al.*, 1965). All values were close to 35,300. The data from the amino acid sequence studies reported later in this chapter indicate a molecular weight near 29,000.

The two enterotoxin C's purified in the Food Research Institute laboratories were isolated from different strains, C_1 from strain 137 and C_2 from strain 361, and classification of both as enterotoxin C is based on the fact that both react with the same antibody. Although they appear to be identical in most respects, their movements in an electrical field are quite different (Avena and Bergdoll, 1967), and it is on this basis that they are designated C_1 and C_2. It is expected that there may be differences in the other enterotoxins produced by different strains if time were taken to purify them and study their properties. However, this is not of great significance since identification is based on the reactions with specific antibodies and small differences in the properties of the molecules would not affect the antigen–antibody reaction. Thus, the specific antibodies to either C_1 or C_2 can be used to identify all C enterotoxins.

The lower isoelectric points of enterotoxins A and C_2 do affect the conditions for adsorption of these enterotoxins by carbolymethylcellulose because they are less readily adsorbed than B and C_1, which have much higher isoelectric points. According to the calculations of Spero *et al.* (1965), there is an apparent excess of eight basic groups in the enterotoxin B molecule, requiring the titration of all the histidine and two of the lysine residues to achieve electrical neutrality. From these data they calculated an isoionic point of 8.70, which is in good agreement with experimental values of 8.6 for the isoelectric point and 8.55 for the isoionic point (Schantz *et al.*, 1965). Chu *et al.* (1966) calculated an excess of four basic groups for enterotoxin A. They assumed that the excess basic groups were due to four imidazole groups of the histidine residues existing in the undissociated form at the isoionic or isoelectric points. They based their assumption on the pK value 6.3-6.9 for the imidazole group of the histidine residue. The amino acid analyses for enterotoxins C_1 and C_2 indicate an excess of eight basic groups for C_1 and an excess of four basic groups for C_2 (Huang *et al.*, 1967), which corresponds to the calculated isoelectric points for these two proteins.

B. Effect of Various Treatments

1. Proteolytic Enzymes

The enterotoxins in the active state are resistant to proteolytic enzymes such as trypsin, chymotrypsin, rennin, and papain. Pepsin destroys their activity at a pH of about 2 (Table VI), but is ineffective at higher pH values (Bergdoll, 1966; Chu *et al.*, 1966; Schantz *et al.*, 1965).

Treatment of enterotoxin B alternately three times with carboxypeptidases A and B resulted in the removal of 18-20 amino acid residues from the C-terminal end of the enterotoxin B molecule before proline appeared in the chain. The enterotoxin residue that was recovered by carboxymethylcellulose chromatography reacted with the specific antibody to enterotoxin B without any observable change and was toxic to monkeys (Bergdoll *et al.*, 1965b).

TABLE VI
EFFECT OF PEPSIN ON ENTEROTOXIN B AT 37°C[a]

Time (hours)	Precipitate band movement in 10 days (mm)						
	pH 6.5	pH 2.0		pH 2.5		pH 3.0	
	Control	Control	Pepsin	Control	Pepsin	Control	Pepsin
1	11.5	9.6	1.5	9.9	10.6	10.7	11.9
2.5	12.0	9.8	0.0	10.2	9.6	10.7	11.2
5.0	11.5	9.8	0.0	10.2	8.6	11.3	10.5

[a] Bergdoll, 1961.

2. Heat

The biological activities of the enterotoxins are affected somewhat differently by heat. The activity of B was retained after heating a solution of the toxin at 60°C and pH 7.3 for as long as 16 hours (Schantz *et al.*, 1965), while a decrease of 50% in the reaction of A with its specific antibody resulted when it was heated at 60°C and pH 6.85 for 20 minutes

(Chu *et al.*, 1966). Heating of C_1 for 30 minutes at 60°C resulted in no change in the reaction of the enterotoxin with its specific antibody. After 60 minutes, however, the solution became turbid (Borja and Berg- doll, 1967). Solutions of enterotoxin C_2 became turbid when heated at 52°C (Avena and Bergdoll, 1967). Heating of B at 99°C required 87 minutes to destroy its activity (Read and Bradshaw, 1966a), while heating A for only 1 minute at 100°C completely destroyed its activity (Chu *et al.*, 1966). Heating C_2 for 1 minute at 100°C destroyed about 80% of its activ- ity (Avena and Bergdoll, 1967). These results indicate that of the entero- toxins, A is the most sensitive to heat, while B is the least sensitive. It should be pointed out, however, that the purified enterotoxins are more sensitive to heat than the crude toxins or when the purified toxins are in the presence of other substances. Hilker *et al.* (1968) reported that crude enterotoxin A (21 μg/ml) in Veronal buffer (pH 7.2) required heating at 100°C for 130 minutes to reduce the enterotoxin content to less than 1 μg/ml and that the length of time required to reduce the content to below 1 μg/ml depended on the amount of enterotoxin present in the solution, the larger the amount the longer the time required. The enterotoxin in these experiments was determined by the single gel diffusion tube test, whereas in another test using monkey feedings enterotoxin was detect- able after 40 minutes at 100°C, but not after longer heating (Denny *et al.*, 1966b). The enterotoxin could be inactivated by processes used in can- ning foods commercially, although pasteurization or spray drying of milk as currently practiced does not inactivate enterotoxin B (Read and Brad- shaw, 1966b).

3. IRRADIATION

A difference in inactivation of enterotoxin B was observed by Read and Bradshaw (1967) when the toxin was irradiated in Veronal buffer and milk. A dose of 5 Mrad was required to reduce an enterotoxin concentra- tion of 31 μg/ml to less than 1 μg/ml in 0.04 M Veronal buffer (pH 7.2), while 20 Mrad was required when milk was used as the vehicle. Based on this greater resistance of enterotoxin in milk, these authors conclude that irradiation processes now used for pasteurization or sterilization of foods cannot be expected to inactivate enterotoxin B if it is present in the food.

C. COMPOSITION

1. AMINO ACIDS

The amino acid compositions of enterotoxins A, B, C_1, and C_2, as deter- mined in the Food Research Institute laboratories are given in Table VII. Spero *et al.* (1965) also determined the amino acid composition of entero-

TABLE VII

AMINO ACID COMPOSITION OF THE ENTEROTOXINS

Amino acid	Amino acid content (gm/100 gm protein)			
	Enterotoxin A^a	Enterotoxin B^b	Enterotoxin C_1^c	Enterotoxin C_2^c
Lysine	11.32	14.85	14.43	13.99
Histidine	2.86	2.34	2.91	2.87
Arginine	3.99	2.69	1.71	1.75
Aspartic acid	15.75	18.13	17.85	18.38
Threonine	6.28	4.50	5.31	5.80
Serine	3.90	4.05	4.58	4.81
Glutamic acid	11.65	9.45	8.95	8.93
Proline	1.82	2.11	2.16	2.23
Glycine	3.56	1.78	2.99	2.90
Alanine	2.19	1.32	1.85	1.61
Half-cystine	0.62	0.68	0.79	0.74
Valine	4.95	5.66	6.50	5.87
Methionine	1.11	3.52	3.20	3.60
Isoleucine	4.34	3.53	4.09	4.02
Leucine	8.68	6.86	6.54	6.13
Tyrosine	10.09	11.50	9.80	10.27
Phenylalanine	5.12	6.23	5.35	5.25
Tryptophan	1.71	0.95	0.99	0.84
Amide NH_2	1.66	1.66	1.71	1.62
Total	99.94	100.15	100.00	99.99

[a] Tentative.

[b] Bergdoll et al., 1965b.

[c] Huang et al., 1967.

toxin B with essentially the same results as those obtained in the Food Research Institute except that they obtained 20% less half-cystine. Since the amounts are very small, this may not be significant except that when used to calculate the molecular weight, quite different values are obtained. The amino acid sequence studies indicate the Food Research Institute value to be near the true value. The number of amino acid residues for each of the enterotoxins is given in Table VIII. Enterotoxin A contains less lysine, aspartic acid, and methionine, and more arginine, glutamic acid, leucine, and tryptophan than the other toxins. However, it is not known whether these differences are significant as far as the stability and activity of the molecule is concerned. The exact composition of enterotoxin A has not been definitely established as yet since the results have been variable from preparation to preparation.

2. TERMINAL AMINO ACIDS

The terminal amino acids for the enterotoxins are given in Table IX. The value for the C-terminal amino acid for enterotoxin A is tentative since it has been difficult to obtain consistent results with the different purified preparations. The basis for selecting alanine is, that even though the recovery of this amino acid is below what would be expected, it is the only one obtained in more than trace amounts. It is interesting to note that the N-terminal amino acid of B, C_1, and C_2 is the same and that both terminal amino acids for C_1 and C_2 are the same.

3. AMINO ACID SEQUENCE

Determination of the amino acid sequence of enterotoxin B is nearing completion by investigators in the Food Research Institute laboratories.

TABLE VIII
AMINO ACID RESIDUES IN THE ENTEROTOXINS

Amino acid	Amino acid residues			
	Enterotoxin A^a (35,700)	Enterotoxin B^b (30,000)	Enterotoxin C_1^c (34,100)	Enterotoxin C_2^c (34,000)
Lysine	31	35	38	37
Histidine	7	5	7	7
Arginine	9	5	4	4
Aspartic acid	48	47	53	54
Threonine	22	13	18	20
Serine	16	14	18	19
Glutamic acid	32	22	24	24
Proline	7	7	8	8
Glycine	22	9	18	17
Alanine	11	5	9	8
Half-cystine	2	2	2	2
Valine	18	17	22	20
Methionine	3	8	8	9
Isoleucine	13	9	12	12
Leucine	27	18	20	18
Tyrosine	22	21	21	21
Phenylalanine	12	13	12	12
Tryptophan	3	2	2	2
Amide NH_2	37	29	36	34
Total	305	252	296	294

[a]Tentative.

[b]Bergdoll et al., 1965b.

[c]Huang et al., 1967.

TABLE IX
TERMINAL AMINO ACIDS OF THE ENTEROTOXINS

Enterotoxin	N-terminal amino acid	C-terminal amino acid
A	Alanine	Serine
B	Glutamic acid	Lysine
C_1	Glutamic acid	Glycine
C_2	Glutamic acid	Glycine

The resistance of the active toxin to proteolytic enzymes necessitated alteration of the toxin molecule in some manner. The forms found most useful in this work was the reduced carboxymethylated, reduced aminoethylated, and oxidized enterotoxin with the oxidized form most susceptible to enzymatic digestion (Huang *et al.*, 1969). Thirty peptides were obtained after digestion of the oxidized enterotoxin with trypsin by chromatography of Dowex 50 W-X2 and AG1-X2 and with further purification by paper chromatography and electrophoresis (Huang and Bergdoll, 1969). The amino acids in the isolated peptides accounted for 239 (Table X) of the 252 residues reported by Bergdoll *et al.* (1965b) for a molecular weight of 30,000. This gives a molecular weight of near 28,500. Stepwise degradation from the amino-terminal end by modification of the Edman and Sjöquist (1956) procedure, digestion with chymotrypsin, pepsin, papain, carboxypeptidase, and leucine amino peptidase were the principal methods used. Current studies with chymotrypsin should make possible elucidation of the complete structure of enterotoxin B.

D. CONFORMATION

Potentiometric and spectrophotometric titrations of enterotoxin B carried out in 0.16 M potassium chloride give results that indicate the titration curves to be essentially reversible between pH 1.50 and 11.0 (Chu, 1968). All of the ionizable groups found from the titration curves were consistent with the amino acid composition. Spectrophotometric titration reveals that six tyrosyl residues which have a pK_{int} of 10.3 are titrated normally, while eight are titrated between pH 11 and 12, and seven between pH 12.0 and 13.5. Acetylation with acetylimidazole and nitration with tetranitromethane reveal that six "free" tyrosyl residues are present in enterotoxin B. These modifications bring about essentially no loss of biological activity. However, the antigen–antibody reaction was diminished when the abnormal tyrosyl residues were acetylated in 8 M urea or 5 M guanidine hydrochloride. Information obtained about the electrostatic interaction factor indicates enterotoxin B to exist as a very compact, unhydrated molecule over a wide pH range. The observation of a conformational change around pH 11.5 where the dissociation of tyrosine is time-dependent, however, indicate that the abnormal tyrosine groups may play an important role in the structural features of the toxin, such as interaction with other side chain groups to form an internal core to maintain the rigid structure. It is concluded that since enterotoxin B cannot refold to the original conformation after more than 14 tyrosyl residues have been modified, that like most other biologically active proteins, the structure integrity for this toxin is essential for the biological activity.

Studies with enterotoxin C_1 (Borja, 1969; Borja and Bergdoll, 1969) revealed that five tyrosyl residues are titrated normally, while six are titrated between pH 11 and 12, and ten above pH 12. Five tyrosyl residues are acetylated with acetylimidazole, nitrated with tetranitromethane, and oxidized with tyrosinase. Such treatments do not affect the immunological and toxic properties of the enterotoxin molecule. The enterotoxins undergo considerable unfolding in 5 M guanidine hydrochloride, which is indicated by a large change in the intrinsic viscosity and the fact that all

TABLE X
AMINO ACID SEQUENCE STUDIES
ENTEROTOXIN B–TRYPSIN DIGESTION

Amino Acid	Residues found	Residues reported[a]
Lysine	33	35
Histidine	5	5
Arginine	5	5
Aspartic acid	44	47
Threonine	13	13
Serine	14	14
Glutamic acid	20	22
Proline	6	7
Glycine	9	9
Alanine	5	5
Half-cystine	2	2
Valine	16	17
Methionine	8	8
Isoleucine	9	9
Leucine	16	18
Tyrosine	21	21
Phenylalanine	12	13
Tryptophan	1	2
Total	239	252

[a] Bergdoll et al., 1965b.

the tyrosyl residues can be titrated normally. Acetylation of all of the tyrosyl residues in enterotoxin C results in almost complete loss of activity. It would appear that the overall structures of enterotoxins B and C are similar.

Chemical modification of the ϵ-amino groups of 90% of the lysine residues with guanidine did not alter the emetic activity nor the combining power of the antigen-antibody reaction (Chu *et al.*, 1969). The combining power of the acetylated, succinylated, and carbamylated enterotoxin with antibody, however, was reduced, the decrease being proportional to the amino groups modified. The decrease in combining power was proportional to loss in biological activity which was concluded to be due to a decrease in the net positive charge in the protein.

Dalidowicz *et al.* (1966) found the single disulfide bridge in enterotoxin B to be nonessential for biological activity and conformation of the protein. Reduction of the disulfide bridge and alkylation of the sulfhydryl groups with both iodoacetamide and iodoacetate produced derivatives that had the same emetic activity as the native enterotoxin when administered intravenously to monkeys. The physical properties of the alkylated enterotoxins, as measured by viscosity and sedimentation, remained essentially the same as that of the native enterotoxin. Treatment with 6 *M* guanidine hydrochloride had no effect on the biological activity. Avena and Bergdoll (1967) also found that guanidine hydrochloride had no effect on the biological activity of enterotoxin C_2.

From present information about the enterotoxins, it is evident that they are simple proteins composed solely of amino acids. The fact that only one N- and one C-terminal amino acid has been detected for each enterotoxin indicates they are single polypeptide chains. Studies on the conformation of the enterotoxins indicate that they are compact molecules. There are no free sulfhydryl groups and only one disulfide bridge is present, the latter being nonessential for biological activity and conformation of the protein.

VII. Synthesis

A. FACTORS AFFECTING SYNTHESIS

Several papers have been published on the factors affecting enterotoxin B production. This particular enterotoxin has been used for these studies since it is produced in much greater quantities than any of the other enterotoxins, e.g., 200-500 μg per milliliter of culture supernate versus 5-10 μg per milliliter for enterotoxin A. Friedman (1966) reported that enterotoxin B synthesis by *Staphylococcus aureus* strain S-6 in broth cultures was inhibited without appreciable effect on growth by a number of substances including potassium hydrogen phosphate, potassium chloride, sodium fluoride, acriflavine, streptomycin sulfate, chloramphenicol, spermine phosphate, etc. Inhibition varied with the pH of the medium in some cases and in some instances could be reversed by ammonium, magnesium, and calcium salts. The mechanism of inhibition is not known; however, it probably is different for the different inhibitors. For example, it is suggested that the inhibitions by K^+ and sodium fluoride and reversal of each by Mg^{2+} is due to a Mg^{2+} requirement by the enzymatic system controlling enterotoxin synthesis. Inhibitions by chloramphenicol and streptomycin may be due to their effect on protein synthesis. Rosenwald and Lincoln (1966) also reported that streptomycin inhibited elaboration of enterotoxin B without concurrent effect on growth of the microorganisms. They suggest that the inhibition may be due to incomplete synthesis of the protein or failure of release from the cell because of streptomycin-induced alterations in the cell itself.

Friedman (1968) has concluded that the cell surface is very important in the inhibition of enterotoxin B formation by a number of compounds, such as Tween 80, oleic acid, sodium deoxycholate, penicillin, D-cycloserine, and bacitracin, which do not affect the growth of the organism, although none of the mechanisms involved have been elucidated and are likely to vary. The studies with detergent-like compounds and agents blocking cell wall synthesis which were able to inhibit enterotoxin formation serve to strengthen the hypothesis that enterotoxin is associated with the cell surface. Because penicillin, D-cycloserine, and bacitracin affect cell wall synthesis at different sites, it is most likely that they do not act specifically on enterotoxin but affect the cell surface in such a way as to preclude the formation of enterotoxin. The failure of these substances to block α-hemolysin or coagulase production indicates that their activities are not toward bacterial protein in general, but more specifically toward those cellular products whose origin is at or near the cell wall; thus, it is concluded that the outer surface must contain the site(s) of enterotoxin synthesis.

Genigeorgis and Sadler (1966c) determined that enterotoxin B can be produced in brain heart infusion broth at pH 6.9 and 10% sodium chloride, and at pH 5.1 and 4% sodium chloride. Growth and enterotoxin production were better when the pH was increased and the salt concentration decreased. McLean *et al.* (1968) in a later paper demonstrated that sodium chloride has a much greater effect on enterotoxin B production than on growth of the microorganisms, although the same effect on enterotoxin production is not demonstrated with sodium nitrite or nitrate unless they are used in combination with sodium chloride. These investigators also showed that much less enterotoxin is produced when incubations are carried out at 20°C instead of 37°C. Their work showed that maximal enterotoxin B production occurred at the beginning of the stationary phase of growth.

B. Synthesis by Nongrowing Cells

Markus and Silverman (1968) have described a system in which enterotoxin B is produced without cell growth by cells harvested from the latter part of the exponential and early stationary phase of growth. In addition, it was shown that these cells could produce some toxin without an exogenous nitrogen source and with only glucose in the presence of chloramphenicol, a protein synthesis inhibitor, thus indicating the presence of toxin precursors in the cell. Aerobic conditions were essential for toxin formation by the nongrowing cells and the fact that respiration poisons such as 2,4-dinitrophenol or sodium azide inhibited toxin formation suggested that this process was energy-requiring. Cells harvested from the middle of the exponential growth phase did not produce enterotoxin in the non-nitrogenous, glucose-containing medium.

C. Production in Synthetic Media

Another approach to the synthesis of enterotoxin has been taken and that is to study the requirements for its production through the use of synthetic media. Surgalla (1947) reported the first studies using chemically defined media consisting of two to sixteen amino acids, vitamins, inorganic salts, and glucose. The simplest medium that resulted in some enterotoxin production contained arginine and cystine plus nicotinic acid, thiamine, glucose, magnesium sulfate, ferrous ammonium sulfate, and potassium dihydrogen phosphate. Evidence was not obtained that amino acids unessential for growth were necessary for enterotoxin production; both toxin production and growth seemed to be reduced in the simpler media, an observation attributable to the amount of available nitrogen in the media. Since this work was done before reliable methods for analysis were available, it was not possible to compare the effectiveness of the various media. Mah *et al.* (1967) reported a study of the nutritional requirements of *Staphylococcus aureus* strain S-6 for production of enterotoxin B in which a synthetic medium was developed composed of inorganic salts, eleven amino acids (glycine, valine, leucine, threonine, phenylalanine, tyrosine, cysteine, methionine, proline, arginine, and histidine) and three vitamins (thiamine, nicotinic acid, and biotin). Biotin was a growth factor requirement when glutamic acid but not glucose was used as a carbon source. Enterotoxin was produced in this medium, but at about one-seventh the level of that produced in a more complex medium using Protein Hydrolysate Powder (Mead Johnson International) as the nitrogen source even though the growth yields were about the same. Wu (1968) has made some preliminary studies of the effect on enterotoxin B production of various fractions obtained from Protein Hydrolysate Powder (PHP). Certain fractions obtained by fractionation with the ion exchange resin Dowex 50 W-X2 appeared to stimulate enterotoxin production. Analysis of these fractions indicated that certain peptides were the primary stimulating factors.

VIII. Pathogenesis and Mode of Action

A. INTRODUCTION

The readily observable symptoms of staphylococcal food poisoning have been well defined for many years, the two main ones being vomiting and diarrhea which develop 1-6 hours after ingestion of food containing enterotoxin (Dack, 1956). Other symptoms are salivation, nausea, retching, and abdominal cramping. In severe cases there may be headache, muscular cramping, sweating, and marked prostration. In the severe cases fever may occur or the temperature may be subnormal, there may be a drop in blood pressure, and blood and mucus may be observed in the stools and vomitus. The degree to which any of these symptoms appear is related to the amount of enterotoxin ingested and the sensitivity of the individual. In mild cases there may be nausea and vomiting without diarrhea or cramping and diarrhea without vomiting. There are other effects such as enteritis and changes in the blood composition which require other than visual observations to detect.

The complete effect of enterotoxin on humans is not known since the opportunities to study this type of intoxication in man is rather limited. Most victims are not hospitalized and when they are, no one may be around sufficiently interested to make any meaningful tests. Since this disease is seldom fatal, it has been difficult to determine what if any internal effects this toxin may have.

Many papers have been published on studies of the effect of enterotoxin on various animals such as rhesus monkeys, cats, dogs, rabbits, chinchillas, rats, and mice. Although the rodents do not have a vomiting mechanism, they have been useful in studying some of the other effects of the enterotoxins. Animals are less sensitive to enterotoxin than man on a kilogram basis, and in some cases (e.g., the cat and dog) are quite insensitive to intragastric administration of the toxins. This has resulted in using parenteral routes for injection of the enterotoxin which may or may not give comparable reactions to those obtained by the intragastric route.

It has not been proved unequivocally that enterotoxin enters unchanged, if at all, into the circulatory system through the digestive tract, since no one has reported demonstrating the presence of enterotoxin in the blood. The fact that when enterotoxin is injected intravenously, much smaller does are required to produce vomiting and diarrhea than by the intragastric route and results are usually obtained in a shorter period of time may indicate the toxin does enter the circulatory system. Also, animals become resistant to the toxin after repeated oral doses, and since antibodies to the enterotoxin are formed after parenteral injections, it could be assumed that the development of resistance is due to antibody formation. Although the presence of antibodies in serum from monkeys that became resistant to large doses of enterotoxin B (200 minimum emetic doses) after several intragastric injections could not be demonstrated *in vitro*, passive immunization experiments did demonstrate the presence of an enterotoxin neutralizing substance in the serum (Bergdoll, 1966). Felsenfeld and Nasuniya (1964) reported the detection of enterotoxin antibodies *in vitro* in the serum of residents of Thailand, although it is extremely doubtful that any of the antigen-antibody reactions they obtained were due to antibodies to enterotoxin. The possibility that the enterotoxin may be altered in the digestive tract before it enters the circulatory system (if it does) may produce different effects than the toxin injected directly into the blood stream, thus raising the question as to whether the results obtained from intravenous studies can be applied to enterotoxin given intragastrically.

B. Emesis

Sugiyama at the Food Research Institute has been foremost in the investigations of the mode of action of the enterotoxins. Much of his work has been done with the rhesus monkey since this is the animal of choice for enterotoxin research (Surgalla *et al.*, 1951). His first investigations were centered on emesis, which is the symptom most readily observable in monkeys. The available data from his studies on emesis indicate that the site of emetic action of enterotoxin in the monkey is in the abdominal viscera and that the sensory stimulus for this action reaches the vomiting center via the vagus and sympathetic nerves (Sugiyama and Hayama, 1965). Information from these studies, however, did not permit identification of a specific organ as the locus of emetic action.

Monkeys subjected to complete deafferentation of the abdominal viscera (vagotomy plus abdominal sympathectomy) did not vomit even after lethal doses of enterotoxin were administered either *per os* or intravenously. This failure to vomit was not due to nonspecific suppression of the vomiting reflex since the animals still vomited to Veriloid, an emetic acting at an emetic receptor site other than the gastrointestinal tract. Neither intrathoracic vagotomy nor abdominal sympathectomy alone rendered the animal completely refractory to enterotoxin, although vagotomy provided a high degree of emetic tolerance in monkeys given enterotoxin *per os* (100-fold in some animals) (Sugiyama *et al.*, 1961) but only a low degree of tolerance to intravenous injection in these animals (5-10-fold) (Sugiyama and Hayama, 1964) and in cats (5-fold) (Clark *et al.*, 1962). Bayliss (1940) had shown that vomiting was greatly reduced in acutely vagotomized cats when challenged intraperitoneally with heated crude enterotoxin filtrates. Sugiyama and Hayama (1965) concluded that the site of emetic action in the monkey and the cat is similar. Sugiyama and Hayama (1964) suggested that the difference in the results obtained by the intravenous and *per os* injection routes after vagotomy might be explained as follows. Atony and slower emptying time in the upper gastrointestinal tract following vagotomy may increase destruction of the enterotoxin before it reaches the emetic receptor sites that may be situated along the lower part of the gastrointestinal tract. Enterotoxin injected intravenously would reach the receptor sites without destruction, but some increase over the preoperative threshold dose would be required, since vagotomy would interrupt the sensory pathways for emesis for the upper portion of the gastrointestinal tract.

In an earlier investigation, Sugiyama *et al.* (1961) found that in monkeys ablation of the area postrema—medullary emetic chemoreceptor trigger zone (CTZ) of the dog and cat—gave complete protection against intravenous and *per os* administration of enterotoxin. This investigation was suggested from the fact that dihydroergotamine methanesulfonate—a drug closely related to Hydergine which is a CTZ emetic in dogs (but not in monkeys)—increased the vomiting incidence from enterotoxin given to monkeys (Sugiyama *et al.*, 1958) and the fact that perphenazine (Trilafon)—a potent antiemetic in dogs against Hydergine—induced vomiting—effectively inhibited enterotoxin emesis in monkeys (Sugiyama *et al.*, 1960). However, Clark *et al.* (1962) found that CTZ ablation in the cat did not influence the emetic response to intravenous injection of enterotoxin. This difference in cats and monkeys was apparently resolved when it was discovered that the sacro-lumbo-thoraco-bulbar tracts which innervate the abdominal viscera have terminations near the area postrema in monkeys (Kuru and Sugihara, 1955; Kuru, 1956) and that ablation of this area cannot be made in the monkey without affecting the neural elements from the abdominal viscera essential for enterotoxin vomiting (Sugiyama and Hayama, 1965).

C. Diarrhea

Shemano *et al.* (1967) conclude from their experiments with trained dogs that enterotoxin-induced diarrhea may be attributed in part to inhibition of water absorption from the intestinal lumen or to increased transmucosal fluid flux into the lumen or to both. Their work seemed to rule out increased intestinal motility and transport as important factors contributing to diarrhea when intravenous injection of 100 μg/kg of enterotoxin resulted in a marked depression of intestinal tone and contractility in trained dogs with Thiry-Vella loops, Mann loops, or cecostomies. Essentially similar effects on the proximal and distal colon were observed. The relative large doses of enterotoxin were given in order to consistently produce diarrhea and vomiting in these animals. The peak effects usually occurred 90 to 180 minutes after enterotoxin injection with onset in some cases being quick and in others delayed up to 3 hours. There was no consistent time relationship between onset of depressed intestinal contractility and emesis. None of these effects were observed in dogs anesthetized with 30 mg/kg pentobarbital sodium. Tyramine depressed intestinal tone and contractility both in anesthetized and conscious trained dogs. Neither chronic bilateral vagotomy nor chemical sympathectomy (guanethidine and *N, N*-diisopropyl-*N'*-isoamyl-*N'*diethylaminoethylurea pretreatment) markedly influenced the intestinal depressant effects or diarrhea and emetic effects of enterotoxin. Enterotoxin had no effect on the isolated rabbit ileum. Enterotoxin markedly inhibited intestinal transport in dogs as evidenced by charcoal meal, sponge bolus, and X-ray studies in conscious but not in anesthetized dogs. The depressant effect does not appear to be related to a direct action of the enterotoxin on the intestine, an atropine or papaverine-like effect, central vagal inhibition, or peripheral release of catecholamines, or enterotoxin-induced nausea and vomiting.

In an earlier investigation, Hayama and Sugiyama (1964) found that diarrhea could be induced in rabbits after removal of the cecum when given enterotoxin intravenously but not *per os*. Amine antagonists such as atropine and pyribenzamine gave definite but incomplete protection. Although the effect of removal of the cecum is not understood, the fact that it is an important organ of digestion in the rabbit does suggest that the gastrointestinal tract above the cecum may be an important site of action of intravenously administered toxin, although the toxin has no demonstrable effect on the smooth muscle of isolated small intestine preparations. Since the mucoid-watery fecal excretions indicate the importance of increased mucous secretion and net movement of water into the intestinal lumen, these investigators suggest that the absence of the cecum would allow direct movement of the intestinal contents from the small to the large bowel so that hypermotility, excessive mucus, and water secretion along the intestinal tract could result in diarrhea. The suggestion of hypermotility would appear to be ruled out by the experiments on dogs by Shemano *et al.* (1967).

D. ENTERITIS

One of the features of severe food poisoning is enteritis. Although it has not been shown that enteritis from food poisoning in humans is due to the enterotoxins, it has been demonstrated that enterotoxin B given *per os* in monkeys (Kent, 1966), dogs (Kocandrle *et al.,* 1966), and chincillas (also partially purified A) (Warren *et al.,* 1963) does result in the development of enteritis, the severity of which depends on the amount of enterotoxin given. Enteritis also occurred when crude bacterial culture filtrates from enterotoxin producing staphylococci were given to cats and chinchillas (Prohaska *et al.,* 1959) and to dogs (Prohaska, 1963; Warren *et al.,* 1964). In the experiments with dogs the enterotoxin containing filtrates were administered directly into the alimentary tract via a Maydl interostomy. The changes characteristic of acute exogenous gastritis resulting from food poisoning in humans determined by gastroscopic examination by Palmer (1951) appear to be characteristic of the observations made in animals. These findings were: patchy mucosal hypermia, regional edema, muscular irritation, erosions, petechiae, and purulent exudate. Examination after 48 hours showed the stomachs had returned to normal.

In experiments with rhesus monkeys (2-3 kg) acute gastroenteritis was well developed by 2 hours after the *per os* administration of enterotoxin B and reached a maximum at 4-8 hours with the mucosa becoming nearly normal by 72 hours (Kent, 1966). The onset of vomiting and diarrhea correlated well with the time sequence and severity of the lesions with large doses — 150 μg, which was approximately 50 times the ED_{50} — resulting in earlier and more constant clinical signs as well as intestinal lesions. The results with smaller doses (30 μg) were more variable, although the clinical signs and lesions correlated well. The gastric lesions did not correlate well with the dose of enterotoxin which may have been due to variability in gastric emptying. At the height of the reaction the jejunal mucosa exhibited long crypts and short villi which occurred in as little as 4 hours.

The tissue destructive effect and emetic effect of enterotoxin did not always occur together, as it was found that gastritis progressed in some monkeys after daily doses even though the animals became refractory to emesis after the first dose. Some animals receiving daily doses also showed a mild enteritis.

The development of enteritis in monkeys was compared with changes in the enzyme activities of acid and alkaline phosphatase, glucose-6-phosphatase, DPNH and TPNH diaphorases, succinic dehydrogenase, glucose-6-phosphate dehydrogenase, and the hexokinase system (Kent *et al.* 1966). The gastric mucosa exhibited a slight reduction of enzyme activity in the surface mucous epithelium and a slight increase in acid phosphatase activity in chief cells. A rapid decrease and recovery of enzyme activity in the jejunal epithelium correlated well with alterations in the structure of the epithelium; however, in the ileum where the inflammatory reaction was less severe, only slight changes in enzyme activity resulted. The greater changes in the jejunum were apparently due to severe injury to the absorption cells of the villi.

The injection of 0.1–0.5 mg/kg (i.v.) or 1 mg/kg (via a Maydl enterocutaneous fistula in the midportion of the jejunum) in dogs produced salivation, vomiting, and watery diarrhea often mixed with blood (Kocandrle *et al.,* 1966). Autopsy 24 hours after injection revealed acute enteritis with edema, hyperemia, and ulcerations of the mucosa of the duodenum and the proximal jejunum, edema with hypermia in the pancreas, and congestion of the liver. Severe round cell infiltration of the mucosa and destruction of the surface of the epithelium were revealed by microscopic examination.

Merrill and Sprinz (1968) found that after intragastric administration of enterotoxin (150 μg) to monkeys the most pronounced changes were at the villus crest. The surface epithelium otherwise appeared well preserved, except for some slight cytoplasmic vacuolation and flattening which was more pronounced in the crypt cells. Electron micrographs revealed the vacuolation to correspond to degeneration of mitochondria of villus and crypt epithelial cells and of diverse cells of the tunica propria of the jejunal mucosa (to which they attribute a major role) with the intestinal microvilli involved to a lesser degree. These investigators suggest that the rapid development of a discernible lesion and its almost exclusive limitation to the mitochondria indicate the site of action of enterotoxin is centered in these organelles. They propose that cellular integrity is preserved from an alternate energy source and that the damaged mitochondria are capable of reconstruction.

Schaeffer *et al.* (1966) reported that enterotoxin B had a cytotoxic effect on human embryonic intestinal cells (*in vitro*) which was characterized by retraction of the cells from the monolayer followed by clumping and finally sloughing of the clumped cells from the glass surface. The effect was neutralized with specific antisera. No cytotoxicity was evident until after 2 days of growth had taken place when the cell count was approximately 4×10^5 cells per culture. Further studies (Schaeffer et al., 1967) showed that treatment of the cell culture with trypsin rendered the cells resistant to enterotoxin for 48 hours with the time of resistance proportional to the length of trypsin treatment. These investigators suggest that some specific surface configuration of the cell required for the interaction with the toxin is destroyed by trypsin. Whether these studies are indicative of the effect of enterotoxin in the gastrointestinal tract is questionable since the 50% effective dose of enterotoxin in these experiments was 40–60 $\mu g/ml$.

The similarity of pseudomembranous enterocolitis in patients after antibiotic therapy, when essentially pure cultures of staphylococci could be isolated from the intestinal tract, to that in humans suffering from staphylococcus food poisoning suggested that the cause in both cases may be enterotoxin (Dack, 1956; Prohaska et al., 1956). The staphylococci isolated from patients suffering from enteritis after antibiotic therapy were found to be potent enterotoxin producers (Surgalla and Dack, 1955; Hallander and Körlof, 1968). Tan et al. (1959) demonstrated that enteritis developed in chinchillas that were given a suitable antibiotic (oxytetracycline) for several days followed by a pure culture of an enterotoxigenic strain of staphylococcus. Only staphylococci could be isolated from the intestinal tract and they were still potent enterotoxin producers. Attempts in the Food Research Institute laboratories to use monkeys for this type of experiment were unsuccessful.

E. Death

Death rarely occurs in otherwise normal humans as a result of staphylococcus food poisoning, although a few fatalities have been recorded, some in very young children (Kienitz, 1964), some in elderly people suffering from other ailments, and some in instances where improper treatment has been prescribed, for example, the administration of antibiotics (Dack, 1956). Antibiotics may destroy the normal flora of the intestinal tract and result in uninhibited growth of the enterotoxin-producing staphylococci ingested with the contaminated food, thus resulting in additional toxin being added to the system. Weed (1943) reported the death of two children, 3 and 4 years of age, within 24 hours after they drank 125 ml of unrefrigerated milk that had been taken approximately 12 hours earlier from a goat suffering from acute suppurative mastitis. Although this investigator stated that the pathological findings did not reveal anything which could logically be considered the cause of death, he did report the following. The lungs showed a moderate amount of pulmonary edema with marked congestion of the aveolar vessels and in a few areas there appeared to be definite hemorrhages into the aveolae. There was a small amount of leukocytic infiltration in the periportal areas of the liver. These findings might be significant in view of recent observations in animals receiving lethal doses of enterotoxin.

Many patients afflicted with pseudomembranous enterocolitis usually brought about by antibiotic therapy but not always (Prohaska *et al.*, 1956), suffer shock and fatal circulatory collapse following severe diarrhea.

Several studies have been made with rhesus monkeys using large doses of enterotoxin B (up to 1 mg/kg administered intravenously) which resulted in death in many of the animals. The symptoms, usually occurring 30-60 minutes after intravenous injection, were vomiting, diarrhea, anorexia, fever, oliguria, pale mucous membranes, and mild to severe depression with severe shock, dyspnea, and cyanosis in lethal intoxication. Approximately 60% of monkeys (2.3-3.5 kg) died after receiving 25 μg/kg, death occurring 6 hours to 9 days after injection. Although the cause of death was indefinite, a fall in intravascular fluid volume was noted with an increase in lung weights (Crawley *et al.*, 1966b). Feingold (1967) reported that in animals dying between 45 and 55 hours after injection, pulmonary edema was the most important finding, with the lungs being 1.5-2.5 times heavier than in control animals. The fluid was confined primarily to the perivascular and peribronchial interstitial space with the lymphatics in these areas engorged. The primary pathological change was degeneration of the capillary endothelial cells and necrosis with less frequent damage to the endothelium of venules. Also noted were interstitial hemorrhage and edema, a histiocytic infiltrate, and a striking herniation of capillary endothelium into the vascular lumen.

Another study was made dealing primarily with the lethal shock occurring after intravenous injection of enterotoxin (50-1000 μg/kg) (Hodoval *et al.*, 1968). Irreversible arterial hypotension was found consistently at all lethal doses of toxin with arterial blood pressure and cardiac output declining substantially as shock developed. Other observations were made which were consistent with a pooling of blood in the peripheral vascular beds. These investigators suggest the possibility that primary toxicity may involve vascular endothelial permeability although no positive experimental support has been advanced as yet.

In another study on monkeys given lethal doses of enterotoxin, Hodoval *et al.* (1967) found essentially no changes from the base line electroencephalogram (EEG) patterns until shortly before death when with preterminal severe shock, there was a marked decrease in EEG wave frequency and an initial increase in amplitude. These investigators postulate that cerebral anoxia caused by inadequate blood flow was the primary cause of the EEG pattern alterations.

It has been noted that intravenous injection of enterotoxin into monkeys resulted in death without antecedent emesis or diarrhea (Crawley *et al.*, 1966b) and in some cases death did not occur until long after the expected time of vomition. This suggests the possibility that the mechanisms leading to death and vomition may be different. On occasion, administration *per os* of large doses of enterotoxin B to monkeys in the Food Research Institute laboratories has resulted in death of the animals which usually was not preceded by vomiting. Since these deaths occurred during routine feeding experiments, no data are available concerning changes in blood pressure, etc. These observations would indicate that emesis and diarrhea were not essential contributing factors in death caused by enterotoxin.

F. CHANGES AFFECTING THE CIRCULATORY SYSTEM

1. SERUM GLUTAMIC-OXALACETIC ACID TRANSAMINASE

Sugiyama *et al.* (1958) found that administration of enterotoxin *per os* to monkeys resulted in elevation of the serum glutamic-oxalacetic acid transaminase (GOT) activity 2-3-fold within 6-8 hours after administration. Crawley *et al.* (1966a) reported that the only change in enzyme concentration in the blood after intravenous injections of 25 μg/kg of enterotoxin B to rhesus monkeys was a rapid increase in GOT. The rise in GOT may result at least in part from the extensive tissue damage in the gastrointestinal tract which occurs when enterotoxin is given (IV or *per os*).

2. LEUKOCYTOSIS

Leukocytosis is another change observable after the administration of enterotoxin to monkeys, either *per os* (Sugiyama and McKissic, 1966) or intravenously (Crawley *et al.*, 1966a, b). Leukocytosis was observed within 30 minutes after administration *per os* of 5-10 μg of enterotoxin per animal, even though vomiting occurred 1-3 hours later. This suggested an almost immediate toxic reaction upon entrance of the toxin into the gastrointestinal tract. A neutrophilic leukocytosis peak was reached in 3 hours and then subsided to normal leukocyte counts in 28 hours.

Intravenous injections of enterotoxin in doses slightly more than the minimum emetic dose—1-1.5 μg/kg of A, B, and C (Sugiyama and McKissic, 1966)—or in large doses—25 μg/kg of B (Crawley *et al.*, 1966a)—

resulted in a biphasic effect in which leukopenia preceded a neutrophilic leukocytosis with a large number of immature leukocytes after the larger doses. A study using ^{131}I-labeled enterotoxin B (20–200 μg/kg) given intravenously to monkeys (2.3–3.5 kg) showed that some of the enterotoxin was bound by the leukocytes which were removed rapidly from the circulation (Crawley *et al.*, 1966b). In these studies 60% of the toxin was removed from the blood in less than 60 seconds with less than 1% remaining on the buffy coat. These investigators postulated that the lungs removed the leukocyte-bound toxin from circulation since high concentrations of label were found early in these organs and an early severe leukopenia developed. These authors also assumed that part of the enterotoxin was bound to serum albumin, but Normann and Johnsey (1968) reported that if the toxin is bound to plasma proteins, the binding must be of a weak character and easily dissociable.

3. REMOVAL FROM THE BLOOD STREAM

Several papers have been published by the U.S. Army Medical Unit (Fort Detrick, Frederick, Maryland) on the disappearance of enterotoxin B from the blood stream (Crawley *et al.*, 1966b; Rapoport *et al.*, 1966, 1967; Morris *et al.*, 1967; Normann and Johnsey, 1968; Normann and Jaeger, 1969). Radioiodinated enterotoxin B was given intravenously to rhesus monkeys (2–3.5 kg) in large doses (1 mg/kg) for most of these studies. Although this amount of toxin is lethal, it was not possible to reduce the dosage below lethal levels and detect the distribution of the radioactive toxin throughout the animal body.

The enterotoxin disappeared very rapidly from the blood, 60% in less than 60 seconds (Crawley *et al.*, 1966b), with the kidney being the major site of accumulation with approximately one-third of the injected dose being localized in the renal cortex in 30 minutes (Morris *et al.*, 1967). By combining fluorescent labeling of the toxin with fluorescent antibody methods, Normann and Jaeger (1969) were able to show that the proximal convoluted tubules of the kidney are the principal sites of toxin removal (about 75% of injected dose) and that the toxin gains access to these tubules by a process of glomerular filtration and tubular reabsorption. Enterotoxin was present on the luminal side of the proximal convoluted tubules as distinct layer of fluorescence adjacent to the cell surface in 15 seconds after intravenous injection. The toxin appeared to show an affinity only for the brush border of tubular epithelium. A definite gradient of fluorescent intensity from the luminal side of the cell toward the cell base was observed by 15 minutes with the entire cell becoming fluorescent at 30 minutes. The enterotoxin disappeared from the kidney rapidly, essentially all being gone after 8 hours. Although the ^{131}I left the kidney via the blood stream rather than the urine (Morris *et al.*, 1967), the fluorescent antibody technique indicated that the toxin was destroyed by the tubular cells, but it is not known how this was accomplished.

The importance of the kidney in the removal of enterotoxin from circulation was demonstrated by acute renal artery ligation (Rapoport *et al.*, 1967) and nephrectomy (Normann and Jaeger, 1969) which caused a dramatic drop in clearance rate from the bloodstream.

Animals resistant to enterotoxin exhibited a slower disappearance of toxin from the blood and faster and greater excretion of ^{131}I without the clinical signs of lethal intoxication observed in nonresistant animals (Crawley *et al.*, 1966b). Administration of protective antibody before intravenous enterotoxin challenge markedly delayed the clearance of enterotoxin from the blood (Rapoport *et al.*, 1966). Also, therapeutic administration of antiserum actually returned toxin to the circulation and death was delayed or prevented, which indicated that the enterotoxin binding to unidentified tissue sites where it exerts its toxic action is apparently relatively loose, since adherence to the antitoxin appears to be considerably stronger. The delay in clearance of enterotoxin from the blood by antibodies was due at least in part to the inability of the antigen–antibody complex to enter the kidney (Morris *et al.*, 1967). Whether the entrance of enterotoxin into the kidneys is partly responsible for its lethal action is not known, although animals live longer when the toxin is prevented from entering them. The therapeutic effect of antibody administration could be a neutralization of the enterotoxin in the kidney. The return of enterotoxin to the bloodstream must come from tissues other than the kidney, since the antigen–antibody complex is too large to be returned to the bloodstream from that organ. These other tissues, whatever they are, may also be involved in the lethal action of the toxin.

The organ of next importance to the kidney in removing enterotoxin from the bloodstream is the liver. When radioiodinated toxin was used, 20-25% of the total activity was found in the liver within 30 minutes, but dropped off rapidly after that time (Morris *et al.*, 1967). Only small amounts of toxin were found in the liver by the fluorescent antibody technique. In the case of the rat, nephrectomy resulted in an intensification of fluorescence in the liver, revealing it to be an alternative site to the kidney. The majority of the toxin was confined to the Kupffer cells (Normann and Jaeger, 1969).

Less than 5% of the radioactive enterotoxin appeared in the lungs and less than 1% in the heart, spleen, thyroid, or brain (Morris *et al.*, 1967). No evidence is available to indicate any effect of enterotoxin on cardiac action and the failure to find any accumulation in the brain is in agreement with the conclusion of Sugiyama and Hayama (1965) that initiation of vomiting depends on local stimulation of a reflex arc originating in the gastrointestinal tract. Studies on distribution of toxin given by the intragastric route could not be done because of the deiodination of the toxin in the intestinal tract. No attempt was reported to follow the distribution by the fluorescent antibody technique. The question as to whether the same pattern of distribution would be observed if emetic doses (< 1 μg) were used instead of 1 mg/kg may never be answered.

4. OTHER CHANGES

Other changes that have been observed (Crawley *et al.*, 1966a) after intravenous injection of enterotoxin B (25 μg/kg) to rhesus monkeys (2.3–3.5 kg) are initial increases in catecholamine and blood glucose levels followed by decreases. An early increase in blood urea nitrogen occurred possibly as a result of both prerenal azotemia and functional renal failure associated with hypotension. There was a decrease in serum protein, calcium, and chlorine concentrations with time, an increase in inorganic phosphorus levels, but no change in sodium or potassium concentrations.

Parenteral injection of enterotoxins A and B increased the plasma fibrinogen levels of rabbits and monkeys 2–3 times the prechallenge concentration (Sugiyama *et al.*, 1964b). A drop in blood serotonin corresponded to a decrease in number of circulating blood platelets. The dosage required for these responses was close to the minimal emetic dose for monkeys by the intravenous route. Gilbert (1966) reported that results obtained from intravenous administration of enterotoxin B to beagle dogs indicated alterations of the clotting mechanism and that the plasma factors are primarily involved.

G. ENTEROTOXIN SIMILARITY TO ENDOTOXIN

Many of the responses in animals to enterotoxin are similar to those induced by endotoxin which Sugiyama (1966) suggests might be due to the effect of the enterotoxin on the gut in such a manner that the endotoxin of the indigenous microflora of the gastrointestinal tract could exert its toxic action. Other possibilities are that the responses may be due to toxic products resulting from the tissue–enterotoxin interaction that evoke endotoxin-like responses, or it may be a coincidence that the enterotoxic action is similar to that of endotoxin. The similarity certainly cannot be explained on the basis of their being similar compounds, because enterotoxin is a protein and endotoxin is a lipopolysaccharide. The endotoxin-like activities of enterotoxin are discussed below.

The first feeding of enterotoxin to monkeys results in the rapid development of temporary tolerance to a second challenge with the homologous antigenic type of enterotoxin (Sugiyama et al., 1962). A number of investigators have shown that mice given bacterial endotoxins develop a nonspecific resistance against lethal infections by gram-negative bacteria and endotoxin. One might question the similarities of the effect of these two substances, however, since the protection provided by endotoxins apparently is complete, whereas the protection provided by enterotoxin may be only against emesis since many animals are definitely ill although they do not vomit.

Administration of enterotoxin B to cats either intracerebroventricularly or intravenously elicited a monophasic fever pattern by the first route and a biphasic pattern by the second route (Clark and Borison, 1963). Similar results were obtained with intravenous injection of enterotoxin A, the only difference being that A appeared to be 3–6 times as potent as B (Clark and Page, 1968). Tolerance to the pyrogenic effect developed after repeated injections of the enterotoxin. Although there was some similarity to the pyrogenic response resulting from administration of endotoxin, there were differences in the relative peak amplitudes and temporal features of the biphasic fever patterns when the two substances were given intravenously. Intraventricular enterotoxin apparently exerts its pyrogenic effect locally within the central nervous system since a much smaller dose was required to give an effect than intravenously (0.02 μg total versus 1.0 μg/kg). Cross tolerance between lipopolysaccharide (LPS) and enterotoxin was not observed. Martin and Marcus (1964) also observed that both endotoxin and enterotoxin are pyrogenic in rabbits and cats and emeticogenic in cats.

Enterotoxin can be substituted for LPS as the preparative dose for the local Schwartzman reaction in rabbits, although it is ineffective as the provoking agent when either enterotoxin or endotoxin is used as the preparative dose. The altered reactivity to epinephrine induced by enterotoxin resembles that produced by LPS (Bokkenheuser et al., 1963). These investigators suggest that the susceptibilities of rabbits to the two toxins are independently determined. Yagasaki and Sugiyama (1966) found that intravenous injection of rabbits with even 0.2 μg/kg of enterotoxins A and B induced a significant increase in the vasoconstrictive effect of topically applied epinephrine within 3 hours. Maximum sensitivity occurred some 10 hours after toxin administration and persisted for 18 hours with toxin levels of 1–10 μg/kg. These results were similar to those induced by endotoxin except for the much slower evolution of the state of increased responsiveness to epinephrine.

Procedures used for the blockade of the reticuloendothelial system increase the sensitivity of monkeys to the intragastric emetic stimulus of enterotoxin (Sugiyama et al., 1963) as well as the pyrogenic (Beeson, 1947) and lethal effectiveness (Good and Thomas, 1952) of endotoxin. Injection of Thorotrast intravenously 18 hours before intragastric challenge with enterotoxins A and B increased the sensitivity of the monkeys to emetic action approximately 20-fold. Enterotoxin B (1 mg/kg) injected intravenously in rhesus monkeys (2.5–3.5 kg) is rapidly cleared from the blood in a similar fashion to endotoxin clearance in rabbits; however, in contrast to an increased clearance rate of endotoxin from rabbits given immune serum, a marked delay in clearance of enterotoxin occurs in monkeys given protective antibody before challenge (Rapoport et al., 1966). Also, therapeutic administration of antiserum actually returns toxin to the circulation and death is delayed or prevented. This tends to exclude the reticuloendothelial system as a factor in enterotoxin removal. It is postulated that enterotoxin becomes bound to various, as yet unidentified, tissue sites where it exerts its toxic action. The binding is apparently relatively loose, since adherence to the antitoxin is considerably stronger; thus, administration of antisera removes the enterotoxin from these sites and thus relieves the toxic action. When monkeys were pretreated with Thorotrast before intravenous injection of enterotoxin B-^{131}I, no effect was observed on the rapid clearance and metabolic alteration of the enterotoxin (Rapoport et al., 1967). It is not possible to compare these results with the potentiation of the emetic effect of enterotoxin given per os to Thorotrast-treated monkeys (Sugiyama et al., 1963), since the clearance of large doses of enterotoxin from the blood may be unrelated to its emetic effect. When massive doses are given intravenously it is almost impossible to determine the effect on such food poisoning symptoms as emesis and diarrhea which occur from doses less than 1 μg/kg (i.v.).

Sugiyama did show that enterotoxin alters the phagocytic activity of the reticuloendothelial system in the rabbit in a manner comparable to that of endotoxin by demonstrating that carbon clearance was depressed 2 hours after enterotoxin injection (1 and 10 μg/kg i.v.). This was transitory, however, as reticuloendothelial activity was returning to normal after 4 hours and was above normal after 24 and 42 hours.

Parenteral injection of enterotoxin increases the plasma fibrinogen levels of rabbits and monkeys (Sugiyama et al., 1964b), although it differs from the hyperfibrinogenemia following LPS (McKay and Shapiro, 1958) which results in a more prolonged rise in titer. Injection of enterotoxin into rabbits intravenously resulted in a gradual fall in total blood serotonin corresponding to the decrease in number of circulating blood platelets (Sugiyama et al., 1964b) while endotoxin causes a more precipitous decrease (Davis et al., 1961). These differences are sufficiently great to indicate that the action results from two different agents. Endotoxin given intravenously is emetic for cats (Sugiyama *et al.*, 1966) and other suitable animals and the similarity in the site of action of the two toxins in the cat is indicated by denervation studies (Clark *et al.*, 1962). These results are compatible with the abdominal visceral origin of the emetic stimuli, a conclusion supported by similar studies with enterotoxin in monkeys (Sugiyama and Hayama, 1965). Endotoxin and enterotoxin both cause an increase in the total plasma lipid levels in rabbits with the triglyceride fraction showing the greatest proportionate rise (Sugiyama, 1966).

Trasylol, a proteolytic enzyme inhibitor, has a significant protective effect against the emetic stimulus of enterotoxin given *per os* to monkeys. Since this substance can inhibit the local dermal Shwartzman lesion following bacterial endotoxin, and enterotoxin can substitute for endotoxin as the preparative agent for the Shwartzman reaction, the effect of Trasylol on enterotoxin may be significant (Sugiyama, 1966). Trasylol is a solution of polypeptides of molecular weight 11,600 (Kraut *et al.*, 1960) originally isolated from beef paratid gland; it has a marked ability to inhibit proteolytic enzymes such as trypsin and chymotrypsin. Since enterotoxin is a protein, it is possible that its action is inhibited in a similar manner to that of the proteolytic enzymes. It may be coincidental that Trasylol inhibits the development of the Shwartzman lesion and enterotoxin emesis.

Another similarity of enterotoxin to endotoxin noted by Hodoval *et al.* (1967) is the altered electroencephalogram (EEG) patterns that accompany enterotoxin toxicity. After administration of enterotoxin B (1 mg/kg i.v.) to rhesus monkeys no change in EEG patterns was noted until shortly before death when with preterminal severe shock, there was a marked decrease in EEG wave frequency and an initial increase in amplitude.

IX. Immunology and Immunochemistry

A. INTRODUCTION

The possibility of immunizing man against staphylococcal food poisoning was considered as soon as it was demonstrated that the poisoning was due to a substance produced by the staphylococci. Dack *et al.* (1931) attempted to immunize human volunteers by administering crude enterotoxin by mouth, but no significant immunity was acquired. Dolman (1943) was also unsuccessful in a similar attempt. No other attempts to immunize humans by oral administration of enterotoxin have been reported, although the presence of antibodies to enterotoxin in the serum of humans resistant to enterotoxin has been claimed (Felsenfeld and Nasuniya, 1964). However, since partially purified enterotoxin was used as the reference material it is impossible to conclude that any of the precipitation lines obtained was due to the enterotoxin–antienterotoxin reaction. Although antibodies have not been reported definitely to be present in humans resistant to staphylococcal food poisoning, it can be assumed that the resistance is due to antibody formation resulting from repeated exposure to the toxin, since Dolman (1944) did find that after several subcutaneous injections of formalinized crude enterotoxin human volunteers developed a resistance to the toxin.

Monkeys that were fed enterotoxin B *per os* repeatedly became resistant to 200 minimum emetic doses of toxin. Attempts to demonstrate the presence of precipitating antibodies in the serum from these monkeys was unsuccessful, although the use of the serum for passive immunization of other monkeys did give some protection against *per os* administration of 10 emetic doses of enterotoxin (Bergdoll, 1966). This indicated the presence of an antitoxin in the sera of the resistant monkeys. It was also demonstrated that rhesus monkeys could be immunized against 200 emetic doses of enterotoxin B by three intramuscular injections of aluminum hydroxide-adsorbed enterotoxoid at 5-week intervals. Other investigators had reported the immunization of monkeys by several subcutaneous injections of crude enterotoxin (Woolpert and Dack, 1933; Davison *et al.*, 1938), of kittens by several intraperitoneal injections (Dolman, 1936), of kittens by subcutaneous injections of formalinized crude enterotoxin (Minett, 1938), and of cats and kittens by repeated intravenous injections (Dolman, 1944).

Demonstration of the presence of antibodies in the serum from immunized animals was demonstrated when kittens did not react to crude enterotoxin when it was mixed with antiserum from immunized animals (Dolman and Wilson, 1938; Davison *et al.*, 1938). Surgalla *et al.* (1954) obtained negative reactions when monkeys were given *per os* partially purified enterotoxin treated with antisera from rabbits.

Although humans could be immunized against enterotoxin, it would be impractical to do so. Most of the investigations concerning the development of specific antibodies to the enterotoxins in animals have been directed toward the preparation of specific antibodies for their detection and assay.

B. Specific Antibodies

Identification of a specific precipitating antibody to enterotoxin B was accomplished only after the enterotoxin had been purified and the purified toxin used to immunize rabbits and monkeys (Bergdoll *et al.*, 1959b). A single line of precipitate was obtained by various double gel diffusion techniques when the purified toxin was reacted with antiserum prepared with the pure toxin. This antiserum was demonstrated to have enterotoxin-neutralizing properties thus demonstrating that the antigen-antibody reaction was the enterotoxin-antienterotoxin system. Antibodies to this enterotoxin had been prepared using partially purified enterotoxin, but because of the presence of other antibodies it was not possible to relate any particular precipitate band to the enterotoxin-antienterotoxin system (Surgalla *et al.*, 1952, 1954).

The relating of a specific antibody to the enterotoxin produced by one staphylococcus strain (S-6) resulted in the discovery that the enterotoxin produced by another strain (196E) did not react with the antibody to the enterotoxin produced by the first strain (Bergdoll *et al.*, 1959b). Neither did the S-6 enterotoxin react with the antibodies produced by strain 196E enterotoxin. It had been reported (Casman, 1958) that the two enterotoxins reacted with a common antibody; however, after a private discussion on February 3, 1958, between Bergdoll and Casman of the data available, it was concluded that these two strains did indeed produce different enterotoxins. The report of Bergdoll *et al.* (1959a) was the first specific proof of the existence of antigenically different enterotoxins, although Thatcher and Matheson (1955) had reported that immunization of cats with crude enterotoxins from three different strains protected the animals against the homologous crude enterotoxins (boiled 30 minutes) but not against the heterologous toxins. It is difficult to draw conclusions from this study since one of the strains (L.16) produced β-hemolysin and enough remained after heating to cause emesis in cats. One of the strains was the S-6 strain which produces enterotoxin B and a small amount of A, and the other one, 224, was from Casman's laboratory and later was reported to produce enterotoxin A (Casman, 1960). Studies in the Food Research Institute (Bergdoll *et al.*, 1968b) indicated that strain L. 16 produced enterotoxin D and strain 224 produced enterotoxin E. Production of enterotoxin A by 224 was not confirmed.

Casman (1960) reported the identification of a specific antibody for the enterotoxin produced by strain 196E (enterotoxin A) and since that time, specific antibodies have been prepared to enterotoxin C (Bergdoll *et al.*, 1965a), enterotoxin D (Casman *et al.*, 1967), and to enterotoxin E (tentative) (Bergdoll *et al.*, 1968a). Antibodies have been prepared to enterotoxin C produced by two different strains (137 and 361) and information from the Food Research Institute laboratories show that the enterotoxins do cross react with the heterologous antibodies. Close observation indicates slight differences in the reaction of the enterotoxins with the

homologous and heterologous antisera. Initially, complete lines of identification are formed on Ouchterlony plates; however, after longer development, spurs develop with the heterologous antisera. In single gel
diffusion tubes, the density of the precipitate formed is greater with
the homologous antiserum than with the heterologous antiserum.

The preparation of specific antibodies has been done primarily in rabbits although other animals such as the monkey and horse have been used.
The methods for preparation have varied with the different investigators.
Initially, in the Food Research Institute, a series of sixteen injections
were used, the first eight with enterotoxin incubated in 0.4% formalin at
30°C for 18 days and the second eight with untreated antigen. The first
injection was given intramuscularly with Freund adjuvants and the remainder (without adjuvant) by five routes (intraperitoneal, intramuscular,
intradermal, subcutaneous, and intravenous) (Bergdoll et al., 1959a).
Later this was changed to a series of intramuscular injections of untreated
toxin with Freund's complete adjuvant (Difco) (Bergdoll et al., 1965a). A
typical series of injections for purified toxins is 0.005, 0.01, 0.04, 0.2, and
1.0 mg at approximately 1-week intervals, depending on how rapidly the
rabbits regained any weight losses. The amount of toxin used in any one
injection was determined by the effect on the rabbits. It is desirable that
some weight loss (100-150 gm for 2.5-3 kg rabbits) results after each
injection. Five weeks after the 1.0 mg injection, a 2-3 mg injection is
given and bleedings are begun approximately 8 days later. Four to six
bleedings of approximately 50 ml each over a 2-3 week period are made
from an ear vein (Nace and Spradlin, 1962). Booster injections of 2-3 mg
of enterotoxin can be given every 5 weeks indefinitely with 4-6 bleedings
after each injection.

The method used by Casman and Bennett (1964) involved the injections of rabbits at weekly intervals as follows (enterotoxin B): 1 and 2 μg
intracutaneously, 5 μg subcutaneously, and 50, 100, 1000, and 2500 μg
mixed with aluminum phosphate subcutaneously. After 3 weeks, 4000 μg
mixed with aluminum phosphate was given subcutaneously, and after
another month, 1000 μg in saline was given intravenously. After 1 week,
if antibody titers were sufficiently high, 60 ml of blood was removed from
a marginal ear vein. The intravenous injections of 1000 μg was repeated
at monthly intervals for 4 months. The titer of the antiserum was such
that it could be used in the microslide test at 1:50 to 1:100 dilutions. The
potency of the antiserum obtained by the method used in the Food Research Institute is similar to that obtained by Casman and Bennett (1963).
One advantage of the Food Research Institute method is that 200-300 ml
of blood can be obtained after each booster injection.

C. ENTEROTOXOIDS

The immunization of animals against enterotoxin necessitates the inactivation of all biological activities, although it is possible to use purified enterotoxin without treatment with some risk to the animal's welfare. The most common procedure for inactivation of the biological activities is the use of formaldehyde (Bergdoll, 1966). Various procedures involving this reagent have been used (Dolman and Wilson, 1938; Thatcher and Matheson, 1955; Minett, 1938; Dolman, 1944; Burbianka, 1956; Demelová and Součková, 1963; Silverman et al., 1966). The method used by Bergdoll (1966) was incubation of the enterotoxin in 0.7% formalin for 3 weeks at 37°C. All biological activities including enterotoxin were inactivated, and the resulting material proved effective in immunizing rhesus monkeys. Several substances reported in the literature as being effective toxoiding agents for various antigens (ascorbic acid, Thatcher and Matheson, 1955; pepsin, Parfentjen et al., 1941; potassium thiocyanate, Hosoya and Yokoyama, 1956; Miyasaki and Hiraide, 1957; and sodium ricinoleate, Larson et al., 1924) were found to be less than completely effective against enterotoxin. Höhne (1967) reported that he could not demonstrate precipitating antibodies in the antisera from rabbits injected with heated culture filtrates.

Hopper (1961) reported that beta propiolactone effectively inactivated enterotoxin when the toxin was treated with 2.5% of this reagent and allowed to stand overnight before feeding to rhesus monkeys. This reagent may be preferable to formalin, but adequate testing has not been done. Enterotoxoids are used only when immunizing animals or man for protection against staphylococcal food poisoning, since much higher titers for preparation of specific antisera can be obtained by using the untreated toxin for injection.

REFERENCES

Avena, R. M., and Bergdoll, M. S. (1967). *Biochemistry* 6, 1474.
Baird-Parker, A. C., and Joseph, R. L. (1964). *Nature* 202, 510.
Bayliss, M. J. (1940). *J. Exptl. Med.* 72, 669.
Beeson, P. B. (1947). *Proc. Soc. Exptl. Biol. Med.* 64, 146.
Bergdoll, M. S. (1961). Unpublished data.
Bergdoll, M. S. (1962). *Proc. 14th Res. Conf., Am. Meat Inst. Found. Circ.* No. 70, p. 47.
Bergdoll, M. S. (1966). *J. Infect. Diseases* 116, 191.
Bergdoll, M. S. (1968). Unpublished data.
Bergdoll, M. S., Kadavy, J. L., Surgalla, M. J., and Dack, G. M. (1951). *Arch. Biochem. Biophys.* 33, 259.
Bergdoll, M. S., Lavin, B., Surgalla, M. J., and Dack, G. M. (1952). *Science* 116, 633.

Bergdoll, M. S., Sugiyama, H., and Dack, G. M. (1959a). *Arch. Biochem. Biophys.* **85**, 62.
Bergdoll, M. S., Surgalla, M. J., and Dack, G. M. (1959b). *J. Immunol.* **8**, 334.
Bergdoll, M. S., Sugiyama, H., and Dack, G. M. (1961). *J. Biochem. Microbiol. Technol. Eng.* **3**, 41.
Bergdoll, M. S., Borja, C. R., and Avena, R. M. (1965a). *J. Bacteriol.* **90**, 1481.
Bergdoll, M. S., Chu, F. S., Huang, I.-Y., Rowe, C., and Shih, T. (1965b). *Arch. Biochem. Biophys.* **112**, 104.
Bergdoll, M. S., Weiss, K. F., and Muster, M. J. (1967). *Bacteriol. Proc.* p. 12.
Bergdoll, M. S., Borja, C. R., Fanning, E., and Weiss, K. F. (1968a). Unpublished data.
Bergdoll, M. S., Robbins, R., Reiser, R., and Weiss, K. F. (1968b). Unpublished data.
Bokkenheuser, V., Cardella, M. A., Gorzynski, E. A., Wright, G. G., and Neter, E. (1963). *Proc. Soc. Exptl. Biol. Med.* **112**, 18.
Borja, C. R. (1969). *Biochemistry* **8**, 71.
Borja, C. R., and Bergdoll, M. S. (1967). *Biochemistry* **6**, 1467.
Borja, C. R., and Bergdoll, M. S. (1969). *Biochemistry* **8**, 75.
Burbianka, M. (1956). *Acta Microbiol. Polon.* **5**, 245.
Burnet, F. M. (1930). *J. Pathol. Bacteriol.* **33**, 1.
Burnet, F. M. (1931). *J. Pathol. Bacteriol.* **34**, 471.
Casman, E. P. (1958). *Public Health Rept. (U.S.)* **73**, 599.
Casman, E. P. (1960). *J. Bacteriol.* **79**, 849.
Casman, E. P. (1965). *Ann. N. Y. Acad. Sci.* **128**, 124.
Casman, E. P., and Bennett, R. W. (1963). *J. Bacteriol.* **86**, 18.
Casman, E. P., and Bennett, R. W. (1964). *Appl. Microbiol.* **12**, 363.
Casman, E. P., and Bennett, R. W. (1965). *Appl. Microbiol.* **13**, 181.
Casman, E. P., Bergdoll, M. S., and Robinson, J. (1963). *J. Bacteriol.* **85**, 715.
Casman, E. P., Bennett, R. W., Dorsey, A. E., and Issa, J. A. (1967). *J. Bacteriol.* **94**, 1875.
Chang, S. L., and Hall, H. E. (1963). *Appl. Microbiol.* **11**, 365.
Chesbro, W. R., and Auborn, K. (1967). *Appl. Microbiol.* **15**, 1150.
Chu, F. S. (1968). *J. Biol. Chem.* **243**, 4342.
Chu, F. S., Crary, E., and Bergdoll, M. S. (1969). *Biochemistry* **8**, 2890.
Chu, F. S., Thadhani, K., Schantz, E. J., and Bergdoll, M. S. (1966). *Biochemistry* **5**, 3281.
Clark, W. G., and Borison, H. L. (1963). *J. Pharmacol. Exptl. Therap.* **142**, 237.
Clark, W. G., and Page, J. S. (1968). *J. Bacteriol.* **96**, 1940.
Clark, W. G., Vanderhooft, G. F., and Borison, H. L. (1962). *Proc. Soc. Exptl. Biol. Med.* **111**, 205.
Crawley, G. J., Black, J. N., Gray, I., and Blanchard, J. W. (1966a). *Appl. Microbiol.* **14**, 445.
Crawley, G. J., Gray, I., Leblang, W. A., and Blanchard, J. W. (1966b). *J. Infect. Diseases* **116**, 48.
Dack, G. M. (1956). *Am. J. Surg.* **92**, 765.
Dack, G. M., Cary, W. E., Woolpert, O., and Wiggers, H. (1930). *J. Prevent. Med. (Baltimore)* **4**, 167.
Dack, G. M., Jordan, E. O., and Woolpert, O. (1931). *J. Prevent. Med. (Baltimore)* **5**, 151.
Dalidowicz, J. E., Silverman, S. J., Schantz, E. J., Stefanye, D., and Spero, L. (1966). *Biochemistry* **5**, 237.
D'Arca Simonetti, A. (1965). *Nuovi Ann. Igiene Microbiol.* **16**, 291.
Davis, R. B., Meeker, W. R., and Bailey, W. L. (1961). *Proc. Soc. Exptl. Biol. Med.* **108**, 774.
Davison, E., and Dack, G. M. (1939). *J. Infect. Diseases* **64**, 302.
Davison, E., Dack, G. M., and Cary, W. E. (1938). *J. Infect. Diseases* **62**, 219.

Demelová, M., and Součková, J. (1963). *J. Hyg., Epidemiol., Microbiol., Immunol. (Prague)* **7**, 195.

Denny, C. B., and Bohrer, C. W. (1963). *J. Bacteriol.* **86**, 347.

Denny, C. B., Tan, P. L., and Bohrer, C. W. (1966a). *J. Environ. Health* **29**, 222.

Denny, C. B., Tan, P. L., and Bohrer, C. W. (1966b). *J. Food Sci.* **31**, 762.

DeValle, M. R. (1960). M.S. Thesis, University of Wisconsin.

Dolman, C. E. (1934). *J. Infect. Diseases* **55**, 172.

Dolman, C. E. (1936). *Can. J. Public Health* **27**, 494.

Dolman, C. E. (1943). *Can. J. Public Health* **34**, 205.

Dolman, C. E. (1944). *Can. J. Public Health* **35**, 337.

Dolman, C. E., and Wilson, R. J. (1938). *J. Immunol.* **35**, 13.

Dolman, C. E., and Wilson, R. J. (1940). *Can. J. Public Health* **31**, 68.

Dolman, C. E., Wilson, R. J., and Cockcroft, W. H. (1936). *Can. J. Public Health* **27**, 489.

Eddy, C. A. (1951). *Proc. Soc. Exptl. Biol. Med.* **78**, 131.

Edman, P., and Sjöquist, J. (1956). *Acta Chem. Scand.* **10**, 1507.

Ehrenberg, A. (1957). *Acta Chem. Scand.* **11**, 1257.

Evans, J. B., Buettner, L. G., and Niven, C. F., Jr. (1950). *J. Bacteriol.* **60**, 481.

Favorite, G. O., and Hammon, W. McD. (1941). *J. Bacteriol.* **41**, 305.

Feingold, M. J. (1967). *Lab. Invest.* **16**, 912.

Felsenfeld, O., and Nasuniya, N. (1964). *J. Trop. Med. Hyg.* **67**, 300.

Frea, J. I., McCoy, E., and Strong, F. M. (1963). *J. Bacteriol.* **86**, 1308.

Friedman, M. E. (1966). *J. Bacteriol.* **92**, 277.

Friedman, M. E. (1968). *J. Bacteriol.* **95**, 1051.

Friedman, M. E., and White, J. D. (1965). *J. Bacteriol.* **89**, 1155.

Genigeorgis, C., and Sadler, W. W. (1966a). *J. Food Sci.* **31**, 441.

Genigeorgis, C., and Sadler, W. W. (1966b). *J. Food Sci.* **31**, 605.

Genigeorgis, C., and Sadler, W. W. (1966c). *J. Bacteriol.* **92**, 1383.

Gilbert, C. F. (1966). *Thromb. Diath. Haemorrag.* **16**, 697.

Good, R. A., and Thomas, L. (1952). *J. Exptl. Med.* **96**, 625.

Hall, H. E., Angelotti, R., and Lewis, K. H. (1963). *Public Health Rept. (U.S.)* **78**, 1093.

Hall, H. E., Angelotti, R., and Lewis, K. H. (1965). *Health Lab. Sci.* **2**, 179.

Hallander, H. O. (1965). *Acta Pathol. Microbiol. Scand.* **63**, 299.

Hallander, H. O., and Körlof, B. (1968). *Acta Pathol. Microbiol. Scand.* **71**, 359.

Hammon, W. McD. (1941). *Am. J. Public Health* **31**, 1191.

Hayama, T., and Sugiyama, H. (1964). *Proc. Soc. Exptl. Biol. Med.* **117**, 115.

Haynes, W. C., Kuehne, R. W., and Rhodes, L. J. (1954). *Appl. Microbiol.* **2**, 239.

Heidelberger, M., and Kendall, F. E. (1929). *J. Exptl. Med.* **50**, 809.

Herold, J. D., Shultz, J. S., and Gerhardt, P. (1967). *Appl. Microbiol.* **15**, 1192.

Hilker, J. S., Heilman, W. R., Tan, P. L., Denny, C. B., and Bohrer, C. W. (1968). *Appl. Microbiol.* **16**, 308.

Hodoval, L. F., Morris, E. L., Elsberry, D. D., and Beisel, W. R. (1967). *Appl. Microbiol.* **15**, 403.

Hodoval, L. F., Morris, E. L., Crawley, G. J., and Beisel, W. R. (1968). *Appl. Microbiol.* **16**, 187.

Höhne, C. (1967). *Z. Immunitaetsforsch., Allergie Klin. Immunol.* **132**, 12.

Hopkins, E. W., and Poland, E. F. (1942). *Food. Res.* **7**, 414.

Hopper, S. H. (1961). *Bacteriol. Proc.* p. 109.

Hopper, S. H. (1963). *J. Food Sci.* **28**, 572.

Hosoya, S., and Yokoyama, M. (1956). *Nippon Saikingaku Zasshi* **11**, 133.

Huang, I.-Y., and Bergdoll, M. S. (1969). Unpublished manuscript.

Huang, I.-Y., Shih, T., Borja, C. R., Avena, R. M., and Bergdoll, M. S. (1967). *Biochemistry* 6, 1480.

Huang, I.-Y., Schantz, E. J., and Bergdoll, M. S. (1969). *Arch. Biochem. Biophys.* 132, 423.

Hurst, V. (1965). *Health Lab. Sci.* 2, 122.

Johnson, H. M., Hall, H. E., and Simon, M. (1967). *Appl. Microbiol.* 15, 815.

Jordan, E. O., and McBroom, J. (1931). *Proc. Soc. Exptl. Biol. Med.* 29, 161.

Jordan, E. O., and Burrows, W. (1933). *Proc. Soc. Exptl. Biol. Med.* 30, 448.

Joseph, R. L., and Baird-Parker, A. C. (1965). *Nature* 207, 663.

Kato, E., Khan, M., Kujovich, L., and Bergdoll, M. S. (1966). *Appl. Microbiol.* 14, 966.

Kent, T. H. (1966). *Am. J. Pathol.* 48, 387.

Kent, T. H., Jervis, H. R., and Kuhns, J. G. (1966). *Am. J. Pathol.* 48, 667.

Kienitz, M. (1962). *Zentr. Bakteriol., Parasitenk., Abt. I. Orig.* 184, 87.

Kienitz, M. (1964). *Aerztl. Praxis* 16, 872.

Kienitz, M., and Preuner, R. (1959). *Zentr. Bakteriol., Parasitenk., Abt. I. Orig.* 174, 56.

Kienitz, M., and Schmelter, G. (1964). *Zentr. Bakteriol., Parasitenk., Abt. I. Orig.* 193, 447.

Kocandrle, V., Houttuin, E., and Prohaska, J. V. (1966). *J. Surg. Res.* 6, 50.

Kollias, V. A. (1967). Master's Thesis, University of North Carolina.

Kraut, H., Koerbel, W., Scholtan, W., and Schultz, F. (1960). *Z. Physik. Chem. (Leipzig)* 321, 90.

Kuru, M. (1956). *J. Comp. Neurol.* 104, 207.

Kuru, M., and Sugihara, S. (1955). *Japan. J. Physiol.* 5, 21.

Larson, W. P., Evans, R. D., and Nelson, E. (1924). *Proc. Soc. Exptl. Biol. Med.* 22, 194.

McLean, R. A., Lilly, H., and Alford, J. A. (1968). *J. Bacteriol.* 95, 1207.

McIntosh, M., and Duggan, D. E. (1965). *J. Protozool.* 12, 342.

McKay, D. G., and Shapiro, S. S. (1958). *J. Exptl. Med.* 104, 383.

Mah, R. A., Fung, D. Y. C., and Morse, S. A. (1967). *Appl. Microbiol.* 15, 866.

Markus, Z., and Silverman, G. J. (1968). *J. Bacteriol.* 96, 1446.

Martin, W. J., and Marcus, S. (1964). *J. Bacteriol.* 87, 1019.

Matheson, B. H., and Thatcher, F. S. (1955). *Can. J. Microbiol.* 1, 372.

Merrill, T. G., and Sprinz, H. (1968). *Lab. Invest.* 18, 114.

Milone, N. A. (1962). *J. Food Sci.* 27, 501.

Minett, F. C. (1938). *J. Hyg.* 38, 623.

Miyasaki, S., and Hiraide, I. (1957). *Japan. J. Microbiol.* 1, 37.

Morris, E. L., Hodoval, L. F., and Beisel, W. R. (1967). *J. Infect. Diseases* 117, 273.

Morse, S. A., and Mah, R. A. (1967). *Appl. Microbiol.* 15, 58.

Mullet, E., Jr., and Friedman, M. E. (1961). *Bacteriol. Proc.* p. 108.

Munch-Peterson, E. (1963). *J. Food Sci.* 28, 692.

Nace, G. W., and Spradlin, P. (1962). *Turtox News* 40, 26.

Nikodemusz, I., Kanizsai, L., and Sellei, E. (1963). *Acta Med. Acad. Sci. Hung.* 19, 209.

Normann, S. J., and Jaeger, R. F. (1969). *Lab. Invest.* 20, 17.

Normann, S. J., and Johnsey, R. T. (1968). *J. Bacteriol.* 95, 1178.

Omori, G., and Kato, Y. (1959). *Biken's J.* 2, 92.

Palmer, E. D. (1951). *Gastroenterology* 19, 462.

Parfentjen, I. A., Clapp, F. L., and Waldschmidt, A. (1941). *J. Immunol.* 40, 189.

Parker, M. T., and Lapage, S. P. (1957). *J. Clin. Pathol.* 10, 313.

Prohaska, J. V. (1963). *Ann. Surg.* 158, 492.

Prohaska, J. V., Long, E. T., and Nelsen, T. S. (1956). *A.M.A. Arch. Surg.* 72, 977.

Prohaska, J. V., Jacobson, M. J., Drake, C. T., and Tan, T. (1959). *Surg., Gynecol. Obstet.* 108, 73.

Raj, H., and Bergdoll, M. S. (1969). *J. Bacteriol.* 98, 833.

Raj, H., and Liston, J. (1962). *Bacteriol. Proc.* p. 65.

Rapoport, M. I., Hodoval, L. F., Grogan, E. W., McGann, V., and Beisel, W. R. (1966). *J. Clin. Invest.* **45**, 1365.

Rapoport, M. I., Hodoval, L. F., and Beisel, W. R. (1967). *J. Bacteriol.* **93**, 779.

Read, R. B., Jr., and Bradshaw, J. G. (1966a). *Appl. Microbiol.* **14**, 130.

Read, R. B., Jr., and Bradshaw, J. G. (1966b). *J. Dairy Sci.* **49**, 202.

Read, R. B., Jr., and Bradshaw, J. G. (1967). *Appl. Microbiol.* **15**, 603.

Read, R. B., Jr., and Pritchard, W. L. (1963). *Can. J. Microbiol.* **9**, 879.

Read, R. B., Jr., Bradshaw, J., Pritchard, W. L., and Black, L. A. (1965a). *J. Dairy Sci.* **48**, 420.

Read, R. B., Jr., Pritchard, W. L., Bradshaw, J., and Black, L. A. (1965b). *J. Dairy Sci.* **48**, 411.

Ritzerfeld, W., Kienitz, M., and Glodny, H. (1960). *Z. Hyg. Infektionskrankh.* **147**, 144.

Robinton, E. D. (1949). *Proc. Soc. Exptl. Biol. Med.* **72**, 265.

Robinton, E. D. (1950). *Yale J. Biol. Med.* **23**, 94.

Rosenwald, A. J., and Lincoln, R. E. (1966). *J. Bacteriol.* **92**, 279.

Schachman, H. K. (1957). *Methods Enzymol.* **4**, 32.

Schaeffer, W. I., Gabliks, J., and Calitis, R. (1966). *J. Bacteriol.* **91**, 21.

Schaeffer, W. I., Gabliks, J., and Calitis, R. (1967). *J. Bacteriol.* **93**, 1489.

Schantz, E. J. (1966). Private communication.

Schantz, E. J., and Lauffer, M. A. (1962). *Biochemistry* **1**, 658.

Schantz, E. J., Roessler, W. G., Wagman, J., Spero, L., Donnery, D. A., and Bergdoll, M. S. (1965). *Biochemistry* **4**, 1011.

Segalove, M. (1947). *J. Infect. Diseases* **81**, 228.

Shemano, I., Hitchens, J. T., and Beiler, J. M. (1967). *Gastroenterology* **53**, 71.

Silverman, S. J. (1963). *J. Bacteriol.* **85**, 955.

Silverman, S. J., Schantz, E. J., Espeseth, D. A., and Roessler, W. G. (1966). *Bacteriol. Proc.* p. 43.

Silverman, S. J., Knott, A. R., and Howard, M. (1968). *Appl. Microbiol.* **16**, 1019.

Spero, L., Stefanye, D., Brecher, P. I., Jacoby, H. M., Dalidowicz, J. E., and Schantz, E. J. (1965). *Biochemistry* **4**, 1024.

Sugiyama, H. (1966). *J. Infect. Diseases* **116**, 162.

Sugiyama, H., and Hayama, T. (1964). *Proc. Soc. Exptl. Biol. Med.* **115**, 243.

Sugiyama, H., and Hayama, T. (1965). *J. Infect. Diseases* **115**, 330.

Sugiyama, H., and McKissic, E. M., Jr. (1966). *J. Bacteriol.* **92**, 349.

Sugiyama, H., Bergdoll, M. S., and Dack, G. M. (1958). *Proc. Soc. Exptl. Biol. Med.* **97**, 900.

Sugiyama, H., Bergdoll, M. S., and Wilkerson, R. G. (1960). *Proc. Soc. Exptl. Biol. Med.* **103**, 168.

Sugiyama, H., Chow, K. L., and Dragstedt, L. R., II. (1961). *Proc. Soc. Exptl. Biol. Med.* **108**, 92.

Sugiyama, H., Bergdoll, M. S., and Dack, G. M. (1962). *J. Infect. Diseases* **111**, 233.

Sugiyama, H., McKissic, E. M., Jr., and Bergdoll, M. S. (1963). *Proc. Soc. Exptl. Biol. Med.* **113**, 468.

Sugiyama, H., McKissic, E. M., Jr., Bergdoll, M. S., and Heller, B. (1964a). *J. Infect. Diseases* **114**, 111.

Sugiyama, H., McKissic, E. M., Jr., and Hayama, T. (1964b). *Proc. Soc. Exptl. Biol. Med.* **117**, 726.

Sugiyama, H., Hayama, T., and Yagasaki, O. (1966). *Proc. Soc. Exptl. Biol. Med.* **121**, 278.

Surgalla, M. J. (1947). *J. Infect Diseases* **81**, 97.

Surgalla, M. J., and Dack, G. M. (1955). *J. Am. Med. Assoc.* **158**, 649.

Surgalla, M. J., and Hite, K. E. (1945). *J. Infect. Diseases* **76**, 78.

Surgalla, M. J., Kadavy, J. L., Bergdoll, M. S., and Dack, G. M. (1951). *J. Infect. Diseases* **89**, 180.

Surgalla, M. J., Bergdoll, M. S., and Dack, G. M. (1952). *J. Immunol.* **69**, 357.

Surgalla, M. J., Bergdoll, M. S., and Dack, G. M. (1953). *J. Lab. Clin. Med.* **41**, 782.

Surgalla, M. J., Bergdoll, M. S., and Dack, G. M. (1954). *J. Immunol.* **72**, 398.

Tan, T., Drake, C. T., Jacobson, M. J., and Prohaska, J. V. (1959). *Surg., Gynecol. Obstet.* **108**, 415.

Thatcher, F. S., and Matheson, B. H. (1955). *Can. J. Microbiol.* **1**, 382.

Thatcher, F. S., and Simon, W. (1956). *Can. J. Microbiol.* **2**, 703.

Wagman, J., Edwards, R. C., and Schantz, E. J. (1965). *Biochemistry* **4**, 1017.

Warren, S. E., Sugiyama, H., and Prohaska, J. V. (1963). *Surg., Gynecol. Obstet.* **116**, 29.

Warren, S. E., Jacobson, M., Mirany, J., and Prohaska, J. V. (1964). *J. Exptl. Med.* **120**, 561.

Weed, L. A. (1943). *Am. J. Public Health* **33**, 1314.

Weirether, F. J., Lewis, E. E., Rosenwald, A. J., and Lincoln, R. E. (1966). *Appl. Microbiol.* **14**, 284.

Wentworth, B. B. (1963). *Bacteriol. Reviews* **27**, 253.

Wilson, B. J. (1959). *J. Bacteriol.* **78**, 240.

Woolpert, O. C., and Dack, G. M. (1933). *J. Infect. Diseases* **52**, 6.

Wu, C-H. (1968). M.S. Thesis, University of Wisconsin.

Yagasaki, O., and Sugiyama, H. (1966). *Proc. Soc. Exptl. Biol. Med.* **122**, 459.

Zehren, V. L., and Zehren, V. F. (1968). *J. Dairy Sci.* **51**, 635.

CHAPTER 8

Staphylococcal Leukocidin

A. M. WOODIN*

I. Introduction

Leukocidin is an extracellular product of the staphylococcus consisting of two proteins, the F component and the S component. Together, but not alone, these proteins are toxic to the polymorphonuclear leukocytes and macrophages of the rabbit and man. No other cell type has been found to be susceptible.

The two reasons for studying bacterial toxins are, of course, for the information they provide on the pathogenicity of the organisms producing them and on the properties of the cells they attack. The first of these has been studied by Gladstone and Mudd and their collaborators and they have shown that leukocidin production alone is not responsible for the pathogenicity of the staphylococcus. The second has been studied by

*Member of the External Staff, Medical Research Council.

Woodin and Wieneke and has led to the unexpected finding that leukocidin induces changes that mimic those in excitable or secretory cells during membrane depolarization or stimulation with hormones.

The present review incorporates some of the material summarized by Woodin (1968). Earlier reviews on leukocidin and its cytotoxic effect (Woodin and Wieneke, 1964a; Woodin, 1965, 1966a) are out of date and should be disregarded.

II. Historical Review

Van der Velde (1894) and Denys and Van der Velde (1895) observed that the staphylococcus produces toxins lethal to leukocytes and Neisser and Wechsberg (1901) titrated leukocidal activity in staphylococcal filtrates by observing the inhibition of respiration in polymorphonuclear leukocytes. Julianelle (1922) distinguished between the leukocidal and hemolytic activities and this was emphasized by Panton and Valentine (1932). Subsequent work (Wright, 1936; Proom, 1937; Gladstone and van Heyningen, 1957) suggested that the specific leukocidal, α-hemolytic, β-hemolytic, and δ-hemolytic activities were due to distinct substances and now that three of these have been purified (Woodin, 1960; Bernheimer, 1965; Yoshida, 1963) this is established. A summary of the specificity of the hemolysins and leukocidins with regard to cell type and species is given by Gladstone (1966). Following the crystallization of leukocidin, research has been concentrated on the determination of its significance in staphylococcal pathogenicity and the analysis of its cytotoxic effect.

III. Preparation, Purification, and Properties

A. PREPARATION

Good yields can be obtained *in vitro* by culturing the V 8 strain of the staphylococcus in a CCY medium based on that originally described by Gladstone and Fildes (1940). This medium consists of amino acids, salts, lactate, glycophosphate, and a diffusate of yeast extract. None of the components in the medium are precipitated by ammonium sulfate, but many are co-precipitated with proteins. Extensive dialysis or the use of Sephadex is required to free the proteins precipitated from the culture filtrate by ammonium sulfate from components of the medium. The nature and preparation of the yeast diffusate is critical in obtaining high yields of leukocidin. Oxoid yeast extract was found to give 20 times more leukocidin than Difco yeast extract (Woodin, 1959). The diffusate is produced by dialyzing a suspension of 120 gm of Oxoid yeast extract in 85 ml of water in dialysis sacking (1.5 cm flat width) against 770 ml of water in a cylinder (5 × 80 cm) for 24 hours at 4°C. The cylinders are placed on a rocking machine so that the air bubbles placed in the sack and the tube traverse the contents 20 times a minute. The final diffusate should have a dry weight of 75 gm/liter. High concentrations of diffusate are inhibitory to leukocidin production, and as a preliminary to large scale (1000 liters) production, it is advisable to determine the optimum amounts of yeast extract by titration on a small scale.

A chemically defined medium for leukocidin production has not been described. This is not likely to be easily designed, as fractionation of Oxoid yeast extract on ion exchange resins gave material stimulating leukocidin production in different fractions and more than one substance may be involved (Woodin, 1969).

On a small scale, it is convenient to produce leukocidin by a 20-hour culture in rocking T-tubes (van Heyningen and Gladstone, 1953). Production on the 150 liter scale was successfully carried out by Mr. R. Elsworth and Mr. R. Telling at the Microbiological Research Establishment at Porton, England. The medium was that described by Gladstone and van Heyningen (1957) with the substitution of a diffusate of Oxoid yeast extract and Oxoid Casamino acids for the corresponding Difco products. The medium (125 liters) was inoculated with 25 liters of seed (prepared in turn from a 1-liter shake flask inoculated from an agar slope), and the culture was grown in a stainless steel reactor with bottom aeration and stirring. A maximum leukocidin content was found after 8–10 hours when the culture contained 6 gm/liter of organisms and 50 mg/liter of each component of leukocidin. To recover the leukocidin, the organisms were centrifuged off and the culture supernate was transferred to vessels containing sufficient solid ammonium sulfate to ensure saturation at room temperature. With smaller volumes it is convenient to place the culture supernate in dialysis sacs with solid ammonium sulfate outside the sacs. In either case, the precipitated proteins were recovered by centrifugation (some precipitate floats) and the resultant slurry used for purification of leukocidin.

B. PURIFICATION

In preliminary experiments carried out using material obtained with media containing Difco yeast extract, different batches behaved quite differently and a fresh fractionation scheme was required for each batch. It was also observed in these preliminary experiments that while solutions containing leukocidin were stable for days, various mild fractionations led to complete inactivation. After the realization that this was due to the dual nature of leukocidin, and also, that by choice of the appropriate yeast extract, culture filtrates could be produced in which leukocidin represented some 10-20% of the protein, it became possible to fractionate and purify leukocidin without great difficulty. This was greatly aided by the development by others of chromatographic methods for protein separation (Tiselius *et al.*, 1956; Peterson and Sober, 1956; Boman and Westlund, 1956).

To purify the two components of leukocidin, impurities were removed by fractionation with ammonium sulfate and by chromatography on calcium phosphate; then the F fraction of leukocidin was then separated from the S fraction by two-stage chromatography on carboxymethylcellulose. To purify the F component and the S component of leukocidin, each of these fractions was now worked up separately by the same method. Impurities were removed on Dowex 2x8 at low ionic strength, and then each component was purified by gradient elution from the cation exchange resin Amberlite CG 50. Full details of the procedure are given by Woodin (1959, 1960). Crystalization of the purified F component is achieved at low ionic strength and is a valuable method of removing residual impurities. Crystallization of the S component is achieved by salting out with ammonium sulfate, but as residual impurities are also precipitated, it is of little value in purifying.

C. Leukocidin Fractionation for Use in the Assay of Leukocidin.

To determine leukocidin and its antibodies, it is necessary to have preparations of the F component and of the S component of leukocidin fairly free from each other but not necessarily free from other proteins. Woodin (1961a) described a method for preparing these, and Elsworth and Sargent (1969) have described an improved procedure which can be used on a large scale. This method has been used by these two workers to prepare the test toxin for use with the international standard antileukocidin in the determination of antibodies in sera.

D. Chemical Nature of Leukocidin

Following the crystallization of leukocidin, an elementary survey of the physical properties was carried out (Woodin, 1960). The F component crystallizes at pH 7, and because its solubility at this pH is too low for its properties to be determined by conventional methods, the measurements were made in 0.1 M acetate buffer, pH 5. At this pH, sedimentation and diffusion constants determined in the analytical ultracentrifuge gave the values of 32,000 and 38,000 for the molecular weights of the F component and the S component, respectively. Both proteins sedimented with single symmetrical peaks, but the boundary spreading indicated that both proteins were polydisperse, presumably through the adoption of different conformational forms. To determine the sedimentation constants at pH 7, the proteins were labeled with ^{131}I and centrifuged in a sucrose gradient containing 0.15 M sodium chloride and 0.05 M tris buffer, pH 7, with catalase as marker. For both proteins, the mean value of 3 Svedberg units was obtained, the same as that found at pH 5, but again, there was evidence of polydispersity in both proteins (Woodin, 1969). On electrophoresis in free solution, both proteins gave single peaks at pH 5, the S component having the greater charge. It is this difference in charge that is exploited in the purification and separation of the two components of leukocidin on carboxymethylcellulose. Wadstrom (1969) carried out electrophoresis of staphylococcal filtrates containing leukocidin activity in a pH gradient and obtained isolectic points at pH 9; single bands of leukocidin activity were obtained.

At low ionic strength, both the F and the S components of leukocidin undergo partial polymerization, and about 30% of each protein becomes sedimentable at 30,000 g for 30 minutes (Woodin and Wieneke, 1966c). The sedimented material dissolves in solutions of physiological ionic strength, and no difference in the biological activity of this or the leukocidin remaining in the original supernate can be detected. It appears that in solutions of physiological ionic strength, both components of leukocidin exist in different conformational states and that when the ionic strength is lowered, some of these polymerize. The interconversion of the different conformational states must be very slow.

An attempt was made to specify these conformational forms by measuring rates of deuterium exchange. With three samples of glycylglycine the exchangeable hydrogens determined by the method of Hvidt et al. (1960) were found to be 4.05, 4.2, and 4.2 gram atoms per mole, (theoretical is 4.0), and with the F component of leukocidin in concentrated urea solution, 450 gram atoms of exchangeable hydrogen per mole were obtained consistently. However, with different preparations of the F component at physiological ionic strength, consistent results could not be obtained, suggesting that different preparations had different ratios of the postulated conformational forms.

The study of leukocidin as protein is in its infancy. It will be shown below that leukocidin undergoes interactions with phospholipids that might mimic those between proteins and lipids in membranes. An extension to the study of the physical properties of leukocidin could prove very rewarding.

E. Assay of Leukocidin and Its Antibodies

The principle of this assay is based on the following considerations (Woodin, 1961a). The two components of leukocidin act synergistically, not additively; each component is inactive alone but is potentiated by the addition of the other. Thus, to determine the F component in a culture filtrate, serial dilutions are made and an excess of the S component added to each tube. To determine the S component an excess of the F component is added to a further set of dilutions. If the leukocidal activity is now determined, an end point will be reached when the concentration of the diluted component is less than that in a minimal leukocidal dose. Antibody to the two components of leukocidin is determined by an analogous method. Two test toxins are set up, in one of which the F component is in large excess over the S component, and vice versa. Special precautions are required if the antiserum under investigation contains a large excess of one antileukocidin antibody over the other. These precautions are described by Woodin (1961a) and Gladstone et al. (1962) give detailed schedules for the determination of antileukocidin antibodies.

Theoretically end points should be determined by observing the chemical change induced by the toxin, or, the response of the cell that is specific to the toxin. It will be suggested below that for leukocidin these are a conformational change in the triphosphoinositide of the cell membrane and a specific increased permeability to potassium, respectively. There is no possibility of either of these being adapted for routine leukocidin determination. End points are therefore determined from the nonspecific responses of leukocytes or macrophages to leukocidin and distinction from hemolysins having leukocidal activity is made by using different cell types and species.

Now that the response to leukocidin is known in detail, many methods could be used to determine end points. In routine use are the inhibition of respiration in rabbit macrophages (Woodin, 1959) or the observation of morphological changes in human polymorphonuclear leukocytes (Gladstone et al., 1962). The first has the disadvantage that macrophages have to be prepared from peritoneal exudates but the advantage that analysis can be carried out by an unskilled technician. The second requires a little skill with the microscope, and as polymorphonuclear leukocytes are much more fragile than macrophages, all glassware must be scrupulously clean. However, it is ideal for use in pathology laboratories.

In special circumstances, other methods can be employed. Woodin and Wieneke (1966c), for example, used the uptake of ^{45}Ca by injured polymorphonuclear leukocytes as an end point to determine leukocidin in homogenates of leukocytes.

F. ANTIBODY-COMBINING POWER OF LEUKOCIDIN

Initially an antiserum CPP 76/73 obtained from the Wellcome Research Laboratories, Beckenham, England, was used in estimations of leukocidin (Gladstone and van Heyningen, 1957; Woodin, 1959, 1960) and it was assigned the value 240 units of antileukocidin antibody per milliliter. When the two components of leukocidin were separated and purified, it was found that the combining powers for the F component and S component were 270 L$^+$/mg and 1780 L$^+$/mg, respectively. This suggested that the antiserum was deficient in antibodies to the S component of leukocidin. Accordingly, Gladstone et $al.$ (1962) changed the unit value of the antiserum CPP 76/73 to 48 anti-S units per milliliter and 240 units anti-F per milliliter. The units assigned to the international standard antileukocidin correspond to these. On this basis, the F component of leukocidin will have 270 L$^+$/mg and the S component of leukocidin 350 L$^+$/mg.

G. TOXOIDED LEUKOCIDIN

Gladstone (1965) has made a systematic study of the conditions for the preparation of leukocidin toxoid. Partly purified leukocidin (containing about 30% F component of leukocidin and 25% S component) could be effectively toxoided with 0.5% formaldehyde at pH 6.5. Both the F and the S components lost more than 95% of their ability to potentiate each other, but 70% of their combining power was retained. After further purification and separation of the two components of leukocidin, treatment with formaldehyde or with iodine resulted in loss of combining power and therefore of antigenicity. With this more highly purified material, toxoiding was accomplished with 0.2% β-propiolactone, which after 24 hours at 37% reduced the toxicity of both the F and the S component to about 3% of the starting material, while 40-60% of the combining power was retained.

IV. Mode of Action of Leukocidin

A. GENERAL OUTLINE

To determine the mode of action of leukocidin, a systematic study of the response of the leukocyte to leukocidin was made first. The result suggested that the primary response of the cell is an increased potassium permeability due to an alteration in the potassium pump. It was then found that leukocidin is not completely absorbed by the leukocyte, but is mainly converted into an inactive form which remains in solution. This reaction enabled the leukocyte surface membrane to be identified in cell homogenates, and its purification to be achieved. The properties of the cation-sensitive phosphatases of the isolated membrane confirmed that the primary response of the cell is an alteration in the potassium pump. The study of the physical interaction of leukocidin with the membrane suggested that phospholipids are involved. When the interaction of leukocidin with purified phospholipids was examined, it was found that triphosphoinositide, but no other phospholipid, induced an inactivation of leukocidin resembling that induced by the cell membrane. The presence of triphosphoinositide in the leukocyte cell membrane and its conformational alteration by leukocidin were then demonstrated.

The subsequent discovery of the inhibition of the potassium efflux in the leukocidin-treated cell by tetraethylammonium ions suggested that the permeability changes may be relevant to those in peripheral nerve. The utility of a detailed analysis of a cell treated with a toxin was emphasized by the use of the leukocidin-treated leukocyte to identify the action of phosphonates in inhibiting chemotaxis.

B. Character of the Leukocidin-Treated Cell.

Figure 1 summarizes the description of the leukocyte treated with leukocidin (Woodin, 1961b, 1962; Woodin et al., 1963; Woodin and Wieneke, 1963a,b, 1964b, 1966b,c). In the figure, the cell at the top represents the normal leukocyte, and the three cells at the bottom represent leukocytes that have been treated with leukocidin in various environments. The cell in the center is in the hypothetical condition of response to the primary action of leukocidin but not to any peculiarity of the environment. Special features of each cell are listed at their sides and general characteristics of all leukocidin-treated cells at the bottom of the figure. The nuclei of the cells are omitted because their biochemical changes in the leukocidin-treated cells have not been studied in detail. The study of the leukocidin effects has been confined to the first 10 minutes of intoxication. A maximal effect results from treating 10^8 leukocytes per milliliter with 2–4 μg of each component of leukocidin. The two components must be added together, none of the effects shown in Fig. 1 results from treatment with either component of leukocidin alone.

The normal leukocyte has certain distinctive features that might be recalled at this stage. The cytoplasm has no well-defined endoplasmic reticulum, ribosomes are absent, and in the case of leukocytes in peritoneal exudates so are mitochondria. The leukocytes in the bloodstream seem to possess mitochondria (Bessis, 1964). The cytoplasm has numerous granules (lysosomes) of three morphological forms (Florey and Grant, 1961). Metabolic features are the ability to survive anarobically, insensitivity to inhibitors of respiration, and a tendency to respond to changes in behavior with a stimulated pentose phosphate pathway (Karnovsky, 1962). The sodium content of the leukocyte is abnormally high and the maintenance of the intracellular potassium concentration is coupled to glycolysis (Elsbach and Schwartz, 1959). The characteristic physiological function of the leukocyte, of course, is phagocytosis, and the uptake of particles is followed by the extrusion of the proteins of the granule into the phagocytosis vesicle (Hirsch and Cohn, 1960).

The leukocyte treated with leukocidin shows no accumulation in soluble form of amino acids, phosphorus, nucleotides, or carbohydrate. The distribution of nucleic acids in subcellular fractions is not altered and a chromatographic analysis of the lipids of the normal and leukocidin-treated cell showed no major difference. There is no evidence that in the period allowed intracellular hydrolases are active. During a 10-minute treatment with leukocidin, no decrease in the rate of lactate production or glucose-6-^{14}C oxidation can be detected; in the presence of calcium the oxidation of glucose-1-^{14}C is stimulated by leukocidin, in its absence it is unchanged. Longer periods of incubation produce metabolic changes but it is clear that these are not a direct effect of leukocidin.

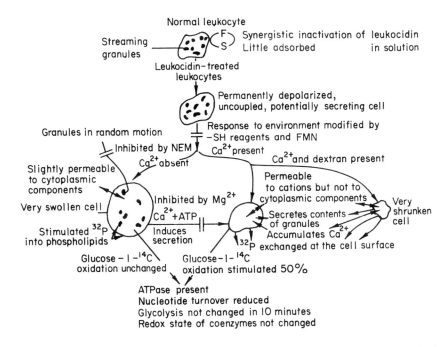

FIG. 1 The changes induced in leukocytes during 10 minutes of treatment with leukocidin.

Electron micrographs of cells treated with leukocidin in the absence of calcium show no gross morphological change, while cells prepared in the presence of calcium are degranulated. Under the light microscope, the leukocidin-treated cell shows a transition of the streaming motion of the granules to random Brownian motion and this leads rapidly to degranulation when calcium is present. When cells are treated with leukocidin in the presence of ethylenediaminetetraacetate (EDTA), the granules also cease to be visible after about 10 minutes, although electron micrographs of cells stained with osmium and lead show them to be intact but swollen. Many of the changes observed under the light microscope can result not from morphological alteration but from a change in the refractive index of the cytoplasm. This can be large, as the leukocidin-treated cell swells considerably.

The permeability changes in the leukocidin-treated cell are very restricted. There is an immediate loss of potassium, but phosphate, nucleotides, amino acids, and reducing sugars are retained in the leukocidin-treated cell at 6–30 times the concentration in the supernate. When calcium is present in the medium, it is accumulated in the cell and magnesium is displaced. If chelating agents are present in the medium, calcium is lost from the cell and further alterations to permeability occur. Judged by the distribution of the cytoplasmic enzyme aldolase, the leukocidin-treated cell prepared in the presence of calcium is not permeable to cytoplasmic protein, but large amounts of protein are present in the cell supernate. This is not found with the macrophage, an observation that, coupled with the degranulation seen under the microscope, led to the discovery that the protein is derived from the cytoplasmic granules. The secretion of the granule protein only happens when calcium is present.

Accompanying the permeability changes are alterations to the phosphorus metabolism. Orthophosphate accumulates at the expense of ATP (other phosphate esters are not affected) and there is a decrease in the rate of nucleotide turnover. If calcium is present in the medium, a new orthophosphate–nucleotide exchange reaction appears at the cell surface; and also dependent upon the presence of calcium is the amount of radioactivity incorporated into phospholipids.

The main features of the leukocidin-treated cell, therefore, are increased permeability to cations, secretion of protein, accumulation of calcium, stimulated ATPase, and stimulated nucleotide − orthophosphate exchange.

An increased permeability of the surface membrane restricted to ions is a characteristic of excitable tissues during membrane depolarization. In some cases it is also associated with an increased rate of exchange of calcium between the tissue and surrounding fluids (Douglas and Poisner,

1962). In the living cell the ion changes are accompanied by increased respiration and are reversed. In the leukocidin-treated cell, respiration does not increase and the ion changes are not reversed. On this basis, the center cell in Fig. 1 can be described as a permanently depolarized, un-coupled, potentially secreting cell.

C. A CLASSIFICATION OF LEUKOCIDIN EFFECTS

In the introduction to this chapter, the responses of cells to toxins and hormones were divided into reactions specific to the reagent and those not so. To detect the nonspecific response of the leukocyte to injury, Woodin and Wieneke (1964b, 1966a) have studied the response of leukocidin to streptolysin O and to excess vitamin A. These reagents hemolyze eryth-rocytes and isolated lysosomes, and these reactions can be prevented by hydrocortisone and cholesterol (for references, see Dingle and Lucy, 1965; Weissman et al., 1963). Hirsch et al. (1963) had reported some observations made with the light microscope on the effect of streptolysin O on leukocytes. Woodin and Wieneke (1964b, 1966a) found that both streptolysin O and excess vitamin A induced the secretion of the granule proteins, not by granule lysis in the cytoplasm followed by diffusion through the cell membrane, but by the same process found with the leuko-cidin-treated leukocyte. Woodin and Wieneke (1969) have also found that streptolysin O induces an intracellular accumulation of calcium and stim-ulates the incorporation of orthophosphate into nucleotides. These phe-nomena are thus not specific effects of leukocidin.

Effects of leukocidin can be subdivided again into those in which leuko-cidin participates directly and those in which it does not but which nevertheless stem exclusively from the action of leukocidin. It will be shown below that the site of action of leukocidin is the outside of the cell membrane and that it remains in solution during its attack on the cell. It is therefore available to antibody during its action. An excess of antileukoci-din antibody added to leukocidin-treated cells prepared in the absence of calcium does not prevent the subsequent secretion of the granule proteins induced by calcium ions. Similarly, neutralization in this way does not prevent or halt the accumulation of calcium or of phosphate or the incor-poration of phosphorus-32 into nucleotides. Leukocidin thus does not participate directly in any of these processes. There is circumstantial evi-dence that the pattern of accumulation of orthophosphate may be peculiar to leukocidin, for it is not dependent upon divalent cations nor is it inhib-ited by fluoride, while the pattern of phosphate accumulation in the strep-tolysin O-treated cell is.

Thus, the study of the leukocidin-treated cell leads to the conclusion that the only unique response to leukocidin is the restricted increased permeability to cations. It is not possible to determine if this can be halted by leukocidin, because the electrolyte changes are too fast. The other cytotoxic effects of leukocidin stem from this altered cation permeability, and as leukocidin does not participate directly in them, the normal cell must have the reagents to bring them about. The relationship of the non-specific responses of leukocidin to the properties of the normal cell are discussed by Woodin (1968).

Some experiments of Elsbach and Schwartz (1959) are relevant to the mechanism of the loss of cations from the leukocidin-treated cell. They found that if leukocytes were cooled to 0°C over a period of some hours, they lost potassium, but that if they were subsequently warmed to 37°C, they regained it. The rate at which potassium is regained is 40 times slower than the rate at which it is lost from the leukocidin-treated cell, showing that this phenomenon is due to an increased permeability and not to an inhibition of active transport. The primary response of the leukocyte to leukocidin is therefore a structural change leading to increased permeability. However, the experiments on cooled leukocytes show that the structural change must immediately lead to something more than an increased permeability to cations, for cells which have changed their electrolytes on cooling do not develop the cytotoxic effects of leukocidin on rewarming. From what has been said above, it is probable that the structural change induced by leukocidin leads directly to a new ATPase. The molecule in which the structural change is induced will be coupled to the phosphorus metabolism of the cell. The experiments of Elsbach and Schwartz (1959) are of importance in a further respect. After cooling to 0°C with accumulation of sodium and loss of potassium, incubation at 37°C does not restore the low sodium content although potassium is accumulated. I have also observed that mere transference of leukocytes from ascitic fluid to Hanks medium results in accumulation of sodium with cell swelling, although the potassium content is little changed (Woodin, 1969). These findings suggest that in the leukocyte the electrolyte balance is maintained by regulation of the potassium content and that the normal leukocyte is highly permeable to sodium.

An increased permeability to electrolyte should manifest itself as a reduced membrane resistance. The resistance of the mammalian cell membrane is about 10,000 Ω/cm^2, and so the sites in the normal cell membrane freely permeable to electrolyte cannot occupy more than about 10^{-6} of the surface, and an increase in their number should be detectable. Some preliminary impedence measurements (Woodin, 1966b) have not given a completely clear-cut result. These measurements were made on centrifuged pellets of normal, leukocidin-treated, and streptolysin O-treated leukocytes and showed that the membrane capacitance of all three was the same. The calculation of the membrane resistance was complicated by the swelling of the cells in the centrifuged pellet at the expense of the extracellular fluid. The qualitative behavior of the three cells was different. Compared with the normal leukocytes, the streptolysin O-treated showed a large, stable increase in conductance, but with the leukocidin-treated cells the conductance of the pellet decreased over about 30 minutes. Leukocidin-treated cells prepared in the absence of calcium then showed a stable conductance, but if calcium was present, the conductance increased again and reached a stable value after about 1 hour. The calculation of the membrane resistance requires a value for the extracellular volume and this cannot be obtained if the cells in the pellet swell. By assuming an infinite resistance at low frequency, the extracellular volume can be calculated from the impedence measurements, and the respective values 18% and 2% for normal and leukocidin-treated cells in the absence of calcium can be calculated from the data of Woodin (1966b). If all the current at 500 cps passed through this extracellular space, the ratio of the conductances should be 9 while the value found is 4. This suggests that the assumption that the membrane resistance of the leukocidin-treated cell is infinite is unsound and that perhaps 1–2% of the surface area is permeable to electrolyte. There are many assumptions in these calculations, but they indicate clearly that the sites in the leukocidin-treated cell membrane permeable to electrolyte are rare. We do not expect leukocidin to act upon lecithin, sphingomyelin, phosphatidylethanolamine, or the structural protein of the cell membrane. Correspondingly, any change that leukocidin induces in these substances must be regarded as irrelevant to the mode of action.

Confirmation of the rarity of the sites of action of leukocidin, their specific effect on the potassium content of the cell, and the coupling of the changes to phosphorus metabolism was provided by studying the cation-sensitive phosphatases of the leukocyte cell membrane (Woodin and Wieneke, 1968b, 1969). There is no sodium-sensitive ATPase in the membrane, correlating with the absence of a sodium pump from the cell. But there is a potassium-sensitive, oubain-sensitive acyl phosphatase. This correlates with the presence of a potassium pump in the cell, and moreover, leukocidin produces a 50% increase in the phosphatase activity. The effect is irreversible; it is not prevented if the leukocidin is neutralized with antibody, it occurs at leukocidin/membrane concentration ratios that lead to inactivation of leukocidin, it is synergistic between the two components of leukocidin, and it is not shown by streptolysin O or vitamin A.

Further evidence for the mode of action of leukocidin has been pro-

vided by the enhancement of some of the leukocidin effects by organo-
phosphates (Woodin and Wieneke, 1969). Diisopropylfluorophosphate,
for example, produces a threefold stimulation of β-glucuronidase secretion, calcium accumulation, and orthophosphate production when leukocidin is present in suboptimal amounts. Phosphonates do not enhance
these cellular reactions if they are induced by streptolysin O or vitamin A.
It was then shown by an independent method that phosphonates act on
the leukocyte by inhibiting the potassium pump. Thus, both leukocidin
and phosphonates affect the potassium pump but in different ways, and
it appears that the enhancement arises from the phosphonates preventing
the cell from reversing the structural change induced by leukocidin.
Since the inactivation of leukocidin by cell suspensions (see below) and
the activation of the acyl phosphatase of the cell membrane are not
enhanced by phosphonates, further evidence is provided that these two
effects precede the production of the potassium channel and the other
cytotoxic effects.

Phosphonates inhibit chemotaxis in leukocytes induced by activated
components of complement. The demonstration that their site of action
is the potassium pump can be regarded as "technological fall-out" from
the study of the cytotoxic action of leukocidin.

D. Interaction of Leukocidin with the Leukocyte Cell Membrane

The site of action of leukocidin is known unambiguously because
when radioactive leukocidin is added to leukocyte suspensions all the biological activity but only very little radioactivity is lost from the supernate
(Fig. 2). The rate of the inactivation excludes the involvement of pinocytosis and establishes that the inactivation occurs on the outside of the
leukocyte membrane. As leukocidin remains in solution, it also follows
that the primary action of leukocidin is on the cell surface membrane.
Whether the inactivation of leukocidin and the action of leukocidin on the
membrane are identical is discussed below. Homogenized leukocytes
also inactivate leukocidin. The reaction is due to a molecular grouping
not dependent on the cells' metabolism and has provided a method of
controlling the purification of the surface membrane by density gradient
centrifugation (Woodin and Wieneke, 1966c).

As a guide to the change induced by leukocidin, the fate of leukocidin
added to isolated surface membranes has been studied (Woodin and Wieneke, 1966c). Three modes of interaction can be distinguished. At physiological ionic strength leukocidin is inactivated by a process which is synergistic between the two components, goes to completion, and leaves

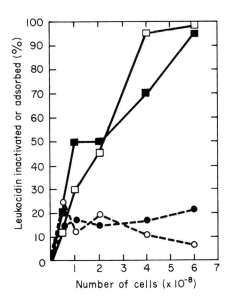

FIG. 2. Inactivation and adsorption of leukocidin by leukocytes. Leukocytes in 0.9 ml Ca^{2+}-free Hanks medium containing 0.1% bovine serum albumin were incubated at room temperature for 15 minutes with 0.1 ml 0.15 M sodium chloride solution containing 6.3 μg of each component of leukocidin. Some mixtures contained the ^{131}I-labeled S component of leukocidin (200,000 cpm) and other mixtures the ^{131}I-labeled F component of leukocidin (150,000 cpm). After incubation, the mixtures were centrifuged at 2000 g, and the radioactivity and biological activity of each component in the supernate were determined. □ = S component activity, ○ = S component radioactivity, ■ = F component activity, ● = F component radioactivity.

most of the leukocidin in solution. The small amount of adsorption involves mainly the S component and does not go to completion with increasing amounts of membrane. The third interaction leads to polymerization of leukocidin and is only observed at low ionic strength. Thus, if mixtures of leukocidin and membrane at low ionic strength are centrifuged, much more leukocidin is sedimented than is adsorbed at physiological ionic strength; but if the membranes are separated by flotation, the leukocidin does not accompany them. The polymerization is synergistic between the two components of leukocidin and as with adsorbtion does not go to completion; 30% of the added leucocidin remains unpolymerized however high the membrane concentration (Fig. 3).

The inactivation of 1 μg of leukocidin requires 500 μg of membrane protein, and this amount of leucocidin is of the same order of magnitude as the cytotoxic dose for the cells from which 500 μg of membrane protein are derived. The inactivation of increasing amounts of leukocidin requires

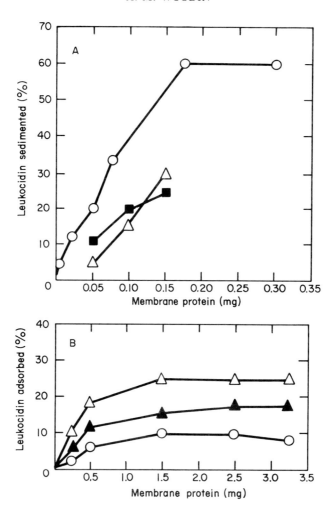

Fig. 3. Elimination of leukocidin by isolated leukocyte membranes. (A) *Sedimentation of leukocidin at low ionic strength.* Membranes were incubated in 0.6 ml of 5 mM sodium chloride and 5 mM phosphate buffer, pH 7.2, for 15 minutes at room temperature with 60 μg of one or both components of leukocidin and centrifuged at 8000 g for 20 minutes. The protein lost from the supernate was determined. O = Both components present. △ = F component only present, ■ = S component only present. (B) *Flotation of leukocidin by membranes.* Membranes were incubated at room temperature in 0.6 ml of 60% sucrose solution, 2 mM EDTA and 5 mM phosphate buffer, pH 7.3, containing 500 μg bovine serum albumin and 15 μg of one or both components of leukocidin. Some mixtures contained the ^{131}I-labeled F component of leukocidin (30,000 cpm) and other mixtures contained the ^{131}I-labeled S component of leukocidin (56,000 cpm). After 30 minutes at room temperature, 5 ml 48% sucrose solution was added on top of the mixtures and the tubes were centrifuged at 105,000 g for 30 minutes. The radioactivity in the top 0.5 cm of the tube was determined. △ = ^{131}I-labeled S component present, O = ^{131}I-labeled F component present.

increasing amounts of membrane; this, therefore, is changed in the process. The polymerization reaction, however, proceeds with a tenfold smaller amount of membrane, and when enough is present (determined by the volume, time of reaction, and association constants of the leukocidin polymers), the same percentage change is induced over a wide range of leukocidin concentrations. In the polymerization reaction, the membrane appears to act as a catalyst and is not changed. Radioactive leukocidin that had been totally inactivated by leukocytes was adsorbed to the same extent as normal leukocidin. The basis of this adsorption has not been studied.

These observations suggested that the inactivation reaction was likely to be more relevant to the primary effect of leukocidin than the others. The basis of the polymerization reaction has also been studied, however, for information on the nature of the synergism between the two components of leukocidin. Degradation of membranes with enzymes and solvents indicated that lipids were involved in both inactivation and polymerization of leukocidin.

E. INTERACTION OF LEUKOCIDIN WITH PURIFIED LIPIDS

Phosphatidylserine, phosphatidylethanolamine, phosphatidylcholine, triphosphoinositide, diphosphoinositide, sphingomyelin, and lysolecithin were purified by chromatography on silicic acid, DEAE-cellulose and a thin layer of Kieselguhr G. Preparations of cerebrosides, gangliosides, tristearin, and monophosphoinositide were partially purified. The interaction of leukocidin with these lipids, suspended ultrasonically in water, was studied by sedimentation, flotation, light scattering, and changes in the biological activity of leukocidin (Woodin and Wieneke 1967).

1. POLYMERIZATION

At low ionic strength, phosphatidylserine, diphosphoinositide, triphosphoinositide, partially pure monophosphoinositide, and phosphatidylcholine convert the F component of leukocidin to a polymeric form. All the other lipids listed above are inactive. The process is reversed at higher ionic strength and inhibited by low concentrations of calcium. Thus, the F component of leukocidin interacts with charged glycerophospholipids containing two esterified fatty acids under conditions that induce electrostatic repulsion between the polar, hydrophilic regions in the micelle. This we take as evidence that the F component of leukocidin interacts with the hydrophobic, fatty acid side chains of the phospholipid. Further evidence for this is that phosphoserine does not prevent phosphatidylserine, nor does triphosphoinositol, prevent triphosphoinositide, from inducing the polymerization of the F component of leukocidin.

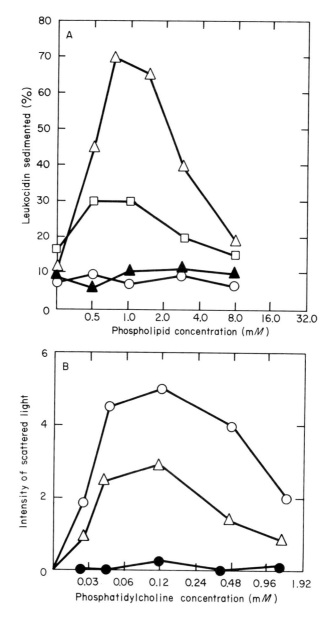

FIG. 4. Polymerization of leukocidin by phospholipids. (A) *Sedimentation.* Phospholipids in 0.6 ml 1 mM EDTA and 10 mM tris buffer, pH 7.2, were maintained at room temperature for 30 minutes with 60 μg of each component of leukocidin labeled with iodine-131 and were then centrifuged at 8000 g for 20 minutes. The radioactivity lost from the supernate was determined. $\triangle$ = Phosphatidylserine, $\square$ = phosphatidylcholine, $\triangle$ = phosphatidylethanol-

The interaction of the F component of leukocidin with the hydrophobic regions of the phospholipids does not result simply in adsorption of the protein on the surface of the micelle. The ratio of the masses of leukocidin and phospholipid producing the aggregates indicates that polymerization of leukocidin also occurs. With high phospholipid concentrations, the aggregation is reversed through adsorbtion of monomeric leukocidin on the phospholipid micelle surface. However, no stable complexes are formed under any conditions. The phospholipids can be separated from leukocidin by flotation. The S component of leukocidin is not polymerized by phospholipids, but it becomes polymerized by interacting with the F component after its modification by phospholipids, and then the S component of leukocidin can increase the amount of the F component polymerized. Figure 4 shows the effect of some phospholipids on the sedimentation and light scattering by leukocidin.

To confirm the conclusion of Woodin and Wieneke (1967), the interaction of the F component of leukocidin with diglycerides prepared from phosphatidylserine by treatment with phospholipase C from *Bacillus cereus* was studied (Woodin, 1969). The light scattered by the diglycerides suspended ultrasonically in water was very much greater than that scattered by corresponding concentrations of phospholipids, but an increase induced by the F component of leukocidin could be detected (Fig. 5). This was reversed at high diglyceride concentrations. If electrolyte was added to the mixtures of diglycerides and the F component of leukocidin, the light scattered was less than that scattered by the diglycerides before addition of leukocidin. This suggests that the F component of leukocidin breaks up the diglyceride micelles into smaller units which adsorb on the polymerized leukocidin. When electrolyte is added, the leukocidin depolymerizes and the smaller diglyceride micelles are released.

The interaction energy between the F component of leukocidin and diglycerides would not be expected to have a high electrostatic component, which indicates that a low ionic strength in the polymerization reaction of the F component of leukocidin and phospholipids arises through the need to change leukocidin. It has already been shown from sedimentation studies that leukocidin alone, at low ionic strength, partially polymerizes. It is possible that at low ionic strength electrostatic repulsion of charged groups on the surface of the leukocidin moleucule produces a more open

amine. $\circ$ = sphingomyelin. (B) *Light scattering*. Phosphatidylcholine was maintained with one or both components of leukocidin (100 μg/ml) at room temperature for 15 minutes in 1 mM EDTA and 10 mM tris buffer, pH 7.2, and the intensity of light scattered at 90° to the incident light was measured on a Locarte fluorimeter. $\circ$ = Both components present, $\bullet$ = S component only present, $\triangle$ = F component only present.

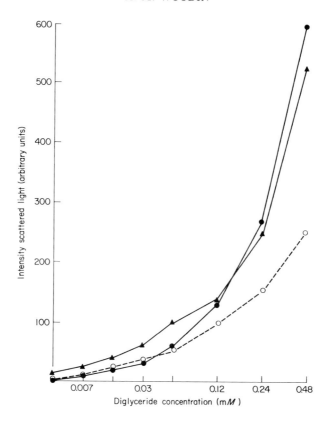

FIG. 5. The interaction of the F component of leukocidin with diglycerides. Diglycerides were prepared from phosphatidylserine by digestion with a phospholipase C followed by chromatography on silicic acid. Mixtures of the diglycerides and the F component of leukocidin (100 μg/ml) were maintained at room temperature for 15 minutes in 1 mM EDTA, 10 mM tris buffer, pH 7.2, and the intensity of scattered light was determined. Then sodium chloride was added to give 0.15 M final concentration and the intensity of scattered light was measured again. Unlike the data recorded in Fig. 4, the light scattered from the diglycerides alone was not subtracted from that of the mixtures. ● = Diglycerides alone, △ = diglycerides with leukocidin, O = diglycerides with leukocidin and sodium chloride.

structure and permits access of the esterified fatty acids to the hydrophobic interior.

The interaction between the F component of leukocidin and phospholipids is thus unique. Neither undergoes a change in covalent structure. The phospholipids act as templates in directing the conformational state of the protein. The chemical nature of these changes is of interest in the general context of the interaction of proteins and lipids and membranes. The observation most relevant to the mode of action of leukocidin is that the F component of leukocidin interacts with the hydrophobic regions of phospholipids and the S component of leukocidin does not.

2. INACTIVATION

The only phospholipid to convert leukocidin to a biologically inactive form is triphosphoinositide. The S component of leukocidin is inactivated at physiological ionic strength. The F component of leukocidin is inactivated at low ionic strength and remains inactive when this is increased to physiological values. This is consistent with the suggestion made above that access to the hydrophobic regions of the phospholipid is required in the interaction with the F component of leukocidin. The inactivation of the S component of leukocidin by triphosphoinositide is inhibited at low ionic strength and impure preparations of triphosphoinositide (where separation would occur of the triphosphoinositide molecules in the micelle) requires traces of calcium. It appears that the interaction of the S component of leukocidin requires clusters of the hydrophilic regions of the phospholipid.

The inactivation of increasing amounts of leukocidin requires increasing amounts of triphosphoinositide. The inactivation thus produces a reciprocal change in the phospholipid. The covalent structure is not altered (triphosphoinositide can be recovered by extraction into organic solvents and then used again to inactive leukocidin), nor are stable complexes produced, the S component of leukocidin and triphosphoinositide sediment separately. The S component of leukocidin induces a conformational change in the triphosphoinositide micelle. The inactivation of the F component of leukocidin also requires increasing amounts of triphosphoinositide, but as this only occurs at low ionic strength, it may not indicate a change in triphosphoinositide other than adsorption.

3. THE PARTICIPATION OF PHOSPHOLIPIDS IN THE INTERACTION OF LEUKOCIDIN AND THE LEUKOCYTE MEMBRANE

It is possible that the polymerization of the F component of leukocidin by phospholipids is involved in the polymerization of leukocidin by the leukocyte membrane. Maximum polymerization of a mixture of 100 μg of each component is induced by an amount of membrane containing 150 μg protein and 0.1 μM phospholipid. This amount of phospholipid is of the same order of magnitude as that which in aqueous suspension would induce a maximum effect. This correlation is fortuitous, for it is improbable that all the phospholipid of the membrane is exposed to the surface, but it is possible that in the membrane individual phospholipid molecules may be more free to interact with leukocidin than in a micelle. The interaction with phospholipids will not account totally for the polymerization of leukocidin by the membrane, for the S component alone is polymerized by membrances at low ionic strength. This does not happen with the lipids we have studied so far, and it is possible that it results from interaction with a protein component. Reasons were put forward above for disregarding the polymerization of leukocidin in the primary action of leukocidin on the cell, and to these reasons can be added the lack of specificity shown by the phospholipids and, in particular, the finding that the ubiquitous phosphatidylcholine is active. The main significance of the interaction of leukocidin with lipids is the demonstration that the F component interacts with the hydrophobic regions of the lipid.

The inactivation of leucocidin by triphosphoinositide can be the basis of the inactivation of leukocidin by the cell membrane. Wieneke and Woodin (1967) found that the leukocyte cell membrane contains enough triphosphoinositide (about 0.1%) to account for the inactivation. Erythrocyte membranes, which do not inactivate leukocidin, contain enough triphosphoinositide to do so, and the specificity of the interaction, if it is due to triphosphoinositide, must lie in accessibility. Both components of leukocidin are inactivated at physiological ionic strength by the cell, and if triphosphoinositide is involved in this, the hydrophobic regions must be available to the F component of leukocidin and the polar regions to the S component of leukocidin simultaneously. This is feasible in the membrane but cannot be reproduced in aqueous systems containing leukocidin and triphosphoinositide only. For this reason, the differences in the synergism of the inactivation reaction in the membrane and with isolated triphosphoinositide are not to be taken as evidence against the participation of triphosphoinositide in the interaction of leukocidin and the cell.

F. PROPERTIES OF LEUKOCYTE TRIPHOSPHOINOSITIDE

At this stage in the investigation of the mode of action of leukocidin, it became necessary to establish the structure of triphosphoinositide in the leukocyte cell membrane. The covalent structure of triphosphoinositide from ox brain has been established by Brockerhoff and Ballou (1961) as 1,2-diacylglyceryl-3-phosphoryl-(1-inositol 4,5-diphosphate) (Fig. 6). The triphosphoinositide content of the leukocyte is twelvefold smaller than that of brain, and its isolation from the leukocyte is not feasible. Woodin and Wieneke (1968a) therefore deduced the structure and stability of leukocyte triphosphoinositide from the properties of labeled triphosphoinositide from leukocyte membranes mixed with unlabeled triphosphoinositide from brain. The distribution of phosphorus and radioactivity after the degradations described by Brockerhoff and Ballou

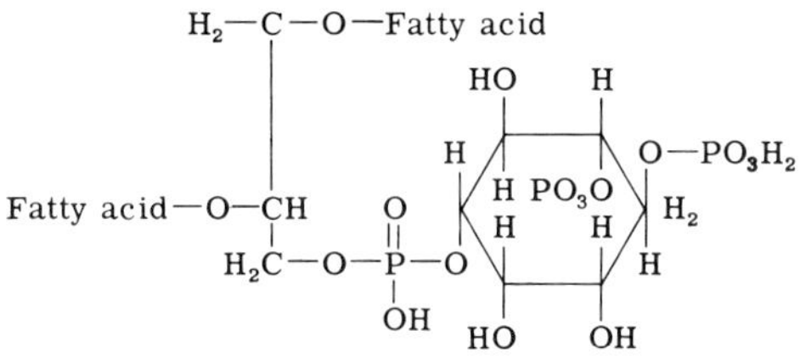

FIG. 6. Structure of triphosphoinositide.

(1961) was determined. By this device it was possible to show that the covalent structure of ox brain and leukocyte triphosphoinositide are identical and that it is not changed by leukocidin. A finding of great interest was that under certain conditions it was possible to partly separate labeled triphosphoinositide from unlabeled triphosphoinositide. This is because triphosphoinositide is able to exist in different states dependent upon the conformation of the inositol triphosphate moiety. Presumably the electrostatic repulsion of the phosphate groups enables the inositol ring of inositol triphosphate to adopt a form different from the "chair" conformation of free inositol.

Subsequently it was shown (Woodin and Wieneke, 1968a) that prolonged chromatography on formaldehyde-treated paper can partly separate the different conformational forms of triphosphoinositide. A method of solubilizing triphosphoinositide from leukocyte membranes without the use of acid conditions or the preparation of calcium salts was then developed, and by this means it was shown that the relative proportions of the triphospoinositide were changed when membranes were treated with leukocidin (Fig. 7).

G. A CONFORMATIONAL CHANGE IN TRIPHOSPHOINOSITIDE AS THE FIRST EFFECT OF LEUKOCIDIN

From the properties of the leukocidin-treated leukocyte, it was concluded that the primary action of leukocidin is to induce a small structural change in a rare, metabolically active component of the membrane. The properties of triphosphoinositide make it an acceptable candidate for this. The high rate of exchange of the phosphate groups of triphosphoinosite in brain was shown by Brockerhoff and Ballou (1962a,b), and Woodin and Wieneke (1969) have found that after 1 hour of incubation with phosphorus-32 the triphosphoinositide of the leukocyte cell membrane is at least 100-fold more radioactive than the bulk of the phospholipid. Triphosphoinositide is closely coupled to the phosphorus metabolism of the cell. The quantities present in the leukocyte cell membrane (between

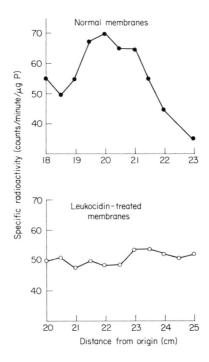

FIG. 7. Chromatographic differences between triphosphoinositide from normal and leu-kocidin-treated membranes. Triphosphoinositide was isolated from normal and leukocidin-treated membranes that had been labeled with phosphorus = 32. It was then purified to-gether with 1 μM of unlabeled triphosphoinositide from ox brain. The mixture was chroma-tographed on formaldehyde-treated paper for 3 days. The specific radioactivity of strips of the triphosphoinositide spot was determined.

1:100 and 1:300 moles per mole of phospholipid) fit the requirement that the substance interacting with leukocidin be rare. The amount is adequate to occupy about 1% of the surface. The inactivation of leukocidin by tri-phosphoinositide micelles resembles that induce by leukocytes. Leukoci-din induces a conformational change in isolated triphosphoinositide and in the triphosphoinositide in the leukocyte membrane. It is therefore highly probable that this is the mode of action of leukocidin.

This theory has not been completely proved. An advance will be made when the inactivation of the F component of leukocidin can be completely simulated in a membrane-free system, when the inhibition of leukocidin by tetraethylammonium ions (see below) is shown to involve triphosphoi-nositide directly, and if it can be shown that the physiological function of triphosphoinositide is the control of potassium permeability (Woodin and Wieneke, 1968a).

H. The Synergism between the Two Components of Leukocidin

This synergism is not yet understood. However, if leukocidin acts as I have suggested above, it is appropriate to consider whether a plausible explanation can be given. If plausible explanations are not available, the mode of action I have postulated will have to be rejected. A speculative scheme which will fit all the facts we have would be:

1. Entry of part of the F component molecule into a region of low dielectric constant in the membrane.

2. Conversion of the F component of leukocidin into the expanded condition analogous to that found in the F component at low ionic strength.

3. Entry of an esterified fatty acid into the hydrophobic regions of the F component of leukocidin, producing a change in the surface of the F component analogous to that produced by phospholipid micelles.

4. Adsorption of the S component onto the altered surface of the F component, analgous to the adsorption found after treatment with phospholipid micelles.

5. Interaction of the S component of leukocidin with the exposed inositol triphosphate moiety of triphosphoinositide altering the conformation of the latter.

6. Creation of a channel permeable to electrolyte with loss of the region of low dielectric constant and return of the F component of leukocidin to the "compact" state.

7. Deadsorption of the inactivated F component from the esterified fatty acid side chains of triphosphoinositide and deadsorption of the inactivated S component of leukocidin from the "compact" F component of leukocidin.

8. Restoration of the conformation of triphosphoinositide in the membrane with expenditure of cellular ATP.

9. Repetition of the cycle with fresh leukocidin molecules.

I. Inhibitors of Leukocidin

The unique character of the mode of action of leukocidin is emphasized by the effect of inhibitors. Cocaine, promethazine, sulfhydryl reagents, membrane stabilizers such as cholesterol, antioxidants such as vitamin E, and inhibitors of glycolysis or respiration do not inhibit leukocidin. Sulfhydryl reagents modify the development of the cytotoxic effects of leukocidin (Woodin and Wieneke 1966b), but this is not due to an effect on the primary action of leukocidin.

Specific inhibition of leucocidin is brought about by tetraethylammonium ions (Woodin and Wieneke, 1968a). At 80 mM concentration, the ions inhibit the efflux of potassium, cell swelling, and secretion of β-glucuronidase by the leukocidin-treated cell. The inhibition is apparently competitive, higher concentrations of tetraethylammonium ions being required to inhibit larger amounts of leukocidin. Inhibition of the action of leukocidin on the macrophage (determined by the dye reduction test) is observed with 40 mM tetraethylammonium ions.

The highly specific action of tetraethylammonium ions suggested to Woodin and Wieneke (1968a) that the physiological function of triphosphoinositide could be to control the passage of potassium across cell membranes.

V. Biological Properties of Leukocidin

A. *In Vivo* PRODUCTION AND ACTION OF LEUKOCIDIN

Gladstone and Glencross (1960) grew various strains of staphylococcus in cellophane sacs inserted in the peritoneal cavities of rabbits and obtained high titers of leukocidin even from strains that produce little *in vitro*. That *in vivo* production of leukocidin is common is also evident from the widespread occurrence of antileukocidin antibodies. The effects of injections of leukocidin into rabbits has been studied by Szmigielski *et al.* (1966) and by Gladstone (1966). With 1 mg/kg a drop in the number of polymorphonuclear leukocytes in the blood and bone marrow was observed 4–8 hours after injection. This was followed by a marked granulocytosis accompanied by an increase in the number of young myeloid cells in the bone marrow. The strong reaction of the granulocytic system was also found after injecting amounts of leukocidin too small to produce detectable changes in the numbers of circulating leukocytes. Histochemical studies by Szmigielski *et al.* (1966) showed that the polymorphonuclear leukocytes which reappear in the blood stream 18 hours after injection of leukocidin have different ATPase and 5-nucleotidase activities. The leukocidin preparation used by these authors was about 70% pure, and they found alterations in the number of circuulating lymphocytes, although *in vitro*, these cells do not respond to purified leukocidin. Nonspecific effects of impure leukocidin preparations could be controlled by injection of the separate components of leukocidin when the effects due to leukocidin, as such, would be absent. Thus, the findings of Szmigielski *et al.* (1966) cannot be ascribed exclusively to the effect of leukocidin. They have established that *in vitro* injections of leukocidin cause death to circulating leukocytes, that these cells are soon replaced, and that these changes occur without death to the rabbit. Alone, it is clear, leukocidin is not a very toxic substance.

B. LEUKOCIDIN IN STAPHYLOCOCCAL PATHOGENICITY

That there is a correlation between *in vivo* leukocidin production and pathogenicity of the staphylococcus was originally suggested by Panton and Valentine (1932). Johanovsky (1958) obtained a negative correlation between the severity of staphylococcal infection and the titer of antileukocidin in patients. Gladstone *et al.* (1962) have also argued that antitoxin production might be a significant factor in resistance to staphylococcal infection. From a survey of the distribution of antibodies to leukocidin and α-hemolysin in human subjects, they concluded that elevated levels of antibody to leukocidin, but not to α-hemolysin, were associated with infection. Mudd *et al.* (1962) found that four commercial staphylococcal toxoids were quite ineffective in stimulating antibody formation to leukocidin. Subsequently, the toxoided leukocidin preparation described by Gladstone (1965) was found to be highly effective in both rabbits and man (Souckova-Stepanova *et al.*, 1965; Mudd *et al.*, 1965). It may well be that pathogenic strains of staphylococcus produce leukocidin *in vivo* and that the assay of antileukocidin antibodies can be of value in diagnosis of deep-seated infection (Towers and Gladstone, 1958), but a protective action of antileukocidin has not been shown. Souckova–Stepanova *et al.* (1965) immunized rabbits with a toxoid containing about 50% leukocidin toxoid and claimed some protection but found that this bore no correlation with the antileukocidin titer.

Implicit in the belief that an extracellular bacterial product such as leukocidin or the hemolysins can influence staphylococcus survival are the assumptions that it is a disadvantage to the host to lose phagocytic cells and that the level of circulating antibody can control staphylococcal invasion. Both these assumptions have been questioned by Rogers (1966). It was found by Rogers and Tompsett (1952) that pathogenic strains of staphylococcus survived phagocytosis, while nonpathogenic strains were rapidly destroyed inside the cell. The intracellular survival protects the staphylococcus against destruction by substances such as antibiotics or antibody in extracellular fluids. It has also been found that if rabbits are rendered granulocytopenic by nitrogen mustards, they can clear injected staphylococci more rapidly than normal rabbits. Leukocidin could have the same effect as the nitrogen mustards, and paradoxically, its production *in vivo* might facilitate staphylococcal clearance. Rogers (1966) also suggests that the levels of circulating antibody to the staphylococcus are at their optimum in the normal healthy adult. It does not appear that antibody to either leukocidin or hemolysin are at their maximum value, however. Mudd *et al.* (1965) obtained considerable increases in these levels, following administration of leucocidin toxoid and α-hemolysin toxoid to patients suffering from staphylococcal infection.

REFERENCES

Bernheimer, A. W. (1965). *Ann. N.Y. Acad. Sci.,* **128**, 112.
Bessis, M. (1964). *Ciba Found. Symp., Cellular Injury* p. 376.
Boman, H. G., and Westlund, L. E. (1956). *Arch. Biochem. Biophys.* **64**, 217.
Brockerhoff, H., and Ballou, C. E. (1961). *J. Biol. Chem.* **236**, 1907.
Brockerhoff, H., and Ballou, C. E. (1962a). *J. Biol. Chem.* **237**, 49.
Brockerhoff, H., and Ballou, C. E. (1962b). *J. Biol. Chem.* **237**, 49.
Denys, J., and Van der Velde, H. (1895). *Cellule* **11**, 359.
Dingle, J. T., and Lucy, J. A. (1965). *Biol. Rev.* **40**, 422.
Douglas, W. W., and Poisner, A. M. (1962). *J. Physiol. (London)* **162**, 385.
Elsbach, P., and Schwartz, I. L. (1959). *J. Gen. Physiol.* **42**, 883.
Elsworth, R., and Sargent, T. (1969). Unpublished results.
Florey, H. W., and Grant, L. H. (1961). *J. Pathol. Bacteriol.* **82**, 13.
Gladstone, G. P. (1965). *Brit. J. Exptl. Pathol.* **46**, 292.
Gladstone, G. P. (1966). *Postepy. Mikrobiol.* **5**, 322.
Gladstone, G. P., and Fildes, P. (1940). *Brit. J. Exptl. Pathol.* **21**, 161.
Gladstone, G. P., and Glencross, E. J. G. (1960). *Brit. J. Exptl. Pathol.* **41**, 313.
Gladstone, G. P., and van Heyningen, W. E. (1957). *Brit. J. Exptl. Pathol.* **38**, 123.
Gladstone, G. P., Mudd, S., Hochstein, H. D., and Lenhart, N. A. (1962). *Brit. J. Exptl. Pathol.* **43**, 295.
Hirsch, J. G., and Cohn, Z. A. (1960). *J. Exptl. Med.* **112**, 1005.
Hirsch, J. G., Bernheimer, A. W., and Weissman, G. (1963). *J. Exptl. Med.* **118**, 223.
Hvidt. A., Johansen, G., and Linderstrom-Lang, K. (1960). *In* "Analytical Methods of Protein Chemistry" P. Alexander and R. J. Block, (eds.), pp. 101–130. Pergamon Press, Oxford.
Johanovsky, J. (1958). *Z. Immunitaetsforsch.* **116**, 318.
Julianelle, L. A. (1922). *J. Infect. Diseases* **31**, 256.
Karnovsky, M. L. (1962). *Physiol. Rev.* **42**, 143.
Mudd, S., Gladstone, G. P., Lenhart, N. A., and Hochstein, H. D. (1962). *Brit. J. Exptl. Pathol.* **43**, 313.
Mudd, S., Gladstone, G. P., and Lenhart, N. A. (1965). *Brit. J. Exptl. Pathol.* **46**, 455.
Neisser, M., and Wechsberg, F. (1901). *Z. Hyg. Infektionskrankh.* **36**, 299.
Panton, P. N., and Valentine, F. C. O. (1932). *Lancet* **1**, 506.
Peterson, E. A., and Sober, H. A. (1956). *J. Am. Chem. Soc.* **78**, 751.
Proom, H. (1937). *J. Pathol. Bacteriol.* **44**, 425.
Rogers, D. E. (1966). *Postepy Mikrobiol.* **5**, 279.
Rogers, D. E., and Tompsett, R. (1952). *J. Exptl. Med.* **95**, 209.
Souckova-Stepanova, J., Gladstone, G. P., and Vareck, P. (1965). *Brit. J. Exptl. Pathol.* **46**, 384.

Szmigielski, S., Jeljaszewicz, J., Wikzynski, J., and Korbecki, M. (1966). *Postepy Mikrobiol.* **5**, 317.

Tiselius, A., Hjerten, S., and Levin, O. (1956). *Arch. Biochem. Biophys.* **65**, 132.

Towers, A. G., and Gladstone, G. P. (1958). *Lancet* **II**, 1192.

Van der Velde, H. (1894). *Cellule* **10**, 401.

van Heyningen, W. E., and Gladstone, G. P. (1953). *Brit. J. Exptl. Pathol.* **34**, 221.

Wadstrom, T. (1969). (unpublished).

Weissman, G., Keiser, H., and Bernheimer, A. W. (1963). *J. Exptl. Med.* **118**, 205.

Wieneke, A. A., and Woodin, A. M. (1967). *Biochem. J.* **105**, 1039.

Woodin, A. M. (1959). *Biochem, J.* **73**, 225.

Woodin, A. M. (1960). *Biochem. J.* **75**, 158.

Woodin, A. M. (1961a). *J. Pathol. Bacteriol.* **81**, 63.

Woodin, A. M. (1961b). *Biochem. J.* **80**, 562.

Woodin, A. M. (1962). *Biochem. J.* **82**, 9.

Woodin, A. M. (1963). *Biochem. Soc. Symp. (Cambridge, Engl.)* **22**, 126.

Woodin, A. M. (1965). *Ann. N.Y. Acad. Sci.* **128**, 152.

Woodin, A. M. (1966a). *Postepy Mikrobiol.* **5**, 163.

Woodin, A. M. (1966b). *Exptl. Cell Res.* **43**, 311.

Woodin, A. M. (1968). *In* "The Biological Basis of Medicine" E. E. Bittar, (ed.), Vol. 2, p. 373. Academic Press, New York.

Woodin, A. M. (1969) (unpublished).

Woodin, A. M., and Wieneke, A. A. (1963a). *Biochem. J.* **87**, 487.

Woodin, A. M., and Wieneke, A. A. (1963b). *Biochem. J.* **87**, 480.

Woodin, A. M., and Wieneke, A. A. (1964a). *Ciba Found. Symp. Cellular Injury* pp. 30-45.

Woodin, A. M., and Wieneke, A. A. (1964b). *Biochem. J.* **90**, 498.

Woodin, A. M., and Wieneke, A. A. (1966a). *Exptl. Cell Res.* **43**, 319.

Woodin, A. M., and Wieneke, A. A. (1966b). *Biochem. J.* **99**, 469.

Woodin, A. M., and Wieneke, A. A. (1966c). *Biochem. J.* **99**, 479.

Woodin, A. M., and Wieneke, A. A. (1967). *Biochem. J.* **105**, 1029.

Woodin, A. M., and Wieneke, A. A. (1968a). *Nature* **220**, 283.

Woodin, A. M., and Wieneke, A. A. (1968b). *Biochem. Biophys. Res. Commun.* **33**, 558.

Woodin, A. M., and Wieneke, A. A. (1969). Unpublished results.

Woodin, A. M., French, J. E., and Marchesi, V. T. (1963). *Biochem. J.* **87**, 567.

Wright, J. (1936). *Lancet* **II**, 1002.

Yoshida, A. (1963). *Biochim. Biophys. Acta* **71**, 544.

Addendum—Production of Test Toxin of P-V Leukocidin

R. Elsworth and K. Sargeant

I. Production of Crude Concentrate

This section describes an established process used periodically since 1958 for the production of filter-sterilized culture filtrates of *staphlococcus* and their conversion into a crude concentrate.

A. The Culture Process

Stock cultures of *Staphlococcus aureus* strain V8 (Panton-Valentine) are grown at 37°C in 4-ounce medical flat bottles containing 20 ml of tryptic meat broth agar. They are stored at 4°C for up to 1 month.

1. Culture Medium.

This medium differs from the formula of Gladstone and van Heyningen (1957) with respect to the following ingredients (the amounts are for a batch of 20 liters).
1. For Bacto casamino acids, substitute 600 gm of Oxoid casein hydrolyzate (L41).
2. Use 3.75 liters of yeast diffusate (nominal Kjeldahl nitrogen value, 7 gm/liter). This is made as follows. A length of Visking dialysis tubing about 54 inches long and 1 inch inflated diameter is knotted at one end. It is charged with 293 gm of light grade Yeatex paste (English Grains Co. Ltd., Burton-on-Trent, Staffs.) and 20 ml of distilled water. Air is excluded by squeezing and the tube is closed by knotting to give a contained length of 50-51 inches. The tube is inserted in a 48-inch piece of 2-inch diameter pipe. The pipe is closed at each end with rubber stoppers, which hold the free ends of the Visking tube. Two liters of distilled water and 2 ml of chloroform are previously added to each pipe. A number of tubes is then rocked about their centers at 14 oscillations per minute so that the end of each tube describes an arc 12 inches long. After 21-23 hours of rocking at room

temperature, the average yield is 1.5 liters of diffusate per tube, to which additional chloroform is added if stored. A typical analysis of the product is:

Specific gravity 15°/15°	1.031
Total N	7 gm/liter
Residue on heating at 100°C to constant weight	70 gm/liter

3. Instead of solid sodium glycerophosphate, 800 ml of a 50% (w/w) solution (B.P.C.) is used.
4. Tap water is substituted for distilled water. Porton water arises from a chalk subsoil and contains a total hardness of 200 ppm calcium carbonate.
5. Adjust the pH value of sterilized medium to pH 7.0–7.2. This is believed to be important. Lower values give lower cell yields and lower leukocidin activity.

2. PRIMARY SEED.

The growth from one bottle of stock culture is washed off with 10 ml of distilled water into 1 liter of culture medium in a 4-liter plugged bottle. This is shaken for 8 hours at 37°C.

3. SECONDARY SEED.

One liter of primary seed is transferred to 20 liters of medium in a 20-liter culture vessel (Elsworth *et al.*, 1957) where it is cultured for 6 hours at 37°C. See Table I for further particulars.

4. MAIN CULTURE.

The secondary seed is transferred to 120 liters of medium in a larger vessel (see Table I). This is operated for 12 hours at 37°C. Leukocidin assays are not carried out during a culture. Instead satisfactory operation is inferred from measurements of optical density and pH value of the culture, together with continuous measurement of the percentage of carbon dioxide in the effluent air. The performance of a typical culture is shown in Table II.

B. ISOLATION OF CRUDE CONCENTRATE

The culture is cooled to below 10°C, clarified by centrifugation, and filtered under aseptic conditions. Ammonium sulfate is dissolved in the sterile filtrate to give a concentration of 3.0 M and the mixture is allowed to stand at 4°C for 16 hours. All subsequent operations are conducted at temperature below 4°C. The precipitate (about 300 gm wet weight from

TABLE I

MAIN FEATURES OF CULTURE VESSELS

Feature	Secondary seed	Main culture
Working volume (liters)	20	140
Vessel diameter (inches)	13	27
Baffles	4 × 1½ inch radial baffles attached to vessel wall	4 × 1½ inch radial baffles attached to vessel wall
Impeller	3 inch diameter disk with 4 vanes, 1 inch long and ½ inch deep, placed radially on underside	7 inch diameter disk with 16 vanes, 2½ inches long and ½ inch deep, placed radially on underside
Impeller speed (rpm)	1420	520
Air rate (liters/minute)	10	70
Sulfite oxidation rate[a] at above air rate (mM O_2/liter/hour)	65	52

[a] Elsworth et al., 1957.

TABLE II

RESULTS OF A TYPICAL MAIN CULTURE

Time (hours)	pH	Bacterial dry weight (gm/liter)	Colony (count/ml)	CO_2 in effluent air (%)	Leukocidin assay (IU/ml)
0	7.0	—	—	0.03	—
4	7.2	6.3	—	1.0	3.8
8	8.0	8.8	—	0.45	5.9
12	8.4	9.4	9.6×10^9	—	6.0

100 liters) is recovered by a combination of centrifugation and filtration. It contains the leukocidin, which is stable in this form during storage at 4°C for several years.

II. Separation of the F and S Components

This section gives a recently developed method of refining the concentrate into the F and S components. These are dispensed into ampoules each containing 150 IU (international units) of an individual component. A pair of ampoules is sufficient for 100 antileukocidin hemagglutination assays (Towers and Gladstone, 1958; Lack and Towers, 1962), a test which may be of value in the diagnosis of deep-seated staphylococcal infections.

A. Extraction and Gel Filtration

The crude concentrate is alternately stirred with 0.1 M phosphate buffer, pH 6.7, and centrifuged until extraction of the leukocidin is complete. The extract (about 1750 ml) is passed through a Sephadex G-50 column (diameter, 10 cm; volume, 10 liters), prepared and eluted in 0.1 M acetate buffer, pH 5.0. The leading fraction (about 2000 ml) contains the leukocidin, which is thus separated from ammonium sulfate and other low molecular weight impurities and transferred to 0.1 M acetate buffer, pH 5.0, and is ready for the next step.

B. Separation of the F and S Components

The whole gel filtration product is passed through a CM-Sephadex C-50 column (diameter, 3 cm; volume, 300 ml), prepared in 0.1 M acetate buffer, pH 5.0. The leukocidin is adsorbed. The column is washed with the acetate buffer and is eluted using a linear gradient from 0.2 M sodium chloride in 0.1 M acetate buffer, pH 5.0, (1 liter) to 0.8 M sodium chloride in the same buffer.

The F and S leukocidin components are partially resolved, and those active fractions which contain less than 3% of the heterologous component are pooled. Less well resolved samples of F and S are rechromatographed.

C. Preparation of Ampoules

The separated F and S components are each dialyzed against 0.01 M phosphate buffer, pH 7.4. The dialyzates are adjusted to contain 60 IU/ml, filtered under aseptic conditions, and distributed in 2.5 ml lots into ampoules, which are stored at −20°C, and exported in solid carbon dioxide. The feasibility of freeze drying the ampoule material is being investigated.

The products are not pure. The ultraviolet absorption values for a recent pair of ampouled products were: F, $E_{280\,m\mu}^{1\,cm} = 2.5$; S, $E_{280\,m\mu}^{1\,cm} = 0.86$.

REFERENCES

Elsworth, R., Williams, V., and Harris-Smith, R. (1957). *J. Appl. Chem.* 7, 261.
Gladstone, G. P., and van Heyningen, W. E. (1957). *Brit. J. Exptl. Path.* 38, 123.
Lack, C. H., and Towers, A. G. (1962). *Brit. Med. J.* II, 1227.
Towers, A. G., and Gladstone, G. P. (1958). *Lancet* II, 1192.

Chapter 9

Anthrax Toxin

Ralph E. Lincoln and Donald C. Fish

I. Introduction

Anthrax has long been of interest to man. It is believed to have been one of the seven plagues suffered by the Egyptians in the time of Moses and was clearly described in ancient Greece. The disease is of historical importance to all microbiologists: Robert Koch used it as the model for his postulates to prove the bacterial etiology of disease; Pasteur used the causative organism *Bacillus anthracis* to develop an effective attenuated live vaccine.

Although anthrax is one of the five major livestock diseases of the tropics (National Academy of Sciences, 1962), the incidence in man is low and it occurs among veterinarians, meat workers, and, in the more developed countries, workers in woolen and goat hair mills. Anthrax is classified (Cecil and Loeb, 1959) as external (carbuncular) or internal (generalized or septicemic). Carbuncular, the most common type, occurs following skin contact with infected materials. This phase of the disease results in a very characteristic, intensely inflamed, yet painless, carbuncle covered with a black eschar. Internal anthrax occurs on a primary basis following respiratory exposure, gastrointestinal challenge, or wound infection, and on a secondary basis (20%) from untreated carbuncular cases. Generalized anthrax is characterized by an incubation period in which clinical symptoms are either nonexistent or minimal and nonspecific followed by acute respiratory distress, shock, and rapid progress to death. There are few recorded recoveries from internal anthrax because of the nonspecific symptoms and the fact that identification of the disease is based on the presence of gram-positive bacilli in the blood. As a consequence, the literature on treatment of generalized anthrax is very small, and most work has been directed toward the development of a vaccine that will protect against infection.

Only since 1954, when the toxigenic nature of this disease was demonstrated (H. Smith and Keppie, 1954), has any real progress been made in understanding the pathophysiology and the bases for treatment and immunity. Although the Porton group showed the marked correlation in the disease syndrome between its toxigenic and bacillary aspects, no general study of the toxemia was published until our 1968 series (Vick *et al.*,

1968; Klein *et al.*, 1968; Remmele *et al.*, 1968; Fish *et al.*, 1968b). Thus, the total literature on the toxin has developed since 1954. Studies on the immunogen, since shown to be the toxin or its components, started in 1946, although aggressin, also presumably the toxin, was demonstrated as early as 1904.

Several recent reviews have emphasized immunity (Ginsburg, 1964; Stamatin, 1964a,b), pathophysiology (Lincoln *et al.*, 1964a), and various general and medical aspects of anthrax (Nungester, 1967). In this chapter, (the literature review for which was completed in July 1968), we will focus on anthrax toxin, and after discussing its purification and properties, we will deal with its mechanism of action and its use as an immunogen. In each section we have attempted to cite essentially all publications relating to toxin, its pathophysiology, and immunogenic reactions.

Because anthrax toxin can act as an aggressin, an antigen, an immunogen, or a toxin, depending upon the particular assay system used, it is very difficult to find a rational basis for its nomenclature. Nevertheless, we will attempt to discuss this problem and then, although current knowledge indicates that anthrax toxin is not related to capsule formation or lysogeny, we will include a paragraph on each. Both affect virulence, and they may be related at some future time to toxin production or mechanism of action.

A. NOMENCLATURE

Bonventre *et al.* (1967a) suggested a rational scheme for toxin nomenclature based on either (1) the function of the toxin in the bacterium, (2) the mechanism of action of the toxin, or (3) the structure of the toxin molecule. We admit ignorance as to the function, if any, of the toxin in the bacterium, although energetically it appears to be a wasteful process if the toxin is merely a waste product of the cell. Although we do know that the toxin affects the central nervous system, we do not know enough about its molecular action to name it by this method. Therefore, we can only name the toxin according to its structure and here, again, we suffer from a distinct lack of facts.

Anthrax toxin appears to act both as a toxic mixture and as a complex toxin (Bonventre *et al.*, 1967a), and three components have been isolated and identified. The nomenclature, interrelationship, and biological activity of the various components are given in Fig. 1. All the components are serologically active and distinct. Protective antigen (PA) and lethal factor (LF), and probably edema factor (EF), are immunogenic. PA and LF occur in different molecular configurations or aggregates, although their exact interrelationship is unknown. Some biological activity can be demonstrated upon injection of either PA or LF alone, but full activity (toxic-

Fig. 1. Nomenclature and activities associated with toxin components.
From Fish and Lincoln (1967).

	Components		
American nomenclature	Edema factor (EF) →	← Protective antigen (PA) →	← Lethal factor (LF)
English nomenclature	Factor I	Factor II	Factor III
Combined nomenclature	EF-I	PA-II	LF-III
Described fractions of component	X, Y	C_1, C_2; α, γ	
Immunological activity	Serologically active	Serologically active	Serologically active
	Probably immunizing	Immunizing	Immunizing
Biological activity		Edema	Lethal

ity) does not occur unless the various components are combined. PA and LF must be combined before the toxin is lethal, and PA and EF must be combined before the toxin is dermonecrotic. EF and LF combined have no biological activity. The three components combined are immunogenic, lethal, and dermonecrotic. Perhaps the best way to visualize the toxin molecule is in relation to an enzyme. Although all three components appear to be protein, the PA component may be visualized as a coenzyme, while the EF and LF components may be visualized as apoenzymes. There is also some evidence that the toxin can exist in isoenzyme forms.

In this review, when we discuss a particular component as PA, EF, or LF, we will be referring to its individual activity as distinct from both that of any other component or that when combined with another component. Unfortunately, the literature prior to 1961 does not include any mention of LF because that component was not separated from EF until then (Stanley and Smith, 1961; Beall et al., 1962). When referring to these early papers, the reader must remember that EF, factor I, and filter factor all refer to a mixture of EF and LF.

A second area of confusion exists because one of the components (PA or protective antigen) bears the same name as the immunogen called protective antigen. All anthrax immunogens have been called protective antigen without regard for prior usage of the term or proof of identity of the material and, as illustrated in Section VII, have varied from extracts of animal tissue to an alum-precipitated in vitro material. Unfortunately, the components present in the various immunogens have not been identified and characterized, and it is impossible to present any reasonable conclusions in this regard here. Consequently, when we use the term "protective antigen," we will be referring to an immunogen of unknown composition. In contrast, when we speak of PA, we will be speaking of one of three readily distinguishable components of the toxin. In order to fully understand the interrelationship among the three toxin components and their function in anthrax intoxication, the assay system must be standardized, and as different assays measure different functions, more than one assay should be performed.

B. RELATIONSHIP OF CAPSULE AND TOXIN

The polyglutamic acid capsule, important in the establishment of the infection but probably not in the terminal phase of the disease (Klein *et al.*, 1961), has long been known to be unrelated to toxin (Cromartie *et al.*, 1947a; Thorne, 1960). Meynell and Meynell (1966) isolated metabolic mutants that could synthesize capsule in the absence of carbon dioxide but could not synthesize toxin. Studies with tetracycline further dissociated the process of capsule formation from that of toxin production.

C. LYSOGENY

Ivanovics (1962) isolated two strains of the *B. anthracis*-specific phage W reported by McCloy (1951). The mouse virulence of strains lysogenic for phage WB was not diminished when compared with the nonlysogenic strain. When lysogenic for Wα the capsulogenic strains appeared less virulent because of the competition between prophage induction and capsule formation induced by the high carbon dioxide tension. Altenbern and Stull (1965) reported that lysis of the Sterne strain induced by mitomycin C did not result in the release of phospholipase, EF, or PA into the media. We (Rosenwald *et al.*, 1963) demonstrated lysogeny and transduction of streptomycin resistance and dependence in the Vollum strain of *B. anthracis*.

D. TOXIN AND AGGRESSIN—HISTORICAL REVIEW

The early literature on anthrax toxin is confused because two overlapping but mutually exclusive schools of thought developed as a result of different assay procedures. One school was interested in anthrax toxin as an aggressin responsible for enhancing virulence of the organism, while the other was interested in the isolation of an immunogen for protection. This not only delayed the clear-cut demonstration of a toxin, but many of the early reports appear to contradict each other because the establishment and the development of the disease are quite different (Klein *et al.*, 1963a).

Bail (1904) and Bail and Weil (1911) identified the presence of a "protective antigen" and an aggressin in extracts of skin lesions from animals with anthrax infections. These protective and tissue-damaging activities appeared to be localized in sterile extracts from anthrax lesions (Cromartie *et al.*, 1947b). These extracts produced lesions when reinjected into rabbits and continued injection immunized against spore challenge. This diffusible factor or toxin elaborated during growth (Cromartie *et al.*, 1947b) was fractionated into two substances, "one an inflammatory, tissue-damaging factor and the second a protective antigen" (Watson *et al.*, 1947). The protective antigen was shown to be an effective immunogen (Gladstone, 1946; Heckley *et al.*, 1949; Wright *et al.*, 1951), but the relationship between Cromartie's diffusible factor and the present toxin (Fish and Lincoln, 1967) has not been resolved. With the further observations of a capsular and a somatic polypeptide antigen, it is no wonder that the literature has been divided until quite recently into studies on synthesis and production either of toxin (Section III) or of "protective antigen" (Section VII).

II. Quantitation of Toxin

Quantitation of anthrax toxin and comparison of results among the various groups working on the toxin are quite difficult because the toxin may be and has been assayed on the bases of lethality, edema production, protection against challenge, and antigen–antibody interaction (Fish and Lincoln, 1967). The correlation among these different assay procedures is not constant (Puziss and Wright, 1954, 1963; Thorne, 1960; Haines *et al.*, 1965; Fish *et al.*, 1968a). Because the toxin is a complex one, this problem is further complicated by the fact that the assay for one toxin component, although valid, will not always indicate the extent of contamination by a second or third component.

To date, three components have been identified and described in some detail, but more components probably are present (Wright and Luksas, 1964), and those already identified may exist in different ratios or molecular states (Fish and Lincoln, 1967; Fish *et al.*, 1968a; Buzzell, 1967). Disk electrophoresis has shown that crude preparations of anthrax toxin contain six (Baier, personal communication) or sixteen (Wilkie and Ward, 1967) protein bands, so future study probably will reveal interactions of which we know nothing at this time.

Interpretations of biological assays made prior to 1961 must be made in the light of the data indicating that EF (Stanley and Smith, 1961) and "filter factor" (Beall *et al.*, 1962) were in reality combinations of EF and LF. While none of the components alone or EF and LF in combination produce evidence of lethality or edema formation, the individual components are able to affect host physiology (Vick *et al.*, 1968; Fish *et al.*, 1968b).

A. BIOLOGICAL ASSAY PROCEDURES

1. LETHALITY

a. Whole Toxin. The IV LD_{50} dose of plasma from guinea pigs dying of anthrax was 0.35 ml (20 ml/kg) and 5.0 ml (10 ml/kg) for mice and guinea pigs, respectively (H. Smith *et al.*, 1955b). Fish and Lincoln (1968) showed that serum from monkeys dying of anthrax contained toxin and was lethal for rats.

Using toxin produced *in vitro*, Beall *et al.* (1962) showed that the Fischer 344 rat was quite susceptible to toxin. Lethality is linearly related to toxin concentration through several log_2 dilutions (Table I) and is the basis for the rat lethality test (Haines *et al.*, 1965). All seven animal species tested have proven susceptible to toxin produced *in vitro* and administered IV (Lincoln *et al.*, 1967).

Because the minimum time-to-death in rats injected with toxin produced *in vitro* is 54 minutes, while death has been obtained 10 minutes post injection of toxin produced *in vivo*, it is possible that these two toxins are not completely identical (Fish and Lincoln, 1968). However, this may merely be a reflection of their molecular configuration (Section IV) rather than an expression of a fundamental difference in structure.

b. Components. Although it first appeared that EF and PA combinations were lethal (Thorne *et al.*, 1960), the EF used was later shown to contain both EF and LF (Stanley and Smith, 1961; Beall *et al.*, 1962). Recent work with isolated or partially purified components (Molnar and Altenbern, 1963; Fish and Lincoln, 1967; Fish *et al.*, 1968a; Vick *et al.*, 1968) has indicated that only LF and PA are required for lethality. However, H. Smith and Gallop (1956) and H. Smith (personal communica-

TABLE I

MEAN RESPONSE TIME OF FISCHER 344 RATS TO ANTHRAX TOXIN[a]

Rat units of toxin[b]	Mean time to death (minutes)
512	58
256	54
128	61
64	74.5
32	105
16	223
8	Survive
4	Survive

[a]Based on Haines *et al.* (1965)

[b]Based on the linear portion of the reciprocal response curve for a standardized toxin preparation (1 ml of toxin at the original concentration contained 32 rat units).

tion) believe that EF is required for maximum lethality in the mouse if not in all animals. As determined by Ouchterlony assay, the minimal PA:LF ratios that caused death in a rat were 10:8 (Molnar and Altenbern, 1963) and 32:4 or 16:8 (Fish et al., 1968a).

2. Skin Edema Formation

a. Whole toxin. Toxin has been quantitated by either (1) measuring the diameter and depth of the dermonecrotic, edematous lesion produced, or (2) determining the highest dilution of toxin that will produce such a lesion after ID injection in a guinea pig or rabbit (Belton and Henderson, 1956; Thorne et al., 1960; Beall et al., 1962; Fish and Lincoln, 1968). Terminal serum of guinea pigs dying of anthrax produced lesions 40 and 15 mm in diameter when 0.2 ml of undiluted and a 1:8 dilution, respectively, were injected ID in guinea pigs (H. Smith et al., 1955b). Rabbit skin is five- to eight-fold more sensitive to toxin than guinea pig skin (Belton and Henderson, 1956). When assaying toxin produced *in vivo*, it is quite important that the assay be performed soon after obtaining the sample because activity is lost rapidly, even when stored at $-20°C$ (Fish and Lincoln, 1968).

b. Components. Only EF and PA are required to produce a skin edema and lesion corresponding to that observed following injection of the whole toxin. From material produced *in vivo*, the minimal amounts of purified EF–LF mixture and PA required to produce a detectable edema in rabbit skin are 0.3 and 15 μg, respectively (Stanley et al., 1960). Fish et al. (1968a) reported a minimum requirement of 18 μg protein (EF purified 35-fold from toxin produced *in vitro*) in combination with PA to yield a visible edema response in guinea pigs.

B. Serological Assay Procedures

1. Ouchterlony

Using the Ouchterlony technique (Ouchterlony, 1953), a concentration as low as 4 μg/ml was measured and correlated with the rabbit skin test and rabbit immunization (Thorne and Belton, 1957). The minimal amounts of each component that have been detected by this procedure are: PA, 0.02 μg (Strange and Thorne, 1958); LF, 0.02 μg (H. Smith and Stanley, 1962); and EF, 0.05 μg (Stanley and Smith, 1961). This assay procedure is the most widely used method for quantitation (Strange and Thorne, 1958; Thorne et al., 1960; Fish and Lincoln, 1967) and has remained essentially unchanged, except for a 3 to 4 fold $\log_2$ increase in titer as a result of equipment modification (Ray and Kadull, 1964) and the use of azocarmine stain (Fish *et al.,* 1968a). This procedure indicates the presence of immunologically distinct lines of precipitation associated with each of the three components. Under certain conditions, however, a particular component may be present but not visualized by this method (Fish *et al.,* 1968a).

By the addition of a measured amount of antibody to the antigen and then titration for either antigen or antibody excess some indication of antibody binding by the toxin or its components may be obtained (Fish *et al.,* 1968a).

2. COMPLEMENT FIXATION

This procedure, developed by McGann *et al.* (1961), has had very limited use (Puziss and Howard, 1963). A correlation is reported between complement fixation titers and immunizing activity of "protective antigen." However, this tedious and time-consuming test does not appear to offer any advantage over other assay procedures.

3. HEMAGGLUTINATION INHIBITION

Russian workers (Konikova *et al.,* 1966) showed strong interest in this technique because they felt it was extremely sensitive. However, until specific antiserum for each component is available, this technique will be of limited applicability.

4. ANTHRAXIN ASSAY

This test apparently is based on an immunoallergic response in immunized guinea pigs that is directly related to the amount of anthraxin (anthrax allergin) administered (reviewed by Shliakhov, 1964; Shliakhov and Shroit, 1964; Dieva, 1965; Shliakhov *et al.,* 1965). Because of the lack of detailed methods and data, we cannot evaluate this method as an assay system.

C. COMPARISON AMONG ASSAY PROCEDURES

The biological activity of both the whole toxin and its individual components is lost before either immunological or serological activity is lost (Beall *et al.,* 1962; Molnar and Altenbern, 1963; Fish *et al.,* 1968a). On storage at $0°C$, toxin lost biological activity before it lost serological activity (H. Smith, 1958). Sargeant *et al.* (1960) noted that immunogenic capacity is not always related to Ouchterlony titer. The following generalization seems warranted: the toxin first loses biological activity, then immunogenicity, and finally, serological activity.

D. Summary and Future Research

Biological (lethality, skin edema) and serological (Ouchterlony) assays for the toxin and its three known components exist. Standardization is needed among groups working with these procedures and materials. Because each assay measures some different capacity of the toxin, all workers should use several different assays. More also needs to be done to correlate results from one assay with those obtained by another procedure.

A vital need exists for a monovalent antiserum for each component so that (1) an individual line of precipitation on an Ouchterlony plate can be unambiguously identified with a biological function, (2) the complex molecular configuration of the toxin can be interpreted, and (3) the graded responses of the various assay systems can be standardized as the toxin is progressively inactivated. Use of monovalent antiserum, as well as antiserum other than the equine antiserum prepared against spores of the Sterne strain, will aid in studies of possible differences among toxins produced *in vivo* and *in vitro* and by strains of varying degrees of virulence.

III. Production and Purification

This section covers the production and purification of toxin per se, whereas the production of an immunogen is discussed in Section VII.

The elegant and simple experiments of H. Smith and Keppie (1954) clearly identified a toxin which was later shown to be an aggressin (H. Smith and Gallop, 1956) similar to that produced *in vitro* (Gladstone, 1946) or *in vivo* (Cromartie *et al.*, 1947b; Watson *et al.*, 1947). The work of H. Smith and Keppie (1954) stimulated recent work on isolation and purification of toxin, resulting in our advances in (1) understanding the mechanism of action, (2) the development of an effective vaccine, and (3) better methods of treatment. Toxin purification was reviewed by Fish and Lincoln (1967).

A. *In Vivo* Toxin

1. Production

For large-scale production of *in vivo* toxin, H. Smith *et al.* (1953) infected large guinea pigs with spores of the Vollum NP strain of *B. anthracis*. The thoracic and peritoneal exudates, collected immediately at death, were mixed, centrifuged to remove guinea pig and bacterial cells, and sterilized by filtration before purification.

Both components (EF–LF mixture and PA) recognized and isolated by Smith and colleagues appear to be present in the plasma in approximately equal amounts as no increase in titer (edema) was observed when either of the separated components was added to the crude plasma (H. Smith *et al.*, 1956a). Toxin concentration increases in the lymph (Klein *et al.*, 1962a) and bloodstream (Tempest and Smith, 1957; Klein *et al.*, 1966) of animals infected with anthrax. The titer and number of lines of precipitation visible in Ouchterlony plates also continues to increase until death (Fish and Lincoln, 1968). Toxins produced *in vivo* and *in vitro* appear identical (Belton and Strange, 1954; Harris-Smith *et al.*, 1958; Fish and Lincoln, 1968), although in several instances we found that toxin produced *in vivo* killed more rapidly than *in-vitro*-produced toxin (Fish and Lincoln, 1968). This may be due to the configuration of the toxin as discussed in Section IV. Several different virulent (V1-b and 116) and hypovirulent (770 and Sterne) strains (Fish and Lincoln, 1968) produced the same toxin *in vivo* as assayed by the Ouchterlony method.

2. PURIFICATION

Two fractions, X and Y, were isolated from plasma–exudate mixtures by precipitation with barium acetate and ethanol (H. Smith *et al.*, 1955b; H. Smith and Gallop, 1956). Except that X appeared to be formed during ultracentrifugation of Y, no further identification of these fractions has been made. A deposit, which resembled fraction Y in immunizing and antiphagocytic properties but differed in having virulence-enhancing activity and toxicity when combined with PA, was obtained after ultracentrifugation of plasma-exudate mixtures (H. Smith *et al.*, 1956a). This deposit was purified about 50-fold with 20% recovery by ammonium sulfate precipitation, DEAE-cellulose chromatography, and further ultracentrifugation (Stanley *et al.*, 1960). Yield was about 2 mg from 20 to 30 large guinea pigs, but the material was contaminated with 16% guinea pig plasma components. PA was purified 20-fold with 20% recovery from the initial ultracentrifuge supernate by DEAE-cellulose chromatography, dialysis, and lyophilization (Stanley *et al.*, 1960). It also contained 15% guinea pig serum components, and all preparations proved heterogeneous by Ouchterlony assay (Stanley *et al.*, 1960).

B. *In Vitro* TOXIN

1. PRODUCTION

The importance of size of the inoculum and length of incubation on the production of protective antigen (toxin) was noted by Heckley *et al.* (1949). However, production of toxin *in vitro* was generally unsuccessful until Harris-Smith *et al.* (1958) and others (H. Smith, 1958; Aleksandrov *et al.*, 1961) demonstrated that toxin is present in the medium for the short time during which the bacterial concentration is approximately 5×10^7 to 10×10^7 chains/ml. Additionally, certain factors like bicarbonate (Gladstone, 1946; Puziss and Wright, 1954; Harris-Smith *et al.*, 1958; Puziss and Howard, 1963), charcoal (Strange and Thorne, 1958), and sugar source (Puziss and Wright, 1959) are important. Recent work indicates that bicarbonate is required early in the growth cycle and that it (1) affects cell permeability and release of the toxin from the cell to the medium (Puziss and Howard, 1963) and (2) does not merely slow the rate of bacterial growth so that toxin persists in the culture (Harris-Smith *et al.*, 1958).

The early literature on toxin production is clouded by the uncertainty as to whether a high pH and/or the presence of serum was needed for production, separation, or stability of the toxin (Gladstone, 1948; Wright *et al.*, 1954a; Thorne and Belton, 1957; Strange and Thorne, 1958; Harris-Smith *et al.*, 1958; Thorne, 1960; Stanley and Smith, 1961, 1963). Consequently, serum was added before processing (Thorne *et al.*, 1960; Beall *et al.*, 1962; Mahlandt *et al.*, 1966), after processing (Wilkie and Ward, 1967), or not at all (Mahlandt *et al.*, 1966; Fish *et al.*, 1968a). Additional confusion was added by the assay system because the presence of serum or high pH prevented the separation of the components (Beall *et al.*, 1962).

The hypovirulent Sterne strain has been used most often for the production of toxin because it produces slightly higher concentrations of toxin than the NP mutant of the virulent V1-b strain (Harris-Smith *et al.*, 1958). Apparently identical toxin is produced by both nonproteolytic (NP) as well as proteolytic strains of V1-b (Wright *et al.*, 1951; Harris-Smith *et al.*, 1958); thus, proteolytic activity does not appear to be a prerequisite for toxin production.

A reliable and standardized method exists for producing the toxin from the Sterne strain grown on medium 599 with minor modifications (Haines *et al.*, 1965), and all three components have been isolated from this toxin.

2. PURIFICATION

Because the toxin is composed of several different components, purification may proceed by (1) concentrating the whole toxin, while keeping the molecular configurations and ratios of all components unchanged or (2) purifying the individual components, and then recombining them to make whole toxin.

a. Whole toxin. Only one group has attempted to purify the whole toxin (Wilkie and Ward, 1967). The toxin, sterilized by Millipore filtration, was concentrated 500- to 1000-fold by ultrafiltration. This resulted in a

25–50% loss of lethal activity for Fischer 344 rats and "consistently lower" skin edema and mouse lethal activities. Chromatographs of the crude filtrate and ultrafiltrate showed evidence of changes during processing: (1) whereas EF was found in the PA peak in the crude filtrate, the EF was not accounted for after ultrafiltration and (2) in the crude filtrate, the LF peak was free of PA, whereas PA contaminated LF preparations after ultrafiltration.

  b. Components. Thorne et al. (1960) separated toxin into two factors (EF–LF mixture and PA) by filtration in the presence of serum, and Stanley and Smith (1961) later demonstrated the presence of the third component (LF).

  i. Edema factor component. EF was purified 25-fold with 25% recovery from cultures prepared for production of the Belton–Strange immunizing antigen (Thorne and Belton, 1957; Strange and Thorne, 1958) by filtration, elution with saturated sodium bicarbonate, and DEAE-cellulose chromatography (Stanley and Smith, 1961). Because this material killed mice when mixed with PA, it probably was contaminated with LF. Based on the observation of Beall et al. (1962) that EF is selectively adsorbed onto glass filters and eluted with 0.3 M sodium carbonate, pH 9.3, Fish et al. (1968a) purified EF 197-fold with 38% recovery by filtration, DEAE-cellulose chromatography, and dialysis. Upon Ouchterlony analysis, the final preparation produced one line of precipitation which was distinct from that produced by PA or LF, and, in combination with PA, it produced edema in guinea pigs and was not lethal to rats.

  ii. Protective antigen component. PA has been precipitated by alum (Harris-Smith et al., 1958), trichloroacetic plus citric acids (Strange and Belton, 1954), ammonium sulfate (Thorne et al., 1960), ethanol (Aleksandrov et al., 1963), and ethanol and acid (Aleksandrov et al., 1964). These preparations are quite heterogeneous by Ouchterlony assay (Strange and Thorne, 1958; Stanley et al., 1960), and the studies did not yield values for calculating recovery or the extent of purification. Strange and Thorne (1958) obtained a preparation of unknown but probably high purity with 25% recovery by ammonium sulfate precipitation, precipitation at pH 5, and alumina C gamma gel chromatography. They were unable to resolve fully the two different fractions (C_1 and C_2); however, in light of recent observations on the spatial configuration of the whole toxin and its components (Section IV), they were probably dealing with some aggregate or polymer. This preparation contained some LF (Stanley and Smith, 1961). We have published three different methods for the purification of PA (Fish et al., 1968a). The best method used glass filtration, ammonium sulfate precipitation, and polyacrylamide gel chromatography to yield a 156-fold purification with 78% recovery. This final preparation is not contaminated with EF or LF, is serologically distinct from EF or LF, is immunologically active, is dermonecrotic in combination with EF, and, with LF, is lethal.

iii. *Lethal factor component.* LF was purified 3.5-fold with 24% recovery by glass filtration, DEAE-cellulose and hydroxyapatite chromatography, and ammonium sulfate precipitation (H. Smith and Stanley, 1962). The purified component showed a single peak in the ultracentrifuge and by paper electrophoresis; however, under certain conditions, two bands were observed on Ouchterlony gel plates. We (Fish *et al.*, 1968a) purified LF 1025-fold with 11% recovery by glass filtration, Sephadex chromatography, and absorption and elution from calcium phosphate gel. This purified material was serologically distinct from the other two components.

C. Summary and Future Research

The toxin and its three components are produced *in vivo* and accumulate in the terminal serum of infected hosts. Smith and colleagues purified this material about 20-fold with 20% recovery, but they completed this work prior to the identification of LF, so they had only two factors (an EF–LF mixture and PA). They also were unable to remove more than 85% of the guinea pig plasma components from their final preparations. We have shown that the titer and number of lines of precipitation on Ouchterlony plates continue to increase until the death of the guinea pig. Future research, using a kinetic approach as well as different strains, should contribute greatly to studies on the production of this toxin.

Production of toxin or its components is readily accomplished *in vitro* in complex or synthetic media. EF, PA, and LF have been separated and purified 197-, 156-, and 1025-fold, respectively. These isolated components are immunologically homogeneous and distinct, and they remain biologically, immunogenically, and serologically active.

Although methods now exist for the production, isolation, and purification of the three components from the Sterne strain, more needs to be done to ascertain the correct interaction among these components and their spatial configuration or structure. The possibility of new components and a comparison of toxins produced *in vivo* and *in vitro* are two areas in which future research would be most productive.

Whenever the toxin or its components are purified, the properties of the purified materials must be checked against both the original material and toxin produced *in vivo*.

Although existing information indicates that toxin produced by one strain resembles quite closely that of another strain, only toxin produced by the Sterne strain has been studied in any great detail, and work with other strains is badly needed.

IV. Nature of Toxin

A. EXPERIMENTAL DATA

All three components appear to be nondialyzable proteins or lipoproteins with absorption maxima at 270 mμ and minima at 250 mμ (Gladstone, 1946, 1948; Strange and Belton, 1954; H. Smith and Gallop, 1956; Strange and Thorne, 1958; Thorne *et al.*, 1960; Stanley *et al.*, 1960; Stanley and Smith, 1961; H. Smith, 1964; Fish *et al.*, 1968a). The ratio of absorbance at 280/260 mμ indicates the presence of 3–8% nucleic acid (Stanley and Smith, 1961; Fish *et al.*, 1968a), but as Stanley and Smith (1961) could not demonstrate the presence of RNA or DNA, and in view of the requirements for pyrimidines or nicotinamide for optimal toxin production (Tempest and Smith, 1957), a more exacting chemical study is required. Small amounts of phosphorous and carbohydrate have also been identified (H. Smith and Gallop, 1956; Strange and Thorne, 1958; Stanley and Smith, 1961), and at least one component (EF) has some chelating activity (Stanley and Smith, 1961). Paper electrophoresis has been used to identify and study the various components (Watson *et al.*, 1947; Strange and Thorne, 1958; Wilkie and Ward, 1967), but the bands are not always clear or reproducible (Heckley *et al.*, 1949; Stanley and Smith, 1961; Fish and Lincoln, 1968; Fish, unpublished observations). Stanley and Smith (1963) showed that none of the three isolated components possessed enzymatic activity.

All investigators have indicated the marked thermolability of the toxin or its components (H. Smith *et al.*, 1955b; H. Smith, 1958; Strange and Thorne, 1958; Thorne *et al.*, 1960; Stanley *et al.*, 1960; Sargeant *et al.*, 1960; Stanley and Smith, 1961; Wilkie and Ward, 1967; Fish *et al.*, 1968a). With the exception of two reports on EF isolated from *in vivo* sources (Stanley *et al.*, 1960); Stanley and Smith, 1961) and one early report on "protective antigen" (Wright *et al.*, 1954a), all indications are that the lyophilized toxin and components are quite stable when stored in the cold (H. Smith *et al.*, 1955b; Belton and Henderson, 1956; Strange and Thorne, 1958, Stanley *et al.*, 1960; Ray and Kadull, 1964; Haines *et al.*, 1965; Fish *et al.*, 1968a). The stability of the various components to heat differs markedly (Strange and Thorne, 1958; Stanley *et al.*, 1960). H. Smith and Stanley (1962) report that purified LF retained complete biological activity after 24 hours of incubation at 37°C. H. Smith *et al.* (1955b) reported that toxin was not inactivated by shaking in thin layers at 0°C, thus removing a possible criticism of the temperature stability studies of Fish *et al.* (1968a), who showed that biological activity was lost before serological activity.

As the various components become more purified, they become increasingly labile in the absence of salts (Strange and Thorne, 1958; Stanley *et al.*, 1960; Fish, unpublished observations). Stanley *et al.* (1960) and Stanley and Smith (1961), using toxin produced *in vivo*, reported that crude EF was destroyed by reducing agents but stabilized by mild oxidizing agents, while purified EF was not stable in the presence of either. PA was labile to both oxidizing and reducing agents (Stanley *et al.*, 1960). Fish *et al.* (1968a), using toxin produced *in vitro*, reported that all three components, even when partially purified, appeared to be stable in the presence of oxidizing or reducing agents, but LF and especially PA were quite susceptible to hydrogen bond disrupting reagents.

The pH range for maximum stability of the components is quite narrow, centering at pH 7.4–8.0, and pH becomes more critical as the components are purified (Gladstone, 1946; H. Smith *et al.*, 1955b; Strange and Thorne, 1958; Thorne *et al.*, 1960; Stanley *et al.*, 1960; Stanley and Smith, 1961; Fish *et al.*, 1968a). These results all contradict those of Wright *et al.* (1954b) who report more potent filtrates of "protective antigen" at pH's up to 8.7.

Evidence for molecular heterogeneity (polymerization, aggregation, differential destruction) has been accumulating since H. Smith and Gallop (1956) first observed that "factor X" seemed to be formed by aggregation of "factor Y" as a result of repeated ultracentrifugation. Strange and Thorne (1958) found one peak of PA activity by paper electrophoresis and two peaks by ultracentrifugation. They postulated degradation of the antigen to account for the additional lines appearing on Ouchterlony plates as the culture passed its peak titer and activity was lost. Similar observations were reported by Wilkie and Ward (1967) using disk electrophoresis. Stanley *et al.* (1960) demonstrated that (1) the relative proportion of peaks observed in the ultracentrifuge depended upon the freshness of the toxin, and (2) mild treatment (heating to 37°C) increased the proportion of high molecular weight peaks. On this basis they postulated that EF formed aggregates rather than dissociating to form smaller components. Sargeant *et al.* (1960) reported that EF and PA combined to form mixtures as demonstrated by the presence of additional lines of precipitation in Ouchterlony plates. They also reported that PA was composed of two fractions whose proportions shifted with purification or storage. Stanley and Smith (1961) and Wilkie and Ward (1967) speculated that all three components join in some sort of a loose complex, probably as a result of the chelating action of EF. If the components do exist as a complex, then it must be very loose because (1) all three components can be readily isolated from whole toxin (Stanley and Smith, 1961; Beall *et al.*, 1962; Fish *et al.*, 1968a), and (2) Ouchterlony analyses of toxin produced both *in vitro* and *in vivo* show the presence of several different lines of precipitation (Fish and Lincoln, 1967, 1968; Fish *et al.*, 1968a). Molnar and Altenbern (1963) demonstrated the transient conversion of PA to an inhibitor of toxin lethality, but we were unable to confirm this observation (Fish *et al.*, 1968a). Immunoelectrophoresis of "purified protective antigen" gave three connected arcs of precipitation, indicating closely related serology but different electrophoretic mobility (Wright and Luksas, 1964). The bands, α_1 and γ, were interpreted to be degradation products of PA. The existence in whole toxin of three components in various states of polymerization was demonstrated by similar techniques (Wilkie and Ward, 1967). Mahlandt *et al.* (1966) reported a different immunological response to combinations of components than that observed by the English workers (Stanley and Smith, 1963), and these changes might also be due to differential aggregation.

We have shown (1) aggregation of PA stored at high concentrations or in the presence of ammonium sulfate, and (2) the presence of multiple peaks of PA or LF activity following chromatography on Sephadex (Fish *et al.*, 1968a). Evidence has been presented for the presence of a particular "more lethal" configuration of the toxin molecule and for the dissociation of *in vivo* toxin, loss of biological activity, and increase in the number of lines of precipitation on Ouchterlony plates (Fish and Lincoln, 1968). These observations, when added to those on the marked synergistic interaction of PA and LF when injected into rats (Fish *et al.*, 1968b), indicate that toxin may exist in a variety of aggregate, polymer, or molecular configurations whose properties may vary markedly (Fish and Lincoln, 1967).

Ultracentrifuge studies of whole toxin indicated that (1) four separate peaks were present and (2) the two faster migrating peaks might arise from aggregation of the slower migrating peaks (Buzzell, 1967). Similarly, PA may exist in multiple aggregate structures (monomer to octomer), and based on assumptions of similarity between this protein and that of tobacco mosaic virus, Buzzell (1967) postulated that the polymers were stabilized by bonding to LF, divalent metal ions, or protocatechuic acid.

Further evidence indicating the variable configuration and composition of the components may be implied from the observations of Wilkie and Ward (1967) and Fish (unpublished observations) that phosphate ions disrupt PA. PA also aggregated in high concentrations or in the presence of ammonium sulfate (Fish and Lincoln, 1967; Buzzell, 1967; Fish *et al.*, 1968a). We found that LF was stable during column chromatography only in the presence of 0.1 M pyridine solutions, pH 8.0, and not in the presence of a variety of other routinely used buffers (Fish *et al.*, 1968a).

Buzzell (1967) reported that molecular weights of proteins associated with lethal activity formed a series of 8,500, 17,000, 34,000, and 51,000, while we obtained a value of approximately 100,000 for both PA and LF (Fish and Lincoln, 1967; Fish *et al.*, 1968a). In view of the apparent structural and configurational complexity of these molecules, however, it is apparent that much more work is needed.

Toxoiding of the toxin or components has been shown and suggested repeatedly (H. Smith *et al.*, 1954; Beall *et al.*, 1962; Molnar and Altenbern, 1963; Fish *et al.*, 1968a), and this area must be re-evaluated in the light of new definitions (Bonventre *et al.*, 1967a) for toxins and toxoids.

B. SUMMARY AND FUTURE RESEARCH

Workers are not in full agreement regarding any of the physicochemical properties of the components of toxin, and this area requires more extensive work with purified components. In general, all three components appear to be proteins or lipoproteins that are most stable when stored at 0–4°C and pH 7.4–8.0.

The evidence for molecular heterogeneity is impressive but circumstantial since no knowledge exists as to the molecular configuration of the toxin molecule produced by the organism either *in vivo* or *in vitro*. Consequently, the lack of agreement among workers as to the characteristics of the individual components may be due either to fundamental changes in the structure of the toxin or to artifacts induced by purification procedures.

Undoubtedly, many of the results discussed here will have to be re-evaluated as we learn more of the structure and complexity of this toxin. Much of our present information arose from incidental observations on toxin produced or purified in different ways. With the use of a toxin standard (Haines *et al.*, 1965) and the new techniques for toxin purification now available (Wilkie and Ward, 1967; Fish *et al.*, 1968a), much useful information can be obtained.

V. Synthesis

A. *In Vivo* TOXIN

The relationship between the number of bacilli and the units of toxin present in the terminal blood of six host species is summarized in Table II

TABLE II

RELATIONSHIP BETWEEN UNITS OF TOXIN AND NUMBER OF BACILLI PER MILLILITER
OF TERMINAL BLOOD AND RESISTANCE TO ESTABLISHMENT OF ANTHRAX[a]

Host	Relative resistance to anthrax	Quantitation of terminal blood	
		Units of toxin	No. of bacilli
Mouse	Very susceptible	—	$10^{6.9}$
Chimpanzee	Susceptible	110	$10^{8.9}$
Guinea pig (unimmunized)	Susceptible	50	$10^{8.3}$
Rabbit	Susceptible	—	$10^{8.0}$
Rhesus monkey	Susceptible	35	$10^{6.8}$
Guinea pig (immunized)	Resistant	55	$10^{6.0}$
NIH black rat	Resistant	25	$10^{5.9}$
Fischer 344 rat	Very resistant	<8	$10^{4.0}$

[a] From Lincoln et al., 1967.

(Tempest and Smith, 1957; Klein et al., 1963a; Lincoln et al., 1964a, 1967). Keppie et al. (1955) observed that immunized guinea pigs died with only a slight bacteremia and used this to support their finding that death was due to a toxin. While it does not argue against the conclusion of Keppie et al. (1955), Jones et al. (1967a,b) showed that the total number of organisms per host was higher in immunized than in unimmunized animals; in the former, the bacteria were retained within the host tissue and not released into the blood stream.

The concentration of bacilli and toxin per milliliter of lymph (Klein et al., 1962a, 1966) or blood (Tempest and Smith, 1957; Klein et al., 1962a, 1963a, 1966; Jones et al., 1967a,b) increases with time, and there is a relatively constant growth of bacteria in the blood, as well as a constant relationship between bacterial growth and survival time (H. Smith et al., 1955a; Keppie et al., 1955; Fish and Lincoln, 1968). However, recent observations indicate that the kinetics of production of the individual components may differ (Fish and Lincoln, 1968). Molnar and Altenbern (1963) concluded that in vitro-produced toxin was fixed to host tissue through the PA component. They reported that PA was removed from circulation by 60–90 minutes post injection, while the concentration of LF remained unchanged over a 4-hour period. Tempest and Smith (1957) reported that toxin injected IV decreased 4-fold per hour. This situation, where toxin is injected in relatively large amounts and death is rapid (Remmele et al., 1968), is quite different from the slow and steady buildup of toxin during the actual infection.

Ward et al. (1965) observed the presence of both circulating toxin and antibodies in immunized animals dying from anthrax, and they concluded that toxin may or may not be the causative agent of death. We (Fish and Lincoln, 1968) also have observed the presence of both antibodies and toxin in the blood of animals dying from anthrax but attribute this to different attachment sites for the antiserum and various components of toxin. The coexistence of antigen and antibody in the blood was noted early in the study of immunology (Wells, 1929). These observations (Ward *et al.*, 1965; Fish and Lincoln, 1968) appear best explained by the observation of Opie (1923) that, in the presence of an excess of either antigen or antibody, the Ag–Ab combination is inhibited and both components remain in the free uncombined state.

One of the most interesting pieces of work, which unfortunately has never been pursued, is the amino acid antimetabolite studies of H. Smith and Tempest (1957) and Tempest and Smith (1957). During the terminal 3 hours of bacteremia, the plasma concentration of 4 (glutamine, glycine, threonine, tryptophan) out of 16 amino acids decreased markedly, while the other 12 increased markedly, except serine which was unchanged. When 57 amino acid analogs were injected, one (8-azaguanine) inhibited both bacterial growth and toxin formation at the same rate, some (ethionine, *p*-fluorophenylalanine, and α-amino-*n*-butyric acid) inhibited bacterial growth and toxin formation at different rates, and some (2-thiouracil and pyridine-3-sulfonic acid) inhibited toxin production without decreasing the growth rate. This indicated that various pyrimidines or nicotinamide might be involved in the synthesis or release of toxin or of one component. The ability to divorce toxin production from bacterial growth should greatly aid studies on toxin synthesis, its control, and exploitation.

B. *In Vitro* TOXIN

Initial efforts to demonstrate toxin production were unsuccessful because of its unexpectedly early appearance and rapid destruction (Gladstone, 1948; H. Smith *et al.*, 1956b). Successful production has since been achieved using either bicarbonate in place of serum albumin (Gladstone, 1946), blood aerated with 20% carbon dioxide (Harris-Smith *et al.*, 1958), gelatin in place of serum (Thorne *et al.*, 1960), or a simple salts medium (Haines *et al.*, 1965). Wright *et al.* (1954a) noted the requirement of proline and threonine for "protective antigen" production rather than growth and speculated that its elaboration was associated with a particular type of metabolic activity. Puziss and Wright (1954) noted that omission of isoleucine, leucine, histidine, aspartic acid, glutamic acid, arginine, methionine, proline, tryptophan, or Ca^{2+} from the growth media had no effect on growth of the organism but inhibited "protective antigen" elaboration. Gladstone (1946) reported that bicarbonate was not required for buffering activity and that it could not be replaced as a one-carbon donor by citrate, succinate, fumarate or malate. Puziss and Wright (1954) noted that omission of bicarbonate had no effect on growth of the organism but that toxin production was completely inhibited. They later reported (Puziss and Wright, 1959) that toxin was produced within the cell but that bicarbonate was needed for the release of the toxin from the cell. However, Meynell and Meynell (1966) indicated that carbon dioxide is required for toxin production. Anaerobic cultures, in contrast to aerobic cultures, appeared to retain some metabolic carbon dioxide to meet this requirement. Puziss and Wright (1959) reported that high titers of "protective antigen" production required the presence of a readily utilizable carbon source and that the peak "protective antigen" titer in the culture coincided with the disappearance of the carbon source. Harris-Smith et al. (1958) noted a difference in the infrared spectra between cells producing or destroying toxin and suggested that these shifts indicated some profound change in the organism itself related to these two different functions.

No study of the kinetics of synthesis of the components exists besides that of Wilkie and Ward (1967) and Fish and Lincoln (1968). Techniques for the selective enhancement or inhibition of the synthesis of a particular toxin component are not known for the Sterne strain, let alone for any of the other strains available (Thorne, 1960), and it is known that other strains have different growth requirements (Puziss and Wright, 1954). Gladstone (1946) could not demonstrate edema with the Vollum strain, whereas Cromartie et al. (1947b) could, and in fact, H. Smith et al. (1953) selected Vollum as the strain of ten tested which produced the maximum volume of edematous fluid. Modification of the virulence of the stock used was "adjusted" by growth on different culture media to produce the type of lesion desired for extraction of the crude toxin fluid. Both virulent and avirulent strains produce toxin (Thorne, 1960), but again, more work needs to be directed at these specific problems.

C. *In Vivo* versus *in Vitro* Toxin

Knowledge of the exact relationship between these two toxins is essential. It is clear that, while they are at least quite closely related (Harris-Smith et al., 1958; H. Smith et al., 1956a; Stanley and Smith, 1961), they differ in serological characteristics (H. Smith and Gallop, 1956; H. Smith et al., 1956a; Sargeant et al., 1960; Stanley and Smith, 1961) and rapidity with which they kill (Fish and Lincoln, 1968). The complexity of this problem is further indicated by the observations on the (1) lack of a toxin-destroying system operating *in vivo* (H. Smith, 1958; Fish and Lincoln, 1968), (2) rapid destruction of toxin or some component of toxin following IV injection (Molnar and Altenbern, 1963; Remmele et al., 1968), (3) transient nature of toxin produced *in vitro* (Harris-Smith *et al.*, 1958; H. Smith and Stanley, 1962; Aleksandrov *et al.*, 1964), and (4) instability of *in vivo* toxin after serum is collected from the host (Fish and Lincoln, 1967, 1968).

D. SUMMARY AND FUTURE RESEARCH

A positive correlation exists *in vivo* between the number of bacilli and units of toxin in the serum or lymph. Toxin production is independent of bacterial growth, and selective utilization of this observation should allow for many future kinetic studies.

Toxin can be produced *in vitro* in a variety of media with carbon dioxide being required for production or release of toxin from the cell. Nutritional requirements for the production of toxin or its components are not well understood.

Toxins produced *in vitro* and *in vivo* are closely related; however, important differences have been noted. The kinetics for the production of each component of this toxin need elucidation, considering not only the *in vivo* and *in vitro* situation but also the bacterial strain and supplementary or growth inhibiting substances. The isolation of strains (1) producing a new toxin component, (2) lacking one of the known components, or (3) with widely different ratios of the components (as compared to the Sterne strain) are attractive possibilities for research and immunization.

Understanding the genetic control for the production of these components will be a challenge for many years. The interesting observation that free circulating antigen and antibody coexist in the blood of immunized hosts at death from anthrax needs to be explained with respect to (1) rates of synthesis of components (or the whole toxin), (2) the kinetics of the Ag–Ab binding, and (3) the binding affinity of the antiserum versus host tissue.

VI. Pathogenesis

A. ANTHRAX INFECTION

Anthrax occurs in two forms. The first is a localized or cutaneous infection manifested by an intense, dark, open eschar. This form occurs in only a few species (man, swine, rabbits, horses), and although the eschar is ugly and open, it is surprisingly nonpainful and is readily healed by antibiotics (Cromartie *et al.*, 1947a). The generalized or septicemic form of anthrax (Lincoln *et al.*, 1964a; Stamatin, 1964a; Nungester, 1967) may either arise from the cutaneous form or result from infection via the respiratory route, infection *per os*, gastrointestinal leakage, or infection of a wound. Regardless of how the infection is established, it develops in an orderly and predictable fashion. The spores germinate and then invade the lymph system. From here, they spill into the bloodstream and are picked up by the reticuloendothelial system, but they soon overgrow this defense system and establish secondary foci of infection. The susceptible host exhibits a characteristic massive bacteremia, and bacilli are found throughout the entire body tissue. The level of toxin found in the blood increases quite late in the course of the disease and appears to parallel the bacterial concentration. As described in Section VII, death from anthrax is not due to the bacteremia but rather to the toxin produced by the bacteria. The only difference between infection and intoxication is that the level of free circulating toxin builds up to a maximum at death in the former, whereas the maximum amount is present initially and the concentration decreases as death approaches in the latter.

B. ANTHRAX INTOXICATION

1. CUTANEOUS INJECTION (EDEMATOUS LESION)

The edematous lesion formed after ID injection of toxin develops within 24 hours and essentially disappears by 7 days (Keppie *et al.*, 1953; H. Smith *et al.*, 1955b). It is attributed to vascular damage leading to edema and hemorrhage in the deeper vascular areas of the corium adjacent to the cutaneous muscle. Some of the collagen fibers show hyaline changes and stain with eosin. Polymorphonuclear leukocytes are widely scattered throughout but concentrate in the midzone of the corium to yield a localized abscess. Depth of the lesion as well as surface size are related to concentration of the toxin (Harris-Smith *et al.*, 1958). This lesion closely resembles that caused by *B. anthracis* (Cromartie *et al.*, 1947a). Evans and Shoesmith (1954) reported that injection of old culture filtrates produced an edema that closely resembled that caused by *B. anthracis*, but it is produced and dries out too rapidly to resemble the lesion produced by *in vivo* toxin (H. Smith *et al.*, 1955b).

2. GENERALIZED INTOXICATION

The mode of action of the toxin in causing death during generalized anthrax and its effect on the central nervous system will be discussed in detail in the next section.

VII. Mode of Action

A. General Remarks (Stamatin, 1964a,b; Lincoln *et al.*,
1964a; Nungester, 1967)

Sterne (1961) noted, "Perhaps we know more about the way anthrax bacillus works than we do about almost any other pathogen of similar invasiveness," and H. Smith and Stoner (1967) concluded, "It seems generally accepted now that death in anthrax is due to toxin." The histopathology of the bacillary disease and of the toxemia from sterile toxin are quite dissimilar, yet the pathophysiology is remarkably similar. In some cases, there have been tendencies to (1) extrapolate from observations on the bacillary disease to the action of the toxin, (2) work only with toxin or a single host and extend conclusions generally, and (3) ignore the fact that what is causal in one host is not causal in another. Each group working in this field has reached a different conclusion as to the primary cause of death. The principal theories as to cause of death are blockage of capillaries by bacteria (Vaughan and Novy, 1902), cardiovascular failure (Middleton and Standen, 1961), effect on the reticuloendothelial system (Albrink, 1961), oxygen depletion (Nordberg *et al.*, 1961), "secondary" shock (H. Smith *et al.*, 1955a), increased vascular permeability (H. Smith and Stoner, 1967), and respiratory failure of central nervous system origin (Vick *et al.*, 1968). In this section, we first will review the reported experimental data on the effect of toxin on the host and then follow with a critical discussion of these data as they affect the theories of the cause of death.

Death from anthrax may be sudden and unexpected, and essentially all mammals, as well as some birds and reptiles, are susceptible. Consequently, specific signs or symptoms of internal or generalized anthrax (i.e., temperature and hematological changes, depression, paralysis, or changes in heart rates or patterns) do not exist. Because recognition of anthrax is based principally on the presence of gram-positive bacilli, and septicemia may not occur in some species, many anthrax deaths go undetected (Dordevic, 1951; Sterne, 1959). Signs in the dead host are more characteristic—rigor mortis is delayed, the blood appears dark red and unoxygenated, and bloating is rapid.

A consideration of either the principal hypotheses on mode of action or the diverse pathology and physiology reported for this disease will indicate that it may attack many organs and physiological systems or functions. However, we find only one universal symptom, and it is one that occurs in both the bacterial and toxigenic disease; namely, respiratory failure. But respiratory failure may occur as a result of central nervous system involvement, extraordinary oxygen depression of undetermined origin, fragility of capillaries, "secondary" shock, or pulmonary edema.

We shall discuss and evaluate the data pertaining to the mode of action of this toxin, seeking a universal cause in all species for both the bacillary and toxemic disease. One must recognize that secondary effects may differ widely, depending on the interaction of host and bacterial strain as influenced by genetic constitution and environment. We feel that, if the primary cause is recognized, then survival experiments should be possible, and these in turn will strongly support the hypothesis for primary mode of action.

B. EXPERIMENTAL OBSERVATIONS

1. GROSS SIGNS

Only the mouse, guinea pig, rat, rabbit, chimpanzee, rhesus monkey, and dog have been challenged with toxin, and all are susceptible (Lincoln *et al.*, 1967). The rat responds uniquely and is discussed below. In the remaining species and also in bull frogs (unpublished), most individuals show restlessness, paralysis (Klein *et al.*, 1961) or hypersensitivity (Klein *et al.*, 1966). Death follows a general flaccid relaxation so that the exact time to death is difficult to establish. Although some edema is found in the pleural and peritoneal cavities at death, it is not marked enough to be major pathology, and the lung appears normal in color and texture.

The rat responds uniquely. Toxemia in this species is acute; it results in death soon after IV administration of toxin (1–2 hours) and is accompanied by gross pulmonary edema. With a dose that results in death in 2 hours, hyperactivity and restlessness first become evident about 20 minutes prior to cessation of respiration and increase progressively. Following toxin challenge, progressive hypothermia is evident (Klein *et al.*, 1967). Terminally, as the animal lies still, a small pool of edematous fluid forms around the nose. Although Gray and Archer (1967) describe the fluid as "reddish," blood cells are not present, and it is electrophoretically indistinguishable from serum (Beall and Dalldorf, 1966; Fish *et al.*, 1968b). The mottled grey and purplish-red lungs lie in a pleural cavity more or less filled with clear exudate and are 2½ times heavier than normal lungs (Beall and Dalldorf, 1966). In all species, when respiration ceases, autopsy or physiological tracing showed the heart beating strongly until its anoxic death (Vick *et al.*, 1968; Fish *et al.*, 1968b).

2. CHANGES IN BLOOD CHEMISTRY

Perhaps the most remarkable change is the fall of the blood oxygen level to less than 1% from normal levels of 18–21% and 12–15% (v/v) for arterial and venous blood, respectively (Eckert and Bonventre, 1963; Klein *et al.*, 1966). In all other diseases except anthrax—and including death by drowning or asphyxiation—(Nordberg *et al.*, 1961), the oxygen level at death remains above 5%. The low blood oxygen level was not due to destruction of erythrocytes or to a decreased oxygen-binding capacity of hemoglobin, because gentle agitation changed the color from the dark red of slow-clotting blood characteristic of anthrax to the bright red of normal oxygenated arterial blood (Eckert and Bonventre, 1963).

Following toxin challenge in rats, a marked hyperglycemia occurs (Eckert and Bonventre, 1963), and a hypoglycemia develops as the toxemia progresses, while liver and muscle glycogen are utilized to maintain "normal" serum glucose levels (Fish *et al.*, 1968b). Serum lactate was elevated about 3.5 times at death (Gray and Archer, 1967). In rabbits injected with sublethal doses of toxin, a marked hyperglycemia occurred, which could be mediated by epinephrine and blocked by ergotamine, but no consistent hypoglycemia developed (Slein and Logan, 1960). The hyperglycemia required both PA and EF (later shown to contain LF) (Beall *et al.*, 1962) and was prevented by antiserum. Blood levels of K^+, Cl^-, and PO_4^{-3} rose, while Ca^{2+}, Na^+, carbon dioxide, and pH decreased (Klein *et al.*, 1966). Blood cholinesterase in rabbits increased, then gradually decreased (Klein *et al.*, 1966). Survivors showed inhibition equal to those dying, and the effect of cholinesterase inhibition may simply accentuate signs of toxemia, such as spastic paralysis.

Slein and Logan (1960), using only one 1-kg rabbit per treatment, injected nonlethal doses of toxin IV. They reported no change in serum glycoprotein levels, but increases in serum aldolase, phosphoglucose isomerase, glutamic/oxaloacetic acid transaminase, amylase, alkaline phosphatase, and cholesterol. Antiserum injected with the toxin diminished but did not prevent these changes. Hyperphosphatasemia occurred after injection of PA or PA plus EF, but not EF alone, and this response was not inhibited by antiserum or bilateral nephrectomy. The rabbit is a particularly variable animal as regards response to weal formation (Belton and Henderson, 1956) and demonstrates no dose response to anthrax spore challenge (Walker *et al.*, 1967). Consequently, more observations must be made on this species than are required on other species to gain equal precision and confidence.

3. Blood Cellular Elements

Toxin resulted in a marked shift to the left of blood cellular elements, and the increase in blood leukocytes was correlated with an increase in polymorphonuclear leukocytes (Klein *et al.*, 1966; Fish *et al.*, 1968b). Eosinophiles are not a feature of anthrax intoxication; however, nucleated erythrocytes were found in toxin-challenged rabbits, but not in primates. The individual purified components may also alter the blood cell pattern (Fish *et al.*, 1968b). Hematocrit values change and appear to reflect whether pulmonary edema is characteristic of the species or not, for hematocrit values increased in rats (Eckert and Bonventre, 1963; Fish *et al.*, 1968b) and hemoglobin content of heart blood nearly doubled (Eckert and Bonventre, 1963), whereas there may be a slight decrease in hematocrit values in other species where gross edema is not characteristic (Klein *et al.*, 1966). Erythrocytes from intoxicated rats are more fragile than those from normal rats (Eckert and Bonventre, 1963).

4. TISSUE OXIDATIVE METABOLISM

Oxygen consumption was depressed (26%) and elevated (21%) in rat lung and brain brei, respectively, prior to toxemic death (Gray and Archer, 1966, 1967; Archer and Gray, 1967). Addition of 2-ketogluconate or succinate increased Q_{O_2} values in lung brei. The nicotinamide adenine dinucleotide level was depressed 23% in lung brei.

5. HISTOPATHOLOGY

As with gross changes, histopathological changes occurred in the rat (Beall and Dalldorf, 1966) but in none of the other species examined (Bonventre *et al.*, 1967b; Vick *et al.*, 1968; Dalldorf, personal communication). Electron microscopic examination of lung sections of rats showed hyperemic areas, elevation of the thin endothelial cell membranes lining the pulmonary capillaries as a result of edema, and the presence of granular thrombi. No other organs examined showed morphological changes (Beall and Dalldorf, 1966; Bonventre *et al.*, 1967b).

6. PHYSIOLOGICAL RESPONSES

Responses to toxin in the cardiovascular system of rhesus monkeys and chimpanzees (Vick *et al.*, 1968; Remmele *et al.*, 1968) and of rats (Fish *et al.*, 1968b) were amazingly few, mild, or transitory prior to respiratory hypoxia, after which evidence of progressive myocardial ischemia developed. Heart rate and blood pressure remained within normal limits. The electrocardiogram, although somewhat changed, showed no evidence of inversion or fibrillation.

The significant changes occurred in the central nervous system of these species. Toxin depressed the cerebral cortical electrical activity as shown by electroencephalogram either partially or completely in both anesthetized and unanesthetized animals (Vick *et al.*, 1968; Fish *et al.*, 1968b). In primates, cyclic changes progressing to electrical silence appeared independent of other physiological responses (Vick *et al.*, 1968); however, some associated cycling of respiration occurred with the rat (Fish *et al.*, 1968b). Subcortical changes in electrical activity occurred simultaneously with the surface cortical changes (Vick *et al.*, 1968). All of these changes were prevented by specific antiserum (Klein *et al.*, 1967; Fish *et al.*, 1968b; Vick *et al.*, 1968). Initial changes in electroencephalogram readings were caused by PA but not LF alone (Vick *et al.*, 1968). In the monkey, changes in the respiration rate were associated with repeated and irregular discharges over the phrenic nerve, which did not synchronize with the inspiration phase of respiration. At all times, from challenge until death, the phrenic nerve remained capable of transmitting an electrical discharge, and stimulation of the cut end of the phrenic nerve elicited a hyperactive response in the diaphragm. Thus, there was no indication of a block in the neuromuscular transmission; rather, the brain was depressed and no longer capable of initiating an electrical discharge (Vick *et al.*, 1968).

Whereas 10,000 rat units of toxin injected IV in monkeys caused death at 28–34 hours, injection of 1000 units directly into the cerebrospinal fluid produced death in 6–10 minutes (Remmele *et al.*, 1968). An immediate tetanic paralysis and cessation of respiration followed injection of toxin, and the central venous and arterial pressures rose sharply. In spite of a heart rate that initially decreased but immediately returned to normal, aortic blood flow dropped precipitously and remained low until death. Electrocardiogram changes were consistent with myocardial hypoxia. Intensive muscle fasciculation developed, and blood pressure and heart rate decreased, progressing to prolonged hypotension, loss of rigidity, and death. Introduction of toxin into the cerebrospinal fluid resulted in a great stimulation of central nervous system discharges as indicated by muscle contraction and changes in blood pressure and flow that led rapidly to anoxia and death. In spite of these extreme changes, survival was obtained either by artificial ventilation of only 10 minutes duration or by two injections of the β-adrenergic stimulant isoproterenol at 420 and 650 seconds post challenge.

C. Critical Evaluation of Hypotheses on Cause of Death

We feel that the primary cause of death must be identical in all hosts whether one considers the bacillary disease or the injection of sterile toxin. For this reason, attributing death to blocking of the capillaries by bacilli (Vaughan and Novy, 1902) may be rejected outright because no bacilli or particulate material is injected with the toxin, yet, the general physiological signs of disease are the same (H. Smith and Keppie, 1955; Klein *et al.*, 1966, 1968). Six other hypotheses are considered below.

1. CARDIOVASCULAR CHANGES

Heart rate, blood pressure, and electrocardiogram readings remain remarkably constant until shortly before death in both primates (Klein *et al.*, 1966, 1968) and rats (Fish *et al.*, 1968b), and lysis of erythrocytes is minor (Eckert and Bonventre, 1963).

2. PRINCIPAL EFFECT ON THE RETICULOENDOTHELIAL SYSTEM

Albrink (1961) speculated that the cells of the reticuloendothelial system are the main target for the toxin, but no experimental support for this proposition is available.

3. ABNORMALLY LOW OXYGEN CONTENT IN BLOOD

Nordberg *et al.* (1961) reported an abnormally low oxygen content in terminal blood of animals dying of anthrax, and Eckert and Bonventre (1963) confirmed this result in animals dying from toxin. Despite the criticism of H. Smith and Stanley (1962), Nordberg's observation appears to be valid (Eckert and Bonventre, 1963; Klein *et al.*, 1966), and acute terminal anoxia is a common secondary phase of death in all hypotheses of cause of death discussed below.

4. SECONDARY SHOCK

Studies of blood chemistry, physiology, and histopathology indicate that a state of secondary shock occurs in guinea pigs dying of anthrax (H. Smith *et al.*, 1955a). Less extensive supporting observations were made on toxin (H. Smith *et al.*, 1955b). H. Smith and Stoner (1967), influenced by the work of Beall and Dalldorf (1966), amend the secondary shock hypothesis to state that the primary cause of death is fluid loss due to increased permeability of blood vessels. As massive edema and increased hematocrit changes are found only in the rat, secondary shock does not seem likely to be the cause of death in all animals (Lincoln *et al.*, 1964a).

5. INCREASED VASCULAR PERMEABILITY

The only significant histological changes reported are in the rat (Beall and Dalldorf, 1966; Bonventre *et al.*, 1967b). In the rat, the toxin appears to increase permeability of the pulmonary, peritoneal, and subcutaneous beds, thereby causing death, which is accompanied by terminal anoxia, edema, shock, and other signs. Gray and Archer (1967) postulated that, as gas exchange in the lung is depressed, a shift to an anaerobic type of respiration ensued resulting in the increased utilization of nicotinamide adenine dinucleotide. While this hypothesis explains the decrease in Q_{O_2} observed in the lung, it does not explain the 21% increase in Q_{O_2} observed in the brain. However, this and similar work should be pursued with more careful attention paid to the use of controls, other host species, and recognition that the response of nervous tissue to toxins can be very selective. For example, botulinum neurotoxin does not affect oxygen consumption of brain slices nor does it show any significant central nervous system effects *in vivo* (Stevenson, 1962), whereas cobra venom, which can affect the central nervous system, modifies oxygen consumption of brain slices *in vitro* (Quastel, 1957). Thus, it is possible that the 21% increase in oxygen consumption of brain brei noted by Gray and Archer (1967) is a modification of cellular respiration directly attributable to toxin.

6. RESPIRATORY FAILURE OF CENTRAL NERVOUS SYSTEM ORIGIN

This model was proposed by Lincoln *et al.* (1964a), criticized by Smith and Stoner (1967), and supported by Vick *et al.* (1968), Remmele *et al.* (1968), Klein *et al.* (1968), and Fish *et al.* (1968b). Respiratory failure is a sign observed for all hosts and frequently is so acute as to cause death which is repeatedly described as "sudden" or "unexpected." The wide range of changes in physiology, enzymatic activity, blood chemistry, and blood cellular elements are nonspecific and believed to be consistent with central nervous system interaction. We (Vick *et al.*, 1968) have demonstrated depression of electroencephalogram tracings and a lack of conductance over the phrenic nerve without detectable effect on neuromuscular and diaphragm function. Lack of demonstrable histological changes in neural elements or in other organs (Bonventre *et al.*, 1967b; Vick *et al.*, 1968) does not necessarily imply lack of physiological involvement. We (Remmele *et al.*, 1968) have shown that survival occurs if respiratory failure is overcome by either forced ventilation or isoproterenol. Specific antiserum prevents depression of electroencephalogram activity and symptoms of respiratory distress.

D. SUMMARY OF CURRENT STATUS ON MODE OF ACTION OF TOXIN

Most of the hypotheses presented to explain the mode of action of toxin deal with secondary effects, and while these may cause death, they are not the primary "mode of action" of the toxin. Gross pulmonary edema appears to be restricted to toxin-challenged Fischer 344 rats; it is not marked in any of the other species in which anthrax has been described or the other six species challenged with toxin. Pulmonary edema may be caused directly by central nervous system injury (Reynolds, 1963), and in fact, Reynolds' description of rats dying from pulmonary edema resulting from electrolytically induced lesions of the hypothalmus is remarkably similar to the signs in rats following lethal toxin challenge. The absence of marked abnormalities in the cardiovascular system indicates that this is not the primary site of toxin action. Recent experiments all indicate a rapid and profound effect on the central nervous system (electroencephalogram) following administration of anthrax toxin. The marked increase in central nervous system discharge followed by electrical silence could account for all the signs and symptoms of anthrax infection or intoxication. Respiratory failure and anoxia are the only common feature in all species challenged with both bacilli and toxin, and it could be brought about by (1) a direct effect of toxin on the respiratory center, (2) neuromuscular blockage, or (3) decreased blood flow mediated by central nervous system involvement.

E. Correlation between Pathophysiology of Anthrax Intoxication and Infection

With the exception of our work with primates (Klein *et al.*, 1962a, 1966, 1968; Lincoln *et al.*, 1964a; Walker *et al.*, 1967) and of H. Smith *et al.* (1955b) with guinea pigs, little has been done to correlate host response to either sterile toxin or bacillary infection. The disease syndromes produced by both toxin and organism are orderly, progressive, and predictable (Lincoln *et al.*, 1964a), and most signs and changes are nonspecific, occurring late in the course of infection, whereas the same changes occur relatively early in the toxemia. These differences are consistent with both the dynamics of toxin development during infection and the results following challenge of a host with sterile toxin. During infection, toxin builds up gradually to a maximum at death, and, in fact, does not become free and detectable in the blood until shortly before death (Fish and Lincoln, 1968), whereas with sterile toxin the full dose is introduced at challenge.

The rat is unique with respect to response to toxin (pulmonary edema and hemoconcentration), and the histopathology following toxin challenge does not resemble that produced by the bacillus (Beall and Dalldorf, 1966; Dalldorf and Beall, 1967). Nevertheless, the central nervous system aspects of toxemia in the rat (Fish *et al.*, 1968b) are identical to those observed in the primate during both toxemia (Vick *et al.*, 1968) and infection (Klein *et al.*, 1968).

F. Dynamics of Toxic Action

There is agreement (Molnar and Altenbern, 1963; Fish *et al.*, 1968a) that changes in the ratio of PA to LF affects lethality and time to death;

however, because the methods used to obtain the components varied with each group, the optimum PA:LF ratio has not been established. As greater amounts of PA are added to a constant amount of LF, the time to death reaches a minimum, then increases to survival; however, as more LF is added to a constant amount of PA, the time to death continues to decrease (Molnar and Altenbern, 1963; Fish *et al.*, 1968a). Injection of toxin via the carotid artery or via the tail or femoral vein did not change the time to death of rats (Bonventre *et al.*, 1967b). Regardless of dose, 55 minutes is the minimum time to death for rats challenged with *in vitro* toxin (Haines *et al.*, 1965; Beall and Dalldorf, 1966; Fish and Lincoln, 1968); however, toxin produced *in vivo* may kill in a much shorter time period (Fish and Lincoln, 1968). Generally, the more resistant a host is to the establishment of bacillary infection, the more susceptible it is to toxin (Table III) (Klein *et al.*, 1963a; Lincoln *et al.*, 1967).

Toxin action is dependent upon (1) the kinetics of attachment to the host tissue, (2) the amount and configuration of each component, (3) the host and any stress conditions, and (4) pharmacological treatment of the host.

G. TREATMENT

Medical treatment of anthrax, except Russian use of antiserum (Mashkov, 1958), ignores the toxin and attempts to remove the bacillus and perhaps give symptomatic support. It is notable, too, that Russian recommendations specifically exclude symptomatic cardiac support (Yablokov, 1950). Prior to antibiotics, "Hyperimmune serum and neosalvarsan were the most rational items of clinical use" (Sterne, 1959), and the case re-

TABLE III

RELATIONSHIP BETWEEN THE NUMBER OF ANTHRAX BACILLI REQUIRED TO ESTABLISH INFECTION AND THE UNITS OF TOXIN REQUIRED TO CAUSE DEATH[a]

Host	Spores required to establish infection	Dose required to cause death (units/kg)	Time to death (hours)
Mouse	5	1000	24
Guinea pig	50	1125	24
Rabbit	5000	2500	72
Rhesus monkey	3000	2500	28
Chimpanzee	—[b]	4000	60
Rat, Fischer 344	0.7×10^6	15	2
Rat, NIH Black	1.5×10^6	280	20
Dog, beagle	5×10^7	60	20

[a] From Lincoln *et al.* (1967).

[b] No data; considered susceptible.

ported by Nilsson (1934) is an example of the heroic use of antiserum. Following extensive experimentation on anthrax, we (Lincoln *et al.*, 1964a,b; Klein *et al.*, 1967; Jones *et al.*, 1967a,b) expressed the view that antitoxin as well as antimicrobial agents and other drug therapy must be used for maximum recovery (i.e., the latest stage at which treatment may be initiated with survival). Antiserum neutralizes circulating toxin and may, as with staphylococcal enterotoxin B (Rapoport *et al.*, 1966), reduce the toxin still reversibly fixed. Hypothermia in rats following challenge with a lethal dose of toxin extended time to death; however, the lethal dose was decreased compared with that required to kill at higher temperatures (Klein *et al.*, 1967). Antiserum administered prior to and for a certain time following toxin challenge prevented death, while its administration at a later time merely extended time to death (Klein *et al.*, 1967; Vick *et al.*, 1968). No drug thus far tested has resulted in survival following IV injection (Beall and Dalldorf, 1966; Klein *et al.*, 1967), and in fact, only Nembutal extended time to death or reduced edema. Even barbiturate was ineffective when the additional stress of 4°C was added. This rules out any significant effect either (1) of endogenous histamine or serotonin on vascular response, or (2) of antistress agents of the steroid class. Use of isoproterenol resulted in survival following toxin injection into the cerebrospinal fluid (Remmele *et al.*, 1968).

Molnar and Altenbern (1963) reported limited data indicating that large doses of PA injected within 5 minutes after toxin challenge prevented death, but merely extended time to death when administered beyond this time. They speculated that PA competitively occupied toxin attachment sites. We also have shown that addition of increasing amounts of PA to a constant amount of LF causes the time to death to reach a minimum and then increase (Fish *et al.*, 1968a). However, any proposal to use an aggressin for treatment lacks appeal because (1) it has been observed that the addition of PA to whole toxin decreases time to death (Fish, unpublished), (2) PA itself lowers by 100-200 times the bacillary dose (hypovirulent strains) required to establish infection (Keppie *et al.*, 1955; Lincoln *et al.*, 1964a), and (3) effective use would require early identification of the disease (before toxin attachment). Use of a PA toxoid that is immunologically active but nonlethal when combined with LF (Bonventre *et al.*, 1967a) has more possibilities, especially if combined with antisera specific for EF and LF.

PA had no effect on treatment of respiratory anthrax in monkeys (Gochenour *et al.*, 1961). However, injection of the Thorne–Belton antigen (probably all components) following treatment and cure of septicemic anthrax to generate an amnestic response is one step in obtaining animals refractive to large challenge doses of spores (Lincoln *et al.*, 1964b).

H. Miscellaneous Responses to Toxin

Toxin (1) is virulence-enhancing, (2) inhibits phagocytosis of *B. anthracis* cells by guinea pig polymorphonuclear leukocytes, (3) is anticomplementary, and (4) inhibits the action of anthracidal substances in normal serum and in extracts of leukocytes (H. Smith and Gallop, 1956; H. Smith *et al.*, 1956a; Kashiba *et al.*, 1959; Lincoln *et al.*, 1964a). Toxin (aggressin) also may play a role in invasiveness (Bail, 1904; H. Smith, 1958), although this conclusion is based on *in vitro* observations with relatively high concentrations of toxin. The latter may not reflect toxin action as an aggressin *in vivo*, where few bacterial cells occur and toxin must be dilute, localized, and follow rather than precede cell growth. In addition to the capsule and toxin, other chemical substances may act as aggressins (Sterne, 1948a,b; Young and Zelle, 1946; Ivanovics, 1964).

Toxin containing an unknown amount of guinea pig serum produced a granuloma in rats which had a high fluid content and appeared histologically as a very loose cell structure. Antiserum prevented formation of the granuloma. When this toxin was instilled into the eye of the rabbit, a nonspecific vasodilation but not chemosis was observed. This toxin neither promoted nor inhibited migration of leukocytes from chicken blood clots (Desaulles *et al.*, 1956).

There is no visible cytopathological effect of toxin on three tissue cell lines (Bonventre, 1965). However, crude toxin liberated β-glucuronidase but not acid phosphatase from large granules derived from rabbit livers. When anthrax bacilli were grown in human embryo cell cultures (Ginsburg and Maslova, 1963; Ginsburg and Fedotova, 1963), the virulent bacilli grew attached to the tissue cell and caused a cytopathogenic effect, whereas hypovirulent bacilli grew free in the medium and caused no cytopathogenic effect. Although toxin was not demonstrated, this response was attributed to the "toxic factor of virulence" (toxin). Crude toxin did not decrease turbidity of suspensions of lysosomes (Bernheimer and Schwartz, 1964). Kashiba *et al.* (1959) noted that the terminal serum of guinea pigs dying of anthrax produced changes in the phagocytic and anthracidal activity of white blood cells from ten host species. Those species whose leukocytes were most readily prevented from phagocytizing killed staphylococcal cells were the guinea pig, cow, man, rabbit, sheep, horse, and mouse, whereas the rat, dog, and swine were resistant or refractive to the serum. Although unable to repeat these observations, Lincoln *et al.* (1967) noted that their data showed an inverse correlation between maximum dilution of terminal serum to inhibit phagocytosis and susceptibility of the host to establishment of anthrax.

EF is reported as virulence-enhancing, antiphagocytic, and anthracidal at low concentrations and as having a direct harmful effect on phagocytes (Keppie *et al.*, 1963).

A 200-fold enhancement of virulence was noted when sterile plasma exudate collected from guinea pigs dying of anthrax was injected with the spore challenge (Keppie *et al.*, 1953). A temporal, 100-fold reduction in the lethal dose of hypovirulent Sterne strain spores was noted in BALb strain mice after receiving PA (Lincoln *et al.*, 1964a).

Contrary to the observations with several other toxins, irradiated rabbits were not more susceptible to toxic plasma than nonirradiated rabbits (Vancurik, 1964). Because the functional capacity of the reticuloendothelial system is weakened by irradiation, Albrink's speculation (1961) that cells of the reticuloendothelial system are the main target of the effect of anthrax toxin is further repudiated.

I. Summary and Future Research

Anthrax toxin affects the central nervous system, causing respiratory failure and anoxia, and central nervous system involvement occurs in both infection and intoxication. Monkeys survived when placed on a positive pressure respirator or given isoproterenol.

More kinetic experiments must be performed with the individual purified components and their factorial combinations to indicate the role and attachment of each component in affecting the host and to separate the primary from secondary effects of the toxin. A radioactive or fluorescent-tagged toxin would prove useful for such work. Survival experiments with toxin-challenged hosts should furnish the basis for the treatment and cure of anthrax in experimental hosts and man. The late diagnosis and sudden death syndrome of anthrax makes treatment difficult, requiring a rapid specific response both with respect to neutralizing the toxin and its effects and providing symptomatic support.

VIII. Immunology and Immunochemistry

Classically, immunity to anthrax is associated with the live, hypovirulent strain developed by Pasteur. However, sterile edematous fluid taken from the host immediately at death was shown quite early to be an effective if variable immunogen (Bail, 1904; Bail and Weil, 1911). Later investigators succeeded in purifying this immunogen, which they called "protective antigen," from *in vivo* and *in vitro* sources.

It is unfortunate that one component of anthrax toxin was named "protective antigen," not only because of the confusion in nomenclature but also because of the attendant connotation that it is the one antigen which protects against challenge. Not only has this connotation proved erroneous (Stanley and Smith, 1963; Mahlandt *et al.*, 1966), but the name itself also had prior use both for the complete toxin (Gladstone, 1946) and for anthrax lesion extracts and exudates from animals dying of anthrax (Cromartie *et al.*, 1947b).

At least six "protective antigens" have been introduced into the literature: (1) edematous extract, (2) Gladstone's antigen, (3) Boor–Tresselt's antigen, (4) Belton–Strange's antigen, (5) aerobic antigen, and (6) anaerobic antigen. These may be classified as those derived from body fluids (1, 2, 3), that produced in a complex undefined medium (4), and those produced in defined synthetic media (5, 6). In none of the "protective antigens" has the component composition and ratio or molecular state of the components been determined; however, there is little doubt that the antigen is related to the toxin.

A. EDEMATOUS FLUID AND TISSUE EXTRACTS

Bail (1904) demonstrated the efficacy of edematous extracts as a vaccine. Salisbury (1926) immunized range animals with "aggressin" (edematous fluid) and found that 27% of the 2684 unimmunized but only 0.32% of the 10,814 immunized animals died. This antigen immunized rabbits, guinea pigs, mice, hamsters, and sheep against various, mostly low, challenge doses of spores (Cromartie *et al.*, 1947b; Watson *et al.*, 1947).

Although effective, production of this vaccine remained an art (Cromartie *et al.*, 1947b), and therefore, potentially more readily controllable methods were developed.

B. GLADSTONE PROTECTIVE ANTIGEN

Gladstone (1946) reported production of a "protective antigen" in static cultures containing the plasma or serum of various species. Its immunizing properties were similar to those of anthrax edematous fluid. Rabbits, monkeys, and sheep were immunized against a spore challenge of about 100 lethal doses. Extended time to death for guinea pigs indicated some immunity, whereas mice were not immunized. Extensive tests conducted with rabbits (Table IV) showed excellent protection if two or more administrations of antigen were given. Passive immunity could be transferred. Later, Gladstone (1948) increased the yield of this antigen about 25 times by growing the culture in cellophane bags continuously perfused with serum and aerated broth. The observations of Gladstone were verified (Heckley *et al.*, 1949) and extended to growth in a synthetic medium containing 20% serum (Wright *et al.*, 1951).

TABLE IV

RESISTANCE TO ANTHRAX CHALLENGE PROVIDED BY IMMUNIZATION WITH FIVE DIFFERENT ANTIGENS

Antigen	Host	Antigen administration protocol				Days after immunization completed	Virulent challenge protocol			Reference
		Route[a]	Amount		Number of injections	Interval (days)	Route[a]	Dose (spores)	Survival[b]	
Gladstone	Rabbit	IC	1.0	ml	3	7	7	IC	100 LD[c]	31/31	Gladstone, 1946
	Rabbit	IV	0.125	ml	3	7	7	IC	100 LD	13/18	Gladstone, 1946
Boor–Tresselt	Rabbit	ID	1.0	ml	3	6	7	ID	1.2×10^3	92%	Boor, 1954
	Guinea pig	ID	1.0	ml	3	6	14	ID	1.2×10^3	100%	Boor, 1954
	Monkey	SC	20	ml	3	6–7	7–23	ID	1.2×10^5	7/7	Tresselt and Boor, 1954
	Sheep	ID	40	ml	3	6	9–10	ID	1.2×10^4	2/2	Tresselt and Boor, 1954
		ID	240	ml	1	6	63–84	ID	1.2×10^5	4/4	Tresselt and Boor, 1954
Belton–Strange	Rabbit	SC	6.5	mg	5	2	7	ID	5.0×10^2	79/79	Belton and Strange, 1954
		SC	3.25	mg	5	2	7	ID	5.0×10^2	30/31	Belton and Strange, 1954
		SC	1.25	ml	2	10	7	ID	5.0×10^2	10/10	Belton and Strange, 1954
	Monkey	SC	1.25	ml	2	10	7	RP	$4-6 \times 10^5$	9/9	Belton and Strange, 1954
	Monkey	SC	1.25	mg	2	10	7	RP	7.0×10^5	10/10	Henderson et al., 1956
Aerobic	Guinea pig	–	1.5	ml	5	2	7	IC	1.0×10^3	8/24[d]	Wright and Puziss, 1957
		–	7.5	ml	5	2	7	IC	1.0×10^3	18/24[d]	Wright and Puziss, 1957
	Rabbit	IC	0.5	ml	5	2	7	IC	1.0×10^4	47/50[e]	Wright et al., 1954b
	Monkey	SC	1.0	ml	2	16	16	RP	$3-8 \times 10^5$	3/4	Wright et al., 1954b
		SC	1.0	ml	2	16	34	RP	$0.8-3 \times 10^6$	4/4	Wright et al., 1954b
	Cattle	SC	5.0	ml	2	30	30,105,210	OR	1.5×10^8	17/24[d]	Jackson et al., 1957
		SC	5.0	ml	2	11	90	OR	1.5×10^8	12/25	Jackson et al., 1957
		SC	5.0	ml	2	11	180	OR	1.5×10^8	7/20	Jackson et al., 1957
Anaerobic	Guinea pig	–	1.5	ml	5	2	7	IC	1.0×10^3	10/24[d]	Wright and Puziss, 1957
		–	7.5	ml	5	2	7	IC	1.0×10^3	21/24[d]	Wright and Puziss, 1957

[a] IC = intracutaneous; IV = intravenous; ID = intradermal; SC = subcutaneous; RP = respiratory; OR = oral.
[b] Given either as (1) total survivors/total tested or (2) as percent.
[c] LD = lethal doses.
[d] Summation of 3 tests.
[e] Summation of 16 tests with 12 preparations.

Further refinement of the protective antigen was achieved by gradual substitution (1) among the medium ingredients, ultimately resulting in a defined medium with no added protein, (2) in strains, (3) in fermentation procedures, and (4) in processing procedures. Each was a minor change, but overall, this development of an effective vaccine was "undoubtedly among the most interesting and important achievements of experimental microbiology in the present century" (Ginsburg, 1964).

C. BOOR-TRESSELT ANTIGEN

Boor and Tresselt (Boor, 1954; Boor and Tresselt, 1954a,b; Tresselt and Boor, 1954) produced and tested the first practical vaccine (Table IV). The final vaccine was produced with the CD-2 strain (intermediate virulence) and a medium consisting of serum albumin (homologous for the species of animal to be immunized), a fractionated yeast extract, phosphate buffer, and bicarbonate. Fermentation was static. Processing consisted of centrifugation and Seitz filtration followed by precipitation (with either alcohol or ammonium sulfate), dialysis, and lyophilization.

D. BELTON-STRANGE ANTIGEN

A nonprotein complex medium containing activated charcoal was used to produce the Belton–Strange antigen (Belton and Strange, 1954). This antigen was grown in static culture, sterilized by filtration through sintered glass, and then concentrated either by (1) lyophilization or (2) alum precipitation. This vaccine gave good protection (Table IV), and although the circulating antibody level was low, a marked amnestic response of "at least" 64-fold occurred following challenge. Simpson (1966) used this antigen in cattle in North Africa and found that immunity, as assayed by Ouchterlony agar gel diffusion, was too variable to evaluate.

E. AEROBIC ANTIGEN OF WRIGHT AND COLLEAGUES

Initially, this immunogen was produced in the chemically defined medium of Brewer et al. (1946) at $\frac{1}{5}$ concentration and with 0.03 M sodium bicarbonate added. Aerobic (thin layer, static culture) growth (Wright et al., 1954a,b; Puziss and Wright, 1954) distinguishes this immunogen from that produced under anaerobic conditions (described in Section F).

The aerobic "protective antigen" was developed in five media (528, 555, 599, 687, and 968) utilizing nonproteolytic (NP) and NP-nonencapsulated (R) strains selected from seven stocks (Vollum, V770, 116, 107, 108, 1062, and 1133). In conducting the research on this immunogen, medium and strain interchanges were made on the assumption that "only protective antigen, a relatively labile filtrate factor readily separable from the bacterial cells and not demonstrable by *in vitro* reactions with antibody, is capable of inducing significant acquired resistance" (Wright *et al.*, 1954a,b). Wright (1965) maintains that "protective antigen" is the substance primarily responsible for the development of immunity to anthrax. This conclusion is held in spite of (1) not knowing the composition of "protective antigen" or having proven whether EF or LF alone, mixed or in combination with "protective antigen" are immunogenic, (2) not having a quantitative assay system (Wright and Wedum, 1954), (3) antigenic activity being "profoundly" affected by processing conditions (Wright *et al.*, 1954a,b), (4) evidence (Stanley and Smith, 1963) that EF is immunogenic and otherwise interacts in the immune reaction, and (5) the fact that immunity obtained with live vaccine following protective antigen enormously increased antibody titer and resistance to challenge (Klein *et al.*, 1962b, 1963b). The work on this antigen, in contrast especially to that on the Belton-Strange antigen, is characterized by use of a statistically inadequate number of animals, usually two or three. The immunogenicity of EF was verified (Mahlandt *et al.*, 1966) and these authors extend the conclusion to LF, thus, as philosophically expected, demonstrating that all components of the whole toxin contribute to immunity. In fact, the observation of Mahlandt *et al.* (1966), that LF in contrast to PA protects rats against toxin challenge, leaves the decision as to the optimum immunogen very much in question.

This immunogen, which has been tested by many different groups and produced with many modifications, undoubtedly confers some protection against challenge (Table IV). However, it does not appear to protect as well as do the previous antigens against ID and IC challenge, although it does protect against respiratory challenge. Protection, as evidenced by the presence of circulating antibody, is of very short duration. Even after receiving the primary series of three injections, 18 of 33 persons were negative before the booster at 6 months (Norman *et al.*, 1960); they also cited unpublished data of Norman, Ray, and Kadull that titers "declined rather rapidly after a booster in studies being done on vaccinated persons at Fort Detrick." Actually, the whole question of titers and the meanings of recorded observations are in confusion (Ray and Kadull, 1964).

These observations explain the early and transient immunity noted in animals (Schlingman *et al.*, 1956; Jackson *et al.*, 1957) and man (Norman *et al.*, 1960; Brachman *et al.*, 1962). The data suggest that (1) immunity is not developed in any definite pattern and (2) in fact, resistance may be lower in partially immunized than in nonimmunized persons. In mice, injection of PA increased susceptibility by about 100-fold (Keppie *et al.*, 1953; Lincoln *et al.*, 1964a).

It does not appear that the aerobic protective antigen produced from the seven strains or their variants in the five growth media differed among themselves, and there was no evidence of antigenic heterogeneity based on challenge of guinea pigs.

Two antigens prepared with different strains and media were used by Schlingman *et al.* (1956) for yearling cattle, sheep, and hogs. The statistical design of the cattle experiment was confounded so that one lot of antigen appeared to immunize, the other not to immunize, against oral challenge. Sheep were partially immunized against a 20,000-spore dose. Swine tests were inconclusive because even controls could not be infected.

An antigen produced with a different medium and strain combination was used by Jackson *et al.* (1957) with cattle challenged orally (Table IV). Partial immunity was obtained, but its development required two injections of antigen and a 30-day interval prior to challenge. Persistence of immunity was short. It is of interest that all six cattle immunized with live vaccine survived challenge at 3 months.

Brachman *et al.* (1960, 1962) used a similar antigen in tests on humans employed in four goat-hair processing mills. These mills employed 1249 people, of which 379 were vaccinated with three injections of antigen. Twenty-six cases of anthrax occurred; one was in vaccinated and two in incompletely vaccinated individuals. Statistical evaluation based on person–months of exposure (excluding the two incompletely vaccinated cases) indicated the antigen was 92.5% effective. However, the confidence limits (65–95%) were very questionable because of (1) several assumptions, (2) few anthrax cases, and (3) changes from the original experimental design. It is true that the Manchester epidemic (9 cases) was stopped (Brachman *et al.*, 1960) simultaneously with the immunization of all employees; however, the goat-hair lot believed to be the source of infection also was removed. As noted by Zhdanov (1961), such results cannot be considered conclusive because of nonuniform exposure.

F. ANAEROBIC ANTIGEN

Stirred anaerobic cultures (Wright and Puziss, 1957; Puziss and Wright, 1959; Wright *et al.*, 1962; Puziss *et al.*, 1963) also produce an immunogen (Table IV). This process uses a vegetative inoculum of the V770-NP1-R strain, and harvest is based on glucose utilization. Antigen is precipitated with preformed aluminum hydroxide gel (the alum process used for the aerobic antigen did not work), and benzethonium chloride (1:40,000) replaces merthiolate as a preservative. Although no data are given, this antigen is reported to be tolerated as well as the aerobic antigen (Puziss and Wright, 1963).

G. ANTIGENS DEVELOPED BY RUSSIAN WORKERS

Because the Soviet medical and veterinary professions have concentrated on using live anthrax vaccine, they have contributed little to the development of a chemical vaccine. The STI-1 vaccinal strain (acapsular, nonproteolytic) was grown in a skim milk, glucose, and inorganic salts medium (Aleksandrov et al., 1961). The alum-precipitated antigen was sterilized with 0.5% β-propiolactone (Aleksandrov et al., 1963). An alcohol-precipitated antigen was prepared (Aleksandrov et al., 1962), but its use has not been reported. The Russian vaccine is effective, and in contrast to practice in the United States, is used in large amounts. When used in multiple vaccines administered simultaneously, the immunity to anthrax was depressed.

H. ANTIGEN INTERACTIONS AS IMMUNOGENS

Anaerobic growth conditions produced four times as much antigen (by serological assay) as aerobic growth, and equal amounts of each conferred equal protection against challenge (Wright and Puziss, 1957; Puziss and Wright, 1963).

Klein et al. (1963b), compared immunities produced by the Belton–Strange, aerobic, and anaerobic antigens. Their results (Table V) show that the immunity index (resistance to a high dose challenge) of the aerobic antigen was 1 $\log_{10}$ less, while the anaerobic antigen was 1 $\log_{10}$ greater, than that observed with the Belton–Strange antigen after primary immunization. The Belton–Strange and anaerobic antigens both developed about the same mean and maximum titers, which were significantly above those of the aerobic antigen. Following a booster, the Belton–Strange and aerobic antigens significantly increased resistance to challenge, while the anaerobic antigen did not. The proportion of positives and the mean titers were both much higher with the Belton–Strange antigen than with either of the other two.

Two "protective antigen" preparations have been made available by government agencies for limited use in men working in high-risk occupations. The British vaccine (Anonymous, 1965) is the Belton–Strange antigen, of which Riemann (1966) says, "An anti-anthrax vaccine is available

TABLE V

MEASURE OF IMMUNITY OF GUINEA PIGS BY THREE ANTHRAX
ANTIGENS WITH AND WITHOUT BOOSTER INJECTIONS[a]

	Antigen type					
	Aerobic		Anaerobic		Belton–Strange	
Measures	Primary	Booster	Primary	Booster	Primary	Booster
Mean immunity index[b] ± σ	1.3 ± 1.4	5.2 ± 0.70	3.3 ± 0.41	3.8 ± 0.47	2.4 ± 0.25	4.8 ± 0.52
Coefficient variation (%)	107	14	12	12	10	11
Positive titers						
Percentage	17	50	42	100	25	100
Range	1:2 – 1:4	<1:2 – 1:16	<1:2 – 1:8	1:4 – 1:16	<1:2 – 1:8	1:8 – 1:128
Mean	<1:2 ± 1:13	1:4 ± 1:15	1:20 ± 1:08	1:83 ± 1:08	1:13 ± 1:06	1:45 ± 1:10
Coefficient variation (%)	7	38	41	11	44	27

[a] From Klein et al. (1963b).
[b] Immunity index is the $\log_{10}$ increase in dose required to cause the immunized host to respond (die) at the same time as the control.

for distribution. One wonders how reliable it is." Simpson (1966) reported that its use in field tests with cattle were inconclusive. The American vaccine is the aerobic antigen developed by Wright and colleagues. Of this vaccine, Matz and Brugsch (1964) state that, "The program developed in the Communicable Disease Center of the U.S. Public Health Service seems to meet the requirements of safety and effectiveness." More specific reservations as to the efficacy of a "protective antigen" vaccine may be based on the following: (1) immunity does not protect against all strains (Auerbach and Wright, 1955; Ward *et al.*, 1965), (2) all three toxin components are required for maximal immunity, and the use of live vaccine after the chemical antigen greatly augments the immunity produced (Klein *et al.*, 1963b; Mahlandt *et al.*, 1966), and (3) no field tests have been conducted paralleling those of Sterne *et al.* (1942) with the live vaccine or of Salisbury (1926) with edematous fluid.

I. IMMUNITY PRODUCED BY INDIVIDUAL COMPONENTS AND INTERACTIONS

Because most antigens used as vaccines were not analyzed to determine which components were present and in what proportions, it became necessary to determine the contribution of each component and the interactions among them.

With three components tested at two levels (+ and −), there are eight factorial combinations. PA was the only single component that produced immunity in guinea pigs. EF plus PA and EF plus LF combined synergistically, while PA plus LF produced no interaction, and EF plus PA plus LF decreased immunity (Stanley and Smith, 1963). These results are contrary to those of Mahlandt *et al.* (1966), who tested both guinea pigs and Fischer rats in 27 factorial combinations. Five criteria were used to evaluate the efficacy of the immunogen against challenge by either spores (guinea pig and rat) or toxin (rat): (1) development of serum antibody level (Ouchterlony assay), (2) protection against challenge [immunity index = the $\log_{10}$ increase in dose required to cause the immunized host to respond (die) at the same time as the unimmunized host], (3) level of toxin in the blood at death, (4) number of bacilli in the blood at death, and (5) units of *in vitro* toxin neutralized per milliliter of serum. The results showed: (1) PA protected both the guinea pig and rat against spore challenge but did not protect the rat against toxin challenge, (2) LF protected both the guinea pig and rat against spore challenge and the rat against toxin challenge, (3) EF was nonimmunogenic in either the guinea pig or rat, (4) LF and PA were additive, (5) EF interacted both with LF alone and LF plus PA to increase resistance in the rat but was not additive in the guinea pig, and (6) the number of bacilli and units of toxin per milliliter in the blood decreased as immunity increased and were therefore inversely related to host resistance. Essentially, only LF-immunized guinea pigs developed antigen–antibody precipitin lines on Ouchterlony plates, while rat sera were all negative. Serum antibody binding titers were not conclusive. Fish *et al.* (1968a) showed that greatly increased immunization was produced by equivalent amounts of purified PA compared to crude culture filtrates.

J. ANTIGEN-LIVE VACCINE INTERACTION

Consistent, tremendously increased resistance has been noted following booster with live vaccine (Table VI) (Klein *et al.*, 1962b, 1963b). The injection of additional antigen or of live vaccine results in a 2.5 or 5.0 $\log_{10}$ increase, respectively, in resistance to challenge. This suggests that the present antigen and/or procedure is incomplete regarding development of full immunity in experimental animals and presumably in man.

When immunity is developed with the PA_5 (5 injections of PA) plus live vaccine, guinea pigs were not killed by doses of 1×10^9 spores (Klein *et al.*, 1962b) or rhesus monkeys by 1×10^{10} spores (Lincoln *et al.*, 1964a).

K. VARIATION IN IMMUNITY PROTOCOLS

The rabbit, which was used by essentially all early workers for immunization studies, does not demonstrate a dose–response curve through an 8-log spore dose (Walker *et al.*, 1967) and is heterogeneous to edema test

TABLE VI

RESPONSE OF GUINEA PIGS IMMUNIZED BY DIFFERENT PROTOCOLS
USING BELTON-STRANGE OR 30R LIVE VACCINE[a]

Immunization protocol[b]	Day of injection of antigen			Mean time to death (hours)	Immunity index[c]
	PA (0.1 ml)	PA (1.0 ml)	10^7 spores		
Control	0	0	0	22	0
PA_5	1,3,5,9,11	0	0	32	3.2
PA_5+PA_1	1,3,5,9,11	22	0	48	5.8
PA_5+LV_1	1,3,5,9,11	0	22	91	8.2
PA_1	0	1	0	32	3.2
LV_1	0	0	1	23	0

[a] From Klein *et al.* (1962a).

[b] The subscript number refers to the number of injections of the indicated component.

[c] Immunity index is the $\log_{10}$ increase in dose required to cause the immunized host to respond (die) at the same time as the control.

response (Belton and Henderson, 1956). Rabbits, rhesus monkeys, and sheep appear to respond readily to immunization—guinea pigs less so, and rats and mice the least. The Fischer 344 rat, which is highly resistant to anthrax, has several unique features that make it an excellent and necessary host in immunization studies: (1) it immunizes readily to LF (Mahlandt *et al.*, 1966); (2) it is killed rapidly by low doses of toxin; and (3) it responds uniformly to toxin (Haines *et al.*, 1965). Because no model exists for extrapolation from experimental hosts to man, it is essential that a variety of species be used before generalization as to antigen (kind, quantity, and ratio) or route of challenge is made. Another aspect of experimentation generally overlooked is that almost all animals used are very young—rats and guinea pigs usually are about one-half and rhesus monkeys one-eighth of the adult weight. The immunological competence of young animals may not be fully developed and may differ from mature animals not only in response to antigens but also in the persistence of immunity. Finally, it should be noted that immunization increases the statistical variance of a test (DeArmon *et al.*, 1961) because the variance in immunological response is superimposed on the variance attributable to challenge.

The same amount of antigen given as a series is more effective than when given as one injection. This is probably part of the reason why the live vaccine results in high immunity, as toxin is released over a period of time. It is possible, too, that the antigens when released from the bacterial cell *in vivo* are in a different molecular configuration than those exposed to the stresses of processing *in vitro.* The ID, SC, IP, and IM routes of administration have been used and probably affect immunity relatively little. No detectable difference was found in immunity to challenge of guinea pigs immunized either IP or IM (Klein *et al.*, 1963b) or IC, IP, or SC (Wright *et al.*, 1954b).

Apparently, the development of immunity confers resistance against all routes of challenge—respiratory, oral, and parenteral—but quantitative resistance varies with the route of challenge. The natural challenge of man is respiratory (woolen and goat-hair factories) or cutaneous (contact with infected materials), or in a few areas, oral (incompletely cooked food), whereas challenge of grazing animals probably is chiefly oral, with respiratory and cutaneous challenge being minor. The most significant and applicable information concerning protection for man will result from studies on aerosol and oral challenge, and much more work needs to be done along these lines. The work with cattle (Schlingman *et al.*, 1956) using oral challenge should be noted for the problems involved in developing a satisfactory challenge for a species not in general experimental use.

L. Collection of Multiple Data

It is unfortunate that more data are not obtained from each experiment as this is largely a matter of planning and concentration of effort. The need to be highly efficient seems obvious when certain species are used; i.e., chimpanzee (critically scarce and verging on extinction) or horses or cattle (unusually expensive). Even with the small, easily raised species, man has a moral obligation while experimenting to obtain as humanely as possible as much useful information as possible. We suggest that the customary observation of whether an animal is alive or not at the beginning and end of the working day is not only inefficient but also scientifically questionable. Continuous observations can be obtained with time-lapse photography, and temperature changes and other physiological parameters can be monitored electronically. The problem of determining the optimum concentration of antigen and the best protocol for immunization is difficult, and Stanley and Smith (1963) and H. Smith (1964) have called it unsolvable because of the large number of animals needed. However, Mahlandt et al. (1966), state that the problem can be solved by using (1) modern statistical design, such as the factorial experiment, (2) quantitative methods, such as the immunity index, and (3) multiple criteria of evaluation, such as five criteria rather than one to evaluate immunity.

M. Summary and Future Research

Six types of "protective antigen" vaccine have been developed; however, only "chemical" antigens (those produced in media lacking serum or tissue extracts) have been developed extensively. While the chemical antigens undoubtedly increase resistance to anthrax challenge, it remains to be seen if their use can control anthrax in a high-risk area. Immunity developed by the chemical vaccine does not equal that obtained with either the living vaccine (Sterne strain) or protective antigen plus live vaccine, and antibody titer is low and transitory. It is quite likely that large amounts of antigen, more frequent boosters, and the addition of more components or live, attenuated spores would greatly enhance the potency of the vaccine.

Brachman (1966) reviewed industrial inhalation anthrax, presented data showing the cases of anthrax for the past 52 years, noted that anthrax is becoming extinct in the United States; he attributed this to the introduction of the chemical vaccine in 1955. However, the long-term trend has not changed slope, and it is possible that other factors (e.g., better ventilation, dust control, cleaner sources of wool or hair) are more important than immunization (Gold, 1967).

Now that methods are available for the purification of each component, the vaccine composition (i.e., number, ratio, and molecular state) as well as the protocol used (i.e., number and interval between injection and amount of antigen used) should be carefully reevaluated. Russian workers (Aleksandrov *et al.*, 1960) have given live vaccine by the aerosol route with high effectiveness. A parallel study immunizing with toxin components would be tremendously interesting. The need for still other general ways to immunize was brought to our attention by Pienaar (personal communication), who notes that anthrax is a very grave threat for the continued existence of the magnificent game preserves or parks in Africa and that consideration has been given to the possibility of immunizing *per os*. Such a method would be feasible because the number of watering holes are few during the dry season. Results of *per os* administration would be fully as interesting as those of the aerogenic route. No large-scale field tests have been conducted with any of the chemical vaccines.

The most difficult problem is to develop a model for man. Extrapolation from animals is dangerous, and, in contrast with other diseases, so few cases occur in those parts of the world where adequate records are maintained that little useful data accumulates. We must develop more sophisticated approaches, using material readily available from man (blood, serum, white blood cell count, circulating antibody) to determine the correct status of any person's immunity.

IX. General Summary

The general nature of anthrax toxin may be considered from three aspects: (1) its function in the bacterial cell, (2) its use as a research tool in toxicology, and (3) its unique host–parasite interaction.

The recent separation and purification of each component of toxin opens the way for more critical studies on all aspects of this toxin than has thus far been possible. The literature on anthrax and its toxin is confused by a lack of specific quantitation so that use of better materials and multiple assay procedures is quite desirable.

Bacillus anthracis produces a compound toxin composed of at least three proteins or lipoproteins. Little is known concerning the chemical composition of the components or of the pathway(s) leading to their synthesis. There is ample evidence that the molecular configuration and/or extent of aggregation of the individual components as well as of the whole toxin, can vary depending upon purity and/or physical environment; however, we have no real understanding of this phenomena. Since the organism is not an obligate parasite and since synthesis of toxin requires expenditure of a significant amount of energy by the cell, it is logical to suppose that the toxin is somehow useful in the organism. Some knowledge concerning the kinetics of toxin production and its function in the cell is desperately needed. We suggest that this information might form a basis for understanding the larger problems of evolution among species and the development of pathogenicity or saprophyticity. Why is a complex toxin evolutionarily selective; why not a simple toxin or a still more complex one? Perhaps the molecular heterogeneity of the toxin molecule gives it some selective advantage. It is intriguing that, in the sporogenic *Bacillus-Clostridium* complex, many species produce either toxins, antibiotics, or pigments. Are these apparently different materials related in some fashion? If so, antibiotic production might reflect a mutational event leading to a slightly altered toxin. *Bacillus anthracis* and *B. cereus*, held by some (N. R. Smith *et al.*, 1952) to be the same species, produce toxins giving distinctly different host responses, use of which Bonventre and Eckert (1963) have suggested as a means of species identification.

As a research tool in toxicology, anthrax toxin is not an ideal agent since it causes multiple responses; however, certain unique responses suggest its use until simpler material becomes available. Because it is composed of three components, each of which is nonlethal in purified form, this toxin offers the chance to study certain interactions not possible with other toxic materials. It is one of the few materials of rather large molecular weight that can affect the central nervous system rapidly and should prove useful in studying the "blood–brain" barrier and possibly, when employed in sublethal concentrations, for effecting the passage of other drugs into the central nervous system. A pulmonary edema of controlled time and possibly intensity can be developed in the Fischer 344 rat. This edema probably is of central nervous system origin and makes anthrax toxin a new tool for research in this area. Another phenomenon which warrants investigation is the extraordinarily low level of oxygen in the arterial blood at death. What mechanism operates which results in depletion of essentially all oxygen, whereas with drowning, suffocation, and certain diseases (Nordberg *et al.*, 1961), the oxygen level does not fall below 5–6%? The fact that either time to death or time for the development of edema cannot be reduced below a minimum period, even with increased toxin concentration, indicates that its action is not enzymatic. Whether the epinephrine-like material recently described in culture filtrates (Williams *et al.*, 1967) is related to toxin is not known, since the absence of toxin or components was assumed.

The interaction of this pathogen or its toxin with the host is of particular interest because establishment or treatment of the disease and the terminal toxemia can be studied separately. The inverse relationship between the dose of spores required to establish anthrax and the level of bacilli or toxin in the blood of the host at death from anthrax has been presented in this paper and treated more fully elsewhere (Lincoln *et al.*, 1967). Susceptible hosts requiring a low dose of spores to establish anthrax die only after a high level of toxin (or bacilli) is reached in the blood, whereas resistant hosts die with much lower levels of toxin. The relationship is so strong that coincidence does not seem likely, and a study based on this relationship should determine whether man reacts as a susceptible or resistant host.

With increased demand for meat and the general lack of research interest on anthrax, the worldwide incidence of anthrax is likely to increase. If so, the need for a field-tested vaccine proven to produce a long-lasting, high level of immunity and administerable by a simple protocol adaptable for massive use will be increased. Likewise, since the incidence of human cases tend to change directly in relation to the incidence of anthrax in the animal population, the treatment of anthrax infection and toxemia, both of which have been successfully accomplished experimentally, must be extended and applied to man. We hope that the fact that anthrax is a toxigenic disease and must be treated as a toxigenic disease will be recognized more widely and that quantitative data on man will increase.

REFERENCES

Albrink, W. S. (1961). *Bacteriol. Rev.* **25**, 268.
Aleksandrov, N. I., Gefen, N. E., Egorova, N. B., Sergeev, V. M., Matyuk, P. D., and Smirnov, M. S. (1960). *Zh. Mikrobiol., Epidemiol. i. Immunobiol.* **31**, 1307.
Aleksandrov, N. I., Gefen, N. E., Budak, A. P., Ezepchuk, Yu. V., Filippenko, A. I., and Runova, V. F. (1961). *Zh. Mikrobiol., Epidemiol. i. Immunobiol.* **32**, No. 5, 42.
Aleksandrov, N. I., Gefen, N. E., Ezepchuk, Yu. V., Budak, A. P., and Runova, V. F. (1962). *Zh. Mikrobiol., Epidemiol. i. Immunobiol.* **33**, No. 4, 63.
Aleksandrov, N. I., Gefen, N. E., Budak, A. P., Runova, V. F., Ezepchuk, Yu., V., and Bachinov, A. G. (1963). *Zh. Mikrobiol., Epidemiol. i. Immunobiol.* **34**, No. 3, 32.
Aleksandrov, N. I., Gefen, N. E., Runova, V. F., and Ezepchuk, Yu. V. (1964). *Zh. Mikrobiol., Epidemiol. i. Immunobiol.* **35**, 119.
Altenbern, R. A., and Stull, H. B. (1965). *J. Gen. Microbiol.* **39**, 53.
Anonymous. (1965). *Brit. Med. J.* **II**, 717.
Archer, L. J., and Gray, I. (1967). *Broteria* **35**, 169.
Auerbach, S., and Wright, G. G. (1955). *J. Immunol.* **75**, 129.
Bail, O. (1904). *Zentr. Bakteriol. Parasitenk., Abt. I. Orig.* **37**, 270.
Bail, O., and Weil, E. (1911). *Arch. Hyg. Bakteriol.* **73**, 218.
Beall, F. A., and Dalldorf, F. G. (1966). *J. Infect. Diseases* **116**, 377.
Beall, F. A., Taylor, M. J., and Thorne, C. B. (1962). *J. Bacteriol.* **83**, 1274.
Belton, F. C., and Henderson, D. W. (1956). *Brit. J. Exptl. Pathol.* **37**, 156.
Belton, F. C., and Strange, R. E. (1954). *Brit. J. Exptl. Pathol.* **35**, 144.
Bernheimer, A. W., and Schwartz, L. L. (1964). *J. Bacteriol.* **87**, 1100
Bonventre, P. F. (1965). *J. Bacteriol.* **90**, 284.

Bonventre, P. F., and Eckert, N. J. (1963). *J. Bacteriol.* **85**, 490.

Bonventre, P. F., Lincoln, R. E., and Lamanna, C. (1967a). *Bacteriol. Rev.* **31**, 95.

Bonventre, P. F., Sueoka, W., True, C. W., Klein, F., and Lincoln, R. E. (1967b). *Federation Proc.* **26**, 1549.

Boor, A. K. (1954). *J. Infect. Diseases* **96**, 194.

Boor, A. K., and Tresselt, H. B. (1954a). *J. Infect. Diseases* **97**, 203.

Boor, H. B., and Tresselt, A. K. (1954b). *J. Infect. Diseases* **97**, 207.

Brachman, P. S. (1966). *Antimicrobial Agents Chemotherapy* p. 111.

Brachman, P. S., Plotkin, S. A., Bumford, F. H., and Atchison, M. M. (1960). *Am. J. Hyg.* **72**, 6.

Brachman, P. S., Gold, H., Plotkin, S. A., Fekety, F. R., Werrin, M., and Ingraham, N. R. (1962). *Am. J. Public Health* **52**, 632.

Brewer, C. R., McCullough, W. G., Mills, R. C., Roessler, W. G., Herbst, E. J., and Howe, A. F. (1946). *Arch. Biochem. Biophys.* **10**, 65.

Buzzell, A. (1967). *Federation Proc.* **26**, 1522.

Cecil, R. L., and Loeb, R. F. (1959). *In* "Textbook of Medicine" (R. L. Cecil and R. F. Loeb, Eds.) 10th ed., Vol. I, pp. 170-178 and 733-737. Saunders, Philadelphia, Pennsylvania.

Cromartie, W. J., Bloom, W. L., and Watson, D. L. (1947a). *J. Infect. Diseases* **80**, 1.

Cromartie, W. J., Watson, D. W., Bloom, W. L., and Heckly, R. J. (1947b). *J. Infect. Diseases* **80**, 14.

Dalldorf, F. G., and Beall, F. A. (1967). *Arch. Pathol.* **83**, 154.

DeArmon, I. A., Jr., Klein, F., Lincoln, R. E., Mahlandt, B. G., and Fernelius, A. L. (1961). *J. Immunol.* **87**, 233.

Desaulles, F., Schar, B., and Meier, R. (1956). *Schweiz. Z. Allgem. Pathol. Bakteriol.* **19**, 639.

Dieva, N. N. (1965). *Zh. Mikrobiol., Epidemiol. i. Immunobiol.* **36**, No. 2, 143.

Dordevic, B. (1951). *Veterinaria, Sarajevo* **1**, 111.

Eckert, N. J., and Bonventre, P. F. (1963). *J. Infect. Diseases* **112**, 226.

Evans, D. G., and Shoesmith, J. G. (1954). *Lancet* **I**, 136.

Fish, D. C., and Lincoln, R. E. (1967). *Federation Proc.* **26**, 1534.

Fish, D. C., and Lincoln, R. E. (1968). *J. Bacteriol.* **95**, 919.

Fish, D. C., Mahlandt, B. G., Dobbs, J. P., and Lincoln, R. E. (1968a). *J. Bacteriol.* **95**, 907.

Fish, D. C., Klein, F., Lincoln, R. E., Walker, J. S., and Dobbs, J. P. (1968b). *J. Infect. Diseases* **118**, 114.

Ginsburg, N. N. (1964). *In* "Anthrax: Problems of Immunology, Clinque and Laboratory Diagnosis" (E. N. Shliaknov, ed.), pp. 4-21. "Kartia Moldoveniaske" State Press, Kishinev.

Ginsburg, N. N., and Fedotova, Yu. M. (1963). *Zh. Mikrobiol., Epidemiol. i. Immunobiol.* **34**, No. 11, 3.

Ginsburg, N. N., and Maslova, T. N. (1963). *Zh. Mikrobiol., Epidemiol. i. Immunobiol.* **34**, No. 4, 62.

Gladstone, G. P. (1946). *Brit. J. Exptl. Pathol.* **27**, 394.

Gladstone, G. P. (1948). *Brit. J. Exptl. Pathol.* **29**, 379.

Gochenour, W. S., Jr., Gleiser, C. A., Gaspar, A., Overholt, E. L., Kuehne, R. W., Byron, W. R., and Tigertt, W. D. (1961). *U. S. Army Med. Unit, Ann. Rept.* 3405.5, Part 2.

Gold, H. (1967). *Federation Proc.* **26**, 1563.

Gray, I., and Archer, L. J. (1966). *Am. J. Physiol.* **210**, 1313.

Gray, I., and Archer, L. J. (1967). *J. Bacteriol.* **93**, 36.

Haines, B. W., Klein, F., and Lincoln, R. E. (1965). *J. Bacteriol.* 89, 74.

Harris-Smith, P. W., Smith, H., and Keppie, J. (1958). *J. Gen. Microbiol.* 19, 91.

Heckley, R. J., Goldwasser, E., and Kefauver, D. (1949). *J. Infect. Diseases* 84, 91.

Henderson, D. W., Peacock, S., and Belton, F. C. (1956). *J. Hyg.* 54, 28.

Ivanovics, G. (1962). *J. Gen. Microbiol.* 28, 87.

Ivanovics, G. (1964). *Ann. Microbiol. Enzimol.* 14, 59.

Jackson, F. C., Wright, G. G., and Armstrong, J. (1957). *Am. J. Vet. Res.* 18, 771.

Jones, W. I., Jr., Klein, F., Walker, J. S., Mahlandt, B. G., Dobbs, J. P., and Lincoln, R. E. (1967a). *J. Bacteriol.* 94, 600.

Jones, W. I., Jr., Klein, F., Lincoln, R. E., Walker, J. S., Mahlandt, B. G., and Dobbs, J. P. (1967b). *J. Bacteriol.* 94, 609.

Kashiba, S., Morishima, T., Kato, K., Shima, M., and Armans, T. (1959). *Biken's J.* 2, 97.

Keppie, J., Smith, H., and Harris-Smith, P. W. (1953). *Brit. J. Exptl. Pathol.* 34, 486.

Keppie, J., Smith, H., and Harris-Smith, P. W. (1955). *Brit. J. Exptl. Pathol.* 36, 315.

Keppie, J., Harris-Smith, P. W., and Smith, H. (1963). *Brit. J. Exptl. Pathol.* 44, 446.

Klein, F., Mahlandt, B. G., Lincoln, R. E., DeArmon, I. A., Jr., and Fernelius, A. L. (1961). *Science* 133, 1021.

Klein, F., Hodge, D. R., Mahlandt, B. G., Jones, W. I., Jr., and Lincoln, R. E. (1962a). *Science* 138, 1331.

Klein, F., DeArmon, I. A., Jr., Lincoln, R. E., Mahlandt, B. G., and Fernelius, A. J. (1962b). *J. Immunol.* 88, 15.

Klein, F., Haines, B. W., Mahlandt, B. G., DeArmon, I. A., Jr., and Lincoln, R. E. (1963a). *J. Bacteriol.* 85, 1032.

Klein, F., Haines, B. W., Mahlandt, B. G., and Lincoln, R. E. (1963b). *J. Immunol.* 91, 431.

Klein, F., Walker, J. S., Fitzpatrick, D. F., Lincoln, R. E., Mahlandt, B. G., Jones, W. I., Jr., Dobbs, J. P., and Hendrix, K. J. (1966). *J. Infect. Diseases* 116, 123.

Klein, F., Lincoln, R. E., Mahlandt, B. G., Dobbs, J. P., and Walker, J. S. (1967). *Proc. Soc. Exptl. Biol. Med.* 124, 678.

Klein, F. G., Lincoln, R. E., Dobbs, J. P., Mahlandt, B. G., Remmele, N. S., and Walker, J. S. (1968). *J. Infect. Diseases* 118, 97.

Konikova, R. Ye., Noskov, F. S., and Syagayev, A. O. (1966). *Zh. Mikrobiol., Epidemiol. i. Immunobiol.* 43, 45.

Lincoln, R. E., Walker, J. S., Klein, F., and Haines, B. W. (1964a). *Advan. Vet. Sci.* 9, 327.

Lincoln, R. E., Klein, F., Walker, J. S., Haines, B. W., Jones, W. I., Jr., Mahlandt, B. G., and Friedman, R. H. (1964b). *Antimicrobial Agents Chemotherapy* p. 759.

Lincoln, R. E., Walker, J. S., Klein, F., Rosenwald, A. J., and Jones, W. I., Jr. (1967). *Federation Proc.* 26, 1558.

McCloy, E. W. (1951). *J. Hyg.* 49, 114.

McGann, V. G., Stearman, R. L., and Wright, G. G. (1961). *J. Immunol.* 86, 458.

Mahlandt, B. G., Klein, F., Lincoln, R. E., Haines, B. W., Jones, W. I., Jr., and Friedman, R. H. (1966). *J. Bacteriol.* 96, 727.

Mashkov, A. V. (1958). *In* "Siberskaya Yazva," pp. 1–36. Min. Public Health USSR, Moscow.

Matz, M. H., and Brugsch, H. G. (1964). *J. Am. Med. Assoc.* 188, 115.

Meynell, G. G. and Meynell, E. (1966). *J. Gen. Microbiol.* 43, 119.

Middleton, G. K., and Standen, A. C. (1961). *J. Infect. Diseases* 108, 85.

Molnar, D. M., and Altenbern, R. A. (1963). *Proc. Soc. Exptl. Biol. Med.* 114, 294.

National Academy of Sciences. (1962). "Tropical Health," Publ. No. 999, p. 161. Natl. Acad. Sci.—Natl. Res. Council, Washington, D.C.

Nilsson, G. M. (1934). *Nebraska State Med. J.* 19, 457.

Nordberg, B. K., Schmiterlow, G. G., and Hansen, H.-J. (1961). *Acta Pathol. Microbiol. Scand.* 53, 295.

Norman, P. S., Ray, J. G., Jr., Brachman, P. S., Plotkin, S. A., and Pagano, J. S. (1960). *Am. J. Hyg.* 72, 32.

Nungester, W. J. (1967). *Federation Proc.* 26, 1483.

Opie, E. L. (1923). *J. Immunol.* 8, 55.

Ouchterlony, O. (1953). *Acta Pathol. Microbiol. Scand.* 32, 231.

Puziss, M., and Howard, M. B. (1963). *J. Bacteriol.* 85, 237.

Puziss, M., and Wright, G. G. (1954). *J. Bacteriol.* 68, 474.

Puziss, M., and Wright, G. G. (1959). *J. Bacteriol.* 78, 137.

Puziss, M., and Wright, G. G. (1963). *J. Bacteriol.* 85, 230.

Puziss, M., Manning, L. C., Lynch, J. W., Barclay, E., Abelow, I., and Wright, G. G. (1963). *Appl. Microbiol.* 11, 330.

Quastel, J. H. (1957). *In* "Metabolism of the Nervous System" (D. Richter, ed.), pp. 267–285. Pergamon Press, Oxford.

Rapoport, M. I., Hodoval, L. F., Grogan, E. W., McGann, V., and Beisel, W. R. (1966). *J. Clin. Invest.* 45, 1365.

Ray, J. G., Jr., and Kadull, P. J. (1964). *Appl. Microbiol.* 12, 349.

Remmele, N. S., Klein, F., Vick, J. A., Walker, J. S., Mahlandt, B. G., and Lincoln, R. E. (1968). *J. Infect. Diseases* 118, 104.

Reynolds, R. W. (1963). *Science* 141, 930.

Riemann, H. A. (1966). *Postgrad. Med.* 42, 247.

Rosenwald, A. J., Felkner, I. C., and Lincoln, R. E. (1963). *Bacteriol. Proc.* p. 138.

Salisbury, C. E. (1926). *J. Am. Vet. Med. Assoc.* 68, 755.

Sargeant, K., Stanley, J. L., and Smith, H. (1960). *J. Gen. Microbiol.* 22, 219.

Schlingman, A. S., Devlin, H. B., Wright, G. G., Maine, R. J., and Manning, M. C. (1956). *Am. J. Vet. Res.* 17, 256.

Shliakhov, E. N., ed. (1964). "Anthrax: Problems of Immunology, Clinique and Laboratory Diagnosis," "Kartia Moldoveniaske" State Press, Kishinev.

Shliakhov, E. N., and Shroit, I. G. (1964). *J. Hyg., Epidemiol., Microbiol., Immunol. (Prague)* 8, 307.

Shliakhov, E. N., Shroit, I. G., and Burdenko, T. A. (1965). *Zh. Mikrobiol., Epidemiol. i. Immunobiol.* 36, No. 3, 106.

Simpson, R. M. (1966). *Bull. Epizootic Disease Africa* 14, 391.

Slein, M. W., and Logan, G. F., Jr. (1960). *J. Bacteriol.* 80, 77.

Smith, H. (1958). *Ann. Rev. Microbiol.* 12, 77.

Smith, H. (1964). *Symp. Soc. Gen. Microbiol.* 14, 1.

Smith, H., and Gallop, R. C. (1956). *Brit. J. Exptl. Pathol.* 37, 144.

Smith, H., and Keppie, J. (1954). *Nature* 173, 869.

Smith, H., and Keppie, J. (1955). *Symp. Soc. Gen. Microbiol.* 5, 126.

Smith, H., and Stanley, J. L. (1962). *J. Gen. Microbiol.* 29, 517.

Smith, H., and Stoner, H. B. (1967). *Federation Proc.* 26, 1554.

Smith, H., and Tempest, D. W. (1957). *J. Gen. Microbiol.* 17, 731.

Smith, H., Keppie, J., and Stanley, J. L. (1953). *Brit. J. Exptl. Pathol.* 34, 471.

Smith, H., Keppie, J., Ross, J. M., and Stanley, J. L. (1954). *Lancet* II, 474.

Smith, H., Keppie, J., Stanley, J. L., and Harris-Smith, P. W. (1955a). *Brit. J. Exptl. Pathol.* 36, 323.

Smith, H., Keppie, J., and Stanley, J. L. (1955b). *Brit. J. Exptl. Pathol.* 36, 460.

Smith, H., Tempest, D. W., Stanley, J. L., Harris-Smith, P. W., and Gallop, R. C. (1956a). *Brit. J. Exptl. Pathol.* 37, 263.

Smith, H., Zwartouw, H. T., and Harris-Smith, P. W. (1956b). *Brit. J. Exptl. Pathol.* 37, 361.

Smith, N. R., Gordon, R. E., and Clark, F. E. (1952). *U. S. Dept. Agr., Agr. Monograph* No. 16, 1.

Stamatin, N. (1964a). *Rec. Med. Vet. Ecole Alfort* 140, 639.

Stamatin, N. (1964b). *Rec. Med. Vet. Ecole Alfort* 140, 735.

Stanley, J. L., and Smith, H. (1961). *J. Gen. Microbiol.* 26, 49.

Stanley, J. L., and Smith, H. (1963). *J. Gen. Microbiol.* 31, 329.

Stanley, J. L., Sargeant, K., and Smith, H. (1960). *J. Gen. Microbiol.* 22, 206.

Sterne, M. (1948a). *Onderstepoort J. Vet. Res.* 23, 157.

Sterne, M. (1948b). *Onderstepoort J. Vet. Res.* 23, 165.

Sterne, M. (1959). *In* "Infectious Diseases of Animals. Diseases Due to Bacteria" (A. W. Stableford and J. A. Galloway, eds.), Vol. I, pp. 16–52. Butterworth, Toronto.

Sterne, M. (1961). *In* "The Veterinary Annual" (W. A. Pool, ed.), pp. 70–73. Wright, Bristol, England.

Sterne, M., Nicol, J., and Lambrecht, M. C. (1942). *J. S. African Vet. Med. Assoc.* 13, 53.

Stevenson, J. W. (1962). *In* "Neurochemistry" (K.A.C. Elliott, I. H. Page, and J. H. Quastel, eds.), 2nd ed., pp. 813–839. Thomas, Springfield, Illinois.

Strange, R. E., and Belton, F. C. (1954). *Brit. J. Exptl. Pathol.* 35, 153.

Strange, R. E., and Thorne, C. B. (1958). *J. Bacteriol.* 76, 192.

Tempest, D. W., and Smith, H. (1957). *J. Gen. Microbiol.* 17, 739.

Thorne, C. B. (1960). *Ann. N. Y. Acad. Sci.* 88, 1024.

Thorne, C. B., and Belton, F. C. (1957). *J. Gen. Microbiol.* 17, 505.

Thorne, C. B., Molnar, D. M., and Strange, R. E. (1960). *J. Bacteriol.* 79, 450.

Tresselt, H. B., and Boor, A. K. (1954). *J. Infect. Diseases* 97, 207.

Vancurik, J. (1964). *Folia Microbiol.* (*Prague*) 9, 164.

Vaughan, V. C., and Novy, F. G. (1902). *In* "Cellular Toxins," 4th ed. Lea Bros., New York.

Vick, J. A., Lincoln, R. E., Klein, F., Mahlandt, B. G., Walker, J. S., and Fish, D. C. (1968). *J. Infect. Diseases* 118, 85.

Walker, J. S., Lincoln, R. E., and Klein, F. (1967). *Federation Proc.* 26, 1539.

Ward, M. K., McGann, V. G., Hogge, A. L., Jr., Huff, M. L., Knode, R. G., Jr., and Roberts, E. O. (1965). *J. Infect. Diseases* 115, 59.

Watson, D. L., Cromartie, W. J., Bloom, W. L., Kegeles, G., and Heckly, R. J. (1947). *J. Infect. Diseases* 80, 28.

Wells, H. G. (1929). "The Chemical Aspects of Immunity," 2nd ed. Chem. Catalog Co., New York.

Wilkie, M. H., and Ward, M. K. (1967). *Federation Proc.* 26, 1527.

Williams, R. P., Hill, H. R., Hawkins, D., Jr., Chao, K.-W., Neuenschwander, J., and Lipscomb, H. S. (1967). *Federation Proc.* 26, 1545.

Wright, G. G. (1965). *In* "Bacterial and Mycotic Infections of Man" (R. J. Dubos and J. G. Hirsch, eds.), 4th ed., pp. 530–544. Lippincott, Philadelphia, Pennsylvania.

Wright, G. G., and Luksas, A. J. (1964). *Federation Proc.* 23, 191.

Wright, G. G., and Puziss, M. (1957). *Nature* 179, 916.

Wright, G. G., and Wedum, A. G. (1954). *In* "A Symposium on Anthrax in Man," pp. 136–144. Univ. of Pennsylvania Press, Philadelphia, Pennsylvania.

Wright, G. G., Hedberg, M. A., and Feinberg, R. J. (1951). *J. Exptl. Med.* 93, 523.

Wright, G. G., Hedberg, M. A., and Slein, J. B. (1954a). *J. Immunol.* **72**, 263.

Wright, G. G., Green, T. W., and Kanode, R. O., Jr. (1954b). *J. Immunol.* **73**, 387.

Wright, G. G., Puziss, M., and Neely, W. B. (1962). *J. Bacteriol.* **83**, 515.

Yablokov, N. A. (1950). *In* "Profilaktika Zabolevaniy Sibirskoy Yaznoy na Proizrodstre (Prophylaxis of Malignant Anthrax in Production)," pp. 1–31. Moscow.

Young, G. A., Jr., and Zelle, M. R. (1946). *J. Infect. Diseases* **79**, 266.

Zhdanov, W. M. (1961). *In* "The Role of Immunization in Communicable Disease Control," Public Health Paper No. 8. World Health Organ., Geneva.

CHAPTER 10

Bacillus cereus Toxin

PETER F. BONVENTRE AND CHARLES E. JOHNSON

I. Historical Background

The fact that *Bacillus cereus* synthesizes materials which might be considered toxins has been appreciated only within the recent past. This aerobic spore-forming bacillus has been considered almost exclusively as one of the ubiquitous, saprophytic members of the Bacillaceae. Were it not for the fact that *B. cereus* presented a diagnostic problem by virtue of its similarity to *Bacillus anthracis*, it probably would have been ignored within the context of clinical medicine. As will be pointed out in the discussion which follows, *B. cereus* is not always a benign bacterium. On the contrary, it can be associated with disease processes of man and animals. From the limited amount of information available to us at the present time, it appears that any virulence which this bacterial species exhibits is associated with one or more of its extracellular products.

With a few significant exceptions, investigations concerned with the toxicity of *B. cereus* products have been carried out with crude culture filtrates. Therefore, it is not possible to deduce from the results of these investigations the relative contribution to toxicity of the individual bacterial products in the filtrates. In addition, the use of unpurified filtrates does not allow the calculation of specific activities, nor can precise quantitative estimates of toxicity be made. In view of this situation, the authors are able to document in only a cursory and incomplete fashion the nature and properties of the toxin and other products of *B. cereus*.

It is not possible to discuss the lethal toxin of *B. cereus* without considering several of the other extracellular products of the organism. *Bacillus cereus* synthesizes significant amounts of penicillinase (Pollock, 1956), phospholipases (Slein and Logan, 1963, 1965), hemolysin (Bernheimer and Grushoff, 1967), and proteolytic enzymes (Gorini, 1950), and all of these materials can be detected readily in culture filtrates. Initially it was thought that the phospholipase, hemolytic, and lethal activities of the filtrates were in fact due to one product (McGaughey and Chu, 1948; Chu, 1949). This assumption was not unreasonable since a precedent for such a situation in the case of *Clostridium perfringens* α-toxin (lecithinase) had been established (Macfarlane and Knight, 1941). In the case of the clostridial toxin, the hemolytic, phospholipase, and lethal properties are exhibited by one protein. As will be seen, these three properties which are exhibited by *B. cereus* culture filtrates are in fact elicited by three distinct extracellular products of the organism (Johnson and Bonventre, 1967).

II. Production, Purification, and Synthesis

The importance of specific nutritional factors for the synthesis of microbial toxins is well documented; eg., *C. perfringens* α-toxin (Adams and Hendee, 1945; Adams *et al.*, 1947; Lichstein and Jayko, 1959; Hauschild, 1965; Nakamura *et al.*, 1968), tetanus toxin (Mueller and Miller, 1949), and diphtheria toxin (Mueller and Miller, 1940) are produced in significant amounts only if the proper nutritional environment is provided. Most investigations which have concerned themselves with the production of *B. cereus* toxin described culture media which supported toxin synthesis, but no attempts were made to elucidate specific nutritional and environmental factors which might influence toxin production by the microorganism (Thorne and Belton, 1957; Bonventre and Eckert, 1963a; Thorne *et al.*, 1960). Johnson (1966) attempted to define the nutritional requirements for toxin production by *B. cereus*. Excellent growth was obtained in all of the complex culture media tested; these included trypticase soy broth (BBL), nutrient broth (Difco), beef infusion broth (Difco), bacto peptone (Difco), and beef infusion broth prepared from fresh beef. Only the latter (fresh beef infusion), however, supported toxin synthesis consistently. The dehydrated commercially prepared beef infusion lacked essential requirements for toxin synthesis (Table I). Seitz filtration or dialysis of fresh beef infusion broth rendered the medium incapable of supporting toxin production. These observations suggested the presence in this medium of "toxigenic factor(s)" of low molecular weight. The fact that addition of the ashed dialyzate back to the dialyzed medium did not restore the ability to support toxin synthesis indicates that the factor is not a trace metal(s). As yet the chemical nature of the materials removed by dialysis and Seitz filtration from fresh beef infusion have not been identified.

Several semisynthetic and completely synthetic media were tested for their capacity to support growth and toxin production (Johnson, 1966). Media containing acid-hydrolyzed casamino acids (Difco) as the only

TABLE I

GROWTH AND TOXIN PRODUCTION BY *B. cereus* (B-48) IN COMPLEX MEDIA[a]

Time of incubation (hours)	Medium	Growth (optical density)	Toxin MLD/ml
17	Fresh beef infusion	0.260	20
	Beef infusion (Difco)	0.345	0
24	Fresh beef infusion	0.310	20
	Beef infusion (Difco)	0.405	0

[a]From Johnson (1966).

carbon and nitrogen sources allowed the production of toxin by *B. cereus*, but the toxin titers were significantly lower than those obtained by growth of the organism in fresh beef infusion broth. Addition of glucose and/or various peptides to the casamino acids medium or fresh beef infusion broth did not enhance toxin production. A synthetic amino acid–basal salt medium containing 18 amino acids (Tristram, 1953) was also found to support toxin production at a low level. Deletion of amino acids singly or in combination from the synthetic medium showed that proline and cystine were not essential for toxin synthesis (Table II). Amino acid antagonism was demonstrated when proline, cystine, serine, and phenylalanine were deleted from the 18 amino acids synthetic medium. In this medium no growth was observed. If threonine and tryptophan were also deleted,

TABLE II

LETHAL TOXIN PRODUCTION IN VARIOUS AMINO ACID MEDIA BY *B. cereus* (B-48) INCUBATED AT 30° AND 37° C[a]

Number of amino acids in medium	Amino acids deleted	Temperature (°C)	Growth (optical density)	Lethal toxin
18[b]	None (control)	30	0.326	+
		37	0.329	+
16	Proline, cystine	30	0.272	+
		37	0.356	+
14	Proline, cystine, serine, phenylalanine	30	0.038	−
		37	0.082	−
12	Proline, cystine, serine, phenylalanine, threonine, tryptophan	30	0.149	−
		37	0.300	−

[a]From Johnson (1966).
[b]Tristram (1953).

the resulting 12 amino acids containing synthetic medium supported excellent growth of *B. cereus*, but no toxin was detectable. Supplementation
of the complete synthetic medium with glucose, peptones, peptides, or B
vitamins either singly or in combination did not result in enhancement of
toxin synthesis by *B. cereus*.

The effect of the temperature of incubation on toxin synthesis was also
examined by Johnson (1966). He found that when the organism was
grown in fresh beef infusion broth, approximately twice as much toxin
was synthesized at 37° than at 30°C. The influence of temperature on
toxin production in the synthetic amino acids medium was not significant.
Growth of *B. cereus* at 37° and 30°C was comparable in both culture media. It is apparent from these studies that growth and toxin synthesis are
not necessarily concurrent phenomena. The synthesis of lethal toxin of *B.
cereus* is governed by specific nutritional requirements which are not essential for growth. It is not possible to say if the same restrictions apply
in vivo.

Thus far, the synthesis of only one extracellular product of *B. cereus*
has been considered; namely, the lethal toxin. As was mentioned previously, *B. cereus* produces several other substances which may contribute
to toxicity. Among these products are several phospholipases and hemolysins. Slein and Logan (1963) showed that one of the *B. cereus* phospholipase enzymes possessed phosphatasemia activity and designated the
material PF. They found that PF increased blood alkaline phosphatases
after intravenous injection into laboratory animals and also released alkaline phosphatase from epiphyseal bone slices. The original assumption
made by Chu (1949) that the hemolytic, phospholipase, and lethal activities exhibited by culture filtrates were due to one protein has been difficult
to disprove. A major difficulty is due to the fact that all three activities are
very closely associated and are difficult to separate by physical methods.
Molnar (1962) succeeded in fractionating culture filtrates of *B. cereus* on
columns of calcium phosphate gel so that the toxin was separated into two
nonlethal components. Lethality could be restored by combining the two
inactive fractions. Phospholipase activity was associated with only one of
the two nonlethal fractions but was not itself dissociated into inactive
subunits by this fractionation procedure. With DEAE—cellulose column
chromatography, however, separation of both the toxin and the phospholipase into inactive subunits was observed (Johnson, 1966). Toxicity and
enzymatic activities were regained when the DEAE–cellulose column
fractions were pooled. The significance of these observations is not clear.
Slein and Logan (1963) reported the presence of two distinct phospholipases in *B. cereus* culture filtrates which were separated on DEAE-
cellulose columns. The two enzymes possessed different sensitivi-

ties to trypsin, and PF activity was exhibited by only one of the two. The enzyme which did not show any PF activity was neither hemolytic nor lethal, while the enzyme which released alkaline phosphatase hemolyzed erythrocytes and killed mice. Slein and Logan (1965) subsequently reported that a purified *B. cereus* phospholipase was free of hemolytic activity when tested with rabbit and sheep erythrocytes. This corroborates the finding of Ottolenghi *et al.* (1961) that the "phospholipolytic" and hemolytic activities can be differentiated on the basis of differential thermal inactivation. A *B. cereus* hemolysin and egg yolk turbidity factor have also been separated by DEAE–cellulose chromatography (Fossum, 1963). It is not clear whether the egg yolk turbidity factor and the phospholipase are identical. Kushner (1957) found that the turbidity factor and phospholipase C have distinct heat stabilities and thus suggests that they may be separate entities. Bernheimer and Grushoff (1967) studied a potent hemolysin of *B. cereus* which they called "cereolysin." The hemolysin was purified by ammonium sulfate fractionation, density gradient electrophoresis, and Sephadex column chromatography. Cereolysin was devoid of phospholipase C activity but was lethal when injected into mice intravenously. The absence of phospholipase activity as measured by the egg yolk turbidity reaction indicated that the hemolysin (cereolysin) is distinct from the enzyme. This is in agreement with the observations of Johnson and Bonventre (1966) who showed that a partially purified *B. cereus* phospholipase preparation was neither lethal when injected into mice or hemolytic for rabbit or human erythrocytes. The latter authors also provided convincing evidence that the lethal toxin, hemolysin, and phospholipase are distinct proteins. Figure 1 shows that *B. cereus* culture filtrates can be resolved by Sephadex gel filtration and that the lethal toxin, hemolysin, and phospholipase are closely associated but different substances. Johnson (1966) demonstrated by means of thin-layer chromatography of lecithin degradation products that the *B. cereus* phospholipase is a phospholipase C and that the microorganism does not produce any phospholipase A, B, or D.

The temporal synthesis of the extracellular products of *B. cereus* during growth was also investigated as a means of differentiating them (Johnson, 1966). It was observed that the hemolytic, phospholipase C, and lethal activities appeared concurrently in the growth menstruum, but they diminished at different times and at different rates (Fig. 2). The rapid disappearance of phospholipase C activity following the attainment of a maximum after 4 hours of incubation at 37°C has been attributed to surface denaturation (Kushner, 1962). The hemolysin titer in the culture filtrate was at a maximum after 3 hours, while the toxin titer did not reach a maximum until 6 hours of incubation. Maximum titers of all three activities

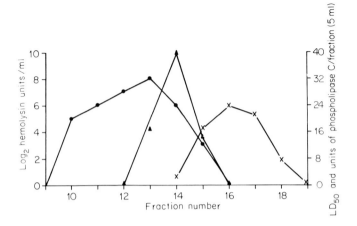

FIG. 1. Separation of toxin, hemolysin, and phospholipase C by gel filtration (Sephadex G-75). X = phospholipase C; 1 unit of enzyme is defined as the amount of enzyme required to liberate 100 μg of acid-soluble phosphorus from an egg yolk lecithin substrate in 45 minutes at 37°C. ▲ = toxin; expressed as $LD_{50}/5$ ml fraction. ● = hemolysin; expressed as $\log_2$ units of hemolysin per milliliter of eluate. From Johnson and Bonventre (1967).

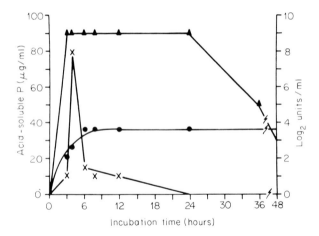

FIG. 2. Temporal synthesis of toxin, hemolysin, and phospholipase C by *B. cereus* cultured in fresh beef infusion at 37°C. ● = lethal toxin; activity expressed as $\log_2$ units per milliliter of culture filtrate (1 unit = 1 LD_{50}). ▲ = hemolysin; activity expressed as $\log_2$ units of hemolysin per milliliter of culture filtrate. X = phospholipase C; activity expressed as micrograms of acid soluble phosphorus per milliliter of trichloroacetic acid filtrate. From Johnson and Bonventre (1967).

were achieved before any evidence of bacterial lysis had occurred and suggests that the products are not associated with any cellular structures nor are they dependent upon lysis for their release. Indeed Bonventre (unpublished observations) found that washed *B. cereus* cells were entirely devoid of cell-associated or intracellular toxin as measured by the mouse lethality test. Altenbern and Stull (1964) reported that the release of *B. cereus* toxin and phospholipase was associated with a phage-mediated lysis of the bacteria and suggested that lysogeny and toxigenicity were related as they are in the case of diphtheria toxin (Freeman, 1951). The apparent discrepancies between Altenbern's and Johnson's observations may be explained by the fact that they used different strains of *B. cereus* as well as different assay methods for detection of toxin and phospholipase. Altenbern and Stull (1964) employed the edema skin test for toxin assay and the lecithovitellin reaction for the detection of phospholipase activity. Neither of these assay methods are quantitative nor are they completely reliable (Johnson, 1966). Figure 2 also shows that the titer of the *B. cereus* hemolysin remained unaltered between 3 and 24 hours and then rapidly diminished between 24 and 48 hours. The lethal toxin in the culture filtrate, in contrast, remained constant between the time it achieved a maximum at 6 hours until the termination of the incubation at 48 hours. The phospholipase enzyme activity declined rapidly so that only 20% of the maximum activity was detectable after 8 hours. These data corroborate the physical findings that the three activities reside in separate and distinct products of *B. cereus*.

The phospholipase C, hemolysin, and lethal toxin behave differently when subjected to various treatments. Slein and Logan (1965) characterized a *B. cereus* phospholipase which utilized both phosphatidylethanolamine and phosphatidylcholine (lecithin) as substrates and which was resistant to the action of trypsin. Johnson and Bonventre (1967) extended these observations by demonstrating that unlike the phospholipase C activity, hemolytic and lethal activities were rapidly inactivated by the proteolytic enzyme (Fig. 3). The three proteins also differ with respect to thermal inactivation. The *B. cereus* phospholipase is relatively resistant to the effects of elevated temperature (Ottolenghi *et al.*, 1961). Johnson (1966) showed that incubation at 56°C for 30 minutes virtually abolished hemolytic and lethal activities but had no significant effect on the phospholipase enzyme. At 45°C, however, the kinetics of inactivation of the hemolysin and the lethal toxin are distinct. Figure 4 shows that the hemolytic activity of *B. cereus* culture filtrates held at 45°C disappears rapidly while the lethal activity is affected only minimally.

The molecular weights of the *B. cereus* extracellular proteins have not

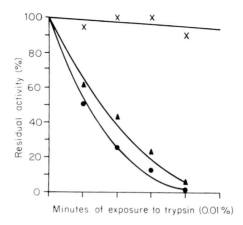

FIG. 3. Inactivation of *B. cereus* extracellular products by trypsin. Trypsin in borate buffer (0.05 *M*, pH 7.5) was added to *B. cereus* culture filtrates to a final concentration 0.01%. Mixtures were incubated at 37°C and samples were removed at the designated intervals. Trypsin was inactivated immediately after removal of the sample by soybean trypsin inhibitor. All three activities were unaltered after 2 hours at 37°C in the filtrate controls not treated with trypsin. ● = lethal toxin; ▲ = hemolysin; X = phospholipase C. From Johnson and Bonventre (1967).

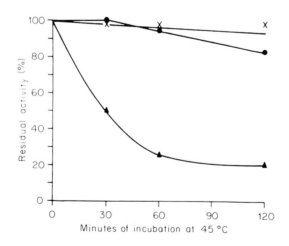

FIG. 4. Inactivation of *B. cereus* extracellular products at 45°C. Lethal toxin, hemolysin and phospholipase C titers were unaltered after 2 hours at 25°C (controls). ● = toxin; ▲ = hemolysin; X = phospholipase C. From Johnson and Bonventre (1967).

been determined precisely. The manner in which they are eluted from the Sephadex G75 columns (Fig. 1) would indicate that the molecular weights of the hemolysin, lethal toxin, and phospholipase C decrease in that order. Bernheimer and Grushoff (1967), on the basis of gel filtration and ultracentrifugation analysis, estimated the molecular weight of the *B. cereus* hemolysin (cereolysin) as about 50,000. No other biophysical characteristics of the toxin or the phospholipase are available at the present time.

The pH of cultures of *B. cereus* is typified by an initial decrease followed by a rise toward the alkaline range. The initiation of the pH rise after reaching a minimum has been shown to be the point at which the bacterial cells become committed to sporulation. The initial decrease in pH is the period of vegetative growth, and the time lapse between the termination of vegetative growth and the initiation of sporulation may be viewed as the transition period from vegetative to spore metabolism (Hanson *et al.*, 1963). As shown in Fig. 5C, the maximum titer of *B. cereus* lethal toxin is achieved during the transitional phase of growth in beef infusion broth (Johnson and Bonventre, 1967). Media which did not support toxin synthesis demonstrated no transition period as measured by the pH plateau at the lowest level (Figs. 5A and 5B) as was apparent with cultures grown in fresh beef infusion broth (Fig. 5C). These observations suggest that the synthesis of *B. cereus* toxin is associated with the transitional phase of growth. It is clear, however, that whatever the relationship between toxin synthesis and the shift in the metabolic pattern from that of

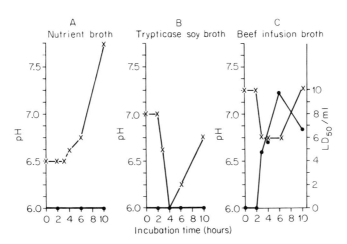

FIG. 5. Toxin synthesis and pH changes in several complex media during the growth of *B. cereus* at 37°C. ● = toxin; X = pH. From Johnson and Bonventre (1967).

the vegetative cell to the spore is, toxin synthesis is not a prerequisite for sporulation. Indeed, sporulation will occur in media which do not support the synthesis of detectable amounts of toxin (Johnson, 1966).

III. Toxicity

Nagler (1939) first described the effect of *Clostridium perfringens* toxic culture filtrates on human serum producing an opalescence and curding (Nagler reaction). Macfarlane and Knight (1941) subsequently showed that the reaction in an egg yolk emulsion (lecithovitellin reaction) was due to a lecithinase in the *Cl. perfringens* filtrates which was identical with the α-toxin. In his initial studies, Nagler (1939) observed a "nonpathogenic" aerobic spore-forming bacillus which caused the opalescence in human serum but which was not inhibited by *Cl. perfringens* antitoxin. Mc-Gaughey and Chu (1948) examined a large number of strains of aerobic bacilli and found that only *B. cereus* and to a lesser extent *B. anthracis* were able to produce the lecithovitellin reaction. As with the α-toxin of *Cl. perfringens*, the reaction was found to be due to the action of a phospholipase which cleaved lecithin into phosphorylcholine and a diglyceride. Such an enzyme is classified as a phospholipase C (Hayaishi, 1955). Chu (1949) compared the biological properties of *B. cereus* and *Cl. perfringens* culture filtrates and presented the first documented evidence that the former contain extracellular materials of a toxic nature. Using ammonium sulfate-precipitated culture filtrates, he found that in addition to giving positive Nagler and egg yolk reactions, they lysed red blood cells, were dermonecrotic when injected into rabbits and guinea pigs, and were lethal when injected into mice. Although it was reasonable for Chu to speculate that like the *Cl. perfringens* α-toxin, the *B. cereus* phospholipase and toxic activities were probably due to one protein, he did state in his paper that " . . . as the enzyme preparation is very crude, it is impossible to say whether its toxicity is due to lecithinase activity exclusively or to some other factors as well." More recent studies have shown that this cautious interpretation of his observations was warranted. Molnar (1962) compared the toxicity of *B. anthracis* and *B. cereus* culture filtrates in an effort to correlate toxicity with phospholipase activity. She found that the potent *B. cereus* phospholipase described by Chu was probably not responsible for toxicity. On the basis of differential precipitation from the culture filtrates of the two activities with ammonium sulfate, differential inhibition by ethanol, and separation of the toxin into two components only one of which was associated with phospholipase activity, she concluded that the toxin and the phospholipase were different molecules. In

Molnar's study, toxicity was measured either by lethality in mice following intravenous injection or by a guinea pig skin reaction which was characterized by an initial inflamatory reaction followed by necrosis after 24
hours. This lesion is similar although not as extensive as the lesion caused
by intradermal injection of viable virulent bacilli (Burdon *et al.*, 1967).
The skin lesion produced by *B. cereus* toxin, however, was found to be
markedly different from the edematous reaction caused by *B. anthracis*
toxin (Thorne *et al.*, 1960). The nature of the skin reaction is only one of
several differences in biological activity which have been documented for
B. cereus and *B. anthracis* culture filtrates. Bonventre and Eckert (1963b)
found that *B. cereus* toxin is extremely rapid in its activity. Mice injected
intravenously with 0.5 ml of a culture filtrate usually died within 5 minutes.
Culture filtrates of virulent *B. anthracis*, however, had no significant lethal activity in mice (Table III). These same *B. anthracis* filtrates, however, were lethal when injected into Fischer 344 albino rats, showing that
anthrax toxin was present (Eckert, 1963). The Fischer 344 rat is the animal of choice for assay of the anthrax toxin, and the potency of toxin
preparations is usually expressed in rat units (Haines *et al.*, 1965). The
difference in the lethal activity for mice of the culture filtrates of *B. cereus*
and *B. anthracis* grown in fresh beef infusion broth can be employed as a

TABLE III

TOXICITY OF CULTURE FILTRATES OF *B. cereus* AND *B. anthracis*[a]

Organism	Number of mice injected	Mortality (%)
B. cereus "X"[b]	300	100
B. cereus B-47[b]	50	100
B. cereus B-48[b]	50	100
B. cereus B-49[b]	50	100
B. cereus Ba-21[c]	50	100
B. cereus Ba-25[c]	50	100
B. cereus ATCC 10987	50	100
B. anthracis VIB[d]	50	0
B. anthracis PM-36[d]	50	0
B. anthracis Sterne[d]	300	1

[a]From Bonventre and Eckert (1963a).
Sterile filtrates of 12-hour infusion broth cultures incubated on a shaker at 37°C. Mice
injected with 0.5 ml of filtrate in caudal vein.

[b]Strain designation of stock collection, Department of Microbiology, University of
Cincinnati, Cincinnati, Ohio.

[c]Obtained from K. Burdon, Department of Microbiology, Baylor Medical School,
Houston, Texas.

[d]Obtained from C. Thorne, Fort Detrick, Frederick, Maryland (VIB and PM-36, virulent
strains; Sterne, avirulent strain).

reliable test for the differentiation of the microorganisms. Bonventre (1965) observed that the crude toxins of *B. cereus* and *B. anthracis* also differed in their toxicity for cultured mammalian cells. The *B. cereus* filtrates rapidly destroyed monolayers of primary and established cell lines, while the anthrax toxin did not exert any cytopathic effect on the tissue cultures (Table IV). Table IV also shows that *B. cereus* toxin is lethal for rats as well as mice. In addition to these animal species, the rabbit is also sensitive to the lethal action of *B. cereus* toxin (Johnson, unpublished observations). The toxicity of the toxin for other animals has not been tested. Intravenous injection into mice is the assay method of choice for the detection of the toxin. *B. cereus* toxin is also lethal when injected intraperitoneally or subcutaneously, but the response is not as consistent and the time to death is much longer (1–24 hours) than when injected intravenously (1–10 minutes) (Johnson and Bonventre, unpublished observations).

The contribution of *B. cereus* toxin, hemolysin, and phospholipase C to the rapidly lethal action of culture filtrates or to the pathogenesis of the cereobacillus disease described by Burdon *et al.* (1967) is still uncertain. The toxin molecule per se is lethal and therefore can be classified as a true microbial toxin as defined by Bonventre *et al.* (1967). There is some evidence that the phospholipase and the hemolysin are not toxic *in vivo*, and

TABLE IV

CYTOPATHIC EFFECT OF *B. cereus* AND *B. anthracis* CULTURE FILTRATES ON TISSUE CULTURE CELLS[a]

Culture filtrate[b]	Dilution	Cytopathic effect			Lethality	
		Guinea pig spleen cells	KB cells	Mouse embryo cells	Rats[c]	Mice[d]
Uninoculated medium A[e]	1:2	−	−	−	−	−
B. anthracis	1:2	−	−	−	+	−
Uninoculated medium B[f]	1:2	−	−	−	−	−
B. cereus	1:2	+	+	+	+	+
	1:4	+	+	+	+	+
	1:8	+	+	+	+	+
	1:16	+	+	+	+	−
B. cereus (heated)[g]	1:2	−/+	−	+	−	−

[a]From Bonventre (1965).
[b]Dialyzed for 2 hours at 4°C against running tap water.
[c]Fischer albino rats (ca. 150–200 gm); 1.0 ml intravenously.
[d]Swiss-Webster mice (ca. 25 gm); 0.5 ml intravenously.
[e]Medium of Thorne *et al.* (1960) for growth of *B. anthracis*.
[f]Fresh beef infusion broth for growth of *B. cereus*.
[g]At 60°C for 2 hours.

if this is ultimately proven to be the case, they should not be considered microbial toxins. Johnson and Bonventre (1967) obtained partially purified preparations of *B. cereus* phospholipase C which exhibited neither lethal nor hemolytic activities. This observation has not been corroborated and further work is required before it can be concluded that the phospholipase molecule is completely nontoxic. The hemolysin purified from cultures of *B. cereus* by Bernheimer and Grushoff (1967) was described as one of the most potent *in vitro* hemolytic agents thus far characterized. However, it is likely that the *B. cereus* hemolysin has little or no significance *in vivo* since normal serum inactivates hemolytic activity quite rapidly (Johnson and Bonventre, 1967). This latter property is in contrast to *Cl. perfringens* α-toxin which retains its capacity to hemolyze erythrocytes in the presence of normal (nonimmune) serum (Macfarlane *et al.*, 1941; Chu, 1949). Bernheimer and Grushoff (1967) observed that their purified hemolysin preparation was lethal for mice. Whether this represents a lethal property of the hemolysin per se or if the hemolysin preparation was contaminated with *B. cereus* toxin is not known. The hemolysin and the toxin are very difficult to separate and appear to be proteins of similar molecular weight and electrophoretic mobility (Johnson, 1966).

IV. Mode of Action

Little can be said concerning the mode of action of *B. cereus* toxin. If this microorganism has any potential as a pathogen, it is likely that the toxin contributes significantly to the pathophysiology of *B. cereus* infections. As already noted, it may be that the phospholipase C per se is of minor significance to disease in view of its lack of apparent toxicity when tested *in vivo* (Johnson, 1966). It may, however, act as an auxiliary virulence factor (Miles, 1954). The hemolysin acts on rabbit, rat, mouse, chicken, and human erythrocytes *in vitro* (Johnson, 1966). Bernheimer and Grushoff (1967) observed that the purified *B. cereus* hemolysin (cereolysin) is similar to streptolysin O in being inhibited by cholesterol, in causing a rapid hemolysis, and in the signs and symptoms preceding death of mice following intravenous injection. These authors speculate that the mode of action of *B. cereus* hemolysin is probably similar to that of streptolysin O. The significance of cereolysin *in vivo* is unknown. The fact that it is inhibited by normal serum and that hemolysis is not prominent in mice injected with *B. cereus* culture filtrates (containing hemolysin, phospholipase, and lethal toxin) suggests that the role of the hemolysin *in vivo* is minimal (Johnson, 1966).

The effect of culture filtrates of *B. cereus* in mice has been described by

Bonventre and Eckert (1963b). Following intravenous inoculation of toxic culture filtrates, mice become immobile and develop arrhythmic breathing within 1 minute. Respiration then becomes increasingly labored and death ensues in a few minutes postinjection. The average survival time of mice injected with 0.5 ml of filtrate was slightly less than 2 minutes. The lungs at necropsy were congested and extensive thrombus formation was evident in the large blood vessels and capillaries (Fig. 6). No pathological change in tissues other than the lungs was observed. The same clinical and pathological effects were produced in albino rats. Whether the lung lesion is produced by the *B. cereus* toxin or other materials in the filtrate such as the phospholipase, proteases, etc., or by a combination of all of them is not known. It may be significant that snake venom, which contains a variety of phospholipases and proteolytic enzymes, when injected intravenously into mice produces lung lesions which are similar although not identical to those caused by *B. cereus* culture filtrates (Bonventre, unpublished observations).

In spite of the marked similarity between *B. cereus* and *B. anthracis*, their respective toxins are not related. In addition to the differences in biological activities already noted (see Section III), they are immunologically distinct (Molnar, 1962) and differ in their molecular composition. *Bacillus cereus* toxin is a simple protein toxin, while the anthrax toxin is a

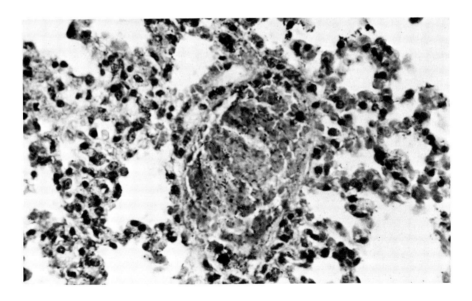

Fig. 6. Mouse lung after injection with *B. cereus* culture filtrate. A capillary is occluded by a thrombus. Hematoxylin and eosin stain, × 562. From Bonventre and Eckert (1963b).

multicomponent toxin (Bonventre *et al.*, 1967). The anthrax toxin consists of three components (lethal component, edema component, and protective antigen component) and all three are necessary before full biological activity of the toxin is expressed (Stanley and Smith, 1961; Beall *et al.*, 1962). In an effort to establish whether the *B. cereus* toxin and phospholipase C were related to the components of the anthrax toxin, the *B. cereus* products were tested for their ability to replace any of the anthrax components. Neither the *B. cereus* toxin nor the phospholipase when mixed with two of the anthrax toxin components in any combination restored full biological activity associated with the three components of anthrax toxin (Lincoln, Klein, Bonventre and Johnson, unpublished observations). These observations suggest that the two toxins are unique with respect to chemical composition and biological activities.

In view of the fact that *B. cereus* culture filtrates and *Cl. perfringens* α-toxin exhibit comparable biochemical and/or biological activities, it is conceivable that they may have a similar mode of action *in vivo*. Several differences, however, have been noted. The *in vitro* phospholipase C and hemolytic activities of *Cl. perfringens* α-toxin are dependent upon the presence of divalent cations in the reaction mixtures (Oakley *et al.*, 1948). No divalent cation requirement for the activity of *B. cereus* phospholipase C and hemolysin was found (Johnson and Bonventre, 1967). The lethal activity of *Cl. perfringens* α-toxin is probably also cation dependent since animals can be protected from lethal doses of the toxin by chelating agents (Moskowitz, 1956, 1958; Lynch and Moskowitz, 1968). In contrast, the activity of the lethal toxin of *B. cereus* cannot be prevented by administration of chelating agents either subsequent to or concomitant with the toxin (Johnson and Bonventre, 1967).

The biological and biochemical similarities exhibited by the α-toxin of *Cl. perfringens* and the *B. cereus* extracellular products, coupled with the taxonomic relationship of the two species, prompted Johnson and Bonventre (1967) to examine the immunological specificity of the respective bacterial products. The immunospecificity of antisera prepared against *Cl. perfringens* α-toxin and partially purified *B. cereus* products were compared in homologous and heterologous antigen–antibody systems. Antisera against partially purified *B. cereus* phospholipase C and toxin did not cross react with the phospholipase C and lethal activities of the *Cl. perfringens* α-toxin. Similarly, anti-α-toxin had no neutralizing effect on either *B. cereus* phospholipase or toxin. Both the *Cl. perfringens* α-toxin and the *B. cereus* products were neutralized when tested with homologous antisera. It can be concluded from these observations that in spite of apparent similarities, the *Cl. perfringens* and *B. cereus* toxins are unrelated.

V. Pathogenesis

Bacillus cereus is not under normal circumstances considered a pathogenic bacterial species. In view of its marked similarity to *B. anthracis*, however, *B. cereus* has been studied more extensively as a potential agent of disease than might have been the case if the similarity between the two organisms did not exist. The similarities were at one time considered to be so striking that N. R. Smith *et al.* (1952) suggested that *B. anthracis* may be a pathogenic variety of *B. cereus*. More recent studies have disavowed this possibility since several reliable criteria can be employed to differentiate the two organisms (Burdon and Wende, 1960; Bonventre and Eckert, 1963a; Knisely, 1965), and thus, *B. anthracis* and *B. cereus* can be classified as separate and distinct bacterial species. A clue to the reason for the striking similarities exhibited by these two organisms is in their DNA composition. McDonald *et al.* (1963) determined the guanine plus cytosine percentages of the deoxyribonucleic acids of several *Bacillus* sp. and found that the base ratios of *B. cereus* and *B. anthracis* strains were very nearly the same. However, the guanine plus cytosine percentages of *Bacillus licheniformis* and *Bacillus subtilis* were much higher. The suggested genetic homology of *B. cereus* and *B. anthracis* indicates that they are closely related species, and one would expect, therefore, that their biochemical and immunological characteristics would overlap.

In spite of the fact that *B. cereus* is not an overt pathogen, it has been incriminated in several human and animal infections. Clark (1937) recovered a bacillus from the blood of a patient diagnosed as having scarlet fever. The bacillus isolated was fatal for guinea pigs and was identified as a strain of *B. cereus*. Stopler *et al.* (1964) isolated *B. cereus* from the blood of a patient with bronchopneumonia. The course of the infection was rapid and fatal and *B. cereus* was isolated from the heart, lung, and spleen in pure culture. A fatal *B. cereus* septicemia as a complication of blood dialysis has also been documented (Curtis *et al.*, 1967). The bacillus has been incriminated in several outbreaks of food poisoning (Hauge, 1950, 1955; Nygren, 1962). In one of these outbreaks (Hauge, 1955), the investigator inoculated the strain of *B. cereus* isolated from the contaminated food product into sterile vanilla sauce which was then incubated at room temperature for 24 hours. He then consumed a hearty portion (200 ml) of the contaminated sauce, and after a 13-hour incubation period, developed abdominal pain and diarrhea. Dack *et al.* (1954), however, reported failure to induce food poisoning in man by *per os* administration of *B. cereus* cultures to human volunteers. The observations of Hauge (1955) and Dack *et al.* (1954) suggest that *B. cereus* food poisoning is a food intoxication rather than a food infection. It is likely that an extracellular toxin(s) is produced by the organism during its growth as is the case in staphylococcal and botulinum food poisoning. Apparently *B. cereus* cannot set up an infection in the enteric tract under normal circumstances as do certain strains of *Cl. perfringens* and *Salmonella* sp. It is not possible to identify the toxic product(s) responsible for *B. cereus* food poisoning. It could be the lethal toxin or the phospholipase, a combination of the two, or still another bacterial product. In view of the fact that the extracellular products of *B. cereus* can now be separated and purified to some degree (Johnson and Bonventre, 1967), such a study either in laboratory animals or human volunteers is feasible.

Bacillus cereus can also cause overt infection in animals. An adult tiger at the Cincinnati Zoo suffered a fatal infection and at autopsy, *B. cereus* was isolated from the blood and viscera in pure culture (E. Bell, personal communication). The range of animal species in which pathogenicity of *B. cereus* has been evaluated is not extensive. Thus far, information is available only for the mouse, guinea pig, and rabbit. Burdon (1947) and Brown *et al.* (1958) reported that stock cultures of *B. cereus* transferred only periodically are generally of low virulence when tested in mice. Cultures can be converted to full virulence by repeated transfer every few hours on blood agar plates. Burdon and Wende (1960) showed that these rapidly growing organisms injected into mice subcutaneously at a concentration of 3×10^5 bacilli resulted in the death of 70% of the animals within 13 hours. In view of the inconsistent recovery of bacilli from the blood and the rapid mortality, a toxemia rather than a generalized infection was suggested as the cause of death (Burdon *et al.*, 1961). The 50% lethal dose (LD_{50}) of *B. cereus* (vegetative cells) was established by Lamanna and Jones (1963) as 3.2×10^7 organisms, and more recently Burdon *et al.* (1967) reported an LD_{50} of the same order of magnitude. This rather large number of bacilli required to produce lethal infections would suggest that *B. cereus* is capable of only limited reproduction *in vivo* before effective host defenses come into play to inhibit bacterial cell division. What appears to be important is that enough toxin be produced *in vivo* before the bacilli are inactivated and destroyed by the humoral and cellular defense mechanisms of the host. In this respect, *B. cereus* infection is comparable to anthrax infections where it has been established that eradication of the infectious agent with antibiotics does not prevent death after the accumulation of a critical amount of anthrax toxin *in vivo* (H. Smith *et al.*, 1955; Lincoln *et al.*, 1964). This is not to imply that the two infections are in any way related or that the two agents are comparable in virulence. Small numbers of virulent anthrax bacilli are capable of establishing infection, resisting phagocytosis, and rapid multiplication in body fluids (Lincoln *et al.*, 1964) by virtue of a polyglutamic acid capsule and other still undefined virulence factors (Watson *et al.*, 1947; Ivanovics *et al.*, 1968). *B. cereus*, however, is readily phagocytized and apparently does not possess the virulence mechanisms which would ensure its survival *in vivo* for any length of time. Thus, in spite of the fact that the toxin of *B. cereus* is lethal in small quantities, the organism probably does not express overt virulence except under abnormal circumstances (i.e., large inoculum or debilitated host). Several observations have been made which suggest that spores of *B. cereus* germinate *in vivo* and are then subject to the same restriction in multiplication as are vegetative cells. Lamanna and Jones (1963) estimated an LD_{50} of 3×10^8 spores for mice. This is one order of magnitude greater than the LD_{50} obtained with vegetative cells. In view of the large number of organisms required for killing, the possibility exists that cell-associated toxin is responsible for death rather than *in vivo* synthesis of the protein. This is unlikely, however, since Bonventre (unpublished observations) found that sonic disintegration of *B. cereus* cultures did not release any intracellular or cell-associated toxin. Furthermore, Molnar (1962) found that antiserum prepared in animals vaccinated with viable spores neutralized both the toxin and phospholipase activities of *B. cereus* culture filtrates. In the absence of cell-associated toxin, Molnar's observations cannot be explained except by assuming that the spores germinated and limited vegetative growth ensued. During the period of vegetative cell production, a sufficient antigenic stimulus was probably provided by the synthesis of the extracellular toxin and phospholipase *in vivo*. This hypothesis could be tested by utilizing nonviable spore and vegetative cell preparations as the immunizing agents and subsequently testing the antisera for their neutralizing activity when tested with the extracellular products of *B. cereus*. To date such experiments have not been attempted.

In addition to the lethal infection of mice, which has been termed "cereobacillus disease" (Burdon and Wende, 1960), virulent strains of *B. cereus* produce necrotic skin lesions in guinea pigs and rabbits injected subcutaneously. The lesion develops rapidly into a hemorrhagic ulcer which at times extends through the entire thickness of the skin (Burdon and Wende, 1960). The cutaneous infection of guinea pigs and rabbits does not result in death as is the case with mice, which when injected by the same route, develop the typical skin ulcer and ultimately succumb to the infection. The LD_{50} values have not been established for *B. cereus* in animal species other than mice.

Very little is known concerning the role of toxins in *B. cereus* infections. All of the evidence for a significant role of toxins in natural or induced infections is primarily circumstantial and few experimental data are available. The possible role of toxin in outbreaks of food poisoning in which *B. cereus* was incriminated has not been substantiated experimentally. Johnson and Bonventre (unpublished observations) attempted to assess the oral toxicity of *B. cereus* phospholipase C and lethal toxin in mice but the results were equivocal. A transient illness was induced, but the animals recovered without exhibiting gastrointestinal symptoms. In view of species variation, a controlled investigation with other laboratory animals is warranted but thus far has not been conducted. The only investigation in which an attempt was made to assess the role of toxin in cereobacillus disease showed that the course of the infection was modified by the lethal toxin (Burdon *et al.*, 1967). Table V shows the results of their experiment. The addition of a sublethal quantity of toxin ($\frac{1}{3}$ MLD) to a 4-hour culture of *B. cereus* increased the mortality for mice at all dilutions of the culture tested. Specific antitoxin prepared in rabbits against crude toxin afforded significant protection, and in the few cases where mice succumbed to the infection, antitoxin prolonged the time to death. In spite of this clear evidence for a significant role of the lethal toxin, attempts to demonstrate the toxin in the blood of infected mice were unsuccessful. Inactivation of the toxin cannot explain the apparent discrepancy since normal rabbit and mouse sera (Johnson, 1966) and mouse plasma (Burdon *et al.*, 1967) do not inactivate the toxin either *in vivo* or *in vitro*. It may be that the toxin is bound very quickly to tissues and an assayable quantity does not accumulate in the bloodstream during infection.

TABLE V

EFFECTS OF ADDED TOXIN OR ANTITOXIN ON VIRULENCE OF *B. cereus* CULTURES FOR MICE[a]

Dilution (0.25 ml)	Estimated number of bacilli	Other material (0.25 ml)[b]	Number of deaths per number inoculated	Time of death (hours)
Undiluted	4.5×10^7	Broth	18/18	2,3–25
	4.5×10^7	Antitoxin	3/12	3,5, 20
1:2	2.5×10^7	Broth	9/12	3–9
	2.5×10^7	Toxin	11/12	2.75–5.75
	2.5×10^7	Antitoxin	0/12	
	1.25×10^7	Broth	0/12	
1:4	1.25×10^7	Toxin	5/12	3–10
	1.25×10^7	Antitoxin	0/12	
	0.6×10^7	Broth	0/12	
1:8	0.6×10^7	Toxin	5/12	8.5–20
	0.6×10^7	Antitoxin	0/12	

[a]From Burdon *et al.* (1967).
[b]Injected intraperitoneally immediately after the culture.

REFERENCES

Adams, M. H., and Hendee, E. D. (1945). *J. Immunol.* **51**, 249.

Adams, M. H., Hendee, E. D., and Pappenheimer, A. M., Jr. (1947). *J. Exptl. Med.* **85**, 701.

Altenbern, R. A., and Stull, H. B. (1964). *Can. J. Microbiol.* **10**, 717.

Beall, F. A., Taylor, M. J., and Thorne, C. B. (1962). *J. Bacteriol.* **83**, 1274.

Bernheimer, A. W., and Grushoff, P. (1967). *J. Gen. Microbiol.* **46**, 143.

Bonventre, P. F. (1965). *J. Bacteriol.* **90**, 284.

Bonventre, P. F., and Eckert, N. J. (1963a). *J. Bacteriol.* **85**, 490.

Bonventre, P. F., and Eckert, N. J. (1963b). *Am. J. Pathol.* **43**, 201.

Bonventre, P. F., Lincoln, R. E., and Lamanna, C. (1967). *Bacteriol. Rev.* **31**, 95.

Brown, E. R., Moody, M. D., Treece, E. L., and Smith, C. (1958). *J. Bacteriol.* **75**, 499.

Burdon, K. L. (1947). *Bacteriol. Proc.* p. 58.

Burdon, K. L., and Wende, R. D. (1960). *J. Infect. Diseases* **107**, 224.

Burdon, K. L., Wende, R. D., and Davis, J. S. (1961). *Bacteriol. Proc.* p. 119.

Burdon, K. L., Davis, J. S., and Wende, R. D. (1967). *J. Infect. Diseases* **117**, 307.

Chu, H. P. (1949). *J. Gen. Microbiol.* **3**, 255.

Clark, F. E. (1937). *J. Bacteriol.* **33**, 435.

Curtis, J. R., Wing, A. J., and Coleman, J. C. (1967). *Lancet* **I**, 136.

Dack, G. M., Sugiyama, H., Owens, F. J., and Kirsner, J. B. (1954). *J. Infect. Diseases* **94**, 34.

Eckert, N. J. (1963). M.S. Thesis, University of Cincinnati, Cincinnati, Ohio.

Fossum, K. (1963). *Acta Pathol. Microbiol. Scand.* **59**, 400.

Freeman, V. J. (1951). *J. Bacteriol.* **61**, 675.

Gorini, L. (1950). *Biochim. Biophys. Acta* **6**, 237.

Haines, B. W., Klein, F., and Lincoln, R. E. (1965). *J. Bacteriol.* **89**, 74.

Hanson, R. S., Srinivasan, V. R., and Halvorson, H. O. (1963). *J. Bacteriol.* **85**, 451.

Hauge, S. (1950). *Nord. Hyg. Tidskr.* **31**, 189.

Hauge, S. (1955). *J. Appl. Bacteriol.* **18**, 591.

Hauschild, A. H. W. (1965). *J. Bacteriol.* **90**, 1793.

Hayaishi, O. (1955). *Methods Enzymol.* **1**, 660-672.

Ivanovics, G., Marjai, E., and Dobozy, A. (1968). *J. Gen. Microbiol.* **53**, 147.

Johnson, C. E. (1966). Ph.D. Thesis, University of Cincinnati, Cincinnati, Ohio.

Johnson, C. E., and Bonventre, P. F. (1966). *Bacteriol. Proc.* p. 41.

Johnson, C. E., and Bonventre, P. F. (1967). *J. Bacteriol.* **94**, 306.

Knisely, R. F. (1965). *J. Bacteriol.* **90**, 1778.

Kushner, D. J. (1957). *J. Bacteriol.* **73**, 297.

Kushner, D. J. (1962). *Can. J. Microbiol.* **8**, 673.

Lamanna, C., and Jones, L. (1963). *J. Bacteriol.* **85**, 534.

Lichstein, H. C., and Jayko, L. G. (1959). *J. Infect. Diseases* **104**, 142.

Lincoln, R. E., Walter, J. S., Klein, F., and Haines, B. W. (1964). *Advan. Vet. Sci.* **9**, 327.

Lynch, K. L., and Moskowitz, M. (1968). *J. Bacteriol.* **96**, 1925.

Macfarlane, M. G., and Knight, B. C. J. G. (1941). *Biochem. J.* **35**, 884.

Macfarlane, R. G., Oakley, C. L., and Anderson, C. G. (1941). *J. Pathol. Bacteriol.* **52**, 99.

McDonald, W. C., Felkner, I. C., Turetsky, A., and Matney, T. S. (1963). *J. Bacteriol.* **85**, 1071.

McGaughey, C. A., and Chu, H. P. (1948). *J. Gen. Microbiol.* **2**, 334.

Miles, A. A. (1954). *In* "Lectures on the Scientific Basis of Medicine," Vol. 3, pp. 192–213. Oxford Univ. Press (Athlone), London and New York.

Molnar, D. M. (1962). *J. Bacteriol.* **84**, 147.

Moskowitz, M. (1956). *Proc. Soc. Exptl. Biol. Med.* **92**, 706.

Moskowitz, M. (1958). *Nature* **181**, 550.

Mueller, J. A., and Miller, P. A. (1940). *J. Immunol.* **40**, 21.

Mueller, J. A., and Miller, P. A. (1949). *J. Biol. Chem.* **181**, 39.

Nagler, F. P. O. (1939). *Brit. J. Exptl. Pathol.* **20**, 473.

Nakamura, M., Cross, J. A., and Cross, W. R. (1968). *Appl. Microbiol.* **16**, 1420.

Nygren, B. (1962). *Acta Pathol. Microbiol. Scand.* Suppl. 160, 13.

Oakley, C. L., Warrack, G. A., and Warren, M. E. (1948). *J. Pathol. Bacteriol.* **60**, 495.

Ottolenghi, A., Gollub, S., and Ulin, A. (1961). *Bacteriol. Proc.* p. 171.

Pollock, M. R. (1956). *J. Gen. Microbiol.* **15**, 154.

Slein, M. W., and Logan, G. F., Jr. (1963). *J. Bacteriol.* **85**, 369.

Slein, M. W., and Logan, G. F., Jr. (1965). *J. Bacteriol.* **90**, 69.

Smith, N. R., Gordon, R. E., and Clark, F. E. (1952). *U.S. Dept. Agri., Agr. Monograph* **559**, No. 16.

Smith, H., Keppie, J., Stanley, J. L., and Harris-Smith, P. W. (1955). *J. Exptl. Pathol.* **36**, 323.

Stanley, J. L., and Smith, H. (1961). *J. Gen. Microbiol.* **26**, 49.

Stopler, T. R., Camuescu, B., and Voiculescu, M. (1964). *Microbiol., Parazitol. Epidemiol.* (*Bucharest*) **9**, 457.

Thorne, C. B., and Belton, F. C. (1957). *J. Gen. Microbiol.* **17**, 505.

Thorne, C. B., Molnar, D. M., and Strange, R. E. (1960). *J. Bacteriol.* **79**, 450.

Tristram, G. R., (1953). *In* "The Proteins" (H. Neurath and K. Bailey, eds.), Vol. 1, Part A, pp. 181–233. Academic Press, New York.

Watson, D. W., Cromartie, W. J., Bloom, W. L., Kegeles, G., and Heckly, R. J. (1947). *J. Infect. Diseases* **80**, 28.

CHAPTER 11

Bacillus thuringiensis Toxins — The Proteinaceous Crystal

MARGUERITE M. LECADET

I. Introduction

Bacillus thuringiensis is a gram-positive sporeforming bacterium which was isolated from dying silkworm larvae by Ishiwata (1902) (as *Bacillus sotto*) and slightly later on, from sick larvae of *Anagasta kuhniella* by Berliner (1915) (as *B. thuringiensis berliner*). This bacterium, which is pathogenic for lepidoptera larvae, is characterized by a rhomboid parasporal body which Berliner called "Restkorper." These observations were confirmed by Mattes (1927) and then by Hannay (1953) who characterized the bipyramidal-shaped inclusion as a crystal.

Since then, and especially during the last 15 years, numerous strains with the same characteristics (parasporal inclusion and pathogenicity for lepidoptera larvae), were isolated under similar conditions (Toumanoff and Vago, 1951; Toumanoff, 1953). For a long time, these different bacterial species were considered (Toumanoff and Lecoroller, 1959) varieties of *Bacillus cereus* to which they are closely related by several morphological and biochemical characteristics. Yet Delaporte and Beguin (1955) and then Heimpel and Angus (1958) had already suggested that all the crystal-forming strains be grouped under the name of *Bacillus thuringiensis*, the strain isolated by Berliner being the type strain. These problems of taxonomy seem to have been conclusively resolved by the very thorough study of the serological and biochemical characteristics of a great number of *B. thuringiensis* strains by de Barjac and Bonnefoi (1962, 1967). These authors proposed a classification with six and then nine serological groups characterized by different flagellar antigens. This very useful classification, which also involves biochemical criteria, and which, moreover, coincides exactly with the pattern of esterase activities suggested by Norris (1964), is generally accepted at the present time and used in the identification of unknown strains of *B. thuringiensis* (Table I).

Thus, all these strains form a parasporal body. It has been known for a long time (Hannay, 1953; Steinhaus and Jerrel, 1954; Angus, 1954, 1956a) that the proteinaceous crystal formed during sporulation and released in the culture medium after bacterial lysis is the main factor responsible for the pathogenicity of lepidoptera larvae. However, the crys-

TABLE I

KEY FOR THE DETERMINATION OF *B. thuringiensis* SPECIES[a]

Serotype	*B. thuringiensis* var. (common name)	Esterase type[b]
1	*berliner*	*berliner*
2	*finitimus*	*finitimus*
3	*alesti*	*alesti*
4	*kenyae*	*kenyae*
4	*sotto*	*sotto*
4	*dendrolimus*	*dendrolimus*
5	*galleriae*	*galleriae*
6	*subtoxicus*	*entomocidus*
6	*entomocidus*	*entomocidus*
7	*aizawai*	*galleriae*
8	*morrison*	*morrison*
9	*tolworth*	*tolworth*

[a]Data from de Barjac and Bonnefoi (1967). In the case of serotypes 4 and 6, the authors reported several biotypes differing by their biochemical characteristics.
[b]According to Norris (1964).

tal, which might be considered an endotoxin, is not the only toxic entity produced by *B. thuringiensis*. Several exotoxins released in the culture medium during bacterial growth have been described in recent years. For these toxins, Heimpel (1967) suggested the following nomenclature: α-exotoxin, lecithinase C, or phospholipase C; β-exotoxin, or heat-stable toxin; γ-exotoxin (an enzyme that clears egg yolk agar, not yet identified); δ-endotoxin, proteinaceous crystal, or the crystalline parasporal body.

The phospholipase was detected in *B. cereus* by Chu (1949). Toumanoff (1953, 1954) and Heimpel (1955) reported its presence in *B. thuringiensis*. The role and mode of action of this enzyme in the process of the intoxication of lepidoptera with *B. thuringiensis* are still not clear and have not been systematically studied. In this section, we will only consider the endotoxin or proteinaceous crystal which is at present the best known, and which is of great theoretical as well as practical interest since it is a crystalline protein and since *B. thuringiensis* crystal-containing preparations are industrially used as microbial insecticides.

II. Preparation and Purification

Bacillus thuringiensis crystalline endotoxin is a bipyramidal-shaped inclusion formed in the bacterium at the same time as the spore (Fig. 1). The inclusion, or crystal, is easily seen by phase-contrast microscopy. Bacterial lysis, which takes place in the last stage of sporulation, releases the crystalline inclusions into the culture medium; they are theoretically produced in the same number as the spores. After lysis, spores, crystals, and cell fragments remain. Techniques for extraction and purification of toxin then consist either in the elimination of the spores and cell fragments so as to recover the inclusion in its crystal form, or in the selective solution of the crystalline inclusion.

Bacillus thuringiensis is grown on rich media, either liquid medium with peptone or casamino acids, or solid medium with Difco nutrient agar.

A. Methods for the Preparation of Pure Crystal Suspensions

The first techniques for isolating the crystals consisted in the elimination of the spores from the mixture harvested in the last stage of culture, either through mechanical disruption (Fitz-James, 1953), or through spontaneous germination followed by autolysis (Hannay and Fitz-James, 1955). The crystals were then freed from the debris through repeated washings and differential centrifugation. These techniques, time consuming and difficult, gave a very poor yield.

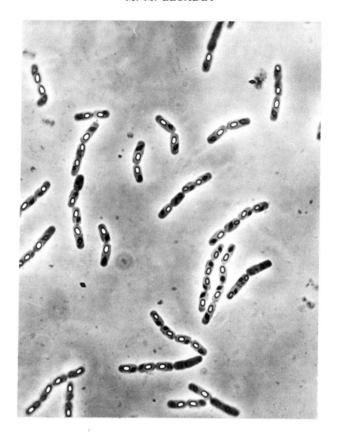

FIG. 1. A culture of *B. thuringiensis* var. *berliner* at the end of sporulation.

Since then, several methods have been perfected which involve the preparation of an emulsion of an aqueous suspension of spores and crystals in suitable organic solvents. The crystals remain in the aqueous phase. Other techniques based on phase systems have been described recently.

1. EMULSION IN ORGANIC SOLVENTS

The first of these techniques was devised by Angus (1959), who used a fluorocarbon (trifluorotrichlorethane). The aqueous suspensions of spores and crystals, harvested after 14 days of culture on Difco agar at 28°C were added to the solvent at a ratio of 9:1 (volume) and emulsified in a high speed mixer. After shaking, the emulsion separates into two phases, the aqueous upper phase which contains almost exclusively crystals, and the lower organic phase which contains hydrophobic spores. Treatment of the aqueous phase must be repeated several times until less than 1% of spores remains. The residual spores are eliminated through germination and autolysis before a final treatment with the solvent. This technique, theoretically very effective, involves several extractions, one after the other, with the solvent, and its yield is low. It has been modified by Bateson (1965), who added 1% sodium sulfate to the aqueous phase and *n*-butyl citrate to the fluorocarbon of the emulsion. With this method it is possible to obtain preparations with 99% of the crystals after only one solvent treatment.

Other techniques, based on the same principle but with solvents more common than trifluorotrichloroethane, have been described. Lecadet (1965) used tetrabromoethane and Pendleton and Morrison (1966a) used carbon tetrachloride after previous filtration on Whatman paper to obtain more crystals. They obtained a yield of 25–40% of the crystals in the initial mixture. Murray and Spencer (1966) obtained a very satisfactory yield by emulsifying with chloroform and filtering through Millipore filter membranes. Their crystal preparations contain approximately one spore per three thousand crystals.

All these techniques are in general use at the present time, but treatment with solvents can have drawbacks as it may modify the crystals; thus it must be strictly controlled.

2. SEPARATION OF SPORES FROM CRYSTALS BY MEANS OF A DIPHASIC SYSTEM

The phase system described by Albertsson (1960) using dextran sulfate and polyethylene glycol is frequently used to free the preparation of formed elements: bacteria, bacteriophages, spores, etc. Goodman *et al.* (1967) perfected a very elegant method for freeing the crystals from the spores. Dextran sulfate 500 and polyethylene glycol 6000 are distributed into two phases in a previously determined proportion so that the spores go preferentially into the phase richer in polyethylene glycol. Through the repetition of this procedure, followed by repeated washings and differential centrifugation, the investigators obtained very pure preparations with 99.94% of crystals and a yield of 250 mg/10 gm of the spore–crystal mixture. This yield is rather low, but the method avoids the risks associated with treatment with solvents.

B. PREPARATION AND PURIFICATION OF THE SOLUBLE TOXIN

The crystalline toxin is insoluble in water or organic solvents. However, it is soluble in alkaline solutions of pH equal to or higher than 11 (Angus, 1954; Hannay and Fitz-James, 1955). It is possible to obtain a solution of the toxin without removing the spores by treating the spore–crystal mixture with sodium hydroxide of molarity between 0.01 and 0.05. Angus (1956b) devised a technique of extraction and purification of B. thuringiensis var. sotto toxin. A first extraction by 0.05 N sodium hydroxide is followed by dialysis against water and precipitation at pH 4.4. The precipitate is redissolved in 0.01 N sodium hydroxide and the solution is reprecipitated through continued dialysis against distilled water. The final precipitate is freeze dried. With this method it is relatively easy to obtain large quantities of toxin. Yet the purification is not sufficient to ensure that protein contaminants from spores do not exist.

Recently Cooksey (1968) described a technique of purification in which the solution in sodium hydroxide and the precipitation at pH 4.4 are followed with fractionation on Sephadex G 200, precipitation with ammonium sulfate, and a second fractionation on Sephadex. The preparation thus obtained contained only the soluble components from the crystal; the purification is followed by electrophoresis on polyacrylamide gel. This time-consuming technique can evidently be used only to provide small amounts of product for structural studies.

It is necessary to point out that all the methods for preparing the crystals or the soluble protein that we have described can only be used for research work in the laboratory and not for industrial preparations as biological insecticides. In such cases, spore-crystal mixtures harvested at the end of the culture are used, and they are generally added to an inert material which makes their spreading easier. At the present time, several preparations are commercially available as powder formulations or in oil emulsions.

III. Nature

A. Morphology of the Crystalline Inclusion

Before considering the problem of the nature of the B. thuringiensis parasporal inclusion, I would like to give a succinct account of its morphology and to stress the rather exceptional aspect of this organized molecule, the size of which approximates that of the spore. Figure 2, obtained by Norris and Watson (1960), discloses a quite characteristic structure in which one will note the repetition of a great number of identical patterns according to a precise periodicity. Several electron microscopic investigations have confirmed these observations. Vankova and Kralik (1966) sum up a study on crystals from several strains as follows, "the crystalline protein inclusions were found to have a bipyramidal shape, ridged on the sur-

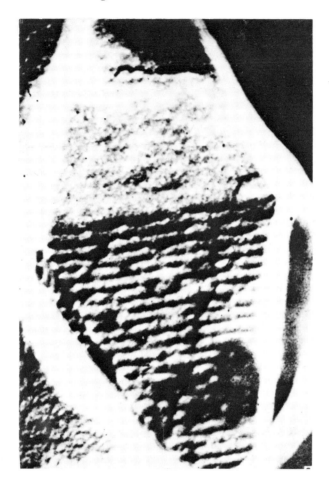

FIG. 2. Electron micrograph of a crystal from *B. cereus* var. *alesti* (*B. thuringiensis* sero-type III according to the new classification). Platinum shadowed carbon replica, × 113,000. From Norris and Watson (1960).

face and composed of rows of spherical formation. The number of units per row and the number of rows were not constant not even in one strain. . . . The average size of the globules varied in the different strains."

More detailed studies have been published by Labaw (1964) and by Holmes and Monro (1965). The investigations of Labaw are presented by Monro as follows, "The crystals are nonregular octahedra, the interfacial angle at the apex is about 38°, the faces are marked with obvious striations of spacing about 260Å, at right angles to the long axis of the particle, and each striation is marked at 87Å intervals along its length . . ." Holmes and Monro's crystallographic studies (1965) with X-ray diffraction bear out these conclusions and suggest that the crystal has a tetragonal symmetry and that the dimensions of the tetragonal unit cell are $a = 89.7$Å and $C = 269$Å.

Recently, Grigorova *et al.* (1967) examined by electron microscopy the shape and structure of the crystals of two strains of *B. thuringiensis*. The authors found two types of crystals — diamond-shaped crystals of bipyramidal shape and cubic crystals which are crystals of biprismatic shape. They suggested that the molecules which form both types have the form of a rotary ellipsoid.

These remarkable studies clearly demonstrate the complexity of this structure and the importance of this inclusion which we will show to be a crystalline protein.

B. CHEMICAL COMPOSITION AND NATURE OF THE CRYSTAL

First studies on the crystal chemical composition pointed clearly to the proteinaceous nature of the toxin. Hannay and Fitz-James (1955) and Angus (1956b) found that pure suspensions of crystals from *berliner* and *sotto* strains contained 16.5-17.8% nitrogen and traces of phosphorus (<0.05%, possibly due to spore contaminants). Similar results were obtained by Holmes and Monro (1965) and Lecadet (1965). These results favored an exclusively proteinaceous composition, but are not absolute proof of this. According to Holmes and Monro, it is not impossible that small amounts of other material are present (0.5% carbohydrates). Be that as it may, ultraviolet spectrophotometry of the solution in 0.01 *N* sodium hydroxide shows an absorption peak at 280 mμ which is characteristic of proteins (Hannay and Fitz-James, 1955; Angus, 1956b).

Table II gives the amino acid composition of the crystals from *berliner* and *anduze* strains obtained by Lecadet (1965) with the Moore and Stein amino acid analyzer, after hydrolysis in 6 *N* hydrochloric acid in vacuum sealed tubes for 18 hours, as well as that of the *sotto* strain crystals, analyzed by Angus (1956b) with the less sensitive paper chromatography method. We obtained all the amino acids usually found in proteins, and we noted that the dicarboxylic amino acids accounted for 25% of all the amino acids present. The basic amino acids represented 13% of the total. The total sum of the amino acids amounted to 95 or 98% of the weight of the analyzed product. The general characteristics of the amino acid composition did not differ much from one strain to another. Similar results have been reported by Holmes and Monro (1965) for crystals from the *berliner* strain.

Ripe, full-grown crystals are stable within large limits of pH and are insoluble in water or organic solvents. Their formed elements can be en-

TABLE II

AMINO ACID COMPOSITION OF CRYSTALS OF *B. thuringiensis*[a]

Amino acids	Var. *berliner* (serotype I)[b] (%)	Var. *anduze* (serotype III)[b] (%)	Var. *sotto* (serotype IV)[c] (%)
Aspartic acid	12.57	11.0	9.5
Threonine	5.76	5.1	5.2
Serine	4.37	5.6	5.6
Glutamine	12.0	14.3	12.9
Proline	4.37	4.9	6.7
Glycine	4.25	4.5	2.7
Alanine	3.80	4.1	3.2
Cystine	1.35	1.34	1.1
Valine	5.0	5.1	5.0
Methionine	1.53	1.65	0.6
Isoleucine	4.40	5.1	—
Leucine	7.65	7.93	10.4
Tyrosine	6.62	5.9	3.9
Phenylalanine	6.77	5.2	7.4
Lysine	3.4	4.0	4.2
Histidine	2.65	3.3	1.7
Arginine	7.81	7.5	9.4
Tryptophan	2.05	1.76	2.1

[a]Data from Lecadet (1965).
[b]Results obtained by automatic analysis.
[c]Results obtained by Angus (1956b); quantitative technique by paper chromatography.

tirely dissociated by various means: through alkalinization above pH 11.5; through disulfide bond reducing agents (Young and Fitz-James, 1959a; Lecadet, 1965); and through the action of several proteolytic enzymes, especially of the proteases extracted from *Pieris brassicae* (Lecadet and Martouret, 1962; Lecadet and Dedonder, 1966a) and from *Bombyx mori* (Lecadet and Martouret, 1967a) (that is, obtained from larvae susceptible to the crystal toxin). The native crystal resists the attack of higher vertebrate proteases such as trypsin and chymotrypsin. Of these, only pepsin in strongly acid medium (pH 1.6) can dissociate the inclusion. These various properties further support the evidence that the molecule is protein in nature.

C. STRUCTURE

We have seen that there is nothing remarkable about the amino acid composition of pure crystal preparations. Then what are the components and the type of bonds which build such a dense and strongly organized structure? Are there one or several proteins? What are the number and the nature of the constitutive chains? Such are the questions to which we will try to give an answer, taking into account all the information contained in the literature.

The various ways by which crystal solution can be obtained seem to point to the presence of several types of covalent and noncovalent linkages in the inclusion structure. Young and Fitz-James (1959a) suggest that the crystal becomes insoluble during its synthesis *in vivo* due to the formation of disulfide bonds. This hypothesis has been restated and confirmed by Lecadet (1966, 1967a), who described the action of reducing agents on the *berliner* strain crystals and demonstrated that dissolution in thioglycolate is possible whatever the pH (down to 7.5) but that it is all the more rapid as the pH increases (Fig. 3). The action of reducing agents is manifested by loss of the crystal's refractility and then by swelling and the gradual disappearance of the structure. The influence of pH on dissolution by reducing agents and solubility in highly alkaline medium point to the important role of linkages other than the disulfide bonds in molecule stability — ionic bonds between charged groups and, probably, hydrogen bonds. The effect of treatment with urea strongly suggests that hydrogen bonds play an important part (Lecadet, 1967a). Urea causes important modifications of structure — loss of refractility, swelling of the inclusion, but no liberation of the protein constituent chains occurs. The process is almost entirely reversible, for when urea is eliminated through dialysis or dilution, the original structure reappears. Moreover, the action of urea quickens dissolution by reducing agents which are then active at very low concentrations. Thus, a number of factors and types of linkages take part in the buildup of this complexly organized structure, but it is not yet possible to determine the respective roles of the various elements.

Other investigators, Estes and Faust (1966) and Heimpel (1967), have suggested that other elements — for instance silicon, which was found in crystals from several *B. thuringiensis* strains (0.3–0.4%) — might be factors in the cohesion of the structure by forming "the basic lattice on which the protein molecules are fixed." According to these authors, the presence of this framework of silicon would explain the slight dissolving effect that bicarbonate buffer exerts in mild alkaline conditions (pH $\geqslant$ 9). Such an hypothesis cannot be systematically put aside, although it is not as yet proved.

The types of linkages that bind the constituent protein chains of the crystal still bring up numerous problems. What are these basic units? Numerous investigations are now being carried on. The facts hitherto known are as follows: Holmes and Monro (1965) reported that ultracentrifugation analysis of the solution in alkali reveals the presence of two main components, which have sedimentation constants of 4.1 S and 0.4–

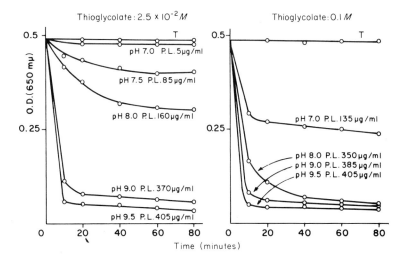

FIG. 3. The action of thioglycolate on pure suspensions (420 μg/ml) of crystals (*B. thuringiensis* var. *berliner*) in 0.05 *M*. borate buffer. From Lecadet (1967a). P. L.: concentration of soluble proteins liberated after 80 minutes at 30°C and measured in the supernates.

0.8 S, in equal concentration. He suggests that "such heterogenicity may reflect the presence of more than one protein in the crystals, hydrolysis of a labile linkage during alkali treatment, or existence of the same protein in two conformations or states of association."

By treatment with thioglycolate at pH 9.5 to release constituent protein chains, followed by alkaline treatment, Lecadet (1966) found at least three components by ultracentrifugation with sedimentation constants at 20°C of 9.6, 4.8, and 0.83 S. The last component is formed in proportions varying from 30 to 80%, according to the conditions of the reduction and the strains studied.

On one hand these results lead us to think that the dissociation is not complete under the described conditions; on the other hand, these alkaline conditions might involve the breakdown of some covalent bonds at random.

Treatment by mercaptoethanol in the presence of guanidinium hydrochloride at neutral pH is a better way of obtaining native protein chains. With this treatment Glatron *et al.* (1969) obtained total solubilization of crystals giving a single component as seen by ultracentrifugation analysis. The molecular weight of the subunit calculated by means of sedimentation equilibrium is about 80,000, the N terminal amino acid is phenylalanine, and the C terminal amino acid is arginine. Therefore the crystal might result from the association of identical subunits.

The problem of the number and nature of the basic units is, at the present time, very important, not only to the study of the inclusion structure, but also to the elucidation of the problem of crystal biosynthesis during sporulation. It will be necessary, moreover, to know the respective roles played by the various types of linkages we have been considering.

IV. Synthesis

Synthesis, or more exactly biosynthesis, of the toxin as a crystal, brings up numerous and very interesting problems for the following reasons: (1) this synthesis is related to sporogenesis and is the result of metabolic processes brought about by sporulation; (2) the crystal represents an important fraction of proteins formed during sporulation; and (3) the biosynthesis of this organized molecule brings up the more general problem of formation of insoluble protein structures in a cell. This question has hitherto been the subject of several *in vivo* studies, exclusively, since the possibility of such a synthesis *in vitro* cannot be as yet considered.

The problem of biosynthesis of this crystalline protein can be considered from the points of view of biogenesis of the main components or condensation of these components during sporulation. That is the reason why the biochemical study of the crystal formation cannot be dissociated from the problems of morphogenesis which must themselves be considered in their relation to sporogenesis.

A. Morphogenesis of the Crystalline Inclusion

In the course of events which characterize sporulation, important morphological changes have been observed in these bacteria, and these have brought about numerous cytological studies and electron microscopic observations on several species of the genus *Bacillus*. These morphological changes can be summarized in six main stages, described by Schaeffer *et al.* (1965) and Ryter (1965) in *Bacillus subtilis*:

1. Condensation of nuclear chromatin into an axial filament.
2. Formation of a spore septum and distribution of the chromatin on each side of the septum.
3. Appearance of the forespore.
4. Formation of the spore wall.
5. Formation of protein spore coats.
6. Fixation of calcium dipicolinate on the cortex which acquires refractibility and thermostability.

The same processes have been described in *B. cereus* by Fitz-James (1965) and more recently by Ellar and Lundgren (1966).

As for *B. thuringiensis,* the cytological investigations of Young and Fitz-James (1959b) by phase-contrast microscopy, with appropriate stains (in particular, fuchsin for the crystal), have shown that the very first indication of an inclusion appears in close proximity to the forespore after the spore septum is completed, and, therefore, at the beginning of stage 3. The crystal develops during the following stages, moves away from the spore, and is fully grown when the spore is ripe. In an electromicroscopic investigation now under way, we have been able to observe that the crystal forms at the end of stage 2 in a septum fold and looks closely apposed to the forespore wall in stage 3. So it is throughout the early stages of sporulation, when the morphological changes become irreversible, that crystal formation starts. Its growth continues between stages 3 and 5 (Fig. 4).

Toxin formation seems to be closely bound to spore formation, and it looks as if it were a secondary phenomenon of sporulation. Yet, in some cases, the two mechanisms can be dissociated; several investigators report that they have observed and obtained strains which have lost the

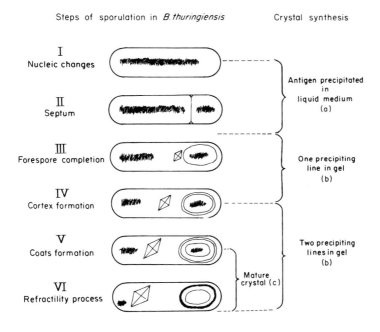

FIG. 4. The steps of sporulation and concomitant formation of parasporal inclusion in *B. thuringiensis.* (a) Data from Lecadet (1967b), (b) data from Monro (1961a) and Lecadet (1967b), (c) mature crystal soluble in thioglycolate according to Young and Fitz-James (1959a).

ability to form the crystal (Fitz-James and Young, 1959; Toumanoff *et al.*, 1955; Smirnoff, 1965), and, even more occasionally, strains which form a crystal but have their sporulation stopped at stage 3 have been reported (Fitz-James, 1965). These different phenotypes are obtained either through spontaneous mutation or through the action of mutagenic agents (Young and Fitz-James, 1959b) or even by modifications of growth medium conditions (Smirnoff, 1964; Vankova, 1957). There are even strains which form two or several crystals in each sporangium (Steinhaus and Jerrel, 1954; Hannay, 1956). It is quite certain that the study of various *B. thuringiensis* mutants will be more and more essential to the knowledge of the mechanisms implied in the crystal formation.

B. Characterization of the Crystal Protein throughout Sporulation

One of the questions brought up by crystal toxin biosynthesis is whether formation of the constitutive proteins occurs at the time of morphological differentiation of the inclusion or precedes it during the early stages of sporulation. Young and Fitz-James (1959a), in an elegant study on *B. thuringiensis* serotype III sporulation, tried to extract the crystal proteins at different pH values throughout sporulation. They showed that the amount of protein extracted with thioglycolate at pH 11.5 increased considerably in the last stage of sporulation; they concluded, "during development the crystal protein remains in a form which can be extracted at a lower pH value or without the aid of a disulfide reducing agent, and a maturation process confers on the crystal the solubility properties associated with the natural form." This maturation process takes place during the last stages of sporulation when the spore and the crystal acquire their refractility.

Monro (1961a) proposes two hypotheses: (1) The inclusion forms through crystallization or modification of protein precursors present at the onset of the stationary phase. (2) The crystal protein is synthesized *de novo* from amino acids when the crystal becomes evident as a structure during sporulation. By means of serological techniques, Monro attempted to identify throughout sporulation the first antigenic structures characteristic of the crystal after transferring the bacteria to a mineral medium at the beginning of the stationary phase. Their results can be summed up in this way: (1) The crystal antigens are not present in the vegetative cells and are formed during sporulation. (2) There are at least two main antigens, one of which appears between 2 and 3 hours after the transfer at about the beginning of stage 3. The other is present 4 hours later, that is to say during the last stages of sporulation at the time when the inclusion is grown and quite discernible. Therefore, there would be no forerunner with the antigenic properties of the crystal in the earliest stages of sporulation.

Lecadet (1967b) found similar results as to the characterization of the crystal antigens with the gel diffusion technique (Ouchterlony) on bacterial extracts during sporulation. Nevertheless, by means of more sensitive techniques of precipitation in liquid medium she obtained positive reactions with specific antisera at the onset of sporulation before the crystal started to form and before it could be detected with the microscope (Fig. 4). The crystal components do not seem to pre-exist during the growth of the culture, and they start accumulating after the sporulation process has begun.

Thus, the first antigenic structures of the crystal form before the structure is fully organized, and one may wonder whether the appearance of the other antigenic structures is not the result of associations of the basic subunits, mentioned in the study of the crystal structure.

C. ORIGIN AND SYNTHESIS OF THE CRYSTAL COMPONENTS

If the protein of the crystal is, in fact, entirely synthesized during sporulation, the question arises as to which cell constituents it is synthesized from. The fact that the formation of the crystal as well as that of the spore can occur in a strictly mineral medium (Monro, 1961a) without the addition of other nutrients suggests that important changes and a general protein turnover take place at the time of sporulation. Young and Fitz-James (1959a) noted that "The considerable synthesis which occurs during sporogenesis in *B. cereus* var. *alesti* (serotype III) was apparently associated with degradation of some pre-existing cell proteins."

In a study on the protein turnover and the formation of protein inclusions in *B. thuringiensis*, Monro (1961b) reported that the main part, if not the whole, of the crystal protein is synthesized from amino acids during sporulation and that these amino acids come from the breakdown of the vegetative cell proteins. Thus, it looks as if the still poorly understood processes that regulate the biological events inducing sporulation condition the formation of the spore proteins as well as those of the crystal at the same time.

In the present state of things, we wonder whether the crystalline toxin cannot be considered a normal product of bacterial metabolism the synthesis of which would normally be derepressed at the time of sporulation. The fact that this protein is produced in large amounts and that the basic components tend toward easy aggregation might suggest that they are structural proteins. The possibility of their being akin to the protein compounds of the spore envelopes is not to be excluded. It is interesting to note that the excretion and aggregation of the initial crystal components take place near the septum and the forespore wall.

In any case, the production of protein or bioactive material during sporulation is rather common. Such is the case with some toxins (Sebald and Schaeffer, 1965), some antibiotics found in *B. subtilis* (Schaeffer *et al.*, 1965), and sporulation proteases (Balassa, 1966).

V. Immunology and Immunochemistry

The study of the antigenic properties of the crystalline toxin proves of basic interest and shows itself to be a valuable tool in research work and in the characterization of the constituent protein chain. Moreover, there are a great variety of *B. thuringiensis* strains of different toxicities. Therefore, comparisons of the immunochemical properties of crystals from different strains should help identify them and eventually allow the establishment of relationships between structure and toxicity. Since 1960, several investigations have been conducted along these lines. In all the cases we will consider, the antiserum preparations have been effected either with pure crystals suspensions or with the proteins obtained through alkaline dissolution, and the analyses have been performed by the usual gel precipitation techniques (Ouchterlony and immunoelectrophoresis).

The first data in this field of research are given by Krywienczyck and Angus (1960). These investigators showed that the crystals from *berliner* (serotype I), *sotto* (serotype IV), and *entomocidus* (serotype VI) have several antigenic determinants. At the same time, de Barjac and Lecadet (1961) studied *berliner* (serotype I), *anduze* (serotype III), and *subtoxicus* (serotype VI) strains and observed that the crystals of these three strains have a common antigen-antibody system, while a second precipitation system is common only to the *berliner* and *subtoxicus* strains.

In their studies on the *berliner, entomocidus,* and *sotto* strains, Krywienczyck and Angus (1965) found that the crystals of these strains also have a common antigen, as the several antisera inactivate *in vitro* and *in vivo* the toxin liberated from the *sotto* strain crystals. These same authors (1966) reported that crystals from the *entomocidus* strain have another antigen which does not exist in *sotto* strain crystals. These experiments thus have demonstrated similarities as well as differences in the structure of the crystals from various strains.

Taking these data into account, Pendleton and Morrison (1966b) made a systematic examination of the antigenic properties of crystals from a great number of *B. thuringiensis* strains using anticrystal sera only. Working on identity or nonidentity criteria of the precipitation systems observed in gel immunodiffusion, the authors have found 28 different serotypes containing 9 different antigens (called a, b, c, d, e, f, g, h, and i) distributed according to different patterns.

In Table III the serotypes of some of the most common and most often studied strains in different laboratories are given as proposed by Pendleton and Morrison (1966b). The authors suggest using these properties as complementary taxonomic criteria of the classification already established by de Barjac and Bonnefoi (1962). Pendleton and Morrison (1967) looked for these different antigens in the products of the enzymatic lysis of the crystals in the regurgitated chyle from *Pieris brassicae* larvae. They showed that enzyme digestion leads to the loss of some antigens and to the appearance of new antigenic patterns.

These few examples demonstrate the complexity of the problem and the difficulties of an immunochemical study comparing crystals of different strains. In effect, the number and the nature of the antigenic determinants which have been brought to light depends, in part, on the strains used, but they also differ according to whether the immunization has been produced with pure crystals or with solutions of crystals. At present, however, and for a given strain, in research work on structure and biosynthesis, the immunochemical techniques can be an effective tool in isolating and characterizing crystal protein chains. For example, Cooksey (1968) purified, from an alkaline solution of Tolworth (serotype IX) crystals, a protein which essentially corresponds to one of the two antigens

TABLE III

PRECIPITIN REACTIONS IN GEL DIFFUSION OF SOLUBLE CRYSTAL PROTEIN
OF *B. thuringiensis* STRAINS AGAINST NINE DIFFERENT ANTISERA[a]

Isolate strains	Esterase type	Crystal antigens a b c d e f g h i	Crystal serotype
berliner	*berliner*	+ − − + − − − − +	adi
steinhaus 1715	*berliner*	+ − − + − − − + +	adhi
finitimus	*finitimus*	− + − − − − − − −	b
alesti	*alesti*	− − − − − − − + +	hi
anduze	*alesti*	+ − − + − − − − −	ad
T-84-A	*sotto*	− − + − − − − − −	c
dendrolimus	*dendrolimus*	− − − + − − − − +	di
kenya	*kenya*	− − − − + − − − −	e
galleriae russi	*galleriae*	− − − − − + − + −	fh
entomocidus	*entomocidus*	+ − + − − − − − −	ac
subtoxicus	*entomocidus*	+ − − − − − − − −	a
92	*morrison*	− − − + − − + − +	dgi
tolworth	*tolworth*	− − − − + − − − −	e

[a]Data from Pendleton and Morrison (1966b); a part of their classification.

present in the initial preparation. By a gentle treatment of the crystals in bicarbonate buffer at pH 8.9, he isolated another component corresponding to the second antigen, which is common to several other strains. Similar studies are currently being carried on in many laboratories.

As for biosynthesis, we have seen (Section III) that the successive appearance of different components can be followed throughout sporulation with these same immunochemical techniques. Nevertheless, the existence of several antigenic patterns is not absolute proof of the presence of several distinct proteins. We have already pointed out that protein chains of different molecular weight might correspond to associative products of the same basic component.

VI. Toxicity

Aoki and Chigasaki (1915) describe the bacterium isolated from silkworm larvae by Ishiwata and the disease which follows when it is ingested by the larvae; they were the first to state that only the old sporulated cultures were pathogenic when ingested by the insect. One must wait for the observations of Steinhaus (1951) Steinhaus and Jerrel (1954), and of Hannay (1953) to link pathogenicity for lepidoptera larvae to the presence of the parasporal inclusion. Angus (1954, 1956a) demonstrated very satisfactorily that crystals alone or their alkaline solutions are toxic for *Bombix mori* larvae, that the spores alone are not toxic, and that crystals are actively toxic only when ingested by the larvae.

A. Species Susceptible to *B. thuringiensis* and to the Endotoxin Alone

Numerous species of insects, especially those among the lepidoptera, are susceptible to the crystallophore bacteria (Steinhaus, 1957; Martouret, 1963; Vankova, 1964). To date, according to Heimpel (1967), their number is about 140, and approximately 100 are among the lepidoptera (Heimpel and Angus, 1960). Among other susceptible species we find some of the order hymenoptera, more rarely diptera (Hall and Dunn, 1958), and even coleopterea (Steinhaus and Bell, 1953). All these species are known to be sensitive to the strains experimented with by the authors.

The range of activity of *B. thuringiensis* preparations varies from one strain to another and depends essentially on the ability of the strain to produce the different toxins mentioned above.

Apparently, the crystal endotoxin is active only on lepidoptera larvae. Table IV gives a succinct list of the species sensitive to the *B. thurin-*

TABLE IV

COMPARATIVE SUSCEPTIBILITY OF LEPIDOPTEROUS LARVAE TO
B. thuringiensis berliner[a]

Family	Species	LD_{50}(mg/100 ml)
Pieridae	Alfalfa caterpillar (*Colias eurytheme*)	0.12
Artiidae	Saltmarsh caterpillar (*Estigmene acrea*)	1.14
Noctuidae	Variegated cutworm (*Peridroma saucia*)	1.8
Noctuidae	Cabbage looper (*Trichoplusia ni*)	3.2
Pyraustidae	Celery leaf tier (*Udea profundalis*)	12.0
Notodontidae	Red-humped caterpillar (*Schizura concinna*)	24.0
Pyraustidae	Lucerne moth (*Nomophila noctuella*)	36.0
Noctuidae	Alfalfa looper (*Autographa californica*)	43.0
Noctuidae	Cotton bollworm (*Heliothis zea*)	100.0
Noctuidae	Black cutworm (*Agrotis ypsilon*)	Not susceptible at level tested

[a]Some of the results found and published by White and Briggs (1964). The species were assayed with a *B. thuringiensis* thuricide standard containing spores and crystals.

giensis berliner (serotype I) crystals. Here the pieridae are the most susceptible to this strain. In this connection, we must also state that toxicity of *B. thuringiensis* preparations is manifested throughout larval development.

B. SYMPTOMS OF INTOXICATION IN LEPIDOPTERA

The toxic manifestations induced by the ingestion of *B. thuringiensis* crystal preparations vary from one species to another. Yet the general characteristics of intoxication are anorexia in the first hours, followed in most cases by lethargy, general paralysis, and changes in the gut leading to death. These toxic effects, due to the crystal alone, are accompanied by septicemia, when spores are present or when the insect has ingested old sporulated cultures. Then it is necessary to distinguish between toxemia, brought on by the crystal alone (which we will discuss in this section), and other pathological manifestations related to the presence of spores or other toxic entities produced by the bacteria.

As for the toxic symptoms induced by the crystal endotoxin in lepidoptera, Heimpel and Angus (1959) classify the susceptible species as three groups:

Group I (type *Bombyx mori*) includes a small number of species. The larval gut pH is high (10 or above). Crystal action is very quickly manifested by gut paralysis followed by general paralysis within 60–80 minutes following ingestion.

Group II (type *Pieris brassicae*) is represented by numerous species. The larval gut pH is approximately 9.5. The first symptom seen is cessation of eating due to a buccal paralysis followed by a more or less complete gut paralysis causing debility, which leads to death.

Group III (type *Anagasta kuhniella*) include larvae that have a gut pH lower than 8.4 and that are not affected by either the crystal or the spore alone. The spore must be associated with the crystal endotoxin to bring about the toxemia which leads slowly to death without the symptoms of paralysis described above.

C. Quantitative Evaluation of Toxicity

The toxic action of the crystalline inclusion is generally tested on group I and II larvae, as these species are susceptible to the crystals alone. The insects chosen for the tests are not always the same in all countries. Nevertheless, *P. brassicae* and *B. mori* larvae are very frequently used at the fifth instar stage, since this stage represents the optimal conditions for biological tests (Grison and de Sacy, 1956; Burgerjon, 1957).

In these two types of insects, and especially in group II insects (*P. brassicae*), the primary effect of the crystal toxin is its action on the digestive tract and especially the buccal paralysis which is observed in the first hours following ingestion. The paralysis is at once marked by the cessation of feeding. Burgerjon (1957, 1962) has demonstrated that the decrease in the larval food consumption is directly correlated to the crystal concentration of the preparation. The mortality which occurs between the first and the sixth day following ingestion is a less useful criterion for evaluating the toxicity of preparations because it is delayed and other secondary effects can add to the toxemia making the data difficult to interpret.

For these reasons, Burgerjon (1962) proposed a technique for measuring the decrease of food consumption by quantitative evaluation with a photoelectric cell (Bulger, 1935) of treated cabbage leaf area consumed by batches of larvae, comparing them to batches of controls. Here the toxin can be force-fed to the larvae with a microsyringe (Dutky, 1951; Martignoni, 1957) or injected into the hemocoel.

Toxic doses are expressed in micrograms per gram of larva, the ED_{50} corresponding to the dose which induces a decrease in food consumption of 50%.

D. TOXICITY OF CRYSTAL PREPARATIONS FROM VARIOUS STRAINS

Various species of lepidoptera are not similarly sensitive to all *B. thuringiensis* strains, and a narrow specificity exists which can be correlated with the nature of the crystals and to the host reactions. Burgerjon (1962) demonstrated that *P. brassicae* larvae are more sensitive to *berliner* strain crystals (serotype I) than to those of the *anduze* strain (serotype III). Comparing the toxicity of the crystals from these two strains, Lecadet and Martouret (1964) found that in *P. brassicae* the ingestion of 0.03 μg of crystals from the *berliner* strain had the same effects as the ingestion of 0.3 μg from the *anduze* strain, that is, they were much less susceptible to the latter (Table V). Angus (1967) studied the toxicity of crystals from three different strains on *B. mori* (Table VI) and we can see that, in this case, the *berliner* strain (*thuringiensis* var. thuringiensis) crystals are the least active.

These results clearly show the diversity of crystal toxicity according to the species considered. Since many *B. thuringiensis* strains have been isolated to date, it will certainly be possible to discover the most active strains against each lepidoptera species. Recent studies in this direction have been published by Burgerjon and Biache (1967). Last, it looks as if

TABLE V

TOXICITY OF PURE CRYSTALS OF TWO STRAINS OF B. *thuringiensis* FOR *Pieris brassicae* LARVAE[a]

Amount given[b] (μg/gm of larvae)	*anduze* (Serotype III)				*berliner* (Serotype I)			
	Reduction of eating (RC %)	Mortality[c]			Reduction of eating (RC %)	Mortality[c]		
		3	5	10		3	5	10
15	99	10	—	—	99	10	—	—
3	89	8	9	10	99	10	—	—
0.6	67	8	8	10	99	10	—	—
0.3	40	4	8	9	94	9	10	—
0.15	32	6	9	9	84	7	8	9
0.06	18	3	6	—	68	6	9	10
0.03	0	0	0	—	24	5	6	7

[a]Results obtained and published by Lecadet and Martouret (1964).
[b]By forced ingestion.
[c]Mortality on the third, fifth, and tenth day of the experiment for lots of 10 larvae.

TABLE VI

Toxicity of Parasporal Inclusions for
Bombyx mori Larvae[a]

B. thuringiensis var.	Estimate of ED_{50} $(\mu g)^b$	Estimate of LD_{50} $(\mu g)^b$
thuringiensis (type berliner)	26	5
sotto	0.02	0.015
entomocidus	0.03	0.025

[a]Data from Angus (1967).
[b]Expressed as micrograms per gram of larvae; ED_{50} for paralysis in 6 hours, LD_{50} for death in 48 hours.

the most active doses of a given strain against a given species are very small and always lower than 1 μg/gm of larvae.

E. Toxicity of the Soluble Products

It has been shown that native crystal toxins and their alkaline solutions are only active when ingested (Angus, 1954, 1956a). Angus also observed that sotto strain crystals are soluble in *B. mori* gut content, and he postulated that the crystal might be a protoxin transformed into active toxin when going through the midgut (Angus, 1956b). Martouret (1960), and then Lecadet and Martouret (1962), obtained *in vitro* the dissolution of *berliner* strain crystals in *P. brassicae* regurgitated chyle, and they showed that the supernates are toxic not only when fed, but also when injected into the hemocoel. These authors suggested that an enzymatic lysis unmasks the toxic pattern of the crystal protein chain. Lecadet and Dedonder (1966a) isolated two proteases from *P. brassicae* chyle. These enzymes solubilize the crystal and release several groups of soluble proteins of various dimensions. Some have a molecular weight of 40,000 or above, the others have a lower molecular weight, are dialyzable, and can be retained on Sephadex G-75 (Lecadet and Dedonder, 1967). These hydrolyzates are active by injection into the hemocoel. Table VII gives an indication of the toxic doses.

The ED_{50} can be determined by graphs (Fig. 5) plotting decrease of food consumption against dosage (Lecadet and Martouret, 1967a). The ED_{50} is 0.04 μg/gm of larvae when the hydrolyzates are ingested and 0.6 μg/gm when they are injected into the hemocoel. In this latter case, the ED_{50} is higher but it is always lower than 1 μg/gm of larvae.

An enzymatic system similar to that of *P. brassicae* has been found in *B. mori*. Lecadet and Martouret (1967b) demonstrated that the hydrolyzates of the crystals by these enzymes are toxic when injected into *B. mori* larvae as well as *P. brassicae* larvae; however, the toxic doses are

TABLE VII

COMPARATIVE TOXICITY OF PROTEINACEOUS AND PEPTIDE FRACTIONS OF ENZYMATIC
HYDROLYZATES OF *B. thuringiensis berliner* CRYSTALS FOR *Pieris brassicae* LARVAE[a]

Fraction	Amount given (μg/gm of larvae)	Forced ingestion				Injection			
		RC %[b]	Mortality[c]			RC %[b]	Mortality[c]		
			3	5	10		3	5	10
Nondialyzable	42.5	99	7	10	10	96	10	10	10
proteinaceous	4.25	99	5	7	10	82	6	7	8
fraction excluded	0.425	85	2	8	10	35	1	3	6
by Sephadex G-75	0.075	26	3	4	6	24	6	9	9
Dialyzable peptide	42.5	97	8	100	10	98	10	10	10
fraction included	4.25	96	8	10	10	97	10	10	10
in Sephadex G-75	0.825	96	8	10	10	98	8	10	10
Crystals solubilized by 0.05 *N* NaOH	41.5	100	8	10	10	0	2	3	3

[a]Data from Lecadet and Martouret (1967a)
[b]Toxic activity expressed by the reduction in feeding (RC %) observed after 24 hours.
[c]Mortality on the third, fifth, and tenth day of the experiment for lots of 10 larvae.

higher for *B. mori* than for *P. brassicae*. We will later discuss these differences in susceptibility.

It seems, therefore, that *in vitro* crystal dissolution by the host proteases are common to several species of lepidoptera and that an unmasking of toxic groups active in various species occurs. Recently Heimpel (1967) and then Faust *et al.* (1967) questioned the enzymatic nature of these processes and suggested that the experimental conditions

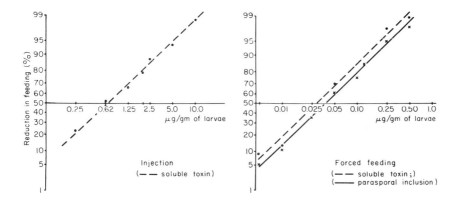

FIG. 5. Quantitative evaluation of the toxicity of the proteinaceous fractions of the enzymatic hydrolyzate (soluble toxin) compared with a suspension of untreated crystals of *B. thuringiensis* var. *berliner*. Dose administered to the *Pieris brassicae* larvae (μg/gm) versus reduction in eating (%). Data from Lecadet and Martouret (1967a).

of hydrolysis made possible a dispersion of the crystalline structure. It is also possible that factors other than the enzymes act *in vivo*. It is equally possible that the alkalinity, which represents an optimum for the enzymes used to solubilize the crystal, increases the efficiency of the proteases. There is, however, no doubt that the lysis of crystals observed *in vitro* is essentially due to proteases (Lecadet and Dedonder, 1966a), since the factors which denature these enzymes (heat, metallic ions, and so on) inhibit crystal dissolution in the same proportions as seen in digestion of soluble proteins.

In any case, one can speculate on the nature of the pattern of toxicity seen in the above experiments. It is as yet premature to tell what it is. One can nevertheless point to the fact that a secondary structure of the molecules is necessary for toxin efficacy. In fact, it has been demonstrated that the crystals, the crystal alkaline solutions (Angus, 1956b), and the preparations which result from enzymatic dissolution of crystal toxins are heat labile. However, low molecular weight peptides (5,000-10,000) isolated from enzymatic lysates (Lecadet and Martouret, 1967a) have a lower toxicity than high molecular weight products.

VII. Mode of Action

The mode of action of crystalline endotoxin has been the subject, since 1959, of numerous investigations which are difficult to interpret because of the diversity of the susceptible species and the observed variations in the efficacy of crystals from different strains of *B. thuringiensis*. The primary site of toxin action as well as the histopathological phenomena which accompany intoxication are still unknown; thus, it is very difficult to explain the processes involved.

A. MOLECULAR LEVEL

There is no longer any doubt as to the proteinaceous nature of the crystalline toxin. The real nature of the active sites, borne by the constituent protein chains, which account for the toxemia, is not yet known, and, thus it is impossible to determine the mechanism of action at the molecular level. Yet the hypothesis of Angus (1956b), who considers the crystal active only *per os* as a protoxin which must be transformed into an active toxin in the host organism, seems to have been confirmed by the investigations of Lecadet and Martouret which pointed to that soluble material released *in vitro* by *P. brassicae* and *B. mori* chyle that is toxic when injected into the hemocoel.

Proteases isolated from the chyle of these larvae, because their action is optimal at a high pH and because they have a large range of specificity (Lecadet and Dedonder, 1966b), dissociate, *in vitro*, the crystalline structure under experimental conditions specified by these authors. The splitting produced by these enzymes yield active fragments—proteins or peptides of various molecular weights—but also inactive fragments that have not had their toxic site unmasked or small peptides that are not toxic.

It is reasonable, therefore, to assume that the reactions obtained *in vitro* can occur *in vivo* in types I and II species sensitive to the crystal alone after ingestion of the crystalline inclusion, as the midgut of these larvae has the pH which corresponds to the optimum of action of the proteases. Moreover, the gut content is rich in reducing agents and is highly buffered (Estes and Faust, 1966), which can only make more effective the action of these enzymes. All the physiological conditions prevailing *in vivo* in the gut of the susceptible species happen to facilitate crystal dissolution and toxin liberation.

Otherwise, the toxemia symptoms, which differ according to the species, might be limited to their power of hydrolyzing the crystalline toxin *in vivo*. As a consequence of this assumption, it is possible to understand that species resistant to the crystals alone could be intoxicated by their hydrolyzates. Such is the case, for instance, for type III insects (*Anagasta kuhniella*). Yamvrias (1962) and then Lecadet and Martouret (1967b) have shown that the hydrolyzates of *berliner* strain crystals obtained with *P. brassicae* and *B. mori* proteases are toxic for *A. kuhniella* larvae when ingested or injected into the hemocoel. For these species there is no hydrolysis *in vivo* when the crystals alone are ingested.

Another consequence of the possibility that enzymatic processes play a part in activating the protoxin is that the variability in the efficacy of the crystals from various strains for various hosts, according to the enzymatic lysis, would be conditioned by two factors—the structure of the crystal as a substrate on one hand and the specificity of the host enzyme on the other hand.

We have already mentioned that *anduze* strain (serotype III) crystals are less active for *P. brassicae* larvae than *berliner* strain (serotype I) crystals. The enzymatic hydrolysis in the latter case is more rapid and more complete than that in the *anduze* strain (Lecadet and Martouret, 1964). These differences might be due to structural differences in the crystals from these two strains. However, *B. mori* is more sensitive to *anduze* strain crystals than to those of the *berliner* strain, and we have observed that *B. mori* proteases hydrolyze *berliner* strain crystals less easily than do *P. brassicae* proteases.

In this case, the specificity of the proteases might explain the differences which have been noted. We can relate these observations to those of Grigorova *et al.* (1967). They have observed that the structures of the two types of crystals — bipyramidal and biprismatic — are probably different, the biprismatic form being the less stable. The differences in toxicity observed by Grigorova (1966) between the crystals of these two types would be due, according to this investigator, to structural differences; the cubic biprismatic crystals, being more toxic, would be the more easily degraded. Investigations in this direction should contribute, in the future, to an elucidation of the crystalline endotoxin mechanism of action. In any case, the isolation of the smallest fragments that are still toxic when they are released *in vivo* will be necessary to explain fully the toxic action of these components.

B. PHYSIOLOGICAL LEVEL

All recent investigations in this field proceed more or less directly from Heimpel and Angus's observations (1959) on the physiological and histopathological manifestations of the toxin in the various groups of lepidoptera already described. These authors show that for type I insects (*B. mori*) general paralysis occurring in the 80 minutes following ingestion results from the pH rise of the hemolymph due to the leakage of the gut juice alkaline materials through the gut wall damaged by the toxin.

In type II insects (*P. brassicae*), the buccal paralysis which occurs immediately after the ingestion of crystals is followed by a more or less complete paralysis of the digestive tract, but there is no modification of the hemolymph pH and no general paralysis. Larval death is attributed to malfunction of the gut and to the invasion of the host hemolymph by the bacteria.

In both cases, in spite of slight differences in symptomatology, important physiological dysfunction is observed in the midgut and modifications of pH occur at this level.

1. ROLE OF pH MODIFICATIONS IN THE MIDGUT AND IN THE HEMOLYMPH

The reason for the general paralysis in type I insects is discussed by Heimpel and Angus (1959, 1960), who noted a decrease in pH in the midgut paralleling the rise of the hemolymph pH and the occurrence of the general paralysis (Fig. 6).

An investigation by Fast and Angus (1965) on gut wall permeability of *B. mori*, with radioactive tracers, showed that glucose-^{14}C transfer into the hemocoel is inhibited by the toxin and that, at the same time, the transfer of sodium carbonate-^{14}C is accelerated. These data suggest that the general paralysis observed in the insect is due to changes in the pH of

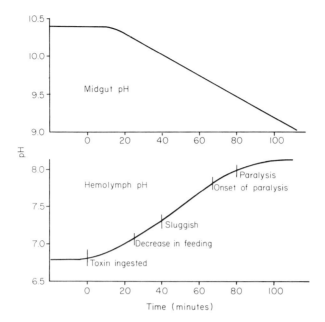

FIG. 6. Changes in pH of the gut contents and blood of *Bombyx mori* larvae after ingesting crystals from *B. thuringiensis* var. *sotto*. Data from Heimpel and Angus (1960).

the hemolymph induced by the alteration of the gut wall permeability. Drilhon and Vago (1960) had already observed in *B. mori*, following intoxication, a change in blood composition (decreased protein content), which, according to these authors, might be correlated with the rise of the hemolymph pH.

As for the type II insects, Martouret (1964) observed a fall of the midgut pH of about two units within 8 hours following the ingestion of the crystals; these modifications of the pH seemed to be related to the intensity of the hydrolysis *in vivo* (Fig. 7). However, the maximum dose of protoxin, over which the reduction of consumption is no longer reversible, would be different and lower than that which limits the reversibility of the pH modifications. This difference indicates, in the author's opinion, that the damage due to pH changes is different from that which induces reduced food intake. Martouret did not observe a significant change in hemolymph pH. More recently, Bentz (1966) indicated that the hemolymph may be more highly buffered than the midgut content.

2. HISTOPATHOLOGY

Histopathological investigations have been carried out by several workers—Mattes (1927) on *A. kuhniella*, Tanada (1953) on *Pieris rapae*,

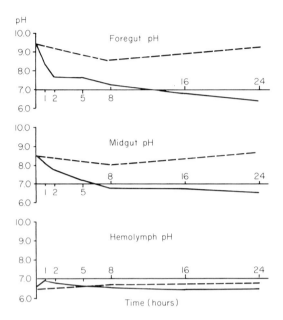

FIG. 7. Changes in pH of the gut contents and hemolymph of *Pieris brassicae* larvae. Solid line = after ingesting 5 μg of crystals from *B. thuringiensis* var. *berliner*; broken line = after ingesting sterile water (control). Data from Martouret (1964).

Heimpel and Angus (1959) on *B. mori*, Hoopingarner and Materu (1964) on *Galleria mellonella*, and Martouret *et al.* (1965) on *P. brassicae.* They agree that the midgut epithelium is seriously damaged by the toxin within the first hours following ingestion.

Heimpel and Angus (1959) suggest that the injuries observed on the midgut epithelium could result from the action of the toxin on cement cells. In this connection, Estes and Faust (1964) observed in *G. mellonella* the release of N-acetylglucosamine in the blood of intoxicated larvae, the presence of N-acetylglucosamine indicating the breakdown of the polysaccharides from cell cementing substances.

Lhoste *et al.* (1964) and then Martouret *et al.* (1965) studied the action of the crystals on the various cell types of the midgut epithelium in *P. brassicae* relative to pH changes of the gut content. These authors demonstrated that the type II cells, which predominate in the epithelium are the most seriously damaged; and this damage may be so severe as to cause complete lysis of the cells, but, in most cases, these phenomena cannot by themselves explain the death of the intoxicated larvae. The authors suggest that the damage observed might result from changes in the gut content pH. They conclude that "we can wonder whether the disintegration of the gut structures, which are observed in the larvae intoxicated with *B. thuringiensis* and generally attributed to the crystalline toxin, is not in fact only a secondary phenomenon. Supporting this hypothesis, Heimpel's works (1955) can be recalled; they have shown that following intoxications of *Pritisphora erichsonii* with *B. cereus*, other organs, especially the muscles and the nervous system, could present pathological manifestations."

Be that as it may, all these symptoms related to the toxemia, and, more particularly, the pH decrease, would facilitate the proliferation of the intestinal gut microflora, in accord with Vago's observations on *B. mori* (1959) or those of Isakova on *Galleria* (1964), and the passage of the bacteria into the hemolymph. The mortality observed in the days following the intoxication would be the result of the sequence of these various processes.

3. INTOXICATION BY INJECTION INTO THE HEMOCOEL

In the context we have just defined, how can we explain the action of the crystal hydrolyzates when they are injected into the hemocoel? Here, the symptoms of intoxication are identical to those we have described for ingestion; cessation of feeding and mortality are observed in the same time period. Moreover, Martouret (1964) also observed a decrease in midgut pH (1 to 2 units), but this change is not permanent and is partly reversible after 24 hours.

Damage to the mesentery has also been observed following toxin injection (Lhoste and Martouret, 1969). However, the damage is not as great as when the toxin is ingested. These results tend to prove that leakage of toxin liberated by the dissolution of the crystals into the hemolymph is, in point of fact, one of the important factors of intoxication; the changes seen in the digestive system induced by injection into the hemocoel would be only secondary phenomena produced, according to Lhoste and Martouret, by a general anoxia, a hypothesis suggested by the experiments of Bentz (1966).

We must also note that the histopathological manifestations and the changes in the pH occur within 6–24 hours following the intoxication, and that in both cases, whether the toxin is ingested or injected, the primary phenomenon is a buccal paralysis observed within the first 2 hours. In a series of experiments involving the use of X-ray photography to trace the movement of barium sulfate, Heimpel and Angus (1959) demonstrated that food ingested with toxin ceases to move through the gut shortly after crystal ingestion (15–20 minutes). This is due to a direct action of the toxin on the foregut observed in the species of types I and II, and one may wonder whether the site of action of the free toxin might not be a nerve center necessary to working of the gut. Such a hypothesis might account for the intoxication induced by the injection of the toxin as well as by its ingestion. In the latter case, the symptoms of paralysis might result from action on the nerve cells.

This is only a hypothesis, and it is premature to adopt it as a conclusion.

In this connection, the nerve blocking effect of *B. thuringienis* protein toxin was investigated by Cooksey *et al.* (1969) by means of *in vitro* studies involving the action of hydrolyzed toxin on a desheathed spinal ganglion preparation of *Periplaneta americana*. The authors suggested that the toxic effect observed might result from a disruption of potassium ion regulation and related this hypothesis to the observation of Angus (1968). The results reported by Angus (1968) pointed out the similarity of effect of valinomycin and crystal protein on *Bombyx mori* larvae (valinomycin is known to affect membrane permeability).

These recent developments might constitute a new approach to elucidate the difficult problem of mode of action of the toxin.

In any case, the study of the intoxication induced by the injection of the free toxin would, in the future, lead to a better understanding of the mechanisms of action at a physiological level.

VIII. Pathogenesis

The toxemia due to *B. thuringiensis* crystalline endotoxin is not the only factor to consider when susceptible species are contaminated by the bacteria under field conditions. Under these conditions, it is important to consider the host-bacillus relationship. According to MacBain Cameron (1967), *B. thuringiensis* is not a primary pathogen in the usual meaning of this word; the primary effect is the toxemia, but in many cases septicemia follows toxemia and is the cause of death. Heimpel (1964) proposes that the crystalliferous bacteria be considered versatile pathogens with a whole arsenal of toxins.

Generally, larval infection by the entomopathogenic bacteria is effected *per os* (Angus, 1961) through the ingestion of contaminated food. Virulence is correlated with the ability of the bacteria to invade the organism, to establish themselves, and to multiply and kill the host (Heimpel, 1964). When pathogenic bacteria, such as *B. thuringiensis*, produce toxic substances, the microorganisms may or may not be present; and if they are present, toxemia will be accompanied by septicemia. Then, what happens when a susceptible species is contaminated by *B. thuringiensis*? If the insect is fed an old, sporulated culture, it succumbs to the toxemia proper, and passage of bacteria into the hemolymph occurs. If the insect ingests spores or still growing cultures, the microorganisms will induce infection only if they find in the digestive tract favorable conditions for their multiplication and their penetration into the hemolymph; this is made easier by the presence of bacterial toxins, especially of the crystalline endotoxin. In this connection, the host-bacteria relationship in susceptible species varies according to the various types of insects, as considered above.

A. INSECTS SUSCEPTIBLE TO THE CRYSTALLINE TOXIN

Type I and II insects present symptoms of toxemia only when crystals or their hydrolyzates are ingested. When bacteria are present, the mode of action of the pathogen is more complex. Heimpel and Angus, (1960) have clearly indicated the sequence of the pathological process. In group I, the ingestion of old, sporulated cultures or of spore-crystal mixtures brings on the toxic symptoms already described. The decrease in gut pH facilitates multiplication and growth of the bacteria, which rapidly invade the hemolymph; at the same time the larvae become paralyzed and their hemolymph pH increases due to the destruction of the gut epithelium. Death occurs through septicemia. If still growing cultures or spores alone are ingested, the growth of the bacteria and the germination of the spores cannot occur in the digestive tract because of its alkalinity.

In type II insects, the sequence of the process is almost identical. The decrease in midgut pH induced by the endotoxin makes possible bacterial or sporal multiplication and development of gut microflora. The digestive syndrome, relative to the toxemia, facilitates bacterial penetration into the hemolymph, and septicemia ensues. Vegetative cells are found in all the tissues.

In all these cases, the role of the digestive tract microflora (Vago, 1959) cannot be denied and varies according to the pathogen dose (Isakova, 1964). Its action adds up to that of the crystals and the spores. Still other factors play a part in *B. thuringiensis* intoxication. When the conditions are favorable for the development of spores or bacteria, the other toxins (phospholipase C or heat-stable toxin), which are secreted by some strains, act to reinforce the toxemia and facilitate bacterial penetration into the hemolymph.

B. GROUP III INSECTS (TYPE *Anagasta kuhniella*)

This group of insects is not sensitive to crystals alone or spores alone, and the sequence of the pathological process due to the ingestion of the spore-crystal mixture is rather complex and manifested differently from that in the cases described above. Intoxication here has been particularly studied by Yamvrias (1961) in *A. kuhniella*. The gut pH of the larvae (approximately 8.0) is not alkaline enough to permit dissolution of the crystals, but it is favorable for spore development. According to Yamvrias, everything happens as if during their germination in the gut the spores created conditions favorable to the action of the crystals or to the production of a toxic pattern, which then facilitates bacterial penetration into the hemolymph. This induces an atypical intestinal disease more or less associated with a chronic toxemia. The disease develops more slowly than in the type I or II insects and the symptoms differ.

The relations among the host, the bacteria, and the pathogenic toxins are complex and still poorly understood. However, the crystalline endotoxin plays a part in the toxemia, since crystal hydrolyzates can produce intoxication (Yamvrias, 1962; Lecadet and Martouret, 1967b).

C. CARPOCAPE (*Laspeyresia pomonella*)

This pathology is as complex as the one just described and is still poorly understood (MacEwen *et al.*, 1960). The disease is also progressive and slow, nonparalytic, and both spores and crystals must be present (Roehrich, 1964). The evolution of the disease evidently depends on the ingested dose and on the physiological conditions which permit the development of the pathogen inside the larva. It looks as if a synergistic action of the various toxins is necessary to prolong the symptoms.

D. CONCLUSIONS

Our examination of the different cases demonstrates the sequence of phenomena implicated in the pathogenesis in the numerous species susceptible to *B. thuringiensis* and the complexity of the infectious process. Under field conditions, the possibility of bacterial development in the host depends not only on physiological conditions, but also on the climate. Ignoffo (1964) has demonstrated that spore viability is related to temperature and humidity. Grison and Wolf (1964) have made similar observations on the susceptibility of *A. kuhniella* to *B. thuringiensis*. Moreover, Angus (1965) suggests "that there is perhaps a degree of adaptation to particular host species" and Grigorova (1964) shows that the strains of *B. thuringiensis* isolated from *Lymantria dispar* are more pathogenic for this insect than apparently identical strains (biochemical and serological criteria) isolated from other insects.

If the crystalline endotoxin is in itself of great interest, its pathogenic action remains restricted to a limited number of lepidoptera species; and the addition of other factors secreted by the pathogen enlarges its range of activity. Today, the *B. thuringiensis* formulations in the fight against noxious insects are in wide use (Grison, 1967); knowledge of the toxin mechanism of action and of the susceptibility of various species will make possible the obtention of highly effective preparations. As for the effects of this bacteria on man and other vertebrates, numerous investigators, and recently Martouret (1967), have demonstrated the complete innocuity of *B. thuringiensis* in the higher vertebrates.

REFERENCES

Albertsson, P. A. (1960). "Partition of Cell Particles and Macromolecules." Wiley, New York.
Angus, T. A. (1954). *Nature* **173**, 545.
Angus, T. A. (1956a). *Can J. Microbiol.* **2**, 111.
Angus, T. A. (1956b). *Can J. Microbiol.* **2**, 416.
Angus, T. A. (1959). *J. Insect Pathol.* **1**, 97.
Angus, T. A. (1961). *Proc. Entomol. Soc. Ontario* **91**, 8.
Angus, T. A. (1965). *Bacteriol. Rev.* **29**, 364.
Angus, T. A. (1967). *J. Invertebrate Pathol.* **9**, 256.
Angus, T. A. (1968). *J. Invertebrate Pathol.* **12**, 145.
Aoki, K., and Chigasaki, Y. (1915). *Mitt. Med. Fac. (Tokyo)* **13**, 419.
Balassa, G. (1966). *Ann. Inst. Pasteur* **110**, 316.
Bateson, J. B. (1965). *Nature* **205**, 622.
Bentz, G. (1966). *J. Insect Physiol.* **12**, 137.
Berliner, E. (1915). *Entomologist* **2**, 29.
Bulger, J. W. (1935). *J. Econ. Entomol.* **28**, 76.
Burgerjon, A. (1957). *Entomophaga* **2**, 129.
Burgerjon, A. (1962). *Ann. Epyhyties* **4**, 663.
Burgerjon, A., and Biache, G., (1967). *Entomol. Exptl. Appl.* **10**, 211.
MacBain Cameron, J. W. (1967). *Insect Pathol. Microbiol. Control, 1967* p. 182. North-Holland Publ., Amsterdam. VI R
Chu, H. P. (1949). *J. Gen. Microbiol.* **3**, 255.
Cooksey, K. E. (1968). *Biochem. J.* **106**, 445.
Cooksey, K. E., Donninger, C., Norris, J. R., and Shankland, D. (1969). *J. Invertebrate Pathol.* **13**, 461.
de Barjac, H., and Bonnefoi, A. (1962). *Entomophaga* **7**, 5.
de Barjac, H., and Bonnefoi, A. (1967). *Compt. Rend.* **264**, 1811.
de Barjac, H., and Lecadet, M. M. (1961). *Compt. Rend.* **252**, 3160.
Delaporte, B., and Beguin, S. (1955). *Ann. Inst. Pasteur* **96**, 680.
Drilhon, A., and Vago, C. (1960). *Antonie van Leeuwenhoek, J. Microbiol. Serol.* **26**, 407.
Dutky, S. R. (1957). *Bull. Entomol. Plant Quart.*, **192**, 10.
Ellar, D. H., and Lundgren, D. G. (1966). *J. Bacteriol.* **92**, 1748.
Estes, Z. E., and Faust, R. M. (1964). *Comp. Biochem. Physiol.* **13**, 443.
Estes, Z. E., and Faust, R. M. (1966). *J. Invertebrate Pathol.* **8**, 141.
Fast, P. G., and Angus, T. A. (1965). *J. Invertebrate Pathol.* **7**, 29.
Faust, R. M., Adams, J. R., and Heimpel, A. M. (1967). *J. Invertebrate Pathol.* **9**, 488.
Fitz-James, P. C. (1953). *J. Bacteriol.* **66**, 312.

Fitz-James, P. C. (1965). *Régulations chez les microorganismes, Marseille, 1963* pp. 529-544. C.N.R.S., Paris.

Fitz-James, P. C., and Young, E. I. (1959). *J. Bacteriol.* 78, 743.

Glatron, M. F., Lecadet, M-M., and Dedonder, R. (1969). *Compt. Rend.* 269, 1338.

Goodman, N. S., Gottfried, R. J., and Rogoff, M. A. (1967). *J. Bacteriol.* 94, 485.

Grigorova, R. (1964). *Entomophaga Colloq. Intern. Pathol. Insectes, Paris, 1962* Mem. Hors Ser. No. 2, p. 179.

Grigorova, R. (1966). *Proc. 9th Intern. Cong. Microbiol., Moscow, 1961* Abstr. Med., p. 308.

Grigorova, R., Kantardgieva, E., and Pashov, N. (1967). *J. Invertebrate Pathol.* 9, 503.

Grison, P. (1967). *Phytiat. Phytopharm.* 16, 63.

Grison, P., and de Sacy, S. (1956). *Ann. Epiphyties* 4, 663.

Grison, P., and Wolf, J. (1964). *Entomophaga Colloq. Intern. Pathol. Insectes, Paris, 1962* Mem. Hors. Ser. No. 2, p. 329.

Hall, I. M., and Dunn, P. H. (1958). *J. Econ. Entomol.* 51, 296.

Hannay, C. L. (1953). *Nature* 172, 1004.

Hannay, C. L. (1956). *Symp. Soc. Gen. Microbiol.* 6, 318-340.

Hannay, C. L., and Fitz-James, P. C. (1955). *Can. J. Microbiol.* 1, 694.

Heimpel, A. M. (1955). *Can. J. Zool.* 33, 311.

Heimpel, A. M. (1964). *Entomophaga Colloq. Intern. Pathol. Insectes, Paris, 1962* Mem. Hors Ser. No. 2, p. 23.

Heimpel, A. M. (1967). *Ann. Rev. Entomol.* 12, 287.

Heimpel, A. M., and Angus, T. A. (1958). *Can. J. Microbiol.* 4, 531.

Heimpel, A. M., and Angus, T. A. (1959). *J. Insect Pathol.* 1, 152.

Heimpel, A. M., and Angus, T. A. (1960). *Bacteriol Rev.* 24, 266.

Holmes, K. C. and Monro, R. A. (1965). *J. Mol. Biol.* 14, 572.

Hoopingarner, R., and Materu, M. E. (1964). *J. Insect Pathol.* 6, 26.

Ignoffo, C. M. (1964). *Entomophaga Colloq. Intern. Pathol. Insectes, Paris, 1962* Mem. Hors Ser. No. 2. p. 294.

Isakova, N. P. (1964). *Entomophaga Colloq. Intern. Pathol. Insectes, Paris, 1962* Mem. Hors Ser. No. 2. p. 175.

Ishiwata-S. (1902). Kyoto Sangyo Ko, hijo Sanji Hokoku 2, 346.

Krywienczyck, J., and Angus, T. A. (1960). *J. Insect Pathol.* 2, 411.

Krywienczyck, J., and Angus, T. A. (1965). *J. Invertebrate Pathol.* 7, 175.

Krywienczyck, J., and Angus, T. A. (1966). *J. Invertebrate Pathol.* 8, 439.

Labaw, L. W. (1964). *J. Ultrastruct. Res.* 10, 66.

Lecadet, M-M. (1965). *Compt. Rend.* 261, 631.

Lecadet, M-M. (1966). *Compt. Rend.* 262, 195.

Lecadet, M-M. (1967a). *Compt. Rend.* 264, 2847.

Lecadet, M-M. (1967b). *Colloq. Biol. Mol. Orsay, 1967* unpublished data.

Lecadet, M-M., and Dedonder, R. (1966a). *Bull. Soc. Chim. Biol.* 48, 631.

Lecadet, M-M., and Dedonder, R. (1966b). *Bull. Soc. Chim. Biol.* 48, 661.

Lecadet, M-M., and Dedonder, R. (1967). *J. Invertebrate Pathol.* 9, 310.

Lecadet, M-M., and Martouret, D. (1962). *Compt. Rend.* 254, 2457.

Lecadet, M-M., and Martouret, D. (1964). *Entomophaga Colloq. Intern. Pathol. Insectes, Paris, 1962* Mem. Hors Ser. No. 2, p. 205.

Lecadet, M-M., and Martouret, D. (1967a). *J. Invertebrate Pathol.* 9, 322.

Lecadet, M-M., and Martouret, D. (1967b). *Compt. Rend.* 265, 1543.

Lhoste, J., and Martouret, D. (1969). In press.

Lhoste, J., Martouret, D., and Roche, A. (1964). *Proc. 12th Intern. Congr. Entomol., Londres, 1964* p. 737.

MacEwen, F. L., Glass, E. H., Davis, A. S., and Spittstoesser, C. M. (1960). *J. Insect Physiol.* **2**, 195.

Martignoni, M. (1957). *Austalt* **32**, 371.

Martouret, D. (1960). *Proc. 11th Intern. Congr. Entomol., Vienna, 1960* Vol. 2, p. 849.

Martouret, D. (1963). *Phytiat.-Phytopharm.* **12**, 71.

Martouret, D. (1964). *Entomophaga Colloq. Intern. Pathol. Insectes, Paris, 1962* Mem. Hors Ser. No. 2, p. 213.

Martouret, D. (1967). *Phytiat.-Phytopharm.* **16**, 75.

Martouret, D., Lhoste, J., and Roche, A. (1965). *Entomophaga* **10**, 349.

Mattes, O. (1927). *Ges. Befoerder. Ges. Naturw. Marburg* **62**, 381.

Monro, R. A. (1961a). *J. Biophys. Biochem. Cytol.* **11**, 321.

Monro, R. A. (1961b). *Biochem. J.* **81**, 225.

Murray, E. D., and Spencer, E. Y. (1966). *J. Invertebrate Pathol.* **8**, 419.

Norris, J. R. (1964). *J. Appl. Bacteriol.* **27**, 439.

Norris, J. R., and Watson, D. H. (1960). *J. Gen. Microbiol.* **22**, 744.

Pendleton, I. R., and Morrison, R. B. (1966a). *Nature* **212**, 728.

Pendleton, I. R., and Morrison, R. B. (1966b). *J. Appl. Bacteriol.* **29**, 519.

Pendleton, I. R., and Morrison, R. B. (1967). *J. Appl. Bacteriol.* **30**, 402.

Roehrich, R. (1964). *Entomophaga Colloq. Intern. Pathol. Insectes, Paris, 1962* Mem. Hors Ser. No. 2, p. 309.

Ryter, A. (1965). *Ann. Inst. Pasteur* **108**, 40.

Schaeffer, P., Ionesco, H., Ryter, A., and Balassa, G. (1965). *Régulations chez les microorganismes, Marseille, 1963* pp. 553–563. C.N.R.S., Paris.

Sebald, M., and Schaeffer, P. (1965). *Compt. Rend.* **260**, 5398.

Smirnoff, W. A. (1964). *J. Invertebrate Pathol.* **5**, 242.

Smirnoff, W. A. (1965). *J. Invertebrate Pathol.* **7**, 71.

Steinhaus, E. A. (1951). *Hilgardia* **20**, 359.

Steinhaus, E. A. (1957). *Univ. Calif. (Berkeley), Lab. Insect Pathol.* Ser. 4, p. 24 (mimeo).

Steinhaus, E. A., and Bell, C. R. (1953). *J. Econ. Entomol.* **51**, 296.

Steinhaus, E. A., and Jerrel, E. A. (1954). *Hilgardia* **23**, 1.

Tanada, Y. (1953). *Proc. Hawaiian Entomol. Soc.* **15**, 159.

Toumanoff, C. (1953). *Ann. Inst. Pasteur* **85**, 90.

Toumanoff, C. (1954). *Ann. Inst. Pasteur* **86**, 570.

Toumanoff, C., and Lecoroller, Y. (1959). *Ann. Inst. Pasteur* **96**, 680.

Toumanoff, C., and Vago, C. (1951). *Compt. Rend.* **233**, 1504.

Toumanoff, C., Lapied, M., and Malmanche, L. (1955). *Ann. Inst. Pasteur* **89**, 644.

Vago, C. (1959). *Ann. Epiphyties* No. 18, 1.

Vankova, J. (1957). *Folia Biol. (Prague)* **3**, 175.

Vankova, J. (1964). *Entomophaga Colloq. Intern. Pathol. Insectes, Paris, 1962* Mem. Hors Ser. No. 2, p. 271.

Vankova, J., and Kralik, O. (1966). *Zentr. Bakteriol., Parasitenk., Abt. I. Orig.* **199**, S380.

White, C. A., and Briggs, J. D. (1964). *Entomophaga Colloq. Intern. Pathol. Insectes, Paris, 1962* Mem. Hors Ser. No. 2, p. 305.

Yamvrias, C. (1961). Thesis, Universite of Paris, Paris.

Yamvrias, C. (1962). *Entomophaga* **7**, 102.

Young, E. I., and Fitz-James, P. C. (1959a). *J. Biophys. Biochem. Cytol.* **6**, 483.

Young, E. I., and Fitz-James, P. C. (1959b). *J. Biophys. Biochem. Cytol.* **6**, 499.

CHAPTER 12

Toxins of *Pseudomonas*

ROBERT J. HECKLY

I. Introduction

Although not as well known for their toxins as the clostridia, many, if not all, of the organisms that have been classified in the genus *Pseudomonas* produce toxin, and some are known to produce several toxins. It is difficult to determine whether a toxin produced by one species is different from or the same as that produced by another because so little comparative work has been done. In some instances, little information has been given by the investigator other than that the filtrate contained a heat-labile toxin. On one hand, toxin was purified and characterized with respect to physical or chemical properties, but not compared with toxins from other species. Purification and characterization studies of enzymes on the other hand, are relevant, even though all of the workers did not test or demonstrate toxicity of their preparations. All enzymes are assumed to be proteins and, since several of the diseases caused by pseudomonads can be directly attributed to the extracellular enzymic action, I will consider all enzymes as potentially toxic. Table I lists some of the enzymes that have been isolated from or identified in culture filtrates of various of the pseudomonads. A considerable amount of work has been done on the production of enzymes *in vitro*, but in some instances, no effort was made to show toxicity. Such studies are being included in this discussion because of their relevance to production and purification. Endotoxins and other nonprotein toxins will not be included in this discussion.

TABLE I
ENZYMES IDENTIFIED IN FILTRATES OF *Pseudomonas* CULTURES

Species	Enzyme
P. aeruginosa	Proteinase, elastase, lipase, collagenase lecithinase, fibrinolysin
P. pseudomallei	Proteinase, lecithinase
P. fluorescence	Lipase, lecithinase
P. fragi	Lecithinase, lipase
P. lachrymans	Protease
P. marginalis	Pectolytic
P. solanacearum	Celluolytic
P. reptilovori	Lecithinase
P. caviae	Lecithinase
P. aureoaciens	Lecithinase
P. chlororaphis	Lecithinase

II. Toxicity

A. *Pseudomonas aeruginosa*

Pseudomonas aeruginosa has received more attention than any of the other *Pseudomonas* species, not so much because it is an important pathogen, but because of its wide distribution. It has been shown to produce extracellular proteins that are toxic, not only to man and the usual laboratory animals, but also to insects, tissue cultures, monocytes, plants and some gram-positive cocci.

The extracellular enzyme fraction obtained from *P. aeruginosa* by Liu *et al.* (1961) was lethal for mice, and following intradermal inoculation, produced necrotic lesions in rabbits. He reported that this fraction also was toxic to mammalian (HeLa) cells in tissue culture. More recently, Wexler *et al.* (1968) described plaque formation in HeLa monolayers by *P. aeruginosa* which resulted from the toxin produced by the organisms (Coleman *et al.*, 1968). The nature of this toxin has not been determined.

Johnson *et al.* (1967) isolated two types of toxin from filtrates of *P. aeruginosa*. Both were lethal for mice, about 50 μg of protein per LD$_{50}$, but one also was proteolytic and produced dermonecrosis with as little as 10 μg of protein. The other type of toxin was nonproteolytic and did not produce dermonecrosis. This latter toxin may be identical with that obtained from a nonproteolytic strain (P-A-103) by Liu (1966b).

Lysenko (1963a) showed that a strain of *P. aeruginosa* was pathogenic for the larvae of the greater wax moth (*Galleria mellonella*). Culture filtrates from this strain contained 250–450 LD$_{50}$ per milliliter when assayed in the larvae (Lysenko, 1963b). Interestingly, Stephens (1959) found that the virulence of *P. aeruginosa* for grasshoppers was increased by mucin. She did not study the presence of toxin, but it is quite possible that mucin in some manner increased toxin production since addition of mucin to culture media markedly increased toxin production by *Pseudomonas pseudomallei* (Colling *et al.*, 1958).

Although production of extracellular deoxyribonuclease by *P. aeruginosa* has been demonstrated (Streitfeld *et al.*, 1962), there is no evidence that this enzyme is a toxin. The enzyme has not been purified and no tests have been made for toxicity.

Elrod and Braun (1942) described *P. aeruginosa* as a possible plant pathogen which also infects animals. Although he did not show the presence of a toxin, he suggested that the phytotoxic factor is not the same as the toxic substance which affects animals. Liu *et al.* (1961), also concluded that the toxin causing necrosis in tobacco leaves infected with *P. aeruginosa* was not the same as that affecting animals, and its low molecular weight would indicate that it is not a protein. *Pseudomonas lachrymans* does produce a proteinaceous toxin which affects plants, but this toxin has not been tested in animals.

B. *Pseudomonas pseudomallei*

Legroux *et al.* (1932) first observed the effect of an exotoxin produced by *P. pseudomallei* (previously classified as *Malleomyces pseudomallei*), but it was not until a number of years later that Nigg *et al.* (1955) demonstrated by intraperitoneal injection of sterile culture filtrate into mice and hamsters that exotoxin was in fact produced by this organism. Nigg *et al.* (1955) also demonstrated that the intradermal inoculation of sterile culture filtrates resulted in necrosis with surrounding edema. The edema production appeared to be due to a heat-stable toxin which was different from the necrotoxin. Unfortunately, no correlation was found between virulence, colonial morphology, and toxin production in over 25 strains of *P. pseudomallei* (Nigg *et al.*, 1955; Colling *et al.*, 1958). However, up to 23 LD_{50} toxin per milliliter (tested intraperitoneally in mice) was obtained in crude culture filtrate and a partially purified toxin contained 22 LD_{50} per milligram (Heckly, 1958). Dermonecrosis could be produced by approximately 2 mg of this purified toxin. As is shown in Table II, this toxin from *P. pseudomallei* was not as potent as the toxin obtained by Johnson *et al.* (1967) from *P. aeruginosa*. Although the *P. pseudomallei* toxin was not pure, it seems unlikely that more than 99% of its dry weight was inactive protein.

TABLE II

Toxicity of Materials Produced by *P. aeruginosa* and *P. pseudomallei*

Organism	Host	LD_{50}	Dermonecrosis
P. aeruginosa	Mice	30 μg	10 μg
P. pseudomallei	Mice	22 mg	—
	Guinea pigs or rabbits	—	2 mg

III. Production, Purification, and Characterization

A. *Pseudomonas aeruginosa*

Various enzymes produced by *P. aeruginosa* have been implicated as toxic proteins. In a general review of bacterial elastases, Oakley and Banerjee (1963) showed that several strains of *P. aeruginosa* and two strains of *Pseudomonas fluorescens* produced elastases which appeared to be identical. Although the enzymes attacked both acid- or alkali-treated elastin, none attacked fresh elastin (aortic arch sections). They showed that the elastase produced by pseudomonads was antigenically different from that produced by *Clostridium histolyticum* which did dissolve fresh aorta. Mandl *et al.* (1962) showed that although there were similarities, the elastase produced by *P. aeruginosa* also differed from elastases produced by *P. pseudomallei* and *Bacillus subtilis*. Fisher and Allen (1958a) demonstrated that the destructive effect of *P. aeruginosa* infections of the cornea was probably due to an extracellular enzyme. A correlation was demonstrated between the proteolytic activity of the organisms and the degree of corneal ulceration. This corneal destruction was not produced by all proteases and Fisher and Allen (1958b) subsequently showed that the cells grown on nutrient agar produced an extracellular collagenase which would digest corneal protein as well as tendon collagen. Recently, Schoellmann and Fisher (1966) separated a collagenase-like material from other proteolytic enzymes of *P. aeruginosa* by column chromatography. To obtain this enzyme, *P. aeruginosa* was grown on 5% peptone for 18 hours at 37°C and a crude enzyme preparation was precipitated by ammonium sulfate (30% saturation). The precipitate was dialyzed and applied to a diethyaminoethyl (DEAE)–Sephadex A-50 column equilibrated with 0.05 M tris (hydroxymethyl)aminomethane (tris) buffer at pH 7.4 and a gradient to 2.0 M sodium chloride was used to elute the enzymes. All caseinolytic activity was associated with the first component and collagenase activity was associated with only the fourth protein component.

In similar studies using culture filtrates from a strongly proteolytic strain of *P. aeruginosa* isolated from a patient, Johnson *et al.* (1967) were unable to separate elastase and caseinase activity. They used liberation of dye from orcein–elastin as a measure of elastase and casein digestion as a measure of protease activity. However, the relative activities in filtrates from various other strains indicate that these two enzymes were distinctly different; the ratio of elastase to protease varied from 2.6 to 12.1. The work of Morihara (1964) also indicated that elastase production varied with the strain of *P. aeruginosa* since many strains produced no elastase, but all of the strains he tested produced a proteinase.

For production of protease, Johnson *et al.* (1967) grew *P. aeruginosa* on agar containing 2% tryptone, 1% glucose, and 0.5% sodium chloride. After 3–5 days at 37°C, they froze the plates to facilitate elution of the extracellular materials from the agar and added 5% manganese chloride to the cell-free extract to remove nucleic acids. After adjusting the pH to 7, ammonium sulfate was added to 30% saturation and the precipitate was discarded. The precipitate obtained at 70% saturation with ammonium sulfate was removed and dissolved in 0.05 M tris buffer at pH 8.6. Additional impurities were precipitated by adding acetone to 44% and the enzyme was then precipitated with 64% acetone. This precipitate was dialyzed against 0.02 M tris buffer at pH 8.6 and applied to a DEAE-Sephadex A-50 column equilibrated against the same buffer. An enzymically inactive protein traveled with the solvent front, whereas the protases were eluted by increasing concentrations of sodium chloride in the buffer. Most of the enzyme activity was eluted at a low salt concentration. A second protease was eluted by about 0.05 M sodium chloride. All three protein fractions were lethal for mice at 30–100 μg/ml. Judging from the purification procedures, the physical and chemical properties of the proteolytic enzymes studied by Johnson *et al.* (1967) were markedly different from those of the enzymes described by Schoellmann and Fisher (1966).

The work of Morihara (1964) is of interest because of the enzyme separations he effected. Cultures of *P. aeruginosa* were grown on a defined medium containing 4% glucose, 0.2% yeast extract, 1% ammonium phosphate, and other salts. Cells were removed by centrifugation after 5 days' incubation with shaking at 28°C. Chromatography on DEAE–cellulose resolved a crude enzyme preparation into three fractions. All three fractions had proteolytic activity but only fraction II had elastase activity. All elastase positive *Pseudomonas* strains produced both enzyme fractions II and III, and all strains produced fraction I, which had little enzymatic activity. Only certain strains produced all three enzymes. Morihara (1965) subsequently showed that the culture conditions were not critical as these same proteinases could be produced using hydrocarbons (heavy oil) as the sole carbon and energy source in the medium.

Morihara *et al.* (1965) obtained crystalline elastase by first precipitating crude enzyme with ammonium sulfate (60% saturation). The precipitate was then dissolved and reprecipitated with 65% acetone to remove a colored oily substance which interfered with crystallization. The partially purified preparation was dialyzed against 0.02 M phosphate buffer at pH 8, and applied to a DEAE–cellulose column, equilibrated with the same dilute buffer. Materials were eluted by stepwise increases in sodium chloride concentration in the dilute buffer. Fraction II, eluted at 0.05–0.1 M sodium chloride, was collected and concentrated and the enzyme was reprecipitated by adding solid ammonium sulfate to 60% saturation. The enzyme was redissolved, insoluble residues removed, and saturated ammonium sulfate was added to the supernatant solution until it became turbid. The crystalline enzyme thus obtained contained 15.5% nitrogen and had an isoelectric point near pH 5.9. On the basis of sedimentation and diffusion measurements, the molecular weight was 39,500. In addition to digesting orcein–elastin, the purified enzyme digested casein, hemoglobin, egg albumin, and fibrin, but not keratin or native collagen. The optimum pH for both the protease (casein substrate) and elastase activity of the enzyme crystallized from fraction II was pH 8; both activities were resistant to heat up to 70°C but not 75°C, and both exhibited the same pH stability curve, being stable between pH 6 and 10. Because of these similarities, and because various inhibitors such as chelating agents or heavy metals inhibited both enzyme activities, they concluded that both enzyme activities were associated with the same active centers on a single enzyme species.

In an earlier series of papers, Morihara (1956, 1957a, 1959a) described the production, purification, and crystallization of a protease from *P. aeruginosa*. He observed that the purified enzyme digested gelatin more effectively than any of the other substrates, such as casein or hemoglobin (Morihara, 1957b), and he concluded that the purified enzyme was a collagenase. However, Morihara (1963) subsequently showed that a similarly purified proteinase did not digest collagen even though it digested gelatin; hence, the term collagenase should not have been applied to the earlier enzyme. Morihara (1963) reported that this enzyme was prepared by adding excess calcium chloride to precipitate calcium phosphate, and therefore, presumably the nucleic acids. The crude enzyme was then precipitated by increasing ammonium sulfate from 0.3 to 0.6 saturation, followed by fractional precipitation with acetone (35–60% acetone). The precipitate at a final concentration of 2% protein was dissolved in 0.01 M calcium chloride and then crystallized by cooling and the slow addition of acetone. This crystalline enzyme had an isoelectric point near pH 4.1 with a pH optimum of 7–9 and a molecular weight of 48,400 (Inoue *et al.*, 1963). The molecular weight, obtained by ultracentrifugal data, was confirmed (Morihara *et al.*, 1964) using amino acid analyses to calculate a minimum molecular weight.

Liu (1964) reported that for the production of extracellular toxin in synthetic media, the most critical factor was phosphate concentration. At 0.003% phosphate, lecithinase was produced whereas at 0.01–0.2% phosphate protease was produced. In a more recent paper, Liu (1966a) used selected strains and growth conditions to obtain either protease or lecithinase because he found it difficult to separate these enzymes by physical or chemical means. For production of lecithinase, he grew strain P-A-103 organisms on tryptone agar enriched with 1% glucose and covered with a sheet of cellophane. After 24 hours at 37°C, the growth was washed off with 3 ml of distilled water. For production of protease, the NCTC 6751 organisms were grown on the same media but without the addition of glucose. The extract from the plate was precipitated by 50% saturation with ammonium sulfate and then dialyzed and concentrated. Of the pseudomonads tested by Esselmann and Liu (1961), only *Pseudomonas fragi* and *Pseudomonas stutzeri* failed to produce lecithinase in trypticase soy agar. However, Alford and Pierce (1963) obtained a lipase from *P. fragi* but they did not test for lecithinase activity.

Arima *et al.* (1967) showed that both *P. aeruginosa* and *Pseudomonas fluorescens* produced a lipoprotein lipase, although an organism identified only as belonging to the genus *Pseudomonas* produced the most lipase. For purification and characterization, the enzyme was produced in beef extract, glucose, and urea medium (Narasaki *et al.*, 1967). The enzyme was precipitated at pH 5 by 60% saturated ammonium sulfate dialyzed against 0.01 *M* acetate buffer, and subjected to Sephadex G-200 gel filtration; fractionation was on DEAE-cellulose at pH 5.0 using gradient elution to 0.4 *M* sodium chloride, in the dilute buffer. A second lipase (LPL-II) was eluted by 1 *M* sodium chloride containing 0.1 *M* sodium hydroxide. The two lipases appear to be similar in chemical composition and enzymatic properties. The enzymes contained 6–10% sugar, 14–20% protein, and 67–79% lipids. They were both stable between pH 4 and 9, with an optimum at pH 7.0, and both were inactivated by heating above 50°C.

According to Liu (1966a), human infection with *P. aeruginosa* involving the skin is characterized by hemorrhagic necrosis surrounded by an area of edema, redness, and induration, indicating the *in vivo* production of toxins. The gross appearance of such skin lesions suggests that hemolysin was involved, and on the basis of his earlier work (Liu, 1957), that such hemolysin might be considered to be a toxin. Using a rather crude separation, Liu *et al.* (1961) divided products of *P. aeruginosa* into broad categories such as pyocyanin, hemolysin, extracellular enzymes, and cell residues. They showed that pyocyanin was not an important factor in the pathogenesis of *Pseudomonas* infection and that while both hemolysin and the extracellular enzyme fraction were toxic, the latter contained most of the toxin. Liu *et al.* (1961) failed to show that the hemolysin fraction was antigenic and, subsequently, Berk (1962, 1964), found that the toxicity of hemolysin preparations was due to protein content (contaminants) rather than the agent responsible for the hemolytic activity. By comparing intracellular hemolysin with that liberated into the medium, Berk (1963) found several differences; however, there was no evidence to warrant considering either hemolysin as a proteinaceous toxin, particularly since these hemolysins were shown to be heat stable. Altenbern (1966) also concluded that hemolysin plays a minor role in *P. aeruginosa* infections.

Rangam *et al.* (1961) demonstrated fibrinolysin in 18-hour broth cultures of *P. aeruginosa* and intradermal inoculation of the sterile culture filtrate resulted in a necrotic lesion. The fibrinolysin was active only within a pH range of 5-9 and a temperature range of 37-40°C. Because the filtrates did not liquefy inspissated serum and the fibrinolytic activity was resistant to heat at 100°C for 30 minutes, they concluded that a proteinase was not responsible for the lytic activity. However, since Keen *et al.* (1967a,b) demonstrated the proteolytic activity of an enzyme produced by *P. lachrymans* as being heat stable, heat stability alone would not preclude a proteolytic enzyme as the cause of fibrin lysis.

Lysenko (1963b) found that a typical protein exotoxin was produced in tryptone broth, but not in chemically defined media, by a strain of *P. aeruginosa* pathogenic for insects. A maximal concentration of between 250 and 450 LD_{50}/ml was obtained in 2 days' growth with shaking at 28°C. The toxin appears to be a protein because it was nondialyzable, precipitated between 0.6 and 0.9 saturation with ammonium sulfate, inactivated in 10 minutes at 60-70°C, and elicited production of antitoxin in rabbits. The toxin was not purified or compared with that of other pseudomonads.

Keen *et al.* (1967a,b) showed that a toxin having proteolytic activity could be obtained from cucumber leaves infected with *P. lachrymans*. This organism also produces a protease in semisynthetic liquid medium with aeration at 26°C. The culture supernatant fluid was concentrated by vacuum evaporation and the protease precipitated by adding ammonium sulfate to 50% saturation. This effected a 2- to 3-fold increase in specific activity. The optimal pH for activity was at about pH 8, but the enzyme was stable from pH 5 to 11. It is an unusual enzyme in that it was heat stable (no significant loss of activity when autoclaved for 10 minutes at 121°C at pH 7-11). In fact, autoclaving at pH 11 slightly increased the proteolytic activity of the preparation. The protease appears to be responsible for the characteristic lesions produced on cucumber leaves, but the enzyme was not purified or shown to be identical with the toxin.

Zyskind *et al.* (1965) described a proteinaceous antibiotic produced by *Pseudomonas*. This material, produced by an unidentified species of *Pseudomonas*, can be considered to be a toxin since it lysed various living gram-positive cells. The staphylolytic substance was produced by growing the *Pseudomonas* in brain-heart infusion broth for 24 hours at 37°C. The toxin was precipitated at 4°C by 75% acetone. Because the material was retained on dialysis, precipitated by acetone or ammonium sulfate, and inactivated at 56°C, they concluded that the staphylolytic substance was a protein possessing enzyme activity. They examined other cultures and found that filtrates of *P. fluorescens* and *P. aeruginosa* exhibited similar staphylolytic activity.

The only *in vivo* production of toxin by *P. aeruginosa* was that described by Liu (1966b) who produced it in rabbits by making numerous intracutaneous injections of living organisms. After 24 hours, the toxin was obtained by extraction of the skin and he further showed that this toxin was similar to that produced *in vitro*. The nonproteolytic strain P-A-103 produced only induration. Less toxin was produced by the proteolytic strains, which elicited extensive necrosis of the skin, than by the nonproteolytic strains.

B. *Pseudomonas pseudomallei*

Colling *et al.* (1958) showed that toxin production by *P. pseudomallei* was markedly influenced by culture conditions. Toxicity of the culture filtrate reached a maximum in 7-10 days of static incubation at 32°C. Toxin production was significantly less when incubated at 37°C, despite excellent growth. Little growth was obtained when air was excluded, and no toxin was produced. However, little or no toxin was produced in aerated cultures or in chemically defined media. When incubated statically, a pellicle is formed, indicating that oxygen tension may be critical. Addition of mucin to 1% in glycerin beef extract broth more than doubled the toxin production. Liu (1957) reported excellent production using cellophane-covered agar, of a toxin that was heat labile and lethal for mice, and is apparently the same toxin as that described by Colling *et al.* (1958). *Pseudomonas aureofaciens* and *Pseudomonas chlororaphis*, as well as *P. pseudomallei* produced similar toxins in Liu's system.

According to the procedure described by Heckly and Nigg (1958), some impurities could be precipitated from the toxic culture filtrate by 20% (w/v) ammonium sulfate, and most of the toxin was precipitated by increasing the concentration of ammonium sulfate to 35%. Analyses of electrophoretically separated material showed that the major component of this ammonium sulfate-precipitated material, with a mobility of about -5×10^{-5} cm²/sec/V, was nontoxic. At pH 6.5, 7.5, and 9.3, the electrophoretic mobility of the toxic component was nearly zero (-0.5×10^{-5} cm²/sec/V). The sedimentation coefficient of the toxin was approximately 2.8 S (Newton and Heckly, 1960).

Despite the low charge and low molecular weight, the toxin is probably a protein as it is antigenic, readily detoxified by formaldehyde or heating at 60°C, and precipitable by ammonium sulfate (Heckly and Nigg, 1958). However, it is an unusual protein in that it is soluble and stable in 80% ethanol at room temperature. Countercurrent dialysis against cold 95% ethanol effected concentration and precipitation of the toxin and provided a convenient method for obtaining partially purified preparations for further studies. The bulk of the biologically inactive substances was then removed by column chromatography. After dialysis against 0.01 M phosphate buffer, only the inactive substances were adsorbed by DEAE-cellulose (Heckly and Klumpp, 1961).

Fractionation of the crude culture filtrate with a nonionic resin, Duolite S-30, indicated that the lethal and necrotoxin may be separable (Heckly and Nigg, 1958), but much of the activity was lost by this procedure. Fractional precipitation with either ammonium sulfate or ethanol failed to separate the toxins. The alcohol-precipitated fraction from culture filtrates of *P. pseudomallei* not only killed mice and produced necrosis when injected intradermally but it exhibited proteolytic activity and inhibited clotting of blood (Heckly, 1964). Neither of the toxins nor the enzyme was adsorbed by DEAE, and all were inactivated at the same rate by heat at 51–53°C at pH 6, 7.5, and 8. Denaturing agents such as phenol, formaldehyde, and urea affected all activities similarly. Although the pH stability curves were nearly identical, there was a slight but significant difference in the rate of inactivation. The enzyme was inactivated slightly more rapidly than the lethal toxin at pH 10.8 or 11, whereas at pH 3.5 the lethal toxin was inactivated more rapidly than the enzyme. By adsorption of crude toxin preparations with antisera prepared against acid- or alkali-treated preparations, it was shown that necrotoxin, with proteolytic activity, could be precipitated leaving the lethal toxin (with anticoagulant activity) in the supernatant fluid. Or, conversely, the lethal toxin could be precipitated leaving the necrotoxin in the supernatant fluid. Such procedures obviously are not suited for large scale purification procedures, but there is no doubt that the lethal toxin and necrotoxin are separate and distinct entities. There was no evidence that the necrotoxin could be separated from the proteolytic enzyme, and the anticoagulant activity appeared to be correlated with lethal toxicity. It is quite possible that the necrotoxin from *P. pseudomallei* is the same as that obtained from *P. aeruginosa* by Liu *et al.* (1961) but no direct comparison has been made.

Evidence that toxins are produced *in vivo* by *P. pseudomallei* is based largely on the similarity of response and pathology of infected mice and mice injected with culture filtrates. The studies of Dannenberg and Scott (1958a,b) on pathogenesis of melioidosis, indicate that toxin produced *in vivo*, particularly the necrotoxin, was a significant factor in producing the observed lesions. Attempts (Heckly and Nigg, unpublished) to demonstrate toxicity of serum taken from animals infected with *P. pseudomallei* have failed. Using crude antitoxin in the Ouchterlony technique of double diffusion in agar, precipitin lines were obtained with the serum from infected animals; however, the lines were extremely faint and could not be identified definitively as being a result of toxin–antitoxin reaction.

IV. Synthesis

No information on synthesis of pseudomonas toxin either *in vitro* or *in vivo* is available. Only one group has considered synthesis of a substance that might be considered to be a toxin. Although they did not test the proteolytic enzyme for toxicity, Morihara (1959b) and Morihara and Tsuzuki (1964) showed that calcium is required for production of a proteinase by *P. aeruginosa* and that the enzyme contained 1–2 gram atoms of calcium per mole of enzyme. Morihara (1959a, 1960) showed that in the synthesis of the active enzyme, the calcium is incorporated immediately after secretion of the preformed calcium-free proteinase. In the absence of calcium, the secreted enzyme undergoes autosplitting, but if calcium is present, the enzyme is stabilized and accumulates in the extracellular fluid.

V. Mode of Action

A. *Pseudomonas aeruginosa*

In some instances, the mode of toxin action is evident, such as for the collagenase described by Fisher and Allen (1958a,b). Toxicity was shown to be directly related to the enzymatic digestion of corneal proteins. Vasculitis, as described by Margaretten *et al.* (1961), is another manifestation of *P. aeruginosa* infection that appears to be due to enzymatic action (elastase activity), which is supported by the conclusions of Mull and Callahan (1965). However, the fact that the enzyme preparations the latter authors obtained from *P. aeruginosa* digested elastin–orcein is in itself not proof that the observed lesions (destruction of the elastic laminae) were caused by that enzyme. Oakley and Banerjee (1963) obtained enzyme preparations from a number of strains of *P. aeruginosa* and *P. fluorescens*, which digested elastin-orcein but not fresh elastin. Admittedly, the elastase obtained by Mull and Callahan (1965) was probably not the same as that described by Oakley and Banerjee (1963); but the ability to digest native elastin is not a general property of enzymes produced by *P. aeruginosa*.

In their studies on the toxicity of *P. aeuruginosa* extracts for mouse monocytes, Berk and Nelson (1961) observed that the extract depressed succinoxidase activity. Subsequently, Berk and Nelson (1962) indicated that hydrolases (acid and alkaline phosphatase and β-glucuronidase) also were inhibited by crude extracts of *P. aeruginosa*, although they did not study the nature of this inhibition.

Lysenko (1963c) also indicated that a toxin produced by *P. aeruginosa* acted as a specific but unidentified metabolic inhibitor. He based his conclusion on the fact that injection of toxin reduced oxygen consumption by the larvae of the moth *Galleria mellonella*. It is quite possible that the enzyme inhibition was a result of proteolytic action of the *P. aeruginosa* extracts on enzymes involved rather than a specific inhibition.

Johnson *et al.* (1967) concluded that the necrosis observed after intradermal injection of *P. aeruginosa* filtrate was due solely to protease activity. However, he noted that lethality for mice was not necessarily a result of the proteolytic activity of the filtrates. Isolation of a lethal toxin which had no demonstrable enzymatic activity (Liu, 1966b) would indicate that lethality is indeed independent of proteolytic activity.

B. *Pseudomonas pseudomallei*

Until it was shown that the proteolytic enzyme was separable from the lethal toxin (Heckly, 1964), it seemed probable that the culture filtrates were toxic (lethal) because of their proteolytic activity. However, since the proteolytic activity has been separated from the lethal toxin, we have no indication of the mechanism of action for the latter. The necrotoxicity appears to be a function of the proteolytic activity because all attempts to separate enzymatic and dermal necrotic activity have failed.

C. PLANT PATHOGENS

There is little information on the elaboration by pseudomonads of protein toxins that affect plants. Various pseudomonads produce toxins which affect plants, and most of these toxins are low molecular weight materials. A notable exception is the protease described by Keen *et al.*

(1967a,b). This enzyme produced by *P. lachrymans* hydrolyzed casein and cucumber protein rapidly, but elastin and gelatin were not affected. Their evidence that the leaf damage is a direct result of proteolytic action included the fact that the enzyme was produced *in vivo* and that the concentration of amino acids increased in direct proportion to the growth of bacteria and production of the enzyme. However, the enzyme was not purified and was not shown to be identical with the toxin.

Ceponis and Friedman (1959) indicated that the browning and spotting of lettuce leaves by *Pseudomonas marginalis* was probably caused by a pectolytic enzyme produced by the organism. The enzyme was rapidly inactivated at 55°C with an optimal pH for activity about pH 8.

The production of cellulase by *Pseudomonas solanacearum* was described by Kelman and Cowling (1965). They concluded that cellulase is involved in pathogenesis as there was a correlation between virulence and cellulase activity of the culture. The enzyme was stable from pH 3 to 10.5 with an optimal pH for activity near pH 7. The enzyme was rapidly inactivated at 60°C.

VI. Immunology

Fisher and Allen (1958b) showed that injection of a partially purified preparation of collagenase from *P. aeruginosa* into rabbits produced antibody that would react with its antigen in Ouchterlony agar gel diffusion. Such antiserum also inhibited the proteolytic activity of collagenase; however, normal serum, especially at low dilutions, was inhibitory to nearly the same extent and the precipitate demonstrated in agar gel diffusion could have involved antigenic components other than the collagenase in the ammonium sulfate-precipitated fraction. Lysenko (1963d), however, demonstrated antitoxin production by ammonium sulfate-precipitated toxin obtained from a strain of *P. aeruginosa* pathogenic for the insect larvae of *G. mellonella*. Sera from nonimmunized rabbits did not significantly decrease toxicity of the filtrates.

Nigg *et al.* (1955) found that mice which survived sublethal doses of toxin were more resistant to infection with *P. pseudomallei* than untreated mice. Subsequently, Heckly and Nigg (1958) showed that mice could be immunized against a partially purified toxin. They reported an immunity index of 15-18 for mice challenged with ammonium sulfate-precipitated toxin. In unpublished studies, I have found that although the toxin could be detoxified with formaldehyde, the antigenic properties were altered such that the toxoid no longer reacted with antitoxin to form precipitin lines in agar diffusion. Furthermore, the antisera produced by injection of toxoid failed to neutralize the toxin *in vitro*.

In a study on identification of pseudomonads, Liu (1961) showed that antibodies could be produced by crude extracts (extracellular antigens) of various pseudomonad species. The crude extracellular antigens from *P. aeruginosa, P. pseudomallei, Pseudomonas caviae,* and *Pseudomonas reptilivora* were toxic, but since the objective of his study was identification, he did not determine which, if any, of the precipitin lines observed in Ouchterlony tests were associated with the toxin. In a subsequent report, Esselmann and Liu (1961) showed that lecithinases of *P. aeruginosa, P. pseudomallei,* and *P. reptilivora* and *P. caviae* were immunologically distinct. Lecithinase of *Pseudomonas aurefaciens* and *Pseudomonas chlororaphis* were serologically related. Furthermore, the lecithinase of many strains of *P. fluorescens* was neutralized by antilecithinase sera of *P. aureofaciens*. An enzymatically inactive but lethal toxin also was neutralized by its antitoxin (Liu, 1966b) but the antitoxin failed to protect mice against intraperitoneal injection of live cultures.

VII. Pathogenesis

As pointed out by Liu and Mercer (1963), conventional methods of testing for virulence of organisms by measuring the LD_{50} are inadequate for comparing virulence of strains of *P. aeruginosa*, because these organisms usually produce localized infections. Since a relatively large number of cells are required to produce death, these deaths may well be the result of a toxin. Therefore, he assessed virulence as the ability to produce necrosis on intradermal inoculation of 0.1 ml of a broth culture of the organisms. This is indeed a large dose when one considers that with virulent organisms such as *Francisella tularensis* or *P. pseudomallei*, only one cell is required to initiate infection. Nevertheless, he showed that virulence of *P. aeruginosa*, as assessed by intradermal inoculation, depended upon both its ability to grow in the animal's serum and its ability to produce exotoxin. No strain lacking either of these attributes was found to be virulent. Inability to grow in serum was related to the presence of specific antibodies, but these antibodies were not necessarily directed against the toxin. He did not test for antitoxic activity in sera that inhibited growth of the organism.

Liu (1966a) then showed that *P. aeruginosa* produced both a lecithinase and a protease and that both were toxic. Each of these enzyme preparations produced characteristic reactions. On intradermal inoculation lecithinase slowly (48 hours) produced a sterile abscess surrounded by edema, redness, and induration, whereas the protease produced an immediate hemorrhagic lesion which was maximal in 2 hours, and within 48 hours, the lesion was necrotic without edema or hemorrhage. This reaction apparently is the same as that produced by *P. pseudomallei* filtrates as illustrated in Fig. 1. Intravenous injection of lecithinase caused necro-

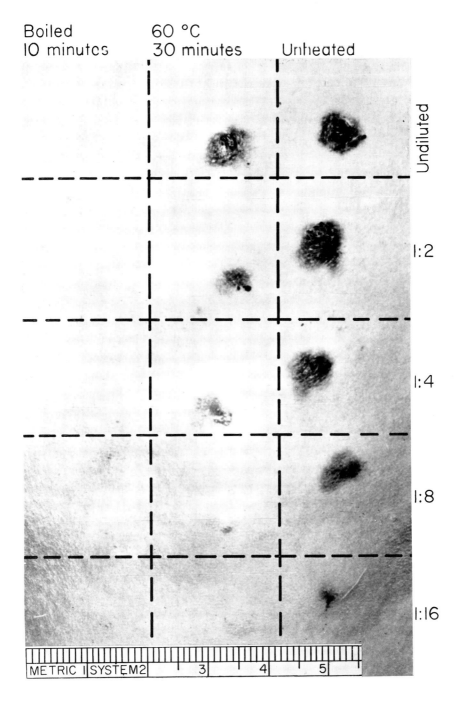

FIG. 1. The effect of heat on the necrotizing action of filtrate from *P. pseudomallei*. The guinea pig was photographed 4 hours after inoculation with 0.1 ml of filtrate of the indicated preparation. From Heckly and Nigg, 1958.

sis of the liver, whereas protease produced hemorrhagic lesions of the intestines and lungs. Intraperitoneal injection of lecithinase produced necrotic spots in the liver within 4-5 hours and no other organs showed any change. Intraperitoneal injection of protease resulted in extensive hemorrhagic lesions of the wall of the peritoneal cavity but no changes in the liver. In contrast, Johnson *et al.* (1967) reported that intraperitoneal injection of a protease isolated from *P. aeruginosa* caused pinpoint blanched areas on the liver. The nonproteolytic toxin isolated by Johnson *et al.* (1967) produced no gross pathological changes in mice and the cause of death was not determined. This was similar to the observation of Liu (1966b), who failed to demonstrate any pathological changes in mice receiving lethal amounts of toxin produced by a nonproteolytic strain of *P. aeruginosa.*

Pseudomonas lecithinase may not actually be a toxin, since the preparations used by Liu (1966a) were crude filtrates and he claimed only that the filtrate contained no protease. It is doubtful that lecithinase is an important factor in natural infection by *P. aeruginosa* because *in vivo* conditions are not favorable for lecithinase production (Liu, 1964). In contrast, appreciable amounts of protease could be produced *in vivo*; thus, the action of protease would be the principal effect (toxicity) of *P. aeruginosa* infections. It seems reasonable that such necrotoxins (proteolytic enzymes) increase the invasiveness of the organisms. Injured tissues are more susceptible to *P. aeruginosa* infection than normal tissue, possibly because the concentration of lactic acid in inflamed skin or other tissue is above normal and, as Liu (1964) has shown, protease production is enhanced by lactic acid.

Intact skin presents an effective barrier to toxin. Even the application of highly active necrotoxin (also a proteolytic enzyme) from *P. pseudomallei* to intact skin failed to produce even the slightest effect (Heckly, unpublished observation). This would explain why *Pseudomonas* is rarely the primary infective agent in disease of healthy individuals.

A review of 14 cases in which *Pseudomonas* infection was considered to be a contributing factor in the death of burned patients (Rabin *et al.*, 1961) indicates that necrosis is a characteristic effect of *Pseudomonas* infection. They did not discuss the pathology in terms of an exotoxin, but the dermal necrosis appears to be similar to that produced by protease from *P. aeruginosa* (Liu, 1966a), and considering the massive growth of organisms in burned areas, it is entirely possible that the organisms also produce lethal amounts of toxin.

Lysenko (1963b) described the effect of a *P. aeruginosa* toxin on caterpillar larvae of *G. mellonella*. Within 60 minutes after injection of concentrated toxin, changes were visible. The caterpillars blackened, lost their turgor and mobility, stopped feeding, and died in 1-2 days. Subsequently, Gupta (1964) showed that the toxin was a cytotoxin for tissue cultures of *G. mellonella* intestinal tissues, producing granulation and vacuolation by the third day. Liu *et al.* (1961) reported that the toxin (extracellular enzyme fraction) from *P. aeruginosa* produced instantaneous dissolution of HeLa cells. They described no morphological changes.

The most striking sign after intraperitoneal injection of mice with *P. pseudomallei* culture filtrates was paralysis of the hind limbs and lachrymation (Nigg *et al.*, 1955). No gross or histological changes were observed in mice killed by the *P. pseudomallei* toxin. The effect of intradermal injection of graded doses of toxin is shown in Fig. 1. The skin became reddened within 5 minutes after injection and the hemorrhagic lesion became evident within 15 minutes. Necrosis was apparent after a few hours.

VIII. Conclusion

The great diversity of *Pseudomonas* toxins makes any general statement regarding them difficult. On the basis of available information based primarily on observations using crude or partially purified preparations, these toxins appear to be relatively low molecular weight proteins — under 50,000. They also seem to have low toxicity, requiring 10-1000 μg to produce an effect. The pH stability range is generally rather narrow (pH 6-9) and the toxins have unusual stability in organic solvents, such as acetone or ethanol. With the exception of some enzymes, which are only presumed to be toxic, none of the extracellular "toxins" have been purified, and hence chemical composition is unknown. Similarly, the observed pathology cannot be ascribed to a particular toxin since all investigators used relatively crude preparations. Except in those diseases characterized by obvious enzymatic degradation of structures, nothing is known about the mode of action of the toxins, and while necrotoxin appears to aid the organisms in maintaining an infection, death of the host may be the result of other undetermined toxins.

More work needs to be done, particularly on the lethal toxins of *Pseudomonas*, with respect to physical and chemical properties, immunochemistry, *in vivo* production, and mode of action.

ACKNOWLEDGMENT

This work was sponsored by the Office of Naval Research under a contract with the Regents of the University of California. Reproduction in whole or in part is permitted for any purpose of the United States Government.

REFERENCES

Alford, J. A., and Pierce, D. A. (1963). *J. Bacteriol.* **86**, 24-29.

Altenbern, R. A. (1966). *Can. J. Microbiol.* **12**, 231-241.

Arima, K., Narasaki, T., Nakamura, Y., and Tamura, G. (1967). *Agr. Biol. Chem.* (*Tokyo*) **31**, 924-929.

Berk, R. S. (1962). *J. Bacteriol.* **84**, 1041-1048.

Berk, R. S. (1963). *J. Bacteriol.* **85**, 522-526.

Berk, R. S. (1964). *J. Bacteriol.* **88**, 559-565.

Berk, R. S., and Nelson, E. L. (1961). *J. Bacteriol.* **81**, 459-463.

Berk, R. S., and Nelson, E. L. (1962). *J. Infect. Diseases* **110**, 1-7.

Ceponis, M. J., and Friedman, B. A. (1959). *Phytopathology* **49**, 141-144.

Coleman, R. G., Janssen, H. J., and Ludovici, P. P. (1968). *Bacteriol. Proc.* p. 95.

Colling, M., Nigg, C., and Heckly, R. J. (1958). *J. Bacteriol.* **76**, 422-426.

Dannenberg, A. M., Jr., and Scott, E. M. (1958a). *J. Exptl. Med.* **107**, 153-166.

Dannenberg, A. M., Jr., and Scott, E. M. (1958b). *Am. J. Pathol.* **34**, 1099-1121.

Elrod, R. P., and Braun, A. C. (1942). *J. Bacteriol.* **44**, 633-645.

Esselmann, M. T., and Liu, P. V. (1961). *J. Bacteriol.* **81**, 939-945.

Fisher, E., Jr., and Allen, J. H. (1958a). *Am. J. Ophthalmol.* **46**, 21-27.

Fisher, E., Jr., and Allen, J. H. (1958b). *Am. J. Ophthalmol.* **46**, 249-254.

Gupta, K. S. (1964). *Current Sci.* (*India*) **33**, 21-22.

Heckly, R. J. (1958). *25th Tech. Progr. Rept. U.S. Naval Biol. Lab.* pp. 71-91.

Heckly, R. J. (1964). *J. Bacteriol.* **88**, 1730-1736.

Heckly, R. J., and Klumpp, M. N. (1961). *31st Tech. Progr. Rept. U.S. Naval Biol. Lab.* pp. 343-355.

Heckly, R. J., and Nigg, C. (1958). *J. Bacteriol.* **76**, 427-436.

Inoue, H., Nakagawa, T., and Morihara, K. (1963). *Biochim. Biophys. Acta* **73**, 125-131.

Johnson, G. G., Morris, J. M., and Berk, R. S. (1967). *Can. J. Microbiol.* **13**, 711-719.

Keen, N. T., Williams, P. H., and Walker, J. C. (1967a). *Phytopathology* **57**, 257-262.

Keen, N. T., Williams, P. H., and Walker, J. C. (1967b). *Phytopathology* **57**, 263-271.

Kelman, A., and Cowling, E. B. (1965). *Phytopathology* **55**, 148-155.

Legroux, R., Kemal-Djemil, and Jeramec, C. (1932). *Compt. Rend.* **194**, 2088-2090.

Liu, P. V. (1957). *J. Bacteriol.* **74**, 718-727.

Liu, P. V. (1961). *J. Bacteriol.* **81**, 28-35.

Liu, P. V. (1964). *J. Bacteriol.* **88**, 1421-1427.

Liu, P. V. (1966a). *J. Infect. Diseases* **116**, 112-116.

Liu, P. V. (1966b). *J. Infect. Diseases* **116**, 481-489.

Liu, P. V., and Mercer, C. B. (1963). *J. Hyg.* **61**, 485-491.

Liu, P. V., Abe, Y., and Bates, J. L. (1961). *J. Infect. Diseases* **108**, 218-228.

Lysenko, O. (1963a). *J. Insect Pathol.* **5**, 78-82.

Lysenko, O. (1963b). *J. Insect Pathol.* **5**, 83-88.

Lysenko, O. (1963c). *J. Insect Pathol.* **5**, 89-93.

Lysenko, O. (1963d). *J. Insect Pathol.* **5**, 94-97.

Mandl, I., Keller, S., and Cohen, B. (1962). *Proc. Soc. Exptl. Biol. Med.* **109**, 923-925.

Margaretten, W., Nakai, H., and Landing, B. H. (1961). *New Engl. J. Med.* **265**, 773-776.

Morihara, K. (1956). *Bull. Agr. Chem. Soc. Japan* **20**, 243-251.

Morihara, K. (1957a). *Bull. Agr. Chem. Soc. Japan* **21**, 11-17.

Morihara, K. (1957b). *Bull. Agr. Chem. Soc. Japan* **21**, 99-106.

Morihara, K. (1959a). *Bull. Agr. Chem. Soc. Japan* **23**, 49-59.

Morihara, K. (1959b). *Bull. Agr. Chem. Soc. Japan* **23**, 60-63.

Morihara, K. (1960). *Bull. Agr. Chem. Soc. Japan* 24, 464-467.

Morihara, K. (1963). *Biochim. Biophys. Acta* 73, 113-124.

Morihara, K. (1964). *J. Bacteriol.* 88, 745-757.

Morihara, K. (1965). *Appl. Microbiol.* 13, 793-797.

Morihara, K., and Tsuzuki, H. (1964). *Biochim. Biophys. Acta* 92, 351-360.

Morihara, K., Yoshida, N., and Kuriyaram, K. (1964). *Biochim. Biophys. Acta* 92, 361-366.

Morihara, K., Tsuzuki, H., Oka, T., Inoue, H., and Ebata, M. (1965). *J. Biol. Chem.* 240, 3295-3304.

Mull, J. D., and Callahan, W. S. (1965). *Exptl. Mol. Pathol.* 4, 567-575.

Narasaki, T., Saiki, T., Tamura, G., and Arima, K. (1967). *Agr. Biol. Chem. (Tokyo)* 31, 993-995.

Newton, N., and Heckly, R. J. (1960). *29th Tech. Progr. Rept., U.S. Naval Biol. Lab.* pp. 41-51.

Nigg, C., Heckly, R. J., and Colling, M. (1955). *Proc. Soc. Exptl. Biol. Med.* 89, 17-20.

Oakley, C. L., and Banerjee, N. G. (1963). *J. Pathol. Bacteriol.* 85, 489-506.

Rabin, E. R., Garber, C. D., Vogel, E. H., Finkelstein, R. A., and Tumbush, W. A. (1961). *New Engl. J. Med.* 265, 1225-1231.

Rangam, C. M., Gupta, J. C., Bhagwat, R. R., and Bhagwat, A. G. (1961). *Indian J. Med. Res.* 49, 232-235.

Schoellmann, G., and Fisher, E., Jr. (1966). *Biochim. Biophys. Acta* 122, 557-559.

Stephens, J. M. (1959). *Can. J. Microbiol.* 5, 73-77.

Streitfeld, M. M., Hoffmann, E. M., and Janklow, H. M. (1962). *J. Bacteriol.* 84, 77-85.

Wexler, S., Moore, M. L., and Ludovici, P. F. (1968). *Bacteriol. Proc.* p. 85.

Zyskind, J. W., Pattee, P. A., and Lache, M. (1965). *Science* 147, 1458-1459.

CHAPTER 13

The Toxins of Mycoplasma

EVANGELIA KAKLAMANIS AND LEWIS THOMAS

Four species of mycoplasma are now known to be toxic for the animals in which they are pathogens. When injected by vein in large enough doses, they produce illness, prostration, and then death, all within a matter of hours after injection. In each case it is the living mycoplasmas that are toxic; organisms killed by heat or disrupted by freezing and thawing are without effect.

Four species out of so many are not enough to warrant any generalization, and yet it is possible that toxicity may be a property of many mycoplasmas, or perhaps all pathogenic mycoplasmas. But if this should be so, there are two great difficulties which stand in the way of establishing this fact. First is the remarkable degree of host specificity to the phenomenon; in this chapter, it will be shown that the organisms are lethal for the animals they infect naturally, but not for others. Second, the property can be lost; within a species some strains are toxic, some are not, and irreversible loss of toxicity has been observed directly for one strain of *Mycoplasma neurolyticum*.

One of the toxic mycoplasmas, *M. neurolyticum*, possesses a soluble exotoxin as well, and the manifestations of toxicity, including the neuro-pathological outcome, are precisely the same for the exotoxin as for the whole organism. This indicates that the toxic property of the whole organism is either the result of production of the exotoxin after the mycoplasmas have been injected, or is due to preformed toxin which the organisms contain at the time of injection. As will be seen, the evidence establishes that the latter is not the case, and that the mycoplasmas are actively at work producing their toxin soon after being injected. The experimental

493

circumstances indicate an analogous process for the other three species, and even though no exotoxin has yet been demonstrated, the resemblances between their behavior and that of *M. neurolyticum* suggest that they are toxic because of their capacity to manufacture a specific toxin *in vivo*.

I. Cytotoxicity of Mycoplasma

There is as yet no clear connection between the manifestations of toxicity for animals and any of the known properties of mycoplasma which lead to their cytotoxicity *in vitro*. There are, however, several mechanisms deserving consideration as possible ways in which mycoplasmas may do damage to cells during infection.

A cytocidal action of mycoplasmas infecting tissue cultures has been noted by several investigators, but no particular species or strain of organism appears to be consistently cytocidal. Gross damage to cells seems to be a nonspecific event when it occurs, perhaps as the result of overwhelming infection of the cultures. Indeed, it is a more remarkable fact that despite the amazing ubiquity of mycoplasmas as contaminants of tissue cultures in laboratories around the world, with 10^6 organisms per milliliter of culture fluid a commonplace observation, so little evidence of injury to cells has been encountered. Gross damage leading to outright cell death is the exception rather than the rule.

More subtle forms of interference with cell function and structure have been observed frequently, and these are most characteristic of infection by arginine-requiring mycoplasmas. Chromosomal abnormalities, consisting of splitting and open breaks, were shown by Aula and Nichols (1967) to be preventable by supplementation of the medium with excess arginine. Copperman and Morton (1967) discovered that *Mycoplasma hominis* I and *M. hominis* II have the property of inhibiting the response of normal lymphocytes to phytohemagglutinin. The inhibitor, a thermolabile protein, was extractable from suspensions of the organisms by freeze–thaw disruption. Its action on lymphocytes was reversible; cells kept in contact with the substance for 48 hours were totally unresponsive to phytohemagglutinin during this time, but when simply washed they regained full reactivity. The addition of arginine to the lymphocyte cultures was found by Aula and Nichols to prevent inhibition. Simberkoff *et al.* (1969) confirmed these observations, and found that the inhibitor also prevents sensitized lymphocytes from responding to antigens, thus suppressing *in vitro* antibody production in explants of lymph node. Canavanine, an analog of arginine, has a similar inhibitory action on lymphocytes. Among ten species of mycoplasmas tested, only the five which possess the arginine deiminase system inhibit lymphocyte inhibition.

Mycoplasmas in general are lacking in catalase, and sufficient quantities of free peroxide are released in cultures to cause methemoglobin formation (Thomas and Bitensky, 1966a) and hemolysis (Somerson *et al.*, 1965) of erythrocytes. It has been suggested that this property may be involved in tissue damage during infection, particularly in view of the known tendency of mycoplasmas to form aggregates on the surface of infected cells. Although direct evidence for this view is lacking at the present time, the affinity of mycoplasmas for a variety of host cells has been well documented (Zucker-Franklin *et al.*, 1966ab; Gesner and Thomas, 1965; Thomas, 1969; Manchee and Taylor-Robinson, 1968; Barile, 1965), and may prove to be an important mechanism in cell damage.

II. Toxicity of *Mycoplasma neurolyticum*

A. PROPERTIES OF THE EXOTOXIN

The exotoxin of *M. neurolyticum*, first noted in 1938 by Sabin, produces in mice the characteristic set of neurological manifestations known as rolling disease. After a latent period, which varies in length depending on the dose of toxin, the animals suddenly begin to roll over and over on the long axis of the body; this may continue for several hours before death, or if a large dose of toxin is given, may last for only a few minutes after which the mice develop generalized convulsions and die. With large doses, a bloody froth at the mouth is frequently seen, indicative of acute pulmonary edema.

Studies of the toxin in this laboratory have yielded the observations below (Thomas *et al.*, 1966b, Aleu and Thomas, 1966; Thomas and Bitensky, 1966b). The toxin is readily obtained from filtrates of broth in which the organisms have grown for about 18–20 hours. In somewhat older cultures, where the pH has dropped below 6.8, the toxin vanishes. It is an extremely labile protein; heating at 45°C for 15 minutes destroys it, and it deteriorates rapidly on standing at room temperature. It is destroyed by trypsin. On G-200 Sephadex columns, it emerges as a single peak immediately following the void fraction, indicating a molecular weight greater than 200,000. It is stable when frozen and can be stored indefinitely as a lyophilized powder.

The toxin produces lesions of spongiform degeneration scattered throughout all parts of the brain but most conspicuous in the cerebellum. Through electron microscopy these are seen to consist of numerous vesicles, measuring 20–40 μ in diameter, which are derived from tremendously dilated astrocytes and their equally swollen processes. These distended cells encroach upon and compress neighboring structures, resulting in neuronal damage and numerous patches of demyelination. Although obviously a neurotoxin, the material is only effective when injected by vein. Even when injected directly into the brain its activity is much less than when given intravenously; intraperitoneal and subcutaneous injections are ineffective. These observations, coupled with the neuropathological findings, suggest an action in the vascular bed of the brain.

The blood–brain barrier is markedly altered by the toxin. Intraperitoneally injected trypan blue rapidly penetrates the brains of animals with rolling disease, and experiments with radioactive glycine (Fig. 1) have shown that the permeability of the brain increases during the latter part of the latent period following injection of toxin, just before the onset of rolling disease (Thomas, 1969). The findings are consistent with an action at the site of attachment of astrocytes to the walls of the brain capillaries, with damage to these membranes leading to the flow of fluid into the whole system of intercommunicating astrocytic processes.

The interaction between the toxin and its target receptors in the central nervous system occurs very rapidly This can be demonstrated by the administration of rabbit antibody against the toxin, at various intervals after intravenous injection of toxin. When given just before toxin, or 1 or 2 minutes after toxin, antibody protects completely against rolling disease

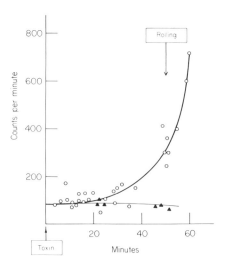

FIG. 1. Permeability of mouse brain to glycine following injection of *M. neurolyticum* toxin. Groups of 6 mice were injected with neurolyticum toxin and tested for blood-brain permeability by injecting glycine-^{14}C at various intervals; the animals were killed 5 minutes after glycine. Open circles indicate glycine uptake by brain following toxin. Triangles show uptake after injection of heat-inactivated toxin; 1000 cpm = 1.2×10^{-5} mM glycine.

TABLE I

PROTECTION BY ANTIBODY AGAINST *M. neurolyticum* TOXIN[a]

Antibody	Dilution	Timing of antibody administration	Incidence of death
Anti-*M. neurolyticum*[b]	1–2	Before toxin	0/6
	1–5	Before toxin	0/6
	1–20	Before toxin	0/6
	1–40	Before toxin	0/6
	1–80	Before toxin	6/6
	1–2	1 Minute after toxin	0/6
	1–2	2 Minutes after toxin	0/6
	1–2	3 Minutes after toxin	6/6
	1–2	4 Minutes after toxin	6/6
Anti-KSA strain[c]	1–2	Before toxin	6/6
Anti-Orale	1–2	Before toxin	6/6
Anti-*M. gallisepticum*	1–2	Before toxin	6/6

[a]Toxin: a lyophilized filtrate of broth culture of "A" strain of *M. neurolyticum*, reconstituted to provide four 50% lethal doses in 0.5 ml. Each mouse given 0.5 ml by tail vein.

[b]Antibody prepared in rabbits against whole, washed suspension of the "A" strain of *M. neurolyticum*. Injections made in tail vein, in 0.5 ml amounts in dilutions indicated.

[c]KSA: a strain of *M. neurolyticum* which has lost its toxicity. Antisera against this strain cause specific growth inhibition of both "A" and KSA strains, but do not protect against neurotoxicity of the "A" strain.

and death. But when delayed until 3 minutes after toxin, antibody no longer protects (Table I). It can be assumed that within this short period the toxin reaches its receptor in the brain and either becomes attached in such a fashion as to be inaccessible to antibody, or completes the injury which later results in rolling disease. In view of the finding that cerebral permeability changes do not take place until 45 minutes after an injection of toxin (Fig. 1), and rolling does not begin until after this, it seems more likely that the toxin is bound to its receptor and becomes invulnerable to antibody.

Binding between the toxin and a constituent of normal brain tissue with irreversible inactivation of the toxin has been demonstrated *in vitro*. The addition of toxin to crude saline homogenates of brain results in complete loss of toxicity after incubation for 5 minutes at 37°C. The component of brain tissue responsible for inactivation is sedimentable at 10,000 g, resistant to heating at 80°C for 1 hour, unaffected by trypsin, and destroyed by treatment with 0.0005 M potassium periodate. Inactivation does not occur at 0°C. Since these properties (Table II) suggest that the receptor for toxin may be a carbohydrate constituent of brain, several preparations of purified ganglioside were tested in the same fashion. Each was found to cause irreversible inactivation of toxin, with a similar degree of temperature dependence (Thomas *et al.*, 1966b).

TABLE II

INACTIVATION OF *M. neurolyticum* TOXIN BY BRAIN EXTRACTS[a]

Tissue extract	Temperature		Protection
Rat brain, 10,000 *g* sediment	37°	10 minutes	+
	0°	1 hour	0
Rat brain, 10,000 *g* supernate	37°	10 minutes	0
	0°	1 hour	0
Rat brain, 10,000 *g* sediment, treated with 0.0005 *M* potassium periodate	37°	10 minutes	0
Rat brain, 10,000 *g* sediment, treated with trypsin	37°	10 minutes	+
Rat brain, 10,000 *g* sediment, heated 80°C for 1 hour	37°	10 minutes	+
Brain ganglioside (0.5 mg/ml)[b]	37°	10 minutes	+
	0°	1 hour	0

[a] Rat brain homogenized in 0.3 *M* sucrose as 10% suspension, centrifuged at 1000 *g* for 10 minutes, and then at 10,000 *g* for 15 minutes. Sediment washed 3 times in 0.3 *M* sucrose and taken up to original volume. Each volume of toxin (4 $LD_{50}/0.5$ ml) and brain suspension mixed and incubated for time indicated, then centrifuged 10,000 *g* to remove brain particles, and supernate tested for toxicity in groups of 6 mice each. Protection of all mice against rolling disease and death indicated by +.

[b] Ganglioside preparation supplied by Dr. A. Bernheimer.

B. TOXICITY OF WHOLE LIVING MYCOPLASMAS

Suspensions of *M. neurolyticum* which have been washed several times and resuspended in Ringer's solution exhibit the same kind of toxicity as the exotoxin. For the organisms to be effective, it is necessary to concentrate them so that 10^{10} or more are contained in 1 ml. The neurological manifestations are identical to those seen with the exotoxin. The latent interval following injection varies from 5 minutes to 2 hours, depending on the dose administered. The pathological alterations in the brain are also the same.

Two possible explanations can account for the toxicity of the whole mycoplasmas: either they contain sufficient amounts of preformed toxin to cause rolling disease, or they produce toxin after being injected. That the latter must be the case is indicated by the following observations. Disruption of the mycoplasmas by 10 cycles of freezing and thawing causes the complete disappearance of toxicity. Since such treatment has no deleterious effect on the activity of solutions of exotoxin, the existence of preformed toxin in the organisms is improbable. Furthermore, pretreatment of mice with rabbit antibody in doses sufficient to protect against large doses of exotoxin yields only slight and inconstant protection against the toxicity of whole mycoplasmas. Exposure of the mycoplasmas to brain homogenates or solutions of purified ganglioside results in no loss of toxicity. Finally, treatment of mice with tetracycline 1 hour before injecting the live mycoplasmas provides solid protection against rolling disease. Since tetracycline has no effect on the action of toxin itself, this finding can only mean that the toxin is actively produced by the organisms after they have been injected.

C. Production of Toxin by Resting Mycoplasmas

It has been observed on many occasions that mice injected with suspensions of whole washed mycoplasmas may begin rolling within as short a time as 5 minutes if a sufficiently large dose is given. This means that the organisms must be able to produce new toxin very rapidly, and the formation of toxin would appear to be independent of replication. This is certainly the case with mycoplasmas *in vitro*. Organisms which have been washed and suspended in Ringer's solution, in the presence of phosphate buffer and glucose, produce detectable amounts of toxin within 15 minutes of incubation at 37°C (Table III). The addition of puromycin suppresses toxin formation, while the aminonucleoside analog of puromycin

TABLE III

PRODUCTION OF *M. neurolyticum* TOXIN BY RESTING MYCOPLASMAS

Medium for suspension of mycoplasma	Time of incubation (minutes)	Toxin in supernatant fluid[a]	
		37°C	0°C
Ringer's solution, in dialysis sac	5	0	0
submerged in PPLO broth	15	++	0
	30	++++	0
	60	++++	0
	120	++	0
	150	0	0
Glucose phosphate buffer[b], pH 7.5	5	0	0
	15	++	0
	30	++++	0
	60	++	0
	120	0	0
Glucose phosphate buffer[b], pH 6.5	30	++	0
Glucose phosphate buffer[b], pH 7.0	30	++	0
Glucose phosphate buffer[b], pH 8.0	30	++	0
Phosphate buffer pH 7.5, no glucose	15	0	0
	30	0	0
	60	0	0

[a]Duplicate tubes incubated for indicated times at 37° and 0°C. Four mice tested for each sample by intravenous injection of 0.5 and 0.1 ml of the supernatant fluid obtained by centrifuging each suspension at 13,000 g for 15 minutes after incubation. Rolling disease and death with 0.1 ml indicated by ++++; with 0.5 ml, but not 0.1 ml, indicated by ++.

[b]Phosphate buffer, 0.1 M, containing 0.5 mg/ml glucose.

does not, indicating that active synthesis of new protein is involved (Table IV).

Thus, it is not surprising that the organisms are able to produce enough toxin to cause rolling disease when sufficient numbers are injected into mice. It is of interest that the route of injection is of less importance for the whole mycoplasmas than for the exotoxin itself. When injected intracerebrally or intraperitoneally they are fully as toxic as when given by vein, while the toxin is only active when injected intravenously. It is probable that the organisms quickly gain entry to the blood, and produce their toxin there; blood cultures taken a few minutes after intracerebral or intraperitoneal injections are usually positive.

D. HOST RANGE OF *M. neurolyticum* TOXIN

Only mice and rats have been found to be vulnerable to the toxin. Guinea pigs, hamsters, rabbits, baby chicks, and turkey poults have been tested with doses 10 times the lethal range for mice with uniformly negative results.

E. LOSS OF TOXIGENICITY BY *M. neurolyticum*

The KSA strain, originally provided for our laboratory by Dr. J. Tully, appears to have permanently lost the capacity to produce toxin. Neither culture filtrates nor highly concentrated suspensions of the whole organisms produce any symptoms when injected in mice or rats. Immunologically, the strain is indistinguishable from the consistently toxic TA strain, as judged by growth inhibition and gel precipitation reactions. However,

TABLE IV

EFFECT OF ANTIBIOTICS ON TOXIN PRODUCTION BY *M. neurolyticum*

Antibiotic[a]	Production of toxin[b]
Puromycin 5 γ/ml	0
Puromycin 1 γ/ml	0
Puromycin aminonucleoside 5 γ/ml	++
Aureomycin 5 γ/ml	0
Kanamycin 5 γ/ml	++

[a]Puromycin and aureomycin obtained from Nutritional Biochemical Corp., Cleveland, Ohio.

[b]Each tube contained 10^{11} thrice-washed mycoplasmas per milliliter suspended in Ringer's solution, with 0.1 M phosphate buffer, pH 7.5, and glucose 0.5 mg/ml. The tubes were incubated for 45 minutes at 37°C, then centrifuged at 13,000 g for 15 minutes, and the supernatant fluid injected into 4 mice in dose of 0.5 ml each. Rolling disease and death indicated by ++.

antibody prepared in rabbits against KSA does not neutralize the TA exotoxin, suggesting that the loss of toxigenicity is a selective event. Attempts to restore toxicity by passage in mice and rats have been unsuccessful.

F. INFECTIVITY OF *M. neurolyticum*

Although this mycoplasma was originally isolated from the brains of mice, and new strains have occasionally been recovered from brain tissue and from the secretions of the paranasal sinus, the organism is surprisingly noninfective for mice. We have tried to establish chronic infections by injecting *M. neurolyticum* intracerebrally, intravenously, and subcutaneously, but without success. If the animals are not killed by the toxin — and this only happens when very large doses are given — they do not become infected for more than 2 or 3 days, after which viable mycoplasmas can no longer be detected in the blood or tissues. The only circumstances in which we have observed anything like a chronic infection has been in mice used for passage of a myeloma tumor by Dr. M. Davidson in Dr. J. Uhr's laboratory. This tumor is itself infected with *M. neurolyticum*, and mice carrying the tumor have a high mortality, with typical manifestations of rolling disease. Cultures of the organs of these animals show that only the tumor is infected. The situation should provide a useful model for study of infection by toxic mycoplasma, with certain interesting implications. Were it not for the available information about *M. neurolyticum* and its exotoxin, the disease would be misinterpreted as one in which a neoplasm causes death because of its own toxic products.

III. Toxicity of Mycoplasma gallisepticum

The whole live organisms of the S6 strain of *M. gallisepticum* are toxic for turkey poults, and there are major points of similarity to the toxicity of *M. neurolyticum* (Thomas *et al.*, 1966a) organisms. The central nervous system is the chief target, and perhaps the only one, for the toxin; the acutely toxic dose range is between 10^{10} and 10^{11} organisms; organisms disrupted by freezing and thawing or killed by heating are no longer toxic; birds are completely protected by pretreatment with tetracycline; brain lesions consisting of spongiform degeneration, caused by fluid-engorged astrocytes and their processes, occur regularly; the toxicity appears to be mediated through an action on the cerebral vascular bed; not all strains are toxic — indeed, only the S6 strain, isolated from turkeys during epidemics of *M. gallisepticum* encephalitis, has thus far been found to be toxic. The toxic effects result from a very rapid and irreversible action on target receptors in the brain, as indicated by the fact that specific antibody is protective only when administered within 5 minutes after injection. Finally, the phenomenon has a high degree of species specificity; no toxicity is demonstrable in adult or baby chickens, pigeons, mice, rats, rabbits, hamsters, or guinea pigs.

There are, however, important differences between the two organisms. No exotoxin can be demonstrated in cultures of *M. gallisepticum*, nor can toxin production be demonstrated in washed suspensions of the organisms. The most conspicuous and constant brain lesions, in turkeys which survive for 24 hours or longer, are those of polyarteritis nodosa, with necrotizing and inflammatory involvement of virtually all arteries in the central nervous system (Thomas *et al.*, 1966a; Cordy and Adler, 1957). Turkeys subjected to sublethal infection and surviving for several weeks often show chronic lesions of granulomatous arteritis.

In addition, the latent interval between the time of injection and the onset of neurological manifestations is not sharply fixed to the first 2 hours or so, as is the case with *M. neurolyticum*. Indeed, latent intervals ranging all the way from 1 hour to a week or longer can be observed simply by varying the dose of organisms (Table V). It is difficult to distinguish between reactions of pure toxicity and the conventional results of infection. For example, 10^{11} mycoplasmas cause convulsions, paralysis, and death within 2 hours after infection — clearly a manifestation of toxin with no likely role for replication and invasion as usually envisioned in an infection. A dose of 10^{10} organisms causes the same symptoms, with the same abrupt onset, but only after an interval of 18–24 hours. With 10^9 mycoplasmas the interval becomes 2–3 days; with 10^8, 5–6 days; with 10^7, a week or longer, and so forth. It is as though the neurotoxicity requires a certain level of toxin. With large doses, this is achieved within a few hours, while smaller numbers need correspondingly longer periods. Whether this represents the accumulation of an exotoxin to a certain

TABLE V

RELATION OF TIME OF ILLNESS IN TURKEYS TO DOSE OF *M. gallisepticum*

	Dose of mycoplasmas[a]					
	10^{11}	10^{10}	10^9	10^8	10^7	10^6
Time of onset of neurological symptoms[b]	1–2 hours	18–24 hours	2–3 days	5–6 days	7–10 days	14–21 days

[a]Number of colony-forming units of S6 strain of *M. gallisepticum* contained in 1 ml inoculum injected in wing vein.

[b]Symptoms denoting onset of disease were usually weakness, torticollis, and paralysis of legs; sometimes generalized convulsions occurred at onset.

threshold level or is dependent upon multiplication of the mycoplasmas until a threshold population is achieved is not known.

The connection between toxicity and the pathogenesis of polyarteritis nodosa of the cerebral vessels remains unclear. When death occurs within the first 24 hours, there are no arterial lesions to be seen either by light or electron microscopy. The lesions begin with fibrinoid necrosis of the arterial walls which is first discernible after 24 hours. Birds with chronic infections produced by experimental infections of the paranasal sinuses may have extensive cerebral arteritis but no manifestations of neurotoxicity; such birds have been observed to survive for as long as 8 weeks without obvious signs of neurological disease. It seems likely that the acute lethal neurotoxicity represents a separate property of the mycoplasma, distinct from whatever it is that causes polyarteritis. Even so, the latter is difficult to explain except by the action of some kind of toxin, since mycoplasmas cannot be visualized by immunofluorescence within or around the walls of affected arteries.

POSSIBLE ROLE OF SIALIC ACID IN TOXIC REACTIONS TO MYCOPLASMAS

As mentioned above, the exotoxin of *M. neurolyticum* becomes bound and irreversibly inactivated by a sedimentable component of normal brain tissue (Thomas *et al.*, 1966b). The active material is thermostable, resistant to trypsin, and destroyed by periodate, and its action can be imitated by purified preparations of brain ganglioside. The findings suggest that the brain receptor for the toxin is a sialic acid component. As a matter of speculation, it is suggested that the toxin itself may be an enzyme which acts on this constituent at the membrane juncture between astrocytic processes and the walls of brain capillaries.

Sialic acid has also been shown to be of importance in the attachment of mycoplasmas to the surfaces of erythrocytes and other cells (Gesner and Thomas, 1965; Thomas, 1969; Manchee and Taylor-Robinson, 1968). Suspensions of washed *M. gallisepticum* cause prompt agglutination of turkey erythrocytes at 37°C, associated with the adherence of dense aggregates of mycoplasmas to the cell surface. Treatment of the erythrocytes with neuraminidase prevents both agglutination and attachment. The presence of sialic acid or substances rich in sialic acid, such as egg white and fetal bovine serum, inhibits agglutination. Similar observations have recently been made in studies of the attachment of *M. gallisepticum* to mammalian lymphocytes and a variety of tissue culture cells. It is conceivable that the neurotoxicity of *M. gallisepticum* involves this affinity between the organism, or a component of the organism, and sialic acid receptors in the central nervous system.

IV. Toxicity of Mycoplasma arthritidis and Mycoplasma pulmonis

Mycoplasma arthritidis and *M. pulmonis* have been found to be toxic for mice and rats (Kaklamanis and Thomas, 1969). The general attributes of the toxins are similar to *M. gallisepticum* except that there are no specific neurological manifestations and no evidence of pathological changes in the central nervous system. The animals become ruffled and ill after an interval ranging from 1–18 hours, depending on the dosage, and then show increasing weakness and lethargy terminating in coma and death, which usually occurs 2–3 hours after the onset of symptoms.

No exotoxin can be demonstrated. The lethal dose range is between 10^{10} and 10^{11} organisms. Animals not killed by the toxin of *M. arthritidis* develop polyarthritis, which usually becomes evident 1–2 days after the injection. Those surviving *M. pulmonis* show no subsequent evidence of disease. Organisms killed by freeze-thawing or by heating are nontoxic. The administration of tetracycline 1 hour before the mycoplasma injection affords partial protection against the lethal effect, and prolongs the time of survival in all animals. Toxicity can only be elicited by the intravenous route; intraperitoneal or subcutaneous injections are without effect. Both mycoplasmas are toxic only for mice and rats.

Mycoplasma arthritidis exhibits a special lethal action on the fetuses of pregnant mice. With doses of mycoplasmas less than those required to kill adults — in the range of 5×10^8 to 5×10^9 organisms — all of the fetuses die *in utero*. Abortion does not occur. Fetuses killed in the early stages of pregnancy are autolysed and absorbed, while those killed near term are delivered stillborn. Mycoplasmas can be consistently cultured from the blood and tissues of the fetuses, indicating that the organisms readily pass the placental barrier. The mechanisms underlying this selective action on the fetus are unknown. It is possible that the phenomenon may be related to the suspected association between mycoplasma infections and abortions during spontaneous infection in other species of animals.

REFERENCES

Aleu, F., and Thomas, L. (1966). *J. Exptl. Med.* 124, 1083–1088.
Aula, P., and Nichols, W. W. (1967). *J. Cellular Physiol.* 70, 281–290.
Barile, M. F. (1965). "Mycoplasma (PPLO), Leukemia and Autoimmune Disease." Wistar Inst. Press, Philadelphia, Pennsylvania.
Copperman, R., and Morton, H. E. (1967). *Proc. Soc. Exptl. Biol. Med.* 123, 790–795.
Cordy, D. R., and Adler, H. E. (1957) *Avian Diseases* 1, 235–245.
Gesner, B., and Thomas, L. (1965). *Science* 151, 590–591.
Kaklamanis, E., and Thomas, L. (1969). Unpublished observations.
Manchee, R. J., and Taylor-Robinson, D. (1968). *J. Gen. Microbiol.* 50, 465.

Sabin, A. B. (1938). *Science* **88**, 575–576.

Simberkoff, M., Thorbecke, J., and Thomas, L. (1969). *J. Exptl. Med.* **129**, 1163.

Somerson, N., Walls, B., and Chanock, R. M. (1965). *Science* **150**, 226–228.

Thomas, L. (1969). *In* "Harvey Lectures," (Series 65), Academic Press, New York.

Thomas, L., and Bitensky, M. (1966a). *Nature.* **210**, 963.

Thomas, L., and Bitensky, M. (1966b). *J. Exptl. Med.* **124**, 1089–1098.

Thomas, L., Davidson, M., and McCluskey, R. T. (1966a). *J. Exptl. Med.* **123**, 897–912.

Thomas, L., Aleu, F., Bitensky, M. W., Davidson, M., and Gesner, B. (1966b). *J. Exptl. Med.* **124**, 1067–1082.

Zucker-Franklin, D., Davidson, M., and Thomas, L. (1966a). *J. Exptl. Med.* **124**, 521–532.

Zucker-Franklin, D., Davidson, M., and Thomas, L. (1966b). *J. Exptl. Med.* **124**, 533–542.

Author Index

Numbers in italics refer to the pages on which the complete references are listed.

A

Abe, Y., 474, 475, 480, 483, *490*
Abelow, I., 406, *412*
Adams, J. R., 459, *469*
Adams, M. H., 416, *434*
Addison, B. V., 92, *97*
Adler, H. E., 502, *504*
Ajl, S. J., 4, 5, 7, 9, 10, 11, 12, 13, 14, 15, 16, 17, 18, 19, 20, 21, 22, 23, 26, 27, 28, 29, 30, 31, 32, 33, *34, 35, 36, 37*, 41, 42, 43, 44, 45, 46, 47, 48, 49, 50, 51, 52, 53, 54, 55, 57, 58, 61, *65, 66, 67*
Akatani, I., 84, *94*
Albert, A., 123, *167*
Albertsson, P. A., 441, *469*
Albrink, W. S., 384, 389, 395, *409*
Aleu, F., 495, 497, *504, 505*
Alexsandrov, N. I., 371, 372, 373, 382, 401, 407, *409*
Alford, J. A., 278, 286, 301, *324*, 479, *490*
Allen, J. H., 476, 483, 484, *490*
Alouf, J. E., 71, 72, 73, 74, 85, 86, 87, 92, *94, 95, 96*
Altenbern, R. A., 365, 367, 368, 369, 377, 378, 379, 381, 391, 392, 393, *409, 411*, 421, *434*, 480, *490*
Ames, G., 28, *34*
Anderson, C. G., 427, *434*
Andrews, P., 13, *35*, 114, *167*
Angeolotti, R., 271, 272, 273, 276, 277, *323*
Angus, T. A., 438, 440, 441, 442, 444, 445, 452, 454, 456, 457, 458, 460, 462, 463, 464, 465, 466, 468, *469, 470*
Anonymous, 401, *409*
Aoki, K., 454, *469*
Arbuthnott, J. P., 193, 194, 195, 196, 197, 198, 199, 201, 202, 204, 206, 207, 208, 209, 210, 211, 212, 214, 215, 217, 218, 219, 220, 222, 224, 227, 228, 230, 232, *232, 233, 234, 235, 236*

Archer, L. J., 385, 386, 387, 389, 390, *409, 410*
Arima, K., 479, *490, 491*
Armans, T., 394, *411*
Armstrong, J., 397, 399, 400, *411*
Arrhenius, 216, 217, *232*
Artenstein, M. S., 198, *232, 235*
Astengo, F., 90, *95*
Atchison, M. M., 400, *410*
Atkins, E. S., 153, 154, 156, *168*
Auborn, K., 287, *322*
Auerbach, S., 403, *409*
Auerbach, T., 72, 73, 91, *96*
Aula, P., 494, *504*
Avena, R. M., 266, 271, 273, 290, 291, 292, 293, 294, 295, 296, 297, 300, 319, 320, *321, 322, 324*
Avigad, L. S., 202, 212, *232*
Azzena, D., 90, *95*

B

Bachinov, A. G., 373, 401, *409*
Badin, J., 87, 88, 89, 90, 92, *95*
Bail, O., 174, *185*, 365, 394, 395, 396, *409*
Bailey, W. L., 316, *322*
Baird-Parker, A. C., 291, *321, 324*
Baker, C. N., 92, *97*
Baker, F. E., 2, 3, 4, *35*, 55, 57, 60, 61, *65*
Baker, H. J., 58, *67*
Balassa, G., 448, 452, *469, 471*
Balat, A., 91, *97*
Baldovin, C., 72, *97*
Baldwin, J. N., 240, 241, 246, 247, 248, 251, *262*
Ball, E. G., 251, *261*
Ballou, C. E., 348, 349, *354*
Bando, Y., 145, *169*
Banerjee, N. G., 476, *491*
Bangham, A. D., 150, 151, 161, *167*, 220, 222, *232*
Barbier, S., 90, *95*
Barbour, S. D., 34, *35*
Barillec, A., 87, 88, 89, 90, *95*

507

Mc

M

Subject Index

A

Acetic acid, plague murine toxins and, 14

Acetylcholine, streptolysin O toxicity and, 79

N-Acetylglucosamine
release, *Bacillus thuringiensis* endotoxin and, 464

Acetylimidazole, enterotoxins and, 298-299

Acetylproline, streptolysin S and, 124

Acid phosphatase,
leakage, streptolysin S and, 162, 164-165

Adenosine triphosphatase, staphylococcal leukocidin and, 338, 339

Adenosine triphosphate,
formation, plague toxin and, 64
mitochondrial ion uptake and, 48-49
mitochondrial swelling and, 48
staphylococcal leukocidin and, 336
streptolysin release and, 126

Adjuvant activity, staphyloccal α-toxin and, 229

Adrenaline, α-toxin and, 225

Aeration, enterotoxin production and, 284

Aerobic antigen, anthrax immunization by, 397, 398-400, 401, 402

Agar, α-toxin production and, 204

Age,
erythrogenic toxins and, 180
scarlet fever and, 176

Aggressin, anthrax toxin and, 365-366, 394

Albumin, streptolysin S formation and, 104-105, 107, 115, 117, 134

Alkaline phosphatase,
release, *Bacillus cereus* toxin and, 418, 419

Allergic concept, erythrogenic toxins and, 175-176, 184-185

Alumina gel, protective antigen and, 373

Amberlite,
enterotoxin concentration on, 277, 289-290
staphylococcal leukocidin and, 330

Amido black, plague murine toxin electrophoresis and, 22

Amino acid(s),
analogs, streptolysin S formation and, 124
Bacillus cereus toxin production and, 417-418
Bacillus thuringiensis endotoxin,
composition, 444-445, 447
synthesis, 451-452
enterotoxin,
composition, 295-296, 297
sequence, 297-298, 299
terminal, 297, 298
plague murine toxin and, 5, 8-10
plasma, anthrax infection and, 380
requirement,
enterotoxin and, 302
plague toxin and, 24, 26
staphylococcal β-toxin, 242-243
α-toxin and, 205
streptolysin O and, 72
streptolysin S,
composition, 113-114
formation, 125-126, 128
α-toxin composition, 213

α-Amino-*n*-butyrate, anthrax toxin and, 380

Anaphylactic reactions, erythrogenic toxins and, 182

Anaerobic antigen, anthrax immunization and, 397, 400-401, 402

Anagasta kuhniella, *Bacillus thuringiensis* and, 456, 461, 467-468

Analgesic(s), streptolysin O toxicity and, 81

Anesthetic(s), streptolysin O toxicity and, 81

Aniline dyes, streptolysin S and, 131-133

Anthranilate,
α-toxin production and, 206
tryptophan analogs and, 28, 29

Anthrax,
historical, 362-363
infection, 382-383
intoxication,
cutaneous, 383
generalized, 383, 384-395

529